Fish Vaccination

Fish Vaccination

Edited by
Roar Gudding, Atle Lillehaug and Øystein Evensen

WILEY Blackwell

Registered office: John Wiley & Sons, Ltd, The Atrium, Southern Gate, Chichester, West Sussex, PO19 8SQ, UK

Editorial offices: 9600 Garsington Road, Oxford, OX4 2DQ, UK
The Atrium, Southern Gate, Chichester, West Sussex, PO19 8SQ, UK
111 River Street, Hoboken, NJ 07030-5774, USA

For details of our global editorial offices, for customer services and for information about how to apply for permission to reuse the copyright material in this book please see our website at www.wiley.com/wiley-blackwell.

Library of Congress Cataloging-in-Publication Data

Fish vaccination / edited by Roar Gudding, Atle Lillehaug, and Øystein Evensen.
pages cm
Includes bibliographical references and index.
ISBN 978-0-470-67455-0 (cloth)
1. Fishes – Vaccination. 2. Fishes – Diseases – Prevention. I. Gudding, Roar. II. Lillehaug, Atle, 1954-
III. Evensen, Øystein, 1959-
SH171.F596 2014
571.9′51 – dc23

2013034537

A catalogue record for this book is available from the British Library.

Wiley also publishes its books in a variety of electronic formats. Some content that appears in print may not be available in electronic books.

Inset photo: Vaccination of fish. Asgeir Østvik. Reproduced with permission.
Cover image: Main photo: Fishing farm. Tiny fishing farm in Ithaka, Greece. Courtesy of Margot Granitsas/Science Photo Library.
Cover design by Design Deluxe

Set in 10/12pt Times by Laserwords Private Limited, Chennai, India

1 2014

MIX
Paper from responsible sources
FSC
www.fsc.org
FSC® C013604

Contents

Contributors

Ofer Ashoulin
Dagon, Maagan Michael fish farm, Kibbutz Ma'agan Michael D.N. Menashe, Israel 37805
E-mail: labmad@mmm.org.il

Stéphane Biacchesi
National Institute for Agricultural Research (INRA), 78352 Jouy en Josas, France
E-mail: stephane.biacchesi@jouy.inra.fr

Eirik Biering
Norwegian Veterinary Institute, Tungasletta 2, 7485, Trondheim, Norway
E-mail: eirik.biering@vetinst.no

Michel Brémont
National Institute for Agricultural Research (INRA), 78352 Jouy en Josas, France
E-mail: michel.bremont@jouy.inra.fr

Andrew Bridle
NCMCRS University of Tasmania, Locked Bag 1370, Launceston 7250, Tasmania, Australia
E-mail: andrew.bridle@utas.edu.au

Jarl Bøgwald
Norwegian College of Fishery Science, UiT The Arctic University of Norway, 9037 Tromsø, Norway
E-mail: jarl.bogwald@uit.no

Duncan J. Colquhoun
Norwegian Veterinary Institute, PO Box 750, 0106 Oslo, Norway
E-mail: duncan.colquhoun@vetinst.no

Roy A. Dalmo
Norwegian College of Fishery Science, UiT The Arctic University of Norway, 9037 Tromsø, Norway
E-mail: roy.dalmo@uit.no

Arnon Dishon
KoVax Ltd, Bynet Build. Har Hotzvim Ind. Park, PO Box 45212 Jerusalem, Israel 90836
E-mail: arnon.dishon@kovax.co.il

Diane G. Elliott
U.S. Geological Survey, Western Fisheries Research Center, 6505 Northeast 65th Street, Seattle, Washington 98115, USA
E-mail: dgelliott@usgs.gov

Øystein Evensen
Norwegian School of Veterinary Science, PO Box 8146 Dep, 0033 Oslo, Norway
E-mail: oystein.evensen@nmbu.no

Knut Falk
Norwegian Veterinary Institute, PO Box 750, 0106 Oslo, Norway
E-mail: knut.falk@vetinst.no

Arne Marius Fiskum
Pharmaq, 7863 Overhalla, Norway
E-mail: arne.fiskum@pharmaq.no

Thomas Goodrich
AquaTactics Fish Health, 12015 115th Avenue NE, Suite 120, Kirkland, Washington 98034, USA
E-mail: tomg@aquatactics.com

Roar Gudding
Norwegian Veterinary Institute, PO Box 750, 0106 Oslo, Norway
E-mail: roar.gudding@vetinst.no

K. Larry Hammell
Atlantic Veterinary College, University of Prince Edward Island, 550 University Avenue, Charlottetown, C1A4P3, Canada
E-mail: lhammell@upei.ca

Anja Holm
Danish Health and Medicines Authority, Axel Heides Gade 1, 2300 Copenhagen S, Denmark
E-mail: anh@dkma.dk

Eva Högfors-Rönnholm
Laboratory of Aquatic Pathobiology, Environmental and Marine Biology, Department of Biosciences, Tykistökatu 6, Biocity, Åbo Akademi University, 20520 Turku, Finland
E-mail: ehogfors@abo.fi

Jorunn B. Jørgensen
Norwegian College of Fishery Science, UiT The Arctic University of Norway, 9037 Tromsø, Norway
E-mail: jorunn.jorgensen@uit.no

Indrani Karunasagar
Department of Fisheries Microbiology, Karnataka Veterinary, Animal and Fisheries Sciences University, College of Fisheries, Mangalore - 575002, India
E-mail: karuna8sagar@yahoo.com

Viswanath.Kiron
Aquatic Animal Health Unit, Faculty of Biosciences and Aquaculture, University of Nordland, PO Box 1490, 8049 Bodø, Norway
E-mail: kiron.viswanath@uin.no

Phillip H. Klesius
USDA-ARS, Aquatic Animal Health Research Laboratory, 990 Wire Road, Auburn, Alabama 36832, USA
E-mail: phillip.klesius@ars.usda.gov

Dag Knappskog
MSD Animal Health, Thormøhlensgate 55, 5001 Bergen, Norway
E-mail: dag.knappskog@merck.com

Erling Olaf Koppang
Norwegian School of Veterinary Science, PO Box 8146 Dep, 0033 Oslo, Norway
E-mail: erling.o.koppang@nmbu.no

Moshe Kotler
Department of Pathology, The Hebrew University–Hadassah Medical School, Jerusalem, 91120, Israel
E-mail: moshek@ekmd.huji.ac.il

Joseph Koumans
MSD Animal Health,Wim de Körverstraat 35, Post code 5381, AN Boxmeer, The Netherlands
E-mail: sjo.koumans@merck.com

Inger Kvitvang
Pharmaq, 7863 Overhalla, Norway
E-mail: inger.kvitvang@pharmaq.no

Atle Lillehaug
Norwegian Veterinary Institute, PO Box 750, 0106 Oslo, Norway
E-mail: atle.lillehaug@vetinst.no

Biswajit Maiti
Department of Fisheries Microbiology, Karnataka Veterinary, Animal and Fisheries Sciences University, College of Fisheries, Mangalore - 575002, India
E-mail: maitibiswajit@yahoo.com

Sergio H. Marshall
Institute of Biology, Faculty of Sciences, Pontifical Catholic University of Valparaiso, PO Box 4059, 2340025 Valparaiso, Chile
E-mail: smarshal@ucv.cl

Emilie Mérour
National Institute for Agricultural Research (INRA), 78352 Jouy en Josas, France
E-mail: emilie.merour@jouy.inra.fr

Paul J. Midtlyng
Norwegian School of Veterinary Science, PO Box 8146 Dep, 0033 Oslo, Norway
E-mail: paul.midtlyng.aquamedic.no

Hetron Mweemba Munang'andu
Norwegian School of Veterinary Science, PO Box 8146 Dep, 0033 Oslo, Norway
E-mail:
hetronmweemba.munang'andu@nmbu.no

Stephen Mutoloki
Norwegian School of Veterinary Science, PO Box 8146 Dep, 0033 Oslo, Norway
E-mail: stephen.mutoloki@nmbu.no

Singaiah NaveenKumar
Department of Fisheries Microbiology, Karnataka Veterinary, Animal and Fisheries Sciences University, College of Fisheries, Mangalore - 575002, India
E-mail: aquas510@gmail.com

Audun H. Nerland
Department of Clinical Science, University of Bergen, 5021 Bergen, Norway
E-mail: audun.nerland@k2.uib.no

Ken Noda
Food Safety and Consumer Affairs Bureau, Ministry of Agriculture, Forestry and Fisheries, 1-2-1 Kasumigaseki Chiyoda-ku, Tokyo 100-8950, Japan
E-mail: ken_noda@nval.maff.go.jp

Barbara Nowak
NCMCRS University of Tasmania, Locked Bag 1370, Launceston 7250, Tasmania, Australia
E-mail: B.Nowak@utas.edu.au

Sonal Patel
Institute of Marine Research, Nordnesgaten 50, 5005 Bergen, Norway
E-mail: sonal.patel@imr.no

Trygve T. Poppe
Norwegian School of Veterinary Science, PO Box 8146 Dep, 0033 Oslo, Norway
E-mail: trygve.poppe@nmbu.no

Julia W. Pridgeon
USDA-ARS, Aquatic Animal Health Research Laboratory, 990 Wire Road, Auburn, Alabama 36832, USA
E-mail: julia.pridgeon@ars.usda.gov

Praveen Rai
Department of Fisheries Microbiology, Karnataka Veterinary, Animal and Fisheries Sciences University, College of Fisheries, Mangalore - 575002, India
E-mail: raiprav@gmail.com

Linda D. Rhodes
Northwest Fisheries Science Center, National Marine Fisheries Service, 2725 Montlake Boulevard East, Seattle, Washington 98112, USA
E-mail: linda.rhodes@noaa.gov

Espen Rimstad
Norwegian School of Veterinary Science, PO Box 8146 Dep, 0033 Oslo, Norway
E-mail: espen.rimstad@nmbu.no

Jesus L. Romalde
Department of Microbiology and Parasitology, CIBUS-Faculty of Biology, University of Santiago de Compostela, 15782 Santiago de Compostela, Spain
E-mail: jesus.romalde@usc.es

Jan H.W.M. Rombout
Aquatic Animal Health Unit, Faculty of Biosciences and Aquaculture, University of Nordland, PO Box 1490, 8049 Bodø, Norway
E-mail: jhwmrombout@gmail.com

Byron E. Rippke
Center for Veterinary Biologics, USDA, 1920 Dayton Avenue, PO Box 844, Ames, Iowa 50010, USA
E-mail: byron.e.rippke@aphis.usda.gov

Kira Salonius
448 Boulter Loop, RR2, Prince Edward Island, Canada COA 1JO
E-mail: ksalonius@bellaliant.net

Craig Shoemaker
USDA-ARS, Aquatic Animal Health Research Laboratory, 990 Wire Road, Auburn, Alabama 36832, USA
E-mail: craig.shoemaker@ars.usda.gov

Krister Sundell
Laboratory of Aquatic Pathobiology, Environmental and Marine Biology, Department of Biosciences, Tykistökatu 6, Biocity, Åbo Akademi University, 20520 Turku, Finland
E-mail: ksundell@abo.fi

Carolina Tafalla
Animal Health Research Center (CISA-INIA), Carretera de Algete a El Casar km 8.1. Valdeolmos 28130, Madrid, Spain
E-mail: tafalla@inia.es

Jaime A. Tobar
Centrovet Ltda, Avenida Salomon Sack 255, 9201310 Cerrillos, Santiago, Chile
E-mail: jaime.tobar@centrovet.com

E. Scott Weber III
University of California, 2108 Tupper Hall, Davis, California 95616, USA
E-mail: sharkdoc01@gmail.com

Gregory D. Wiens
USDA-ARS, National Center for Cool and Cold Water Aquaculture, 11861 Leetown Rd, Kearneysville, West Virginia 25430, USA
E-mail: greg.wiens@ars.usda.gov

Tom Wiklund
Laboratory of Aquatic Pathobiology, Environmental and Marine Biology, Department of Biosciences, Tykistökatu 6, Biocity, Åbo Akademi University, 20520 Turku, Finland
E-mail: twiklund@abo.fi

Rune Wiulsrød
Harbitzalléen 2A, Postbox 267 Skøyen, 0213 Oslo, Norway
E-mail: rune.wiulsrod@pharmaq.no

Preface

Any intensive bioproduction – whether on land or at sea – will experience disease problems. Infections that occur in a wild fish as a sporadic event may cause severe mortality in fish-farming ponds or net-pens. Several regions with aquaculture have experienced great economic losses due to outbreaks of infectious diseases. Treatment with antimicrobials may have a negative impact on human health, the aquatic environment and even the confidence in products from aquaculture. Consequently, the expansion of commercial aquaculture has necessitated more emphasis on biosecurity measures, including disease prevention, in order to obtain a sustainable production.

Vaccination may contribute to both economic as well as environmental sustainability. The prevention of diseases using vaccines has a positive effect on the revenue for the fish farmer and the aquaculture industry by reducing morbidity, mortality and the costs of therapy, and by improving product quality. Vaccination may also improve animal welfare by reducing the suffering of diseased fish. Finally, reduction of the use of chemicals with potentialy detrimental ecological effects may be a prerequisite for further development.

The book aims at a complete coverage of the subject of fish vaccinology. The general part of the book gives science-based information about topics like the immune system of the fish, production and control of vaccines, and vaccination strategies and procedures. The use of vaccines may also have side-effects, and the mechanisms and appearances are described. The specific part includes chapters about vaccination against the most important bacterial and viral diseases in commercial fish species. One chapter about the stimulation of the immune system of crustaceans is also included.

The chapters dealing with specific diseases have a similar structure. These chapters include information that is relevant for vaccination, like the significance and occurrence of the diseases, the etiological agents, the most important antigens, as well as the specific vaccine products, the vaccination procedures, and finally the effects and possible side-effects of vaccination.

The scientific output in fish vaccinology has been substantial, especially during the last 20 years. The lists of references are consequently long, although the chapter authors have been encouraged to use review papers in order to reduce the length of the lists.

Fish vaccinology is a multidisciplinary science. The authors of the different chapters are selected from among leading experts in the different fields. While not compromising on scientific quality, we – as editors – have also placed some emphasis on selecting authors from different geographic regions.

As editors, our aim has been to produce a book that will contribute to the further sustainable development of global aquaculture. Fish farming is a rapidly growing industry in many parts of the world. It is expected that aquaculture will continue to grow both in freshwater and seawater, and contribute to the production of healthy and safe food, the development of local communities, and in some countries, even alleviation of poverty.

Roar Gudding
Atle Lillehaug
Øystein Evensen

1 The History of Fish Vaccination

Roar Gudding[1] and Thomas Goodrich[2]

[1]Norwegian Veterinary Institute, Oslo, Norway
[2]AquaTactics Fish Health, Washington, USA

ABSTRACT

Effective and sustainable disease prevention using vaccines has been an important factor for the successful growth of aquaculture. The first vaccine for aquaculture, a yersiniosis vaccine for salmonid fish in the US, was licensed in 1976. Since then the use of vaccines has expanded to new countries and new species, simultaneous with the growth of the aquaculture industry.

This chapter gives a review of the history of fish vaccinology, including information about the achievements in research and presentation of some of the pioneers of the vaccine industry.

1.1 INTRODUCTION

The knowledge of immunity is many hundreds of years old. Thucydides, a Greek historian living around 400 BC, described plague in his second book of the history of the Peloponnesian war. He noticed that a person who had recovered from plague was protected when exposed a second time (Humphrey and White, 1970).

The modern history of vaccination for prevention of infectious diseases started more than 200 years ago. In 1796, the English physician Edward Jenner inoculated a boy with infectious material from cowpox in order to induce immunity to smallpox. He had noticed that dairy farmers exposed to cowpox had become resistant to smallpox (Jenner, 1798). Jenner used the term "vaccine inoculation", which was gradually changed to vaccination. Vaccine is derived from the Latin word *vacca*, which means cow.

Louis Pasteur and co-workers demonstrated that administration of attenuated and live microorganisms gave protection upon challenge with pathogenic microorganisms (Fenner *et al.*, 1997). Their experiments with prevention of rabies were followed by research on various pathogenic microorganisms with great significance for human and animal health (Humphrey and White, 1970).

roar.gudding@vetinst.no

Fish Vaccination, First Edition. Edited by Roar Gudding, Atle Lillehaug and Øystein Evensen.

In a speech in 1881 Pasteur suggested that the word "vaccination" should be a general word for preventive inoculation of microorganisms as a tribute to the work of Jenner (Fenner *et al.*, 1997). The word "vaccinology" is of more recent vintage. Salk and Salk (1977) introduced the term vaccinology in 1977 to describe the interdisciplinary dimension of disease prevention based upon microorganisms stimulating the immune system to prevent infectious diseases in individuals and populations.

Disease prevention by vaccination is one of the milestones of modern medicine. The use of prophylaxis based on vaccines is expanding in many ways. Vaccination is now considered to be a safe and efficient method for prevention of diseases in human as well as in veterinary medicine.

1.2 AQUACULTURE

Compared with animal husbandry, fish farming is a relatively new method for bioproduction in many countries. When diseases appeared in aquaculture operations with salmonid fish, antibiotics or chemotherapeutics were used for disease treatment, and even for disease prevention. However, the need for efficacious immunoprophylaxis in hatcheries for salmonid fish was expressed as early as the late 1930s.

The first report of disease prevention using vaccines seems to have been by Snieszko *et al.* (1938) who published a paper about protective immunity in carp immunized with *Aeromonas punctata*. However, their paper was written in the Polish language which reduced the availability of the information. The first reports in English seem to have been written by Duff who showed protection against *Aeromonas salmonicida* in trout immunized by parenteral inoculation and by oral administration (Duff, 1939, 1942).

The most important reason for the disinterest in immunoprophylaxis was probably the availability of antimicrobial compounds in the years after World War II. A study by Snieszko and Friddle (1949) concluded that chemotherapy with sulfamerazine was superior to oral administration of a vaccine for the control of furunculosis. It was not until the 1970s that vaccines were applied in commercial aquaculture. Even in the scientific literature there are a limited number of reports about disease prevention by vaccination (Newman, 1993). In aquaculture, the first 30 years after World War II is therefore called the era of chemotherapy (Evelyn, 1997).

1.3 IMMUNOLOGY

Vaccinology includes different disciplines. Immunology is one of them. During the last 150 years there have been various studies of fish immunology and biology with relevance to vaccinology, reviewed by Van Muiswinkel (2008). The background of these scientists has been varied, including biology, anatomy, hematology, physiology, ichthyology, microbiology, pathology, fish diseases and others. Research on the induction of humoral antibodies in immunized fish was published before World War II (Nybelin, 1935; Pliszka, 1939), and continued with studies of immunoglobulins and complement as well as the cellular basis of the immunological response (Ridgway *et al.*, 1966; Cushing, 1970; Corbel, 1975; Press, 1998). Fish were also included in studies of comparative and developmental immunology in order to get a better understanding of the evolutionary development of the immune system (Ambrosius, 1967).

Different fish species, including carp and salmonid fish, were included in the immunological studies, and factors of importance in vaccinology, like temperature and other environmental factors, were also studied (Snieszko, 1974). The role of adjuvants in fish is important for progress in both immunology and vaccinology. Ambrosius and Lehmann (1965) found that adjuvants like aluminum hydroxide and Freund's adjuvant increased the quantity of immunoglobulins, the former slightly and the latter significantly.

The method of administration was also studied. Trout was found to produce a good immune response when injected with antigens from *Aeromonas salmonicida* (Krantz *et al.*, 1963). However, parenteral introduction of antigens seemed to be economically prohibitive and might even be harmful to the fish. Oral immunization was therefore considered to be the only way for practical disease prevention (Snieszko, 1970).

This assessment was also influenced by results from studies on humans and terrestrial animals. The successful vaccination against poliomyelitis in humans and Newcastle disease in poultry by oral administration probably influenced priorities and the direction of research of scientists working with fish immunology and vaccinology (Stone *et al.*, 1969; Sabin and Boulger, 1973). Industrial production of poultry and fish had similarities, and scientists working with different vertebrates shared information.

Experience from the poultry industry was probably also the basis for spray vaccination of fish as a method for administration of antigens. Spray vaccination of fish was given a US patent (Garrison *et al.*, 1980), but the method was not widely used in the field.

1.4 DISEASE PREVENTION

Diseases are the final results of interactions between an agent, a host and the environment of the host and the pathogen (Snieszko, 1974) (see Figure 1.1). In a population of wild fish, diseases have been considered as part of a normal biological process. In cultures of fish this situation gradually changed. The number of fish and the density increased. Diseases that were considered to be a phenomenon in the wild fish population sometimes became a problem in a fish farm.

Disease prevention should be based upon measures including all three interacting factors. However, aquaculture has some disadvantages compared with bioproduction of terrestrial

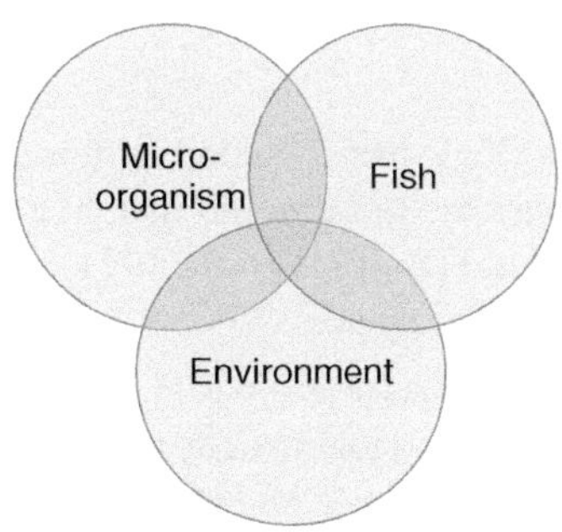

Fig. 1.1 The health triangle. (Source: Adapted from Snieszko 1974. Reproduced with permission of John Wiley & Sons.)

animals. Pathogenic microorganisms may be transmitted through water. Furthermore, disinfection is difficult, or, as in the marine environment, even impossible. Furthermore, the side-effects and risks associated with chemotherapy reduce the use of antibiotics to therapeutic use, and even that should be limited. Some environmental factors might be controlled, but others, like water temperature, could not be influenced. The resistance of the fish, based on natural or acquired immunity, is therefore a crucial factor for the health of farmed fish.

During the short history of modern aquaculture it is accepted that disease prevention based on stimulation of the immune system has become an integrated part of the management of aquaculture operations. The history of fish vaccination consists of both success and failures. Due to scientific efforts and rapid transfer of scientific progress into practical measures, vaccination has become an important part of the development of the global aquaculture industry.

1.5 SCIENTIFIC PRODUCTION – REVIEWS AND CONFERENCES

The scientific production in fish vaccinology and related areas has been considerable. A search on "fish vaccination" in scientific databases showed a total of around 10,000 papers (Science Direct, Blackwell). Most of them have been published during the last 20 years. The total number of publications was slightly above 100 at the end of the 1980s (Newman, 1993).

Fish vaccination has been the subject of many review articles (e.g., Snieszko, 1970; Harrell, 1979; Leong and Fryer, 1993; Newman, 1993; Press and Lillehaug, 1995; Ellis, 1997; Gudding *et al.*, 1999; Vinitnantharat *et al.*, 1999; Sommerset *et al.*, 2005; Toranzo *et al.*, 2009). Several international conferences on fish vaccinology and the proceedings from these have contributed to the progress (Anderson and Hennesen, 1981; de Kinkelin, 1984; Gudding *et al.*, 1997; Midtlyng, 2005). Fish vaccination was also the subject of many dissertations before the turn of the century (e.g., Lamers, 1985; Erdal, 1990; Lillehaug, 1993; Kolb, 1994; Hoel, 1997; Joosten, 1997; Midtlyng, 1998). In addition, there are numerous dissertations on related subjects like fish immunology, fish bacteriology and disease prevention in fish farming. Disease prevention in aquaculture by vaccines has also been reviewed in textbooks and book chapters (e.g., Ellis, 1988; Tatner, 1993; Adams *et al.*, 1997; Midtlyng, 1997).

1.5.1 Salmonids

Whereas research in fish immunology has included different fish species, studies on fish vaccinology have been mainly restricted to salmonid fish. In a chapter about furunculosis, the status in the late 1960s is summarized (Bullock *et al.*, 1971). Under the heading *Prophylactic chemotherapy* the following statement is made:

> "Although the practice of feeding low levels of drugs to control enzootic furunculosis may be useful, it must be done with caution to avoid toxicity to the fishes and alertness to possible appearance of drug resistant strains of *A. salmonicida*".

As for vaccination, the authors concluded that oral immunization against furunculosis with antigens incorporated in the feed was the only feasible way for routine immunization.

However, the authors indicated that the era of chemotherapy in aquaculture should come to an end and vaccination should be used for disease prevention.

An early presentation of vaccination against vibriosis was made by Hayashi *et al.* (1964). Based on immunization studies they concluded that injection of a concentrated vaccine might be a useful prophylactic way to control vibriosis in rainbow trout. One year later, Ross and Klontz (1965) showed that enteric redmouth disease (yersiniosis) could be prevented in fingerling rainbow trout fed pelleted food containing bacterial cells of the redmouth bacterium (*Yersinia ruckeri*).

During the 1970s immunoprophylaxis became recognized as method for prevention of infection caused by fish pathogenic species of *Vibrio* and *Yersinia* in aquaculture. The first product license for a fish vaccine was issued in 1976 when an enteric redmouth bacterin produced by Wildlife Vaccine Inc. was approved (Tebbit *et al.*, 1981). The effect on morbidity and mortality was documented by both scientific studies as well as by experience from commercial operations. Protection could be achieved by inactivated vaccines without adjuvants, administered by injection or immersion (Bullock and Anderson, 1984; Evelyn, 1984).

In the 1980s a new costly disease initially named "Hitra disease" appeared in salmonid aquaculture in Norway. There was some dispute about the etiology of the disease. It was soon concluded that the disease was an infectious disease caused by a new pathogenic bacterium, *Vibrio salmonicida* (Egidius *et al.*, 1986). Since 1988 most Atlantic salmon and rainbow trout in Norway have been vaccinated (initially via immersion) against this disease, which was given the name cold-water vibriosis.

In salmonids the great challenge in disease prevention was furunculosis caused by *Aeromonas salmonicida*. Based on the positive experience with prevention of *Vibrio*-infections using immersion vaccines, there were great expectations for similar effects with a furunculosis vaccine. However, immersion of furunculosis bacterins was found to give insufficient protection. Injection of simple whole-cell culture bacterins stimulated a protective immunity, but the magnitude and duration were less than desired.

In vaccines for terrestrial animals, adjuvants had been added to vaccines for decades. Al-hydrogel, which was used in vaccines for both man and animals, provided improved protection also when used in fish vaccines (Erdal and Reitan, 1992; Lillehaug, 1993). However, in order to achieve a long-lasting effect, oil adjuvants like mineral oils were found to reduce morbidity and mortality to an acceptable level, both in challenge tests as well as in aquaculture operations (Midtlyng, 1998). The local reactions caused by adjuvants were recognized as serious side-effects, but effective disease prevention was considered more important than animal welfare by authorities as well as by the industry and consumers.

Bacterins produced with antigens from *V. anguillarum*, *V. salmonicida* and *A. salmonicida* and added mineral oil adjuvants contributed to effective control of diseases, which without immunoprophylaxis would have caused great losses to the industry. The large amount of antimicrobials for disease treatment before introduction of vaccines was not acceptable for an industry that claimed to be sustainable. The impact of vaccination on the success of Norwegian aquaculture was expressed by a senior in the industry as follows: "The industry might have survived with the economic losses due to high mortality, but it could not survive with the negative effects of high use of antibiotics". Vaccination was consequently one of the factors contributing to the development of the salmonid aquaculture industry. The figures for use of antibiotics in Norwegian aquaculture represent a success story in the history of vaccinology (Gudding, 2014).

The reasons for the success in fish vaccinology in Norway are many. Innovative scientists in public and private institutions and companies deserve to be acknowledged. However, good cooperation between the scientific community, authorities and the industry were also important contributing factors. Vaccines for fish diseases were developed, produced and tested experimentally in the field at a high speed.

Even the approval of vaccines by the authorities was a fast process in Norway with little bureaucracy. During early years of fish vaccination, licensing of fish vaccines was the responsibility of the Ministry of Agriculture. The regulatory requirements were few and approval of fish vaccines was considered to be a part of the learning process. Safety and efficacy in the field were emphasized. The transfer of responsibility to the Norwegian Medicines Agency in 1993 represented a change to a more comprehensive regulatory framework in line with international rules. However, retrospectively it can be stated that the simplistic but effective regulatory work during the first years of aquaculture in Norway contributed significantly to the decrease in antibiotic use in the industry without causing significant negative effects (Midtlyng *et al.*, 2011).

During the early years of aquaculture, major viral diseases included infectious pancreatic necrosis, viral hemorrhagic septicemia and infectious hematopoietic necrosis. For the latter two viral diseases, biosecurity has mainly been based on eradication of diseased populations, and research on vaccination was not prioritized. The first successful experiments on vaccination against these diseases included live vaccines, either avirulent or attenuated strains (Fryer, 1976; Vestergaard-Jørgensen, 1976; Hill *et al.*, 1980). The live vaccines provided acceptable or even good protection under experimental conditions, but safety considerations stopped further work. Some of the vaccines showed residual virulence to groups of vaccinated fish at an unacceptable level. The safety concern for other fish species in the aquatic environment also contributed to limit research on vaccines that could be used in commercial operations.

Inactivated viral vaccines for fish have provided some effect, especially under experimental conditions. However, the protective immunity in the field from inactivated vaccines has been relatively low compared with the protection achieved by most of the bacterial vaccines. Consequently, the aquaculture industry has not been satisfied with the efficacy (Biering *et al.*, 2005).

1.5.2 Non-salmonids

The success with fish farming of salmonids stimulated aquaculture of marine fish species. In the Mediterranean countries, production of sea bass, sea bream and turbot increased, and so did disease-related problems. In the US, bacterial diseases were a challenge for the channel catfish industry. Vaccines were introduced in many countries and continents for disease prevention (Håstein *et al.*, 2005). Some of these were commercial vaccines with national or international licenses, while some were autogenous or experimental vaccines used in a few fish farms.

Two important bacterial diseases for Mediterranean farmed species were vibriosis and pasteurellosis. Inactivated vaccines with the same antigenic composition as the microorganisms causing disease were found to provide acceptable to good protection (Santos *et al.*, 1991; Gravningen *et al.*, 1998). Vaccination against these diseases is now a part of the biosecurity programme in many regions with production of sea bass, sea bream and turbot.

Bacterial diseases were the primary concern in the US channel catfish industry. The primary bacterial pathogens in this industry are *Edwardsiella ictaluri, Flavobacterium columnare* and *Aeromonas hydrophila*. Vaccines have had limited use due to the extensive nature of the husbandry. Current vaccines against infections caused by *E. ictaluri* and *F. columnare* consist of attenuated live immersion vaccines (Shoemaker *et al.*, 2009).

Most of the global aquaculture is located in countries in Asia. So far vaccination has not become an integral part of biosecurity in that region. However, there is a growing interest in disease prevention by vaccines in production of tilapia, pangasius and other species. The first commercial vaccine against a disease in pangasius was licensed in Vietnam in 2011.

1.6 SUCCESSES AND FAILURES

The history of fish vaccination is generally a story of success. The fact that a small fish can be protected against an infectious disease by immersion for a few seconds in a diluted vaccine solution is one example of the remarkable ability of living organisms to cope with biological challenges.

However, there have also been obstacles in the use of the fish immune system for disease prevention. Studies of various fish species have showed that the basic mechanisms of immunity in fish, birds and mammals are similar. However, the history of fish vaccinology also includes results of studies showing differences between species with great influence on the strategy and methods for immunoprophylaxis.

Maternal immunity is a fundamental part of protection against infectious diseases in newborn individuals of mammals and birds. It would be reasonable to believe that a similar mechanism existed for fish. Maternal immunity has been found to be transferred from immunized mothers to offspring in the ovoviviparous guppy (Takahashi and Kawahara, 1987). In salmonid fish the transfer of maternal antibodies seems to be at very low levels and insufficient to provide protection for the offspring against infections (Lillehaug *et al.*, 1996).

The failure of passive immunization is compensated by the early maturation of the immune system. Fish at a size of 2 g were protected after immersion vaccination (Johnson *et al.*, 1982b). The duration of immunity and the development of immunological memory, both crucial in vaccinology, increased with size (Johnson *et al.*, 1982a). Maximum duration of protection was achieved in rainbow trout immersion vaccinated at a size of 4 g. In commercial aquaculture, the duration of protection needed is directly related to the length of the production cycle, that is, the period between vaccination and harvest.

Effective prevention of several bacterial infections in fish by vaccination is well documented in the literature. However, infections caused by intracellular microorganisms are a challenge. This includes both viruses and intracellular bacteria. Attenuated vaccines and/or DNA vaccines seem to be a possible solution.

1.7 THE PIONEERS

The history of fish vaccination includes the achievements by many scientists working in universities and research institutes. Their production is presented and documented in the scientific literature.

Vaccines are also commercial products, developed, produced and marketed by private companies. Manufacturers of fish vaccines were generally small businesses with a few enthusiastic pioneers involved in many parts of the process, from ideas to use of the vaccine in the field.

These industrial entrepreneurs were important for progress in the early days of vaccinology. In addition to know-how about the product, they contributed with knowledge about the correct use of the vaccines.

Many of the early pioneers were excellent scientists who combined theoretical expertise and practical knowledge about disease prevention using vaccines with a commercial interest. A list of companies and pioneers can never be complete and fair for those involved.

The Colorado company Wildlife Vaccines, with Guy Tebbit, John Rohovec and Thomas Goodrich as experts, was the first manufacturer with a licensed fish vaccine. The company produced bacterins for the domestic and international market. Tavolek Inc., a subsidiary of Johnson & Johnson, was the second company with a licensed fish vaccine. Keith Johnson and Don Amend were technical experts involved in most parts of the development and production of the enteric redmouth vaccine and other bacterins. However, Tavolek Inc., and Wildlife Vaccines operated at a time when the market was too small for a profitable business.

In the 1980s Biomed Research Laboratories in Seattle entered the market. Stephen Newman, Tony Novotny, James Nelson and Robert Busch were a competent group of aquaculturists and vaccinologists, with expertise on disease prevention in hatcheries in the Northwestern US and from the manufacture of bacterins.

Two other small companies deserve to be mentioned in the history of vaccinology. Aqua Health Inc., with William Patterson as technical and scientific expert, and Aquaculture Vaccines Ltd., started as a subsidiary of Wildlife Vaccines, with Patrick Smith as expert, played significant roles in the early days of fish vaccination.

The growth of salmon production in Europe was the basis for the establishment of vaccine companies near the markets. Apothekernes Laboratorium, later Alpharma, was an international pharmaceutical company with headquarters in Oslo. The company saw a commercial potential in aquaculture and started fish vaccine production in Tromsø and later in Overhalla. In the early 1990s the company merged with Biomed Research Laboratories as part of the Alpharma group. The aquaculture part of the company was later separated from the parent company under the name Pharmaq.

In Bergen, Norbio was established with the scientists from the university as experts. Norbio was sold to the Dutch company, Intervet, which later merged with Shering-Plough which had also absorbed Aquaculture Vaccines Ltd. The fish vaccine production has from 2011 been a part of Merck Sharp Dome.

Trading of companies is not unusual in the vaccine industry, and some pharmaceutical companies and investors see the economic potential in fish vaccine production. The international pharmaceutical company Novartis has grown in the fish vaccine business, based on competence acquired with the Canadian company Aqua Health Inc.

In countries with a growing aquaculture industry, vaccine companies have been established based on a possible economic potential. Companies like Centrovet in Chile and Kovax in Israel are examples of regional fish vaccine manufacturers with the goal to provide efficacious and safe vaccines for the aquaculture industry.

1.8 CONCLUDING REMARKS

The history of fish vaccinology is a documentation of how the immune system of fish can be stimulated by vaccines to prevent the accidental effects of pathogenic microorganisms. In a few years scientists in universities, research institutes and industry have produced basic and applied knowledge about the biology of microorganisms and the immune system of fish species in aquaculture, and this knowledge has been used for development, production, marketing and use of important products for the aquaculture industry.

Fish vaccinology is still in its infancy. Most of the products are first-generation vaccines, but a comprehensive scientific production and valuable practical experience are a good basis for development of improved products that will contribute to environmental, social and economic sustainability in global aquaculture.

REFERENCES

Adams, A., Thompson, K.D. and Roberts, R.J. 1997. Fish vaccines, in *Vaccine Manual. The Production and Quality Control of Veterinary Vaccines for Use in Developing Countries* (eds N. Mowat and M. Rweyemanu). FAO Animal Production and Health Services No. 35. Rome, FAO, 127–42.

Ambrosius, H. 1967. Untersuchungen über die Immunglobuline niederer Wirbeltiere. *Allerg Asthma* **13**: 111–19.

Ambrosius, H. and Lehmann, R. 1965. Beiträge zur Immunbiologie poikilothermer Wirbeltiere. III Der Einfluss von Adjuvanten auf de Antikörper-produktion. *Acta Biol Med Ger* **14**: 830–44.

Anderson, D.P. and Hennesen, W. (eds) 1981. Fish biologics: serodiagnostics and vaccines. *Dev Biol Stand* **49**: 496 pp.

Biering, E., Villoing, S., Sommerset, I. and Christie, K.E. 2005. Update on viral vaccines for fish. *Dev Biol (Basel)* **121**: 97–113.

Bullock, G.L. and Anderson, D.P. 1984. Immunization against *Yersinia ruckeri*, cause of enteric red mouth, in *Symposium on Fish Vaccination* (ed. P. de Kinkelin). Paris, OIE, 151–66.

Bullock, G.L., Conroy, D.A. and Sniezko, S.F. 1971. Bacterial disease of fishes, in Diseases of Fishes (eds S.F. Snieszko and H.R. Axelrod). Jersey City, TFH Publications 10, 139.

Corbel, M.J. 1975. The immune response of fish: A review. *J Fish Biol.* **7**: 539–63.

Cushing, J.E. 1970. Immunology of fish, in *Fish Physiology*, Vol. 4. (eds W.S. Hoar and D.J. Randall). New York, Academic Press, 465–500.

de Kinkelin, P. (ed.) 1984. *Symposium on fish vaccination: theoretical background and practical results on immunization against infectious diseases*. Paris, OIE.

Duff, D.C.B. 1939. Some serological relationships of the S, R, and G phases of *Bacillus salmonicida*. *J Bacteriol* **38**: 91–100.

Duff, D.C.B. 1942. The oral immunization of trout against *Bacterium salmonicida*. *J Immunol* **44**: 87–94.

Egidius, E., Wiik, R., Andersen, K., *et al.*, 1986. *Vibrio salmonicida* sp. nov., a new fish pathogen. *Int J Syst Evol Microbiol* **36**: 518–20.

Ellis, A.E. (ed.) 1988. *Fish Vaccination*. London, Academic Press.

Ellis, A. 1997. Vaccines for farmed fish, in *Veterinary Vaccinology* (eds P.P. Pastoret, J. Blancou, P. Vannier and C. Verschueren). Amsterdam, Elsevier, 411–17.

Erdal, J.E. 1990. *Immune responses and protection after vaccination of farmed Atlantic salmon against bacterial diseases*. PhD thesis, Norwegian College of Veterinary Medicine, Oslo.

Erdal, J.E. and Reitan, L.J. 1992. Immune response and protective immunity after vaccination of Atlantic salmon (*Salmo salar* L) against furunculosis. *Fish Shellfish Immunol* **2**: 99–108.

Evelyn, T.P.T. 1997. A historical review of fish vaccinology. *Dev Biol Stand* **90**: 3–12.

Evelyn, T.P.T. 1984. Immunization against pathogenic Vibrios, in *Symposium on Fish Vaccination* (ed. P. de Kinkelin). Paris, OIE, 121–50.

Fenner, F., Pastoret, P.P., Blancou, J. and Terre, J. 1997. Historical introduction, in *Veterinary Vaccinology* (eds P.P. Pastoret, J. Blancou, P. Vannier and C. Verschueren). Amsterdam, Elsevier, 3–19.

Fryer, J.L., Rohovec, J.S., Tebbit, G.L., *et al.*, 1976. Vaccination for control of infectious diseases in Pacific salmon. *Fish Pathol* **10**: 155–64.

Garrison, R.L., Gould, R.W., O'Leary, P.J. and Fryer, J.L. 1980. Spray immunization of fish. *US Patent No.* 4, 223,014.

Gravningen, K., Thorarinsson, R., Johansen, L.H., *et al.*, 1998. Bivalent vaccines for sea bass (*Dicentrachus labrax*) against vibriosis and pasteurellosis. *J Appl Ichthyol* **14**: 159–62.
Gudding, R. 2014. Vaccination as a preventive measure, in *Fish Vaccination* (eds R. Gudding A. Lillehaug and Ø. Evensen). Chichester, John Wiley & Sons Ltd., 12–21.
Gudding, R., Lillehaug, A. and Evensen, Ø. 1999. Recent developments in fish vaccinology. *Vet Immunol Immunpathol* **72**: 203–12.
Gudding, R., Lillehaug, A., Midtlyng, P.J. and Brown, F. (eds) 1997. Fish vaccinology. *Dev Biol Stand* **90**: 484 pp.
Harrell, L.W. 1979. Immunization of fishes in world mariculture: A review. *Proc World Maricult Soc* **10**: 534–44.
Hayashi, K., Kobayashi, S., Kamata, T. and Ozaki, H. 1964. Studies on the vibrio disease of rainbow trout. II. Prophylactic vaccination against the vibrio disease. *J Fac Fish Prefect Univ Mie - Tsu* **6**: 181–91.
Hill, B.J., Dorson, D.M. and Dixon, P.F. 1980. Studies on the immunization of trout against IPN, in *Fish Diseases* (ed. W. Ahne). Berlin, Springer Verlag, 29–36.
Hoel, K. 1997. *Adjuvant effects of bacterial components in fish vaccines*. PhD thesis, Norwegian College of Veterinary Medicine, Oslo.
Humphrey, J.H. and White, R.G. 1970. *Immunology for Students of Medicine*, 3rd edn. Oxford, Blackwell Scientific Publications, 1–34.
Håstein, T., Gudding, R. and Evensen, Ø. 2005. Bacterial vaccines for fish – an update of the current situation worldwide. *Dev Biol (Basel)* **121**: 55–74.
Kolb, C. 1994. *Die Vakzination von Fischen*. PhD thesis, Justus-Liebig-Universität, Giessen.
Krantz, G.E., Reddecliff, J.M. and Heist, C.E. 1963. Development of antibodies against *Aeromonas salmonicida* in trout. *J Immunol* **91**: 757–60.
Jenner, E. 1798. *An inquiry into the causes and effects of the variolae vaccinae, a disease discovered in some of the western counties of England particularly Gloucestershire, and known by the name of cow pox*. London, Sampson Low.
Johnson, K.A., Flynn, J.K. and Amend, D.F. 1982a. Duration of immunity in salmonids vaccinated by direct immersion with *Yersinia ruckeri* and *Vibrio anguillarum* bacterins. *J Fish Dis* **5**: 207–13.
Johnson, K.A., Flynn, J.K. and Amend, D.F. 1982b. Onset of immunity in salmonid fry vaccinated by direct immersion in *Vibrio anguillarum* and *Yersinia ruckeri* bacterins. *J Fish Dis* **5**: 197–205.
Joosten, E. 1997. *Immunological aspects of oral vaccination in fish*. PhD thesis, University of Wageningen.
Lamers, C.H.J. 1985. *The reaction of the immune system of fish to vaccination*. PhD thesis, University of Wageningen.
Leong, J.C. and Fryer, J.L. 1993. Viral vaccines for aquaculture. *Annu Rev Fish Dis* **3**: 225–40.
Lillehaug, A. 1993. *Effects and side-effects of vaccination of salmonid fish*. PhD thesis, Norwegian College of Veterinary Medicine, Oslo.
Lillehaug, A., Sevatdal, S. and Endal, T. 1996. Passive transfer of specific maternal immunity does not protect Atlantic salmon (*Salmo salar* L.) fry against yersiniosis. *Fish Shellfish Immunol* **6**: 521–35.
Midtlyng, P.J. 1997. Vaccination against furunculosis, in *Furunculosis – Multidisciplinary Fish Disease Research* (eds E.M. Bernoth, A.E. Ellis, P.J. Midtlyng, G. Olivier and P. Smith). San Diego, Academic Press, 382–404.
Midtlyng, P.J. 1998. *Evaluation of furunculosis vaccines in Atlantic salmon*. PhD thesis, Norwegian College of Veterinary Medicine, Oslo.
Midtlyng, P.J. 2005. Progress in fish vaccinology. *Dev Biol (Basel)* **121**: 335 pp.
Midtlyng, P.J., Grave, K. and Horsberg, T.E. 2011. What has been done to minimize the use of antibacterial and antiparasitic drugs in Norwegian aquaculture. *Aquac Res* 42: 28–34.
Newman, S.G. 1993. Bacterial vaccines for fish. *Annu Rev Fish Dis* **3**: 145–85.
Nybelin, O. 1935. Über Agglutininbildung bei Fischen. *Z Immunitätsforsch* **84**: 74–9.
Pliszka, F. 1939. Untersuchungen über die Agglutininbildung bei Fischen. *Zbl Bakt Abt* 1 143: 262–4.
Press, CMcL. 1998. Immunology of fishes, in *Handbook of Vertebrate Immunology* (eds P.P. Pastoret, P. Griebel, H. Bazin and A. Govaerts). San Diego, Academic Press, 3–62.
Press, C. and Lillehaug, A. 1995. Vaccination in European salmonid aquaculture: a review of practices and prospects. *Br Vet J* **151**: 46–69.
Ridgway, G.J., Hodgins, H.O. and Klontz, G.W. 1966. The immune response in teleosts, in Phylogeny of Immunity (eds R.T. Smith, P.A. Miescher and R.A. Good). Gainesville, FL, University of Florida Press, 199–208.

Ross, A.J. and Klontz, G.W. 1965. Oral immunization of rainbow trout (*Salmo gairdneri*) against an etiologic agent of "red mouth disease". *J Fish Res Bd Can* **22**: 713–19.
Sabin, A.B. and Boulger, L.R. 1973. History of Sabin attenuated poliovirus oral live vaccine strains. *J Biol Stand* **1**: 115–18.
Salk, J. and Salk, D. 1977. Control of influenza and poliomyelitis with killed virus vaccines. *Science* **195**: 834–47.
Santos, Y., Bandin, I., Nunez, S., *et al.*, 1991. Protection of turbot *Scophthalmus maximus* (L.), and rainbow trout, *Oncorhynchus mykiss* (Richardson), against vibriosis using two different vaccines. *J Fish Dis* **14**: 407–11.
Shoemaker, C.A., Klesius, P.H., Evans, J.J. and Aria, C.R. 2009. Use of modified live vaccines in aquaculture. *J World Aquac Soc* **40**: 573–85.
Snieszko, S.F. 1970. Immunization of fishes: a review. *J Wildl Dis* **6**: 24–30.
Snieszko, S.F. 1974. The effects of environmental stress on outbreaks of infectious diseases of fishes. *J Fish Biol* **6**: 197–208.
Snieszko, S.F. and Friddle, S.B. 1949. Prophylaxis of furunculosis in brook trout (*Salvelinus fontinalis*) by oral immunization and sulfamerazine. *Progress Fish Cult* **11**: 161–8.
Snieszko, S., Piotrowska, W., Kocylowski, B. and Marek, K. 1938. Badania bakteriologiczne i serogiczne nad bakteriami posocznicy karpi. Memoires de l'Institut d'Ichtyobiologie et Pisciculture de la Station de Pisciculture Experimentale a Mydlniki de l'Universite Jagiellonienne a Cracovie Nr **38**.
Sommerset, I., Krossøy, B., Biering, E. and Frost, P. 2005. Vaccines for fish in aquaculture. *Exp Rev Vaccines* **4**: 89–101.
Stone, H.D., Ritchie, A.E. and Boney, W.A. 1969. Immunization of chickens against Newcastle disease with beta-propiolactone-killed virus antigen administered in drinking water. *Avian Dis* **13**: 568–78.
Takahashi, Y. and Kawahara, E. 1987. Maternal immunity in newborn fry of ovoviviparous guppy. *Nippon Suis Gakk* **53**: 721–35.
Tatner, M.F. 1993. Fish vaccines, in *Vaccines for Veterinary Applications* (ed. A.R. Peters). Oxford, Butterworth-Heinemann, 199–224.
Tebbit, G.L., Erickson, J.D. and Van de Water, R.B. 1981. Development and use of *Yersinia ruckeri* bacterins to control enteric redmouth disease. *Dev Biol Stand* **49**: 395–401.
Toranzo, A.E., Romalde, J.L., Magariños, B. and Barja, J.L. 2009. Present and future aquaculture vaccines against bacterial fish diseases. *Op Méditerr* **86**: 155–76.
Van Muiswinkel, W.B. 2008. A history of fish immunology and vaccination I. The early days. *Fish Shellfish Immunol* **25**: 397–408.
Vestergaard-Jørgensen, P.E. 1976. Partial resistance of rainbow trout (*Salmo gairdneri*) to viral haemorrhagic septicaemia (VHS) following exposure to non-virulent Egtved-virus. *Nord Vet Med* **28**: 570–1.
Vinitnantharat, S., Gravningen, K. and Greger, E. 1999. Fish vaccines. *Adv Vet Med* **41**: 539–50.

2 Vaccination as a Preventive Measure

Roar Gudding

Norwegian Veterinary Institute, Oslo, Norway

ABSTRACT

Preventive measures have become more and more important as part of biosecurity in agriculture and aquaculture. Disease prevention by vaccination is especially important in aquaculture where the number of individuals at risk is high and where therapy is a challenge from practical, technical and economic points of view. Vaccination contributes to a sustainable aquaculture with low use of antibiotics. One reason for the favourable effect of vaccination in aquaculture is increased resistance to disease in both vaccinated and unvaccinated individuals, or so-called herd immunity. Vaccination is generally a safe and economically acceptable preventive measure. Disease prevention based on stimulation of the immune system of the fish has therefore become fundamental for the development of modern aquaculture. Fish vaccination has been especially successful in production of salmonid fish, but vaccination has also been increasingly utilized for disease prevention in fish species like sea bass, sea bream, carp and channel catfish.

2.1 INTRODUCTION

Aquaculture is the fastest growing food-producing sector in the world (Food and Agriculture Organization, 2012). Globally, production from capture fisheries has levelled off at the same time as the world human population continues to grow. Aquaculture has the potential to make a significant contribution to the increasing demand for aquatic food in many regions of the world. During recent decades there has been significant progress in the aquaculture sector characterized by intensified production and new species.

Scientific achievements in production technology, including breeding and feeding, have been important factors contributing to this progress. A healthy population of farmed fish has also been a decisive factor for increased production. It is more and more accepted that a

roar.gudding@vetinst.no

Fish Vaccination, First Edition. Edited by Roar Gudding, Atle Lillehaug and Øystein Evensen.

favourable health situation is crucial for aquaculture related to food security. One reason for this is recognition of the fact that aquaculture industries in some countries have faced challenges due to microbial infections in aquatic environments. Diseases with high morbidity and mortality have caused significant economic losses in fish farming. This applies to many levels of the industry, from individual fish farms to countries (Barton and Fløysand, 2010).

Sustainability means development that meets the need of the present without compromising the ability of future generations to meet their needs (Brundtland, 1987). Any bioproduction like aquaculture must be sustainable. This means that the fish farming industry should be managed in such a way that negative effects on the environment are acceptable and restorable. There are many indicators of sustainability. Disease prevalence and incidence based on surveillance and monitoring are among these. Bacterial infections in farmed fish are treated with antibiotics or chemotherapeutants, and the total quantities of these compounds used in aquaculture production are another parameter that can be used for documentation of the level of sustainability. A low level and prevalence of residues in aquaculture products, as well as resistant microorganisms in diseased fish, might also be indicative of a sustainable bioindustry (Gudding, 2012).

Aquaculture may even change the ecology of the aquatic environment, including resident fish populations and their pathogens. Diseases that occur as a phenomenon in wild fish populations may become a problem in a densely populated net pen. Farming of salmonids has therefore changed the dynamics of the salmon sector and caused tension and conflicts between stakeholders in farming and angling. It is even postulated that fish farming will lead to evolution of more virulent pathogens (Pulkkinen *et al.*, 2010).

The economic consequences of diseases for the industry and society may be a direct result of reduced production, but may also be indirectly due to the effects of diseases on seafood quality. A good health status is therefore important both for food security and food safety. Low disease prevalence and incidence is also crucial for the welfare of aquatic animals, a factor emphasized by more and more consumers and stakeholders (Turnbull and Kadri, 2007).

Like other methods for food production, aquaculture offers social and economic benefits as well as risks. It is crucial for the future development of the aquaculture industry that bioproduction of farmed fish has credibility in society. However, trust may be unstable, and the public perception of fish farming may change (Schlag, 2010). Biosecurity, contributing to improved health, welfare and economy, is therefore an important part of the long-term efforts towards a sustainable bioproduction with an acceptable "footprint".

2.2 BIOSECURITY AND VACCINATION

Biosecurity includes different activities contributing towards maintenance of a healthy population. As the industry has developed, biosecurity has become an increasingly important part of the management of aquaculture. Prevention, control and eradication are all biosecurity measures used in order to eliminate disease or minimize its frequency and effect on production.

"Prevention is better than cure" is a well-known expression in human as well as veterinary medicine. Preventive measures are especially important in aquaculture where the number of individuals at risk is high and where therapy is a challenge both from practical, technical and economic points of view.

Prevention and control of infectious disease by fish vaccination is becoming increasingly important as a part of aquaculture biosecurity. Vaccinated animals have a reduced risk of disease development and even non-vaccinated animals may be protected due to herd immunity. Prophylaxis based on stimulation of the immune system also reduces the use of antimicrobials. In Norway, all farmed salmonid fish have, for many years, been vaccinated against several diseases before transfer to seawater. Annual antibiotic consumption has, in most years since the beginning of the 1990s, been less than one metric tonne (see Figure 2.1).

Prevention, control and eradication are the three cornerstones of biosecurity. Eradication of diseases in aquatic animals is difficult, sometimes impossible. In contrast to production systems for terrestrial animals, causative agents are not readily destroyed by disinfection procedures in aquatic systems. Vaccines generally protect against disease, but they do not prevent infection. The difficulty in eradicating infectious diseases in the aquatic environment has the consequence that the most realistic alternative is to prevent and control the disease, which means "to live with the disease".

Biosecurity based on prevention and control should be based on the knowledge relating to the so-called health triangle, that is, the host, the microorganism and the environment (Sniezko, 1974). Immunoprophylaxis is primarily based on interactions between the microorganism and host, but a favourable environment also contributes significantly to good resistance in the host. In order to achieve optimal effect, vaccination should always be a supplement to other biosecurity measures that reduce infection pressure or improve environmental factors with an effect upon disease resistance.

Prevention of fish diseases by vaccination is achieved for several bacterial diseases (Press and Lillehaug, 1995; Gudding *et al.*, 1999; Håstein *et al.*, 2005; Sommerset *et al.*, 2005; Bravo and Midtlyng, 2007). Most fish vaccines are inactivated vaccines, and many vaccines provide acceptable protection against disease. However, the fish are not protected against infection, so the vaccines do not provide sterile immunity.

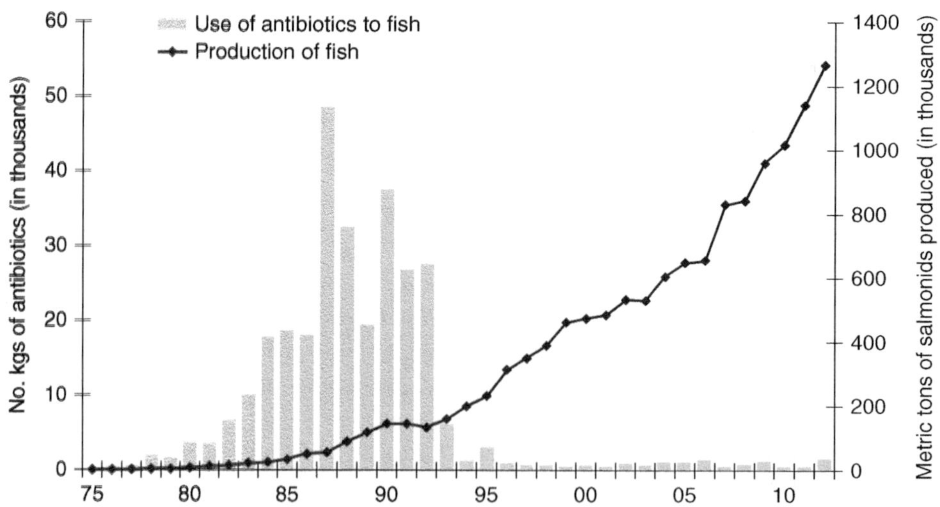

Fig. 2.1 The use of antibiotics in Norwegian aquaculture.

As excretion of microorganisms is significantly reduced, the effect of vaccination is that disease prevalence and incidence is lower in vaccinated groups compared with unvaccinated ones. However, the degree of disease prevention may vary and vaccines may therefore be used with various degrees of success.

2.3 USE OF VACCINATION IN AQUACULTURE

Fish vaccines are primarily used for prevention and control of infectious diseases. Most of the diseases are caused by bacteria. However, vaccines are also used for control of some viral diseases (Biering *et al.*, 2005). So far, there are no fish vaccines for diseases caused by fungi and parasites.

Most vaccines are used for prevention of diseases in anadromous fish like salmonids. However, vaccination programmes are also used in fish farms with species like sea bass, sea bream, cod, tilapia, channel catfish, yellowtail, and turbot (Håstein *et al.*, 2005; Samuelsen *et al.*, 2006; Toranzo *et al.*, 2009). During recent years, aquaculture of pangasius and grouper has increased in some Asian countries, and vaccination has been introduced or is under development (Harikrishnan *et al.*, 2011).

Protection against diseases like vibriosis, yersiniosis and pasteurellosis can be achieved by inactivated vaccines administered by immersion or intraperitoneal injection. For other diseases like furunculosis, adjuvanted, inactivated vaccines are required for protection. Adjuvanted vaccines are up to now administered by injection.

The main reason for the preference for inactivated vaccines is safety. Microorganisms that are attenuated and do not cause disease in one species may be distributed through water to other fish species that are more susceptible. As some diseases, mainly caused by intracellular microorganisms, cannot be prevented by inactivated vaccines, there is a market for vaccines with live, attenuated microorganisms. Live vaccines have been used experimentally, and there are even nationally licensed live vaccines for certain diseases, such as infection caused by *Edwardsiella ictaluri* in channel catfish (Shoemaker *et al.*, 2009).

Competence in vaccinology is generally based on two sciences, microbiology and immunology. During recent years, molecular biology has also become a useful tool in vaccinology, both in production and control of vaccines. Vaccines produced by molecular biological methods include recombinant vaccines, like subunit vaccines where antigens are produced by microorganisms with insertions of genes for certain virulence factors. Some of the vaccines against infectious pancreatic necrosis (IPN) belong to this category (Ramstad *et al.*, 2007).

Genetically modified vaccines are generally live vaccines where a gene has been changed. An experimental attenuated vaccine against *Aeromonas salmonicida* has been constructed as an aromatic-dependent mutant (Marsden *et al.*, 1996). The protection achieved by the vaccine was good. However, as inactivated vaccines already exist with acceptable effects, these alternatives are considered to be more safe.

DNA vaccines have genes coding for certain virulence factors or other factors giving protection against certain microorganisms. DNA vaccines elicit production of an antibody response, as well as cellular immunity. There are many experimental DNA vaccines against fish diseases, and in 2010 a DNA vaccine against infectious hematopoietic necrosis was licensed in Canada and the US. The safety of DNA vaccines has been questioned for some time. The license is therefore an indication that the regulatory authorities accept the documentation of safety.

There are many similarities between the immune system in mammals and birds on the one hand, and fish on the other. One important biological difference with great significance for disease prevention by vaccination is maternal immunity. Vaccination of the mother with subsequent passive transfer of antibodies to the offspring is a well-known method for protecting offspring against infections in many species of terrestrial animals. Transfer of maternal antibodies seems to occur to some extent in some fish species, but practical use of vaccination in brood fish has so far been unsuccessful (Lillehaug *et al.*, 1996).

In aquaculture, stimulation of the immune system is only used for prevention of infectious diseases, that is, immunoprophylaxis. However, in terrestrial animals vaccines are also used for endocrine regulation and manipulation of metabolism and reproduction. One example is vaccination in order to prevent boar taint (Fuchs *et al.*, 2009). This can be done by stimulating the production of antibodies against hormones or other compounds with biological activity. In aquaculture, sterile fish will contribute to reduced genetic interactions with wild fish. One method can be to immunize brood fish with antigens with surface proteins from eggs. Maternal antibodies against egg proteins might hinder germ cells from developing into gonad cells, and the result might be a sterile fish.

2.4 VACCINATION AGAINST DIFFERENT DISEASES

Most fish vaccines have been used against infectious diseases caused by pathogenic microorganisms that are found in the environment, and where eradication cannot be achieved. Microorganisms like *Vibrio*, *Aeromonas*, *Yersinia* and others may cause infections that can be prevented and controlled by vaccination.

Vaccines have not been used to any great extent for control of exotic fish diseases. These are mainly caused by viruses. Inactivated vaccines against viral diseases have generally afforded less protection compared with vaccines against bacterial infections.

Another reason is that vaccination may be an obstacle to trade of live animals or products in a region or a country. This is due to the difficulties in distinguishing between vaccinated and infected animals. The consequence is that it is difficult or impossible to declare freedom for a certain disease if the population is vaccinated. Examples include the regulations of the European Union relating to infectious salmon anemia (ISA). Vaccination against ISA is allowed in areas or countries where the disease is endemic. However, vaccination is prohibited in regions that claim to be free from the disease.

In terrestrial husbandry the difficulties in combining eradication and vaccination have been solved for some diseases by using DIVA (differentiation infectious vaccinated animals) vaccines (Meeusen *et al.*, 2007). Aujeszky's disease in swine is one of the diseases that are controlled by vaccination simultaneously with an ongoing eradication programme.

So far there have been no DIVA vaccines in aquaculture. The first challenge in fish vaccinology is to develop an efficacious viral vaccine. The next one might be a DIVA vaccine. ISA, viral hemorrhagic septicemia (VHS) and infectious hematopoietic necrosis (IHN) are all candidate diseases for which DIVA vaccines might be used in the future.

2.5 HERD IMMUNITY

One of the arguments for vaccination as a preventive measure is increased resistance to disease in vaccinated as well as unvaccinated individuals. This effect, termed "herd immunity", describes a form of immunity that occurs when the vaccination of a significant portion of a population provides protection for individuals without immunity or with low immunity (Anderson and May, 1985).

The number of individuals in a fish farm is very high. Some individuals may be left unvaccinated and some are poor responders. Herd immunity is consequently an important factor for the positive effects of vaccination in aquaculture (Gudding *et al.*, 2013).

Herd immunity is expressed as the proportion of the population that has to be immune or resistant in order to prevent an infection spreading. The effect of herd immunity is determined by factors related to the microorganism causing the disease, and the vaccine that is used for prevention. These variables are the efficacy of the vaccine, φ, and the basic reproduction number of the agent, R_0. Based on these two parameters, the herd immunity can be estimated mathematically by the following equation:

$$\frac{1}{\varphi} \; x \; \left(1 - \frac{1}{R_0}\right)$$

where φ is the vaccine efficacy and R_0 is the basic reproductive number.

Vaccine efficacy is defined as the proportional relationship between mortalities in vaccinated and unvaccinated groups during challenge or disease outbreak. The term "vaccine efficacy" is used interchangeably with "relative percent survival" (RPS). The RPS describes the efficacy of a vaccine as a percentage (Amend, 1981). The RPS can be estimated by the following equation:

$$\text{RPS} = \left(1 - \left(\frac{\%\text{mortality in vaccinated fish}}{\%\text{mortality in non-vaccinated fish}}\right)\right) \times 100\%$$

The basic reproductive number, $R_{0,}$ of an infectious agent is a key factor determining the rate of spread and the proportion of the population affected. R_0 is the average number of secondary infected individuals arising from a single primary infected individual during its entire infectious period in a naïve and susceptible population (Anderson and May, 1991). If R_0 is greater than 1, each primary case will, on average, produce more than one secondary case, leading to an epidemic. On the other hand, when an estimate of R_0 is less than 1, the outbreak is likely not to occur.

The R_0 in aquaculture, similarly to R_0 of diseases of terrestrial animals, depends upon specific characteristics of the diseases, such as transmissibility and infectious period. R_0 also depends upon host density, which has a decisive influence on the frequency of contacts between individuals with potential for disease transmission to occur. There are few data on R_0 for fish diseases. R_0 for infectious salmon anemia (ISA) has been estimated to be in the range of 1.3 to 2.5 (Mardones *et al.*, 2011).

The equation for herd immunity can be used for modelling the effect of vaccination against a disease like ISA. If R_0 for ISA is 2.5 and the RPS for an ISA vaccine is 80%, the threshold for herd immunity is 75%, which means that 75% of the population should be vaccinated and respond immunologically in order to achieve a marginal positive effect of vaccination. A higher percentage of vaccinated fish responding, and the use of a vaccine with a higher RPS, are both factors contributing to an improved result for the vaccination.

2.6 ECONOMIC CONSIDERATIONS

For a fish farmer to vaccinate or not is always an economic consideration of benefits and cost. There are many questions related to economy that should be answered. Among these are: vaccination versus alternative methods for disease prevention; diseases to be included in the vaccination programme; vaccination method; and vaccine to be used. Time of termination of vaccination may also be a relevant issue.

The effect of a vaccination programme is sometimes questioned. The reason can be disease outbreaks despite vaccination, and/or a low RPS value in challenge experiments. However, other parameters may give additional information and a more differentiated picture of the performance of a vaccine in the field. A cohort study of the effect of vaccination against pancreas disease (PD) caused by salmonid alphavirus showed positive effects on several production parameters that are important for the economy (Bang Jensen *et al.*, 2012). The odds for PD were three times lower if the site had vaccinated fish compared with unvaccinated. Furthermore, the overall cumulative mortality was reduced and the growth rate was increased in vaccinated cohorts.

As fish farms may use the same water as their neighbors, considerations about strategy has to include the region where the farm is located. The refusal of vaccination may influence the infection pressure in the region and consequently affect both farmed and wild fish in the region.

There are economic models that can be used to improve the predictability of vaccination decisions (Lillehaug, 1989; Thorarinsson and Powell, 2006). Using these models and mortality level data, cost of vaccination and market prices of fish, it has been demonstrated that vaccination of salmon is economically justified, even when low disease risk and market price applied. The sea bass producer, however, needs market prices and/or a disease risk above a certain level in order to make the vaccination investment affordable.

2.7 RISK ASSESSMENT

Vaccination is generally a safe preventive measure. However, there is increasing concern about side-effects as a result of vaccination. The side-effects can affect the vaccinated fish, the vaccinators and even the environment. The positive effect of vaccination should therefore be assessed against the negative effects associated with immunoprophylaxis (Wooldridge, 2007).

Risk assessment has become a useful tool for quantification of the benefits and risks related to disease management. In some countries, risk assessment is an integral part of the evaluation of medical products. The European Medicines Agency has a use-risk-balance assessment as the final step in the evaluation of vaccines. The animal health authorities in some countries have a final assessment of benefits and risks related to the use of vaccines as a preventive measure. A licensed product may be prohibited if it may be in conflict with or jeopardize other disease prevention and control measures.

Live vaccines may represent a potential source of uncontrolled environmental spread of microorganisms with unpredictable ecological effects. A restrictive policy for use of live vaccines has therefore been justified.

A similar attitude has applied to genetically modified vaccines. However, the risk associated with vaccines produced using molecular biological techniques seems to be negatively correlated with new knowledge of the techniques. Modern techniques of genetic engineering allow the construction of precise genetic modifications for the construction of gene modified organisms with well-defined attenuation. Vaccines attenuated by gene deletions or modifications have consequently higher environmental safety compared with vaccines attenuated by conventional methods (Frey, 2007).

Each risk assessment mainly relates to a country or region. However, it may even apply to a farm. Before using autogenous vaccines or non-licensed products in a farm, an assessment of benefits and risks is especially important.

Administration of alien antigens will trigger biological processes in the vaccinated animals. The side-effects may be systemic or local.

2.8 THE MARKET FOR FISH VACCINES

Disease prevention by vaccination has in the past mainly been applied to salmonid fish. This reflects the costs associated with vaccination. In recent years, however, immunoprophylaxis has become increasingly utilised in non-salmonid fish like sea bass, sea bream, carp and channel catfish. However, vaccination in aquaculture is still in its infancy as a prophylactic method, compared with the use of vaccines in agriculture. In most countries, fish vaccines are produced by commercial vaccine companies. The vaccines are licensed by national and international authorities. Some of the vaccine companies are serving a global aquaculture industry with a variety of products for several species. There are no reliable figures for the value of the market for fish vaccines.

The market for fish vaccines may in some cases be limited, and autogenous vaccines based on strains from a particular farm may be used. Most autogenous vaccines are produced under controlled conditions by commercial vaccine producers. There is reason to believe that the demand for autogenous vaccines will increase. New fish species are being farmed, and new strains or variants of microorganisms may appear. If established vaccine programs do not work, the use of autogenous vaccines may be a solution. A general requirement for autogenous vaccines is that they are produced and controlled according to the guidelines from the regulatory authorities.

The future prospects for fish vaccination are positive. The public demand for an environmentally, socially and economically sustainable aquaculture will probably increase. Together with the scientific achievements in fish vaccinology, this will contribute to further development of the global fish vaccine market.

REFERENCES

Amend, D.F. 1981. Potency testing of fish vaccines. *Dev Biol Stand* **49**: 447–54.

Anderson, R.M. and May, R.M. 1985. Vaccination and herd immunity to infectious diseases. *Nature* **318**: 323–9.

Anderson, R.M. and May, R.M. 1991. *Infectious Diseases of Humans: Dynamics and Control*. Oxford, Oxford University Press.

Bang Jensen, B., Kristoffersen, A.B., Myr, C. and Brun, E. 2012. Cohort study of effect of vaccination on pancreas disease in Norwegian salmon aquaculture. *Dis Aquat Org* **102**: 23–31.

Barton, J.R. and Fløysand, A. 2010. The political ecology of Chilean salmon aquaculture, 1982–2010: a trajectory from economic development to global sustainability. *Global Environ Change* **20**: 739–52.

Biering, E., Villoing, S., Sommerset, I. and Christie, K.E. 2005. Update on viral vaccines for fish. *Dev Biol (Basel)* **121**: 97–113.

Bravo, S. and Midtlyng, P.J. 2007. The use of fish vaccines in Chilean salmon industry 1999–2003. *Aquaculture* **270**: 36–42.

Brundtland, G.H. 1987. Address at closing ceremony of the World Commission on Environment and Development, Tokyo, 27 February 1987. Available at: http://www.regjeringen.no/upload/SMK/Vedlegg/Taler%20og%20artikler%20av%20tidligere%20statsministre/Gro%20Harlem%20Brundtland/1987/Address_at_Eighth_WCED_Meeting.pdf [accessed 3 May 2013].

Food and Agriculture Organization (FAO) Fisheries & Aquaculture. 2012. State of world aquaculture. Available at: http://www.fao.org/fishery/topic/13540/en [accessed 3 May 2013].

Frey, J. 2007. Biological safety concepts of genetically modified live bacterial vaccines. *Vaccine* **25**: 5598–5605.

Fuchs, T., Thun, R., Parvizi, N., *et al.*, 2009. Effect of a gonadotropin-releasing factor vaccine on follicle-stimulating hormone and luteinizing hormone concentrations and on the development of testicles and the expression of boar taint in male pigs. *Theriogenology* **72**: 672–80.

Gudding, R. 2012. Disease prevention as a basis for sustainable aquaculture, in *Improving Biosecurity through Prudent and Responsible Use of Veterinary Medicines in Aquatic Food Production* (eds M.G. Bondad-Reantaso, J.R. Arthur and R.P. Subasinghe). FAO Fisheries and Aquaculture Technical Paper Vol. 547. Rome, Food and Agriculture Organization, 141–6.

Gudding, R., Lillehaug, A. and Evensen, Ø. 1999. Recent developments in fish vaccinology. *Vet Immunol Immunopathol* **72**: 203–12.

Gudding, R., Lillehaug, A. and Tavornpanich, S. 2013. Immunoprophylaxis in biosecurity programs. *World Aquaculture* **44**: 60–63.

Harikrishnan, R., Balasundaram, C. and Heo, M.-S. 2011. Fish health aspects in grouper aquaculture. *Aquaculture* **320**: 1–21

Håstein, T., Gudding, R. and Evensen, Ø. 2005. Bacterial vaccines for fish – An update of the current situation worldwide. *Dev Biol (Basel)* **121**: 55–74.

Lillehaug, A. 1989. A cost-effectiveness study of three different methods of vaccination against vibriosis in salmonids. *Aquaculture* **83**: 227–36.

Lillehaug, A., Sevatdal, S. and Endal, T. 1996. Passive transfer of specific maternal immunity does not protect Atlantic salmon (*Salmo salar* L.) fry against yersiniosis. *Fish Shellfish Immunol* **6**: 521–35.

Mardones, F.O., Perez, A.M., Valdes-Donoso, P. and Carpenter, T.E. 2011. Farm-level reproduction number during an epidemic of infectious salmon anemia virus in southern Chile in 2007–2009. *Prev Vet Med* **102**: 175–84.

Marsden, M.J., Vaughan, L.M., Foster, T.J. and Secombes, C.J. 1996. A live (Δ*aroA) Aeromonas salmonicida* vaccine for furunculosis preferentially stimulates T-cell responses relative to B-cell responses in rainbow trout (*Onchorhyncus mykiss*). *Infect Immun* **64**: 3863–9.

Meeusen, E.N.T., Walker, J., Peters, A., *et al.*, 2007. Current status of veterinary vaccines. *Clin Microbiol Rev* **20**: 489–510.

Press, CMcL. and Lillehaug, A. 1995. Vaccination in European salmonid aquaculture. A review of practices and prospects. *Br Vet J* **151**: 45–69.

Pulkkinen, K., Suomalainen, L.-R., Read, A.F., *et al.*, 2010. Intensive fish farming and the evolution of pathogen virulence: the case of columnaris disease in Finland. *Proc Biol Sci* **277**: 593–600.

Ramstad, A., Romstad, A.B., Knappskog, D.H. and Midtlyng, P.J. 2007. Field validation of experimental challenge models for IPN vaccines. *J Fish Dis* **30**: 723–31.
Samuelsen, O.B., Nerland, A.H., Jørgensen, T., *et al.*, 2006. Viral and bacterial diseases of Atlantic cod *Gadus morhua*, their prophylaxis and treatment: a review. *Dis Aquat Org* **71**: 239–54.
Schlag, A.K. 2010. Aquaculture: an emerging issue for public concern. *J Risk Res* **13**: 829–44.
Shoemaker, C.A., Klesius, P.H., Evans, J.J. and Arias, C.R. 2009. Use of modified live vaccines in aquaculture. *J World Aquac Soc* **40**: 573–85.
Sniezko, S.F. 1974. The effects of environmental stress on outbreaks of infectious diseases of fishes. *J Fish Biol* **6**: 197–208.
Sommerset, I., Krossøy, B., Biering, E. and Frost, P. 2005. Vaccines for fish in aquaculture. *Exp Rev Vaccines* **4**: 89–101.
Thorarinsson, R. and Powell, D.B. 2006. Effects of disease risk, vaccine efficacy, and market price on the economics of fish vaccination. *Aquaculture* **256**: 42–9.
Toranzo, A.E., Romalde, J.L., Magariños, B. and Barja, J.L. 2009. Present and future aquaculture vaccines against fish bacterial diseases. *Op Méditerr* **86**: 155–76.
Turnbull, J.F. and Kadri, S. 2007. Safeguarding the many guises of farmed fish welfare. *Dis Aquat Org* **75**: 173–83.
Wooldridge, M. 2007. Risk modelling for vaccination: a risk assessment perspective. *Dev Biol (Basel)* **130**: 87–97.

3 Non-replicating Vaccines

Hetron Mweemba Munang'andu, Stephen Mutoloki and Øystein Evensen

Norwegian School of Veterinary Science, Oslo, Norway

ABSTRACT

Non-replicating vaccines include killed pathogens, their structures in native or synthetic forms, or their products as antigens. These vaccines will elicit primarily a B-cell response with circulating antibodies as the mode of action. Their main advantage is the safety profile – dead pathogens cannot cause disease. With the advancement of molecular methods and improved knowledge of protective antigens, there are many examples of subunit vaccines eliciting a protective immune response after parenteral delivery. Non-replicating fish vaccines are often formulated with adjuvants which will compensate for the inherent low immunogenicity of these vaccines. Loss of immunogenicity can partly be blamed on the inactivation procedure where chelating or cross-linking chemicals are used. In the years to come, one can foresee that *in vitro* methods will take over from the current *in vivo* methods used for batch release of fish vaccines. Furthermore, this will include antibody-based but likely also antigen-based methods where correlates of protection can be established for the level of antibody responses induced, or simply by quantifying the amount of antigen included in the vaccine.

3.1 INTRODUCTION

Non-replicating vaccines, as the term suggests, are vaccines whose design includes killed pathogens, their structures in native or synthetic forms, or their products as antigens. Safety is the main focus with these vaccines, since dead pathogens cannot cause disease. Nonetheless, they are able to provoke an immune response.

3.2 CLASSIFICATION

The types of non-replicating vaccine in general can be classified into the categories listed below.

oystein.evensen@nmbu.no

Fish Vaccination, First Edition. Edited by Roar Gudding, Atle Lillehaug and Øystein Evensen.

3.2.1 Inactivated vaccines

"Inactivated" is generally preferred to "killed" when referring to viral vaccines of this type, since viruses are not considered to be alive. Inactivated vaccines account for the largest component of prophylactic treatments that led to reduction of bacterial diseases in aquaculture in Norway.

The first generation of inactivated vaccines was developed by Louis Pasteur (Pasteur, 1880), streamlining the process into four basic steps, namely: (i) isolation of the pathogen; (ii) propagation; (iii) inactivation; followed by (iv) administering the inactivated microorganism into the host. Although these steps are still an integral part of modern inactivated vaccines, each of these steps has been streamlined in order to optimize vaccine performance. For example, step one has gone beyond basic isolation and characterization of the pathogen, but it has been expanded into identifying immunogenic components engaged in vaccine protection. Step two, which covers bulk propagation of the pathogen, has also been streamlined using different propagation systems such as bioreactors that enable production of the large quantities of vaccines needed to cope with the increase in demand for vaccines in aquaculture. In the case of step three, there are several procedures used for inactivation of pathogens that do not alter the antigenic structure of microorganisms.

Inactivated vaccines depend upon the inactivation of whole pathogen, and they account for the majority of commercial vaccines currently used in aquaculture. They have the advantage of being easy to make, ecosafe, and are less expensive. Inactivated bacterial vaccines account for the majority of the products on the market, followed by viral vaccines (Tables 3.1 and 3.2). There are no records of commercial vaccines against parasites and fungi at the moment.

Table 3.1 Inactivated bacterial vaccines (licensed and experimental) used in aquaculture.

Disease	Disease agent	Fish species vaccinated
Classical vibriosis	*Listonella/Vibrio anguillarum*	Salmonids, barramundi, grouper, sea bass, sea bream, yellowtail
Cold-water vibriosis	*Vibrio salmonicida*	Salmonids,
Winter ulcer	*Moritella viscosa*	Salmonids
Warm-water vibriosis	*Vibrio alginolyticus, V. vulnificus.*	Barramundi, grouper, sea bass, sea bream, snapper
Edwardsiellosis	*Edwardsiella ictaluri*	Channel fish, pangasius
Furunculosis	*Aeromonas salmonicida*	Salmonids
Yersiniosis	*Yersinia ruckeri*	Salmonids
Pasteurellosis	*Photobacterium damsela subsp. piscicida*	Sea bass, sea bream
Flavobacteriosis	*Flavobacterium columnare*	Salmonids
Flexibacteriosis	*Flexibacter maritimus*	Salmonids
Streptococcosis	*Streptococcus iniae*	Salmonids, tilapia, turbot, yellowtail
Streptococcosis	*Streptococcus agalactiae*	Tilapia
Lactococcosis	*Lactococcus garviae*	Goldstriped amberjack, purplish amberjack, sea bass, sea bream, tilapia
Piscirickettsiosis	*Piscirickettsia salmonis*	Salmonids
Bacterial kidney disease	*Renibacterium salmoninarum*	Salmonids

Table 3.2 Inactivated viral vaccines (licensed and experimental) for use in aquaculture.

Viral disease/ pathogen	Major fish species vaccinated	Immunogenic protein
Infectious pancreatic necrosis virus (IPNV)	Salmonids, various spp	Variable Protein-2 (VP2)
Infectious salmon anemia virus (ISAV)	Salmonids, grouper	Haemagglutinin esterase (HE)
Iridoviral disease	Red sea bream, yellowtail	Whole virus
Grass carp hemorrhagic disease virus (GCHDV)	Grass carp	Glycoprotein (G)
Salmon pancreas disease virus (SPDV)	Salmonids	Fusion protein (E2)

3.2.2 Subunit vaccines

Subunit vaccines rely on the expression of specific immunogenic proteins of pathogens in recombinant vectors. The recombinant proteins are then expressed in large quantities *in vitro* and then purified. Table 3.3 shows some of the immunogenic proteins of viral and bacterial vaccines used in aquaculture. The choice of vectors and cell systems is influenced by: (i) the ability to facilitate the production of large quantities of heterologous proteins *in vitro*; (ii) ease of manipulation; and (iii) the ability to express the conformational structure of the antigenic protein. Consequently, different prokaryotic and eukaryotic cell systems have been used for the production of subunit vaccines for fish diseases. Generally, these vaccines are expected to be less expensive after the initial stages of research development.

3.2.3 Synthetic peptide vaccines

Peptide vaccines use short sequences of amino acids as antigens. Because of their size, they are usually not potent enough thus require coupling to a carrier molecule. One of the earliest synthetic vaccines developed in aquaculture was made by Emmenegger and coworkers (1995) in which the synthetic peptide antigen for infectious hematopoietic necrosis virus (IHNV) was made by coupling the antigens to bovine serum albumin. The vaccine was delivered in Freund's complete adjuvant by intraperitoneal injection. Recently, Lin and coworkers (2002) produced synthetic peptides to be used for protection against freshwater white spot disease by expressing the glycosylated phosphatidylinositol (GPI) anchored membrane protein, known as the immobilization antigen (I-antigen), using an assembly polymerase chain reaction technique to manufacture the peptides. The peptides showed protective responses against the protozoa, *Ichthyophthirius multifilis*. Given that there are few synthetic peptide vaccines developed for use against fish diseases, these are not used in aquaculture.

3.2.4 Particulate vaccines

Bacteria and parasitic cell lysates, sonicated cells and other subcellular materials like lipopolysaccharides (LPS) constitute some of the antigens used in the preparations. However, these vaccines are not yet available for use in aquaculture.

3.3 INACTIVATED VACCINES – METHODS OF INACTIVATION

The main objective of inactivation is simply to render the pathogen unable to cause disease while retaining/preserving the conformational structure so that it is able to stimulate

Table 3.3 Inactivated subunit vaccines (licensed and experimental) showing immunogenic protein and vectors used for the production of fish vaccine.

Classification	Pathogen	Immunogenic protein	Vector	References
Viral	*Infectious pancreatic necrosis virus*	Variable Protein-2 (VP2)	*Escherichia coli*	(Munang'andu *et al.*, 2012)
			Pseudomonas aeruginosa	(Munang'andu *et al.*, 2012)
			Semliki forest virus	(McKenna *et al.*, 2001)
			Yeast	(Allnutt *et al.*, 2007)
			Baculovirus	(Shivappa *et al.*, 2005)
	Infectious hematopoietic necrosis virus	Glycoprotein (G)	*Caulibacter salmonicida*	(Simon *et al.*, 2001)
			Escherichia coli	(Xu *et al.*, 1991)
	Viral hemorrhagic septicemia virus	Glycoprotein (G)	*Escherichia coli*	(Estepa *et al.*, 1994; Lorenzen *et al.*, 1993)
			Aeromonas salmonicida	(Noonan *et al.*, 1995)
			Baculovirus	(Koener and Leong, 1990)
	Spring carp viremia virus (SVCV)	Glycoprotein (G)	*Baculovirus*	(Koener and Leong, 1990)
	Viral nervous necrosis virus	Capsid protein (C)	*Escherichia coli*	(Yuasa *et al.*, 2002)
Bacterial	*Streptococcus iniae*	Iron binding protein - Sip11	*Escherichia coli*	(Cheng *et al.*, 2010)
	Aeromonas hydrophila	Omp48	*Escherichia coli*	(Khushiramani *et al.*, 2012)
	Edwardsiella tarda	Flagella protein	*Escherichia coli*	(Zhang *et al.*, 2012)
	Aeromonas salmonicida	Porin	*Escherichia coli*	(Lutwyche *et al.*, 1995)
	Moritella viscosa	MvOmp1	*Escherichia coli*	(Bjornsson *et al.*, 2011)
	Vibrio alginolyticus	Flagellin (flaA and flaB)	*Escherichia coli*	(Liang *et al.*, 2012)
	Piscirickettsia salmonis	Variable proteins	*Escherichia coli*	(Wilhelm *et al.*, 2006)

Omp, Outer membrane protein; MvOmp, *Moritella viscosa* outer membrane protein.

a protective immune response. Inactivation may target (i) extracellular or outer surface components of microorganisms such as the cell membrane or the lipid bilayer forming the outer coat of viruses, or (ii) intracellular or inner components such as nucleic acids, with the aim of impeding the pathogen's ability to replicate. In principle, inactivation methods fall into two broad categories, namely physical and chemical.

3.3.1 Physical inactivation

Physical inactivation methods for microorganisms include ultraviolet (UV) light, heat and sonication. When genetic material of microorganisms is exposed to UV light, dimerization of the nucleic acids occurs, thereby impeding the ability of these microorganisms to replicate. Thermal inactivation, on the other hand, relies upon the principle that at certain temperatures two basic properties of most microorganisms, namely infectivity and immunogenicity, are lost at the same rate while at other temperatures these properties are lost at different rates. Hence, the paradigm is to find temperatures that do not destroy immunogenicity when infectivity is lost. For most microorganisms, temperatures around 56–60°C for short durations of 10–30 minutes are suitable for destroying infectivity, while immunogenicity is maintained. Thermal inactivation has been used for inactivation of bacterial vaccines under experimental conditions, and has in some studies shown better results than chemical inactivation (Antipa, 1976). Heat inactivation of fish pathogens dates back as far as 1935 when Nybelin (1935) heat-inactivated *Vibrio anguillarum*, which showed high antibody levels in vaccinated trout and carp. Another inactivation approach used for bacteria and parasites is sonication, which disrupts the morphological structure of microorganisms while retaining the immunogenic components essential for evoking adaptive immune responses in vaccinated fish. In fish vaccinology, this approach has mainly been used for bacterial vaccines (Table 3.4) under experimental conditions, and as such there are no licensed commercial vaccines produced using this method.

3.3.2 Chemical inactivation

The most commonly used chemical agent for inactivation of vaccines in both mammals and fish is formaldehyde (formalin). Unlike β-propiolactone (BPL) and binary ethylinimine (BEL), formalin has the ability to alter both the intra- and extracellular properties of different microorganisms, although when used at low concentrations it still maintains its immunogenic properties (Hiatt, 1964). The fact that it is readily available, cheap, easy and relatively safe to use makes it an attractive choice. With very few exceptions, all inactivated vaccines in aquaculture today are inactivated using this method. Table 3.4 shows the compounds used for the inactivation of fish vaccines.

Chemical inactivation can be attained by acidic pH denaturation or through the use of solvents and detergents that disrupt the lipid bilayer covering the outer surface of microorganisms. When molecules from these chemical compounds interact with the lipid bilayer, they render the outer coat dysfunctional, thereby impeding the pathogen's ability to replicate. Although these chemical compounds kill the pathogen, they do not alter the morphological structures that influence the immunogenic properties of microorganisms. Apart from denaturing the outer coat, compounds like BLP and BEL exert their effect by altering the intracellular replication of viruses through irreversible modification of the viral genome while leaving the outer surface morphology unaltered (Bahnemann, 1990; Budowsky, 1991; Budowsky *et al.*, 1993). These

Table 3.4 Examples of inactivation methods used for the preparation of viral and bacterial fish vaccines.

Vaccine category	Inactivation method	Method applied	Pathogen	Reference
Viral vaccines	Physical	Heat	*Infectious hematopoietic necrosis virus*	(Anderson *et al*., 2008)
			Viral hemorrhagic septicemia virus	(Tafalla *et al*., 2008)
			Infectious salmon anemia virus	(Workenhe *et al*., 2008)
	Chemical	BEL	*Infectious hematopoietic necrosis virus*	(Anderson *et al*., 2008)
			Betanodavirus	(Kai and Chi, 2008)
		BPL	*Infectious hematopoietic necrosis virus*	(Anderson *et al*., 2008)
		Formalin	*Infectious hematopoietic necrosis virus*	(Anderson *et al*., 2008)
			Infectious pancreatic necrosis virus	(Munang'andu *et al*., 2013a)
			Crucian carp hematopoietic necrosis virus	(Sato and Okamoto, 2010)
			Rock bream iridovirus	(Seo *et al*., 2013)
			Viral hemorrhagic septicemia virus	(Adelmann *et al*., 2008)
			Wasting spot syndrome virus	(Singh *et al*., 2005)
Bacterial vaccines	Physical	Heat	*Aeromonas hydrophila*	(Song *et al*., 1976)
			Aeromonas salmonicida	(Snieszko and Friddle, 1949)
			Edwardsiella tarda	(Song and Kou, 1981)
			Vibrio anguillarum	(Antipa, 1976a)
		Sonication	*Aeromonas hydrophila*	(Thune and Plumb, 1982)
			Aeromonas salmonicida	(Smith *et al*., 1980)
			Vibrio anguillarum	(Evelyn, 1984)
	Chemical	Chloroform	*Aeromonas salmonicida*	(Duff, 1942)
			Yersinia ruckeri	(Amend *et al*., 1983)
		Formalin	*Aeromonas hydrophila*	(Nayak *et al*., 2004)
			Aeromonas salmonicida	(Santos *et al*., 2005)
			Vibrio anguillarum	(Palm *et al*., 1998)
		Phenol	*Yersinia ruckeri*	(Anderson and Ross, 1972)

BPL, β-propiolactone; BEL, binary ethylinimine.

compounds are widely used for inactivation of different fish viruses under experimental conditions (Table 3.4).

3.4 EVALUATION OF INACTIVATION EFFICACY

It is important to optimize the inactivation steps when developing vaccines for commercial use. Some of the steps included in optimization of the inactivation procedures include:

(i) Determining the concentration of the chemical compound to be used for inactivation.
(ii) Duration of inactivation – time-series collection of samples of the inactivated microorganism can be used to determine the optimal duration required for inactivation.
(iii) Viability test to check that the microorganism is completely inactivated and will not replicate when exposed to conditions that favor its propagation.
(iv) Ensuring that the inactivation method does not destroy the immunogenicity properties of the microorganism.
(v) Determine whether the produced vaccine induces the desired immune response in vaccinated fish. This part requires efficacy trials which should not only evaluate the vaccine's ability to reduce infection rates and mortality, but the evaluation should also include assessment of immune responses induced by the inactivated microorganism.
(vi) Given that fish are food animals used for human consumption, it is important to ensure that inactivation procedures do not pose public health risks. To ensure safety, this calls for testing of drug residues used for inactivation and to determine their public health risk.

3.5 MEASURES OF EFFICACY FOR INACTIVATED VACCINES

In order to optimize vaccine performance, it is important to establish threshold units of immune responses that correlate with protection for use as benchmarks in vaccine production. This calls for identification of biological markers such as signatures of the adaptive immune response that correlate with vaccine protection. A correlate of protection is a biological marker that serves as a cutoff limit at which a vaccine is considered protective. Vaccines that do not measure up to the correlate of protection are considered suboptimal and ideally such vaccines should be not approved for commercial use. Consequently, determining a correlate of protection has become a gold standard upon which new vaccines are certified for use (Plotkin, 2008; United States Food and Drug Administration, 2012).

3.5.1 Relative percent survival (RPS)

Evaluation of vaccine efficacy has traditionally relied upon lethal challenge. Vaccinated fish are exposed to the live pathogen for which the vaccine is being developed in order to induce mortality, while efficacy is measured by the relative percent survival (RPS) of the vaccinated fish compared with the unvaccinated controls (Amend, 1981). The major challenge for this approach is that challenge models used to induce mortality require optimization of the different input variables used in the model, which include: (i) use of a known virulent strain of the pathogen able to cause high mortality; (ii) use of a standardized concentration of the challenge dose; (iii) susceptibility of the test fish; (iv) optimization of experimental conditions in order to avoid exerting undue stress that would alter the outcome of the efficacy trial; and (v) that the experimental designs allow for statistical analyses able to show significant differences between vaccine protected fish and the unvaccinated control fish. For most fish diseases, challenge models are not optimized, and as such they are not easily reproducible. This makes it difficult to compare efficacy data for different vaccine batches. Besides, the approach is not ideal for pathogens known not to cause high mortality in susceptible fish.

3.6 MECHANISMS OF VACCINE PROTECTION

It is important to point out that not all diseases in aquaculture cause mortality. It is evident that some diseases only induce debilitating conditions that lower production without causing significant mortality in the affected animals. Hence, the most plausible approach to measure the efficacy of vaccines against such diseases would be to determine the mechanisms of protective immunity induced by vaccination. For example, pancreas disease (PD) is known to cause pathological conditions that do not always culminate in mortality, and yet its impact on reducing production by slowing growth of infected fish causes significant losses in aquaculture. In mammalia, vaccine development has taken a more functional approach in which vaccines are licensed based on a good understanding of their pathogenesis and mechanisms of protection. For example, the mode of protection for poliovirus and measles vaccines is to prevent viremia (Fox, 1984; Chen *et al.*, 1990), while for rabies it is to prevent virus attachment on acetylcholine, a nerve receptor found on neuronal junctions (Hanham *et al.*, 1993). Hence, the hallmark of vaccination for these diseases is to evoke immune responses that will attain these protective mechanisms. Similarly, it is expected that blocking attachment of infectious salmon anemia virus to the sialic acid receptor (Hellebo *et al.*, 2004; Aamelfot *et al.*, 2012) would prevent establishment of infection, while for PD, protection can be attained by preventing establishment of pathological disease in the pancreas and heart. In the case of *Infectious pancreatic necrosis virus* (IPNV) in Atlantic salmon it has been shown that establishment of pathological disease can be blocked by preventing the seeding of virus in target organs and by ensuring that virus replication does not reach the correlate of pathology (10^7) which is a critical determinant of tissue damage in target organs (Munang'andu *et al.*, 2013a). It is envisaged that as more infection biology studies are carried out for different pathogens in aquatic medicine, efficacy studies will be streamlined to establish threshold endpoints at which protective immunity prevents the progression of infection into disease establishment in vaccinated fish.

3.7 ANTIBODIES AS CORRELATES OF PROTECTIVE IMMUNITY

Traditionally, antibodies are the common correlates of protection used as a measure of the efficacy of most vaccines. As pointed out elsewhere (Pulendran *et al.*, 2010), once antibody levels reach a threshold unit above which they are considered protective, then they are said to have reached a signature of protective immunity. Accordingly, many vaccines for mammals are licensed based upon established antibody titers that serve as correlates of protection. However, this approach is yet to become the basis for the licensure of commercial vaccines in aquaculture. However, current studies focused on this approach in fish vaccinology have made tremendous progress. For example, two independent efficacy studies (Munang'andu *et al.*, 2013b) carried out in Atlantic salmon vaccinated against IPNV showed that antibody levels generated before challenge corresponded with post-challenge survival proportions in fish challenged with the highly virulent Norwegian Sp strain NVI-015. Similarly, Romstad and coworkers (2013) showed high correlations between increase in antibody levels with reduction of post-challenge mortality in Atlantic salmon vaccinated against furunculosis. Hence, it is envisioned that licensure of future vaccines for use in aquaculture will be based upon established threshold units of antibody titers that will serve as correlates of protective immunity.

3.8 ANTIGEN DOSE AS CORRELATE OF PROTECTIVE IMMUNITY

In contrast with human vaccines where efficacy cannot be measured by challenge studies for ethical reasons, in fish vaccinology it has been demonstrated that antigen dose correlates with protective immunity for some disease. Therefore, a threshold unit of antigen dose can be determined that correlates with protective immunity. It has been shown that a suboptimal dose one log (10^1) lower than the protective threshold unit can cause a significant reduction in protective immunity in fish vaccinated against infectious pancreatic necrosis (Munang'andu *et al.*, 2013a). Therefore, it is important that a threshold unit of antigen dose that would serve as a correlate of protection can be established which would in turn serve as a benchmark for vaccine production.

REFERENCES

Aamelfot, M., Dale, O.B., Weli, S.C., *et al.*, 2012. Expression of the infectious salmon anemia virus receptor on Atlantic salmon endothelial cells correlates with the cell tropism of the virus. *J Virol* **86**: 10571–8.

Adelmann, M., Kollner, B., Bergmann, S.M., *et al.*, 2008. Development of an oral vaccine for immunisation of rainbow trout (*Oncorhynchus mykiss*) against viral haemorrhagic septicaemia. *Vaccine* **26**: 837–44.

Allnutt, F.C., Bowers, R.M., Rowe, C.G., *et al.*, 2007. Antigenicity of infectious pancreatic necrosis virus VP2 subviral particles expressed in yeast. *Vaccine* **25**: 4880–88.

Amend, D.F. 1981. Potency testing of fish vaccines. *Dev Biol Stand* **49**: 447–54.

Amend, D.F., Johnson, K.A., Croy, T.R. and McCarthy, D.H. 1983. Some factors affecting the potency of *Yersinia ruckeri* bacterins. *J Fish Dis* **6**: 337–44.

Anderson, D.F. and Ross, A.J. 1972. Comparative study of Hagerman redmouth disease oral bacterins. *Prog Fish Cult* **34**: 226.

Anderson, E., Clouthier, S., Shewmaker, W., *et al.*, 2008. Inactivated infectious haematopoietic necrosis virus (IHNV) vaccines. *J Fish Dis* **31**: 729–45.

Antipa, R. 1976. Field testing of injected *Vibrio anguillarum* bacterins in pen-reared Pacific salmon. *J Fish Res Board Can* **33**: 1291–6.

Bahnemann, H.G. 1990. Inactivation of viral antigens for vaccine preparation with particular reference to the application of binary ethylenimine. *Vaccine* **8**: 299–303.

Bjornsson, H., Marteinsson, V.P., Friojonsson, O.H., *et al.*, 2011. Isolation and characterization of an antigen from the fish pathogen *Moritella viscosa*. *J Appl Microbiol* **111**: 17–25.

Budowsky, E.I. 1991. Problems and prospects for preparation of killed antiviral vaccines. *Adv Virus Res* **39**: 255–90.

Budowsky, E.I., Smirnov, Y. and Shenderovich, S.F. 1993. Principles of selective inactivation of viral genome. VIII. The influence of ß-propiolactone on immunogenic and protective activities of influenza virus. *Vaccine* **11**: 343–8.

Chen, R.T., Markowitz, L.E., Albrecht, P., *et al.*, 1990. Measles antibody – reevaluation of protective titers. *J Infect Dis* **162**: 1036–42.
Cheng, S., Hu, Y.H., Jiao, X.D. and Sun, L. 2010. Identification and immunoprotective analysis of a Streptococcus iniae subunit vaccine candidate. *Vaccine* **28**: 2636–41.
Duff, D.C.B. 1942. The oral immunization of trout against *Bacterium salmonicida*. *J Immunol* **44**: 87–94.
Emmenegger, E., Huang, C., Landolt, M., *et al.*, 1995. Immune response to synthetic peptides representing antigenic sites on the glycoprotein of infectious hematopoietic necrosis virus. *Vet Res* **26**: 374–8.
Estepa, A., Thiry, M. and Coll, J.M. 1994. Recombinant protein fragments from hemorrhagic septicemia rhabdovirus stimulate trout leukocyte anamnestic responses *in vitro*. *J Gen Virol* **75**: 1329–38.
Evelyn, T.P.T. 1984. Immunization against pathogenic vibrios, in *Symposium on Fish Vaccination* (ed. P. de Kinkelin). Paris, OIE, 121–50.
Fox, J.P. 1984. Modes of action of poliovirus vaccines and relation to resulting immunity. *Rev Infect Dis* **6**: S352–5.
Hanham, C.A., Zhao, F. and Tignor, G.H. 1993. Evidence from the antiidiotypic network that the acetylcholine receptor is a rabies virus receptor. *J Virol* **67**: 530–42.
Hellebo, A., Vilas, U., Falk, K. and Vlasak, R. 2004. Infectious salmon anemia virus specifically binds to and hydrolyzes 4-O-acetylated sialic acids. *J Virol* **78**: 3055–62.
Hiatt, C.W. 1964. Kinetics of the inactivation of viruses. *Bacteriol Rev* **28**: 150–63.
Kai, Y.H. and Chi, S.C. 2008. Efficacies of inactivated vaccines against betanodavirus in grouper larvae (*Epinephelus coioides*) by bath immunization. *Vaccine* **26**: 1450–57.
Khushiramani, R.M., Maiti, B., Shekar, M., *et al.*, 2012. Recombinant *Aeromonas hydrophila* outer membrane protein 48 (Omp48) induces a protective immune response against *Aeromonas hydrophila* and *Edwardsiella tarda*. *Res Microbiol* **163**: 286–91.
Koener, J.F. and Leong, J.A.C. 1990. Expression of the glycoprotein gene from a fish rhabdovirus by using baculovirus vectors. *J Virol* **64**: 428–30.
Liang, H.Y., Wu, Z.H., Jian, J.C. and Liu, Z.H. 2012. Construction of a fusion flagellin complex and evaluation of the protective immunity of it in red snapper (*Lutjanus sanguineus*). *Lett Appl Microbiol* **55**: 115–21.
Lin, Y., Cheng, G., Wang, X. and Clark, T.G. 2002. The use of synthetic genes for the expression of ciliate proteins in heterologous systems. *Gene* **288**: 85–94.
Lorenzen, N., Olesen, N.J., Vestergård-Jørgensen, P.E., *et al.*, 1993. Molecular cloning and expression in *Escherichia coli* of the glycoprotein gene of VHS virus, and immunization of rainbow trout with the recombinant protein. *J Gen Virol* **74**: 623–30.
Lutwyche, P., Exner, M.M., Hancock, R.E. and Trust, T.J. 1995. A conserved *Aeromonas salmonicida* porin provides protective immunity to rainbow trout. *Infect Immun* **63**: 3137–42.
McKenna, B.M., Fitzpatrick, R.M., Phenix, K.V., *et al.*, 2001. Formation of infectious pancreatic necrosis virus-like particles following expression of segment A by recombinant semliki forest virus. *Mar Biotechnol (NY)* **3**: 103–10.
Munang'andu, H.M., Fredriksen, B.N., Mutoloki, S., *et al.*, 2012. Comparison of vaccine efficacy for different antigen delivery systems for infectious pancreatic necrosis virus vaccines in Atlantic salmon (*Salmo salar* L.) in a cohabitation challenge model. *Vaccine* **30**: 4007–16.
Munang'andu, H.M., Fredriksen, B.N., Mutoloki, S., *et al.*, 2013a. Antigen dose and humoral immune response correspond with protection for inactivated infectious pancreatic necrosis virus vaccines in Atlantic salmon (*Salmo salar* L). *Vet Res* **44**: 7.
Munang'andu, H.M., Sandtro, A., Mutoloki, S., *et al.*, 2013b. Immunogenicity and cross protective ability of the central VP2 amino acids of infectious pancreatic necrosis virus in Atlantic salmon (*Salmo salar* L.). *PLoS One* **8**: e54263.
Nayak, D.K., Asha, A., Shankar, K.M. and Mohan, C.V. 2004. Evaluation of biofilm of *Aeromonas hydrophila* for oral vaccination of *Clarias batrachus* – a carnivore model. *Fish Shellfish Immunol* **16**: 613–19.
Noonan, B., Enzmann, P.J. and Trust, T.J. 1995. Recombinant infectious hematopoietic necrosis virus and viral hemorrhagic septicemia virus glycoprotein epitopes expressed in *Aeromonas salmonicida* induce protective immunity in rainbow trout (*Oncorhynchus mykiss*). *Appl Environ Microbiol* **61**: 3586–91.
Nybelin, O. 1935. Über Agglutininbildung bei Fischen. *Z Immunitätsforschung* **84**: 74–9.
Palm, R.C., Jr.,, Landolt, M.L. and Busch, R.A. 1998. Route of vaccine administration: effects on the specific humoral response in rainbow trout *Oncorhynchus mykiss*. *Dis Aquat Org* **33**: 157–66.
Pasteur, L. 1880. De l'attenuation du virus du cholera des poules. *CR Acad Sci Paris* **91**: 673–80.
Plotkin, S.A. 2008. Correlates of vaccine-induced immunity. *Clin Infect Dis* **47**: 401–9.

Pulendran, B., Li, S.Z. and Nakaya, H.I. 2010. Systems vaccinology. *Immunity* **33**: 516–29.

Romstad, A.B., Reitan, L.J,. Midtlyng, P., *et al.*, 2013. Antibody responses correlate with antigen dose and *in vivo* protection for oil-adjuvanted, experimental furunculosis (*Aeromonas salmonicida* subsp *salmonicida*) vaccines in Atlantic salmon (*Salmo salar* L.) and can be used for batch potency testing of vaccines. *Vaccine* **31**: 791–6.

Santos, Y., Garcia-Marquez, S., Pereira, P.G., *et al.*, 2005. Efficacy of furunculosis vaccines in turbot, *Scophthalmus maximus* (L.): evaluation of immersion, oral and injection delivery. *J Fish Dis* **28**: 165–72.

Sato, A. and Okamoto, N. 2010. Induction of virus-specific cell-mediated cytotoxic responses of isogeneic ginbuna crucian carp, after oral immunization with inactivated virus. *Fish Shellfish Immunol* **29**: 414–21.

Seo, J.Y., Chung, H.J. and Kim, T.J. 2013. Codon-optimized expression of fish iridovirus capsid protein in yeast and its application as an oral vaccine candidate. *J Fish Dis* 36: 763–8.

Shivappa, R.B., McAllister, P.E., Edwards, G.H., *et al.*, 2005. Development of a subunit vaccine for infectious pancreatic necrosis virus using a baculovirus insect/larvae system. *Dev Biol (Basel)* **121**: 165–74.

Simon, B., Nomellini, J., Chiou, P., *et al.*, 2001. Recombinant vaccines against infectious hematopoietic necrosis virus: production by the *Caulobacter crescentus* S-layer protein secretion system and evaluation in laboratory trials. *Dis Aquatic Org* **44**: 17–27.

Singh, I.S.B., Manjusha, M., Pai, S.S. and Philip, R. 2005. *Fenneropenaeus indicus* is protected from white spot disease by oral administration of inactivated white spot syndrome virus. *Dis Aquatic Org* **66**: 265–70.

Smith, P.D., McCarthy, D.H. and Paterson, W.D. 1980. Further studies on furunculosis vaccination, in *Fish Diseases, Third COPRAQ Session* (ed. W. Ahne). Berlin, Springer-Verlag, 119.

Snieszko, S. and Friddle, S.B. 1949. Prophylaxis of furunculosis in brook trout (*Salvelinus fontinalis*) by oral immunization and sulphamerazine. *Prog Fish Cult* **11**: 161.

Song, Y.L. and Kou, G.H. 1981. Immune response of eels *(Anguilla japonica)* against *Aeromonas hydrophila* and *Edwardsiella anguillimortiferum (E. tarda)* infection. *Proc Rep Chin US Coop ScL Seminar on Fish Dis, Nat- ScL Conn Set* **3**: 107.

Song, Y.L., Chen, S.N. and Kou, G.H. 1976. Agglutinating antibodies production and protection in eel *(Anguilla japonica)* inoculated with *Aeromonas hydrophila (A liquefaciens)* antigens. *J Fish Soc Taiwan* **4**(2): 25–9.

Tafalla, C., Sanchez, E., Lorenzen, N., *et al.*, 2008. Effects of viral hemorrhagic septicemia virus (VHSV) on the rainbow trout (*Oncorhynchus mykiss*) monocyte cell line RTS-11. *Mol Immunol* **45**: 1439–48.

Thune, R.L. and Plumb, J.A. 1982. Effect of delivery method and antigen preparation on the production of antibodies against *Aeromonas hydrophila* in channel catfish. *Prog Fish Cult* **44**: 53.

United States Food and Drug Administration. 2012. *Complete list of vaccines licensed for immunization and distribution in the United States*. US Food and Drug Administration. New Hampshire Avenue, Silver Spring, MD 20993.

Wilhelm, V., Miquel, A., Burzio, L.O., *et al.*, 2006. A vaccine against the salmonid pathogen *Piscirickettsia salmonis* based on recombinant proteins. *Vaccine* **24**: 5083–91.

Workenhe, S.T., Kibenge, M.J., Wright, G.M., *et al.*, 2008. Infectious salmon anaemia virus replication and induction of alpha interferon in Atlantic salmon erythrocytes. *Virol J* **5**: 36.

Xu, L., Mourich, D.V., Engelking, H.M., *et al.*, 1991. Epitope mapping and characterization of the infectious hematopoietic necrosis virus glycoprotein, using fusion proteins synthesized in *Escherichia coli*. *J Virol* **65**: 1611–15.

Yuasa, K., Koesharyani, I., Roza, D., *et al.*, 2002. Immune response of humpback grouper, *Cromileptes altivelis* (Valenciennes) injected with the recombinant coat protein of betanodavirus. *J Fish Dis* **25**: 53–6.

Zhang, M., Wu, H.Z., Li, X.Y., *et al.*, 2012. *Edwardsiella tarda* flagellar protein FlgD: A protective immunogen against edwardsiellosis. *Vaccine* **30**: 3849–56.

4 Replicating Vaccines

Craig A. Shoemaker and Phillip H. Klesius
USDA-ARS, Aquatic Animal Health Research Laboratory, Alabama, USA

ABSTRACT

Early work on fish immunology and disease resistance demonstrated fish that survived infection were usually resistant upon re-infection. The concepts of immune resistance upon re-infection led to the research and development of replicating (live) vaccines. Replicating vaccines are successfully used in human, veterinary, and aquatic animal medicine to prevent disease. Attenuation strategies used to develop live vaccines for fish include laboratory passage, antigen mimicry, physical or chemical mutagenesis and genetic modification using molecular techniques. Laboratory studies have demonstrated the effectiveness of live vaccines in fish; however, regulatory approval in the European Union (EU), Asia and South America has not favored licensure. Replicating vaccines induce mucosal, cellular and humoral immunity. Research has also proven immersion delivery of live vaccines. Today, three live bacterial vaccines have been licensed for use in fish, including a vaccine against bacterial kidney disease (Canada, Chile and the US), one against enteric septicemia of catfish, and one against columnaris disease in catfish (US). A live viral hemorrhagic septicemia virus (VHSV) vaccine is available in Germany. Use of replicating vaccines in aquaculture is an appropriate strategy if potential risks to fish, environment and people are low or negligible. Regulatory authorities should consider the potential release of these vaccines into the environment only with supporting scientific data documenting safety, reversion to virulence potential and the absence of plasmid(s) and/or transmissible genetic elements that encode antibacterial resistance. As with all intensive animal production, vaccines are tools to be used in association with sound health management and biosecurity plans to result in the greatest benefit.

4.1 INTRODUCTION

Early work on fish immunology and disease resistance demonstrated that fish (like animals and humans) that survived infection were typically resistant to re-infection with the same pathogen

craig.shoemaker@ars.usda.gov

Fish Vaccination, First Edition. Edited by Roar Gudding, Atle Lillehaug and Øystein Evensen.

(Fujihara and Nakatani, 1971; Fijan *et al.*, 1977; Shoemaker and Klesius, 1997; Ahne *et al.*, 2002; Panangala *et al.*, 2009; Lorenzen *et al.*, 2010). This concept led to the research and development of replicating (live) vaccines in fish (Hartman and Noga, 1980; Norqvist *et al.*, 1989; Vaughan *et al.*, 1993; Thornton *et al.*, 1994; Lawrence *et al.*, 1997; Hernanz Moral *et al.*, 1998; Marsden *et al.*, 1998; Klesius and Shoemaker, 1999; Thune *et al.*, 1999; Perelberg *et al.*, 2005). Many of the laboratory studies referenced above demonstrated the effectiveness of live vaccines in fish; however, regulatory approval in the European Union (EU), Asia and South America have not favored licensing and use of live vaccines in aquaculture. Replicating vaccines induce both cellular and humoral immunity. Research has also proven the immersion delivery of live vaccines, and thus they are favored in low-value species where injection delivery is not cost-effective. To date, one live bacterial vaccine has been licensed for sale in aquaculture in Canada and Chile (Renogen® only) and three in the US (Shoemaker *et al.*, 2009). These vaccines include Renogen® against bacterial kidney disease, AQUAVAC-ESC® against enteric septicemia of catfish, and AQUAVAC-COL® against columnaris disease of catfish. A live viral hemorrhagic septicemia virus (VHSV) vaccine is available in Germany (Gomez-Casado *et al.*, 2011). This chapter will focus on attenuation strategies for the development of replicating vaccines in aquaculture. Some strategies were initially conceived in human and veterinary medicine (Linde *et al.*, 1990; Schurig *et al.*, 1991; Schnell *et al.*, 1994; Tizard, 1999). Aspects concerning live vaccine safety, delivery and generation of the immune response will also be discussed.

4.2 ATTENUATION STRATEGIES – BACTERIAL VACCINES

4.2.1 Laboratory passage

An early strategy was simple laboratory passage of organisms on media and/or in tissue culture that resulted in attenuation of the pathogenic microorganism. Daly *et al.* (2001) used laboratory attenuated *Renibacterium salmoninarum* strains to immunize Atlantic salmon (*Salmo salar*). Two strains were isolated: one that grew on trypticase soy agar (TSA) and one that grew on brain heart infusion agar (BHIA). Typically, *R. salmoninarum* only grows on KDM-2 (serum and l-cysteine containing media) agar. Following 25 *in vitro* passages, Daly *et al.* (2001) demonstrated limited virulence (8% by the TSA and 0% by the BHIA isolate, respectively) and protection 60–74 days following injection vaccination of Atlantic salmon.

A more recent example was presented by Swain *et al.* (2010). They described the generation of two rough attenuated *Aeromonas hydrophila* variants by simple laboratory passage for 8 years. The rough variants were found to lack the ladder-like lipopolysaccharide (LPS) of the wild-type smooth parent isolates. The rough *A. hydrophila* were about 100,000-fold less virulent than the wild-type *A. hydrophila* by intraperitoneal (IP) injection. Protection following IP injection of the laboratory-passaged *A. hydrophila* in carp (*Labeo rohita*) was also documented (Swain *et al.*, 2010).

4.2.2 Environmental bacterium

A second technique involves passage of the virulent pathogen in an alternative host (i.e., one not susceptible to that pathogen), isolation or use of naturally avirulent isolates or the use of an environmental bacterium that is antigenically similar to the pathogen. The most successful example of this strategy to date is Renogen®. Renogen is based on the use of *Arthrobacter* (*Ar.*) *davidanieli* delivered by injection to protect salmon against bacterial kidney disease caused by *R. salmoninarum* (Griffiths *et al.*, 1998; Salonius *et al.*, 2005). *Ar. davidanieli* is an environmental bacterium phylogenetically and antigenically related to *R. salmoninarum*. Griffiths *et al.* (1998) demonstrated that anti-*Ar. davidanieli* serum cross-reacted with surface carbohydrates of *R. salmoninarium* and suggested that the anti-*Ar. davidanieli* antibody was responsible for protective immunity upon vaccination with replicating *Ar. davidanieli*. Salonius *et al.* (2005) reported relative percent survival (RPS; Amend, 1981) of greater than 80% in injection-vaccinated Atlantic salmon.

Itano *et al.* (2006) used phylogenetic relatedness and antigenic cross-reactivity to identify potential vaccine candidates against *Nocardia seriolae*. In their study, environmental *Nocardia* species were used, and the ability of these isolates (*N. soli* and *N. fluminea*) to induce protective immunity against *N. seriolae* in injection-vaccinated yellowtail (*Seriola quinqueradiata*) was evaluated. Unfortunately, the isolates provided minimal protection upon challenge with virulent *N. seriolae*.

A recent study by Cheng *et al.* (2010) examined the vaccine potential of a naturally avirulent *Edwardsiella tarda* isolate in Japanese flounder (*Paralichthys olivaceus*). The *E. tarda* isolate (ATCC 15947) was originally obtained from human feces and found to be non-pathogenic in blue gourami (*Trichogaster trichopterus)* (Tan *et al.*, 2002). The ATCC 15947 isolate was able to transiently infect the flounder following IP injection and oral delivery, with clearance demonstrated at 8–12 days. Vaccination demonstrated RPS values of 79–81% following IP injection and 21–56% following oral or immersion administration.

4.2.3 Physical or chemical mutagenesis

The third strategy involves chemical or physical mutagenesis that results in random mutation(s) in the pathogen. The vaccine strain is then selected from the one lacking virulence in the host. Ishiguro *et al.* (1981) used physical mutagenesis (e.g. growth at 30°C) to isolate A-layer deficient strains of *A. salmonicida*. Thornton *et al.* (1994) tested A-layer deficient and/or LPS O-antigen lacking strains and demonstrated virulence reduction and vaccine potential of the isolates. They further suggested that an effective vaccine could be generated from A-layer and LPS negative strains, since inclusion of both mutations would aid in vaccine safety.

Probably the most well known and successful chemical mutagenesis strategy is the use of rifampicin. Rifampicin is an antibiotic that inhibits bacterial DNA-dependent RNA polymerase (Wehrli *et al.*, 1968) and typically results in a modified lipopolysaccharide (LPS) (Arias *et al.*, 2003; Zhang *et al.*, 2006) and attenuation of gram-negative bacteria (Norqvist *et al.*, 1989; Schurig *et al.*, 1991; Klesius and Shoemaker, 1999). Norqvist *et al.* (1989) used rifampicin and streptomycin to generate antibiotic resistant *Vibrio anguillarum* that had reduced virulence and was able to protect rainbow trout (*Oncorhynchus mykiss*) when used as a live vaccine. Klesius and Shoemaker (1999) developed the first licensed live vaccine for channel catfish (*Ictalurus punctatus*) using a similar strategy (see Chapter 8). *Edwardsiella ictaluri*, an intracellular pathogen of channel catfish, was cultured on media containing rifampicin until a concentration of 320 μg/ml was reached. The ability of the mutant strain to induce enteric septicemia of catfish disease was then evaluated. Results demonstrated that the isolate was avirulent in channel catfish by immersion exposure and that the isolate did not revert to virulent phenotype either by removing the antibiotic (*in vitro*) or following fish-to-fish passage (5 *in vivo* passages). Vaccine persistence (~14 days) and protective immunity was demonstrated in fingerling catfish (Klesius and Shoemaker, 1999). The live *E. ictaluri* vaccine (AQUAVAC-ESC®), licensed to Intervet/Schering Plough (now Merck Animal Health), underwent rigorous regulatory approval by the US Department of Agriculture Animal Plant Health Inspection Service – Center for Veterinary Biologics. Efficacy has been demonstrated in eyed catfish eggs (Klesius *et al.*, 2000; Shoemaker *et al.*, 2002, 2007), fry (Shoemaker *et al.*, 1999; Wise and Terhune, 2001; Carrias *et al.*, 2008) and fingerlings (Wise *et al.*, 2000; Lawrence and Banes, 2005; Karsi *et al.*, 2009). Bebak and Wagner (2012) reported that 12.3% or $\sim 1.35 \times 10^8$ channel catfish industry fry were vaccinated at about 15 days post-hatch (dph) using the live *E. ictaluri* vaccine in 2009.

Since licensing, other fish pathogens have been passed on rifampicin and were attenuated to be potential live vaccine candidates. Shoemaker and coworkers (2007, 2011; Sundell *et al.*, 2014) demonstrated attenuation and efficacy of a live *F. columnare* vaccine (AQUAVAC-COL®). AQUAVAC-COL® was also shown to be efficacious in largemouth bass (*Micropterus salmoides floridanus*) fry in the laboratory (Shoemaker *et al.*, 2011) and field (Bebak *et al.*, 2009). Bebak and Wagner (2012) reported that 17.0% of channel, blue and channel–blue hybrid catfish fry ($\sim 2.04 \times 10^8$) in the US were vaccinated at around 20 dph in 2009. LaFrentz *et al.* (2008) used rifampicin to attenuate *F. psychrophilum* and demonstrated both safety and efficacy in rainbow trout. This live vaccine candidate is undergoing field trials at the present time in the US (B.R. LaFrentz, personal communication). Other fish pathogens *Aeromonas hydrophila* (Klesius *et al.*, 2011), *E. tarda* (Evans *et al.*, 2006; Sun *et al.*, 2010), and *V. anguillarum* (Yu *et al.*, 2012) have also been attenuated using this strategy, and results demonstrated the vaccine potential of the selected live strains. This strategy has been one of the most practiced to date in the generation of successful veterinary vaccines (Linde *et al.*, 1990; Schurig *et al.*, 1991; Bhatnagar *et al.*, 1994; Klesius and Shoemaker, 1999; Gantois *et al.*, 2006; LaFrentz *et al.*, 2008; Shoemaker *et al.*, 2011).

Recently, novobiocin was used to attenuate *Streptococcus iniae* (Pridgeon and Klesius, 2011a; see Chapter 20) and *E. ictaluri* (Pridgeon and Klesius, 2011b). Novobiocin and rifampicin as two antibiotics in tandem were used to attenuate *A. hydrophila* (Pridgeon and Klesius, 2011c). The vaccine strains were suggested to be safe and provided protection in laboratory trials.

4.2.4 Genetic modification

The fourth strategy uses molecular methods to generate replicating vaccine candidates. Genetic modification is used to disrupt metabolic pathway(s) or virulence gene(s) that result in attenuation. An early strategy was the generation of auxotrophic mutants (Hoiseth and Stocker, 1981; Smith *et al.*, 1984). Typically, the *aro*A gene of the bacteria is inactivated by insertion of a DNA cassette containing an antibiotic resistance gene marker for selection after allelic replacement using a suicide plasmid. Inactivation of this gene does not allow survival within the host because of the failure to synthesize p-aminobenzoic acid which is required for folate biosynthesis. Vaughan *et al.* (1993) were among the first to use this strategy with a fish pathogen and demonstrated attenuation and efficacy of an *aro*A deleted *A. salmonicida* in brown trout (*Salmo trutta*). Following this, a series of *aro*A attenuated vaccine strains against *E. ictaluri* (Thune *et al.*, 1999), *A. hydrophila* (Hernanz Moral *et al.*, 1998; Vivas *et al.*, 2004), and *Yersinia ruckeri 01* (Temprano *et al.*, 2005) were produced and demonstrate to be effective in laboratory studies. However, high doses of these mutants may induce mortality in the host animal (Lawrence *et al.*, 1997; Thune *et al.*, 1999; Grove *et al.*, 2003). Although this strategy creates attenuated vaccine isolates, often the persistence of the attenuated strains is shortlived (24–72 hours) and adequate immunity is not generated in young fish.

Other metabolic pathway gene(s) including cyclic adensosine 3',5'-monophosphate (cAMP) receptor protein (*crp*) and adenylate cyclase (*cya*) have also been targeted. Santander *et al.* (2011) recently generated a *crp* in-frame deletion mutant of *E. ictaluri* based on similar strategies that had been used with other *Enterobacteriaceae* (Curtiss and Kelly, 1987). The *crp* mutant was shown to be attenuated in fingerling channel catfish and conferred protection upon immersion immunization.

Strategies have also targeted virulence genes or virulence regulatory genes (Karsi *et al.*, 2009). Cooper *et al.* (1996) used a mini-transposon to disrupt the production of chondroitin sulfatase (suspected virulence factor) in *E. ictaluri*. Channel catfish exposed to this mutant were shown to be protected following challenge with the parent isolate. Transposon mutagenesis was also used to generate an O polysaccharide-deficient isolate of *E. ictaluri* for use as a live vaccine (Lawrence *et al.*, 2001; Lawrence and Banes, 2005). The authors successfully generated an O polysaccharide-deficient isolate of *E. ictaluri*, but failed to demonstrate protection in immersion-immunized catfish (Lawrence and Banes, 2005). Igarashi and Iida (2002), using a similar technology, reported the development of an attenuated *E. tarda* vaccine by creating an *E. tarda* mutant (transposon mutagenesis) with lower siderophore production that protected tilapia (*Oreochromis niloticus*) upon lethal challenge. Leung *et al.* (1997) also generated mini-Tn5 (transposon mutants) growth- and protease-deficient *A. hydrophila* for use as live vaccines in blue gourami (*Trichogaster trichopterus*). The generated vaccine strains were not completely attenuated (Leung *et al.*, 1997).

Buchanan *et al.* (2005) used random transposon (Tn917) mutagenesis and screening in hybrid striped bass (*Morone chrysops* X *M. saxatilis*) to generate a phosphoglucomutase gene-disrupted *Streptococcus iniae*. The phosphoglucomutase enzyme is important for polysaccharide capsule formation in bacteria. Presence or absence of a capsule is important for virulence (Barnes *et al.*, 2003; Buchanan *et al.*, 2005). This isolate was attenuated in hybrid striped bass and provided protection upon lethal challenge if the live *S. iniae* was delivered by intraperitoneal injection (Buchanan *et al.*, 2005). A recent study by Locke *et al.* (2010) evaluated the phosphoglucomutase mutant and two novel mutants generated by disrupting virulence determinants including the production of capsular polysaccharide (Locke *et al.*, 2007) and m-like protein (Locke *et al.*, 2008). Locke *et al.* (2010) reported on immersion administration of all three *S. iniae* live vaccines compared with a killed vaccine preparation. Interestingly, the m-like protein mutant resulted in 100% protection, but induced a low level of disease in the vaccinated fish. The capsular polysaccharide and phosphoglucomutase mutants were attenuated but provided only partial protection following immersion vaccination.

An important emerging disease of fish is francisellosis caused by an intracellular gram-negative bacterium (Birkbeck *et al.*, 2011). Soto *et al.* (2011) generated *igl*C mutant *Francisella asiatica* and demonstrated protection of tilapia following immersion exposure. *igl*C is one of the genes of the intracellular growth pathogenicity island that aids intracellular survival of *Francisella* sp. in macrophages. The attenuated vaccine resulted in RPS values of 68–87% and protected tilapia against francisellosis in the laboratory.

4.2.5 Vaccination with live recombinant organisms expressing bacterial antigen

A strategy currently being applied to fish bacterial pathogens is use of yeast or bacterial organisms (i.e., *Saccharomyces cerevisiae* or *Lactococcus lactis*), generally regarded as safe, to deliver bacterial antigens. Zhu *et al.* (2006) expressed a *Vibrio harveyi* hemolysin on the surface of yeast cells. They demonstrated safety of the yeast cells displaying the hemolysin via injection experiments. Protective immunity was only seen in turbot, but not flounder injected with high numbers of yeast cells expressing the hemolysin. In a more recent study, Anuradha *et al.* (2010) utilized a live recombinant *Lactococcus lactis* expressing aerolysin genes D1 and D4 from *Aeromonas hydrophila*. In their experiments, tilapia were protected against the homologous strain of *A. hydrophila* following injection and oral administration of the live recombinant *L. lactis*.

4.3 ATTENUATION STRATEGIES – VIRAL VACCINES

4.3.1 Laboratory passage

One of the first reports on laboratory passage to attenuate a fish virus was an early patent describing use of this technique with *Channel catfish virus* (CCV) (Hartman and Noga, 1980) based on the procedure used by Sabin *et al.* (1954) to isolate poliovirus mutants. They created an attenuated CCV (V62) by 62 passages of the virus in a cell line derived from the walking catfish, *Clarius batrachus*. The attenuated virus exhibited distinctly smaller plaque formation on channel catfish cells and was used to vaccinate fish by immersion at 1×10^6 plaque-forming units (PFU)/ml followed by a booster vaccination at day 45–60. Vaccination with booster resulted in 97% survival vs 22% survival in sham vaccinated fish.

Kölbl (1989) patented a strategy to attenuate *Spring viremia of carp virus* (SVCV) and *Viral hemorrhagic septicemia virus* (VHSV). The strategy basically used passage in cell culture using an alternative host cell line (chicken fibroblasts) while at the same time the temperature was increased from 20° to 30°C (~350 passages total) for SVCV. The vaccine strain was shown to be attenuated and confer protection in vaccinated carp (*Cyprinus carpio*). The VHSV vaccine strain was made using a similar strategy with about 250 passages selecting the attenuated virus. Although this appears to be the method employed to produce the approved VHSV live vaccine in Germany (Gomez-Casado *et al.*, 2011), no data are presented on efficacy following vaccination of rainbow trout in the patent. Enzmann *et al.* (1998), however, suggested that the duration of protection in laboratory trials was satisfactory and immunity maintained for about 6 months. Interestingly, prior research from the 1980s employed cell culture passage to generate attenuated VHSV strains that apparently provided protection in young rainbow trout (De Kinkelin and Béarzotti-Le Beer, 1981; Vestergård-Jørgensen, 1982).

A similar strategy was employed by Ronen *et al.* (2003) with *Koi herpesvirus* (KHV). They passaged a virulent isolate for 26 passages in koi fin cells and isolated four clones with reduced virulence. The authors demonstrated protection following intraperitoneal administration of the attenuated virus as compared with sham vaccinated fish. Ronen *et al.* (2003) demonstrated that for efficient vaccination, carp had to be held at a temperature permissive for disease (18–25°C). Carp vaccinated above 27°C failed to develop protective immunity (Perelberg *et al.*, 2005). A specific anti-KHV antibody response was also observed and appeared involved in protective immunity against KHV. To further attenuate the vaccine and reduce the potential for reversion to virulence, Perelberg *et al.* (2005) used ultraviolet (UV) irradiation of the previously isolated vaccine strain. In their study, they selected a vaccine strain following 30 s UV exposure. Carp held at permissive temperature and exposed to 10 and 100 PFU/ml of the attenuated virus acquired protection with 10–20% mortality observed in the vaccinated groups versus 98% mortality in the sham vaccinated fish.

4.3.2 Molecular techniques

Zhang and Hanson (1995) produced a recombinant CCV that was attenuated by deletion of the thymidine kinase (TK) gene. This strategy had been employed with other large DNA viruses like alpha-herpesvirus where it was shown that TK-negative mutants had a reduced capacity to replicate (Wilcox *et al.*, 1992). Zhang and Hanson (1995) were able to show the attenuated CCV maintained infectivity for channel catfish and induced protective immunity following immersion exposure.

A promising approach for the development of a replicating vaccine against VHSV and *Infectious hematopoietic necrosis virus* (IHNV) is reverse genetics. The initial use of this strategy was with the negative-stranded RNA rabies virus (Schnell *et al.*, 1994). Biacchesi *et al.* (2000) detailed the strategy for generation of live recombinant (r) IHNV that was able to express foreign genes. The full-length cDNA of the IHNV RNA genome was generated using reverse transcription (RT)-polymerase chain reaction (PCR) and cloned into a transcription plasmid between a T7 RNA polymerase promoter and the autocatalytic hepatitis delta virus ribosome. Live rIHNV was recovered following transfection of the plasmid into fish cells that had been infected with recombinant vaccinia virus expressing the T7 RNA polymerase. This initial experiment demonstrated proof of concept that the strategy could generate rIHNV that was similar to wild-type virus (i.e., induced cytopathogenic effect (CPE) and mortality in rainbow trout) and thus could potentially be used to engineer new live viral vaccine strains (Biacchesi *et al.*, 2000). Biacchesi *et al.* (2002) generated rIHNV in which the IHNV G protein (external glycoprotein G) gene was replaced with the G protein gene of VHSV and the NV gene was deleted and replaced with a green fluorescent protein (GFP) gene. The recombinant virus was designated rIHNV-Gvhsv-GFP (Biacchesi *et al.*, 2002). The first study examining the potential of rIHNV as a vaccine demonstrated that deletion of the NV gene resulted in irreversible attenuation and high levels of protection in rainbow trout (Thoulouze *et al.*, 2004). Novoa *et al.* (2006), using zebrafish (*Danio rerio*) as a model, studied VHSV infection, immunity and vaccination with rIHNV-Gvhsv-GFP. They were the first to demonstrate protection against VHSV following vaccination with the live recombinant virus. In a more recent study, Romero *et al.* (2008) demonstrated lack of virulence with the live recombinant virus and also protection against both wild-type viruses in rainbow trout with RPS values of 62% and 61% against IHNV and VHSV challenge, respectively. Bootland and Leong (2011) pointed out that although laboratory studies have been successful, scale-up and compliance with regulatory/safety concerns will need to be met prior to commercial use.

4.4 INDUCTION OF IMMUNITY

Replicating vaccines invade and persist in the host and thus stimulate cell-mediated, humoral (antibody) and mucosal immunity (Clark and Cassidy-Hanley, 2005). Survival and replication of the live vaccine in the host result in strong cellular immune responses that typically confer protection of long duration. Cellular immunity (CD4+ and CD8+ T-cell responses) is responsible for providing protection against intracellular infections (Seder and Hill, 2000). Laing and Hansen (2011) reviewed the current information on T-cell immunology in fish. They point out that genomic studies have identified components associated with T-cell function and suggest that T-cell subsets are present in fish (Laing and Hansen, 2011). Studies have demonstrated the presence of relevant major histocompatibility complex (MHC) class I (Antao *et al.*, 2001) and class II molecules (Godwin *et al.*, 2000) in fish. Presentation of antigen with the correct MHC allows for response and recognition by the appropriate subpopulations of T- and B-cells. Seder and Hill (2000) suggested that live vaccines induce Th1 and CD8 T-cell responses. Marsden *et al.* (1996) demonstrated the ability of a replicating *aro*A deleted *A. salmonicida* vaccine to enhance T-cell over B-cell responses in vaccinated rainbow trout. Recent transcriptome analysis of gene expression in catfish liver tissue suggest that upon exposure to live bacteria, MHC class I genes along with other acute phase response genes are upregulated, suggesting active antigen processing and presentation (Peatman *et al.*, 2008; Pridgeon *et al.*, 2012). Induction of MHC class I genes suggests a CD8 T-cell response following infection with intracellular bacteria. Subsequent stimulation of a subpopulation of T-cells may induce interferon gamma production (Milev-Milovanovic *et al.*, 2006) that enhances intracellular pathogen destruction (Seder and Hill, 2000). Macrophage-mediated immunity also appears important in generating protective immunity following administration of replicating bacterial (Russo *et al.*, 2009) and viral (Romero *et al.*, 2011) vaccines. Thus, the general nature of the immune response by fish to live vaccines can be predicted.

Seder and Hill (2000) suggested that killed or subunit vaccines are not effective at stimulating cellular responses. Killed vaccines, or delivery of purified recombinant antigens, results in the induction of humoral (antibody-mediated) immunity. A formalin-inactivated *Edwardsiella ictaluri* vaccine previously used in aquaculture was shown to have a limited ability to enter the fish (Nusbaum and Morrison, 1996). Formalin inactivation may result in the alteration of important surface antigens in some cases (Bader *et al.*, 1997). These two factors can lead to inactivated vaccine failure and no protection in young fish against intracellular pathogens (Thune *et al.*, 1997). Most killed vaccines are delivered by injection in the presence of adjuvant to be effective. Early *Vibrio* bacterins were delivered by immersion (Sommerset *et al.*, 2005); however, the best protective effect has been shown following injection (Norqvist *et al.*, 1989). Duration of immunity induced by killed vaccines is often less than 4 months and only effective on extracellular pathogens or pathogens producing toxins. Extending the length of immunity following administration of killed vaccines often relies upon multiple immunizations and/or use of adjuvant(s). Immunity following exposure to replicating bacterial and viral vaccines has been demonstrated for greater than 4 months (Klesius and Shoemaker, 1997) or 6 months (Enzmann *et al.*, 1998), respectively. Live vaccines are also capable of inducing protection in immunologically immature fish. Protection induced by live vaccination of young fish is believed to result due to vaccine persistence (i.e., until the immune system can respond) and/or the expression of antigens with the correct MHC on host immune cells, thereby activating immunocompetent cells similar to that documented in poultry (Mast and Goddeeris, 1999).

4.5 VACCINE DELIVERY

Replicating vaccines generally have the advantage of being easier to deliver to the animals either through the oral route in feed or water (Frey, 2007), or through immersion of fish in water (Norqvist *et al.*, 1989; Klesius *et al.*, 2004; Perelberg *et al.*, 2005). Replicating vaccines developed for use in warm-water aquaculture are delivered by immersion exposure to young fry (i.e., prior to release into ponds). The vaccine strain(s) retain their ability to colonize and infect the host, which allows for effective immunity to develop following immersion delivery. Live *Vibrio anguillarum* vaccines delivered by immersion were shown to induce high levels of protection using a small dose of vaccine (Norqvist *et al.*, 1989). Norqvist *et al.* (1989) suggested that the ability of the live vaccine to replicate in the host resulted in an increased vaccine signal.

4.6 VACCINE SAFETY CONSIDERATIONS

The concept of safety in the use of replicating vaccines is with respect to the inability of the vaccine strain to cause disease in the vaccinated animal (reversion to virulence) and the potential dissemination of the vaccine strain into the environment. Frey (2007) provides an excellent review of biological safety concepts of genetically modified live bacterial vaccines used in veterinary medicine. The basic principles apply to the use of replicating vaccines in aquaculture. In the US, the Department of Agriculture (USDA) Animal-Plant Health Inspection Service's (APHIS) Center for Veterinary Biologics provides the regulatory authority for licensing and registering veterinary biologics (www.aphis.usda.gov). Safety studies consist of experiments using 10 times the immunizing dose and fish-to-fish passage to assess reversion to virulence. Also, a risk analysis must consider the release of the replicating vaccine into the aquatic environment. Presence of the pathogen in the natural environment, the ability of the pathogen to infect people and the potential of replicating vaccine(s) possessing plasmids or other transmissible genetic elements that may encode antibiotic resistance are important considerations. LaFrentz *et al.* (2011) were among the first to examine a live, replicating fish vaccine for the presence of multidrug resistance plasmid(s). They demonstrated that a live *E. ictaluri* vaccine lacked resistance to common antimicrobials used in aquaculture and did not possess IncA/C or other plasmid incompatibility groups. With the increasing use of molecular techniques, the potential to ensure safer replicating vaccines (e.g. Wang *et al.*, 2013) may lead to the use of this strategy to prevent intracellular diseases that killed vaccines are generally ineffective against.

4.7 ACKNOWLEDGEMENT

The authors gratefully acknowledge Scott LaPatra, Dehai Xu and Ben LaFrentz for critical review and helpful suggestions to the manuscript. Work was supported by the United States Department of Agriculture Agricultural Research Service CRIS Project No. 6420-32000-024D. Mention of trade names or commercial products in this publication is solely for the purpose of providing specific information and does not imply recommendation or endorsement by the United States Department of Agriculture.

REFERENCES

Ahne, W., Bjorklund, H.V., Essbauer, S., *et al.*, 2002. Spring viremia of carp (SVC). *Dis Aquat Org* **52**: 261–72.

Amend, D.F. 1981. Potency testing of fish vaccines. *Dev Biol Stand* **49**: 447–54.

Antao, A.B., Wilson, M., Wang, J., *et al.*, 2001. Genomic organization and differential expression of channel catfish MHC class I genes. *Dev Comp Immunol* **25**: 579–95.

Anuradha, K., Foo, H.L., Mariana, N.S., *et al.*, 2010. Live recombinant *Lactococcus lactis* vaccine expressing aerolysin genes D1 and D4 for protection against *Aeromonas hydrophila* in tilapia (*Oreochromis niloticus*). *J Appl Microbiol* **109**: 1632–42.

Arias, C.R., Shoemaker, C.A., Evans, J.J. and Klesius, P.H. 2003. A comparative study of *Edwardsiella ictaluri* parent (EILO) and *E. ictaluri* rifampicin-mutant (RE-33) isolates using lipopolysaccharides, outer membrane proteins, fatty acids, Biolog, API 20E and genomic analyses. *J Fish Dis* **26**: 415–21.

Bader, J.A., Vinitnantharat, S. and Klesius, P.H. 1997. Comparison of whole-cell antigens of pressure- and formalin-killed *Flexibacter columnaris* from channel catfish (*Ictalurus punctatus*). *Am J Vet Res* **58**: 985–8.

Barnes, A.C., Young, F.M., Horne, M.T. and Ellis, A.E. 2003. *Streptococcus iniae*: serological differences, presence of capsule and resistance to immune serum killing. *Dis Aquat Org* **53**: 241–7.

Bebak, J. and Wagner, B. 2012. Use of vaccination against enteric septicemia of catfish and columnaris disease by the US catfish industry. *J Aquat Anim Health* **24**: 30–36.

Bebak, J., Matthews, M. and Shoemaker, C. 2009. Survival of vaccinated, feed-trained largemouth bass fry (*Micropterus salmoides floridanus*) during natural exposure to *Flavobacterium columnare*. *Vaccine* **27**: 4297–301.

Bhatnagar, N., Getachew, E., Straley, S., *et al.*, 1994. Reduced virulence of rifampicin-resistant mutants of *Francisella tularensis*. *J Infect Dis* **170**: 841–7.

Biacchesi, S., Thoulouze, M.-I., Béarzotti, M., *et al.*, 2000. Recovery of NV knockout infectious hematopoietic necrosis virus expressing foreign genes. *J Virol* **74**: 11247–53.

Biacchesi, S., Béarzotti, M., Bouguyon, E. and Brémont, M. 2002. Heterologous exchanges of the glycoprotein and the matrix protein in a *Novirhabdovirus*. *J Virol* **76**: 2881–9.

Birkbeck, T.H., Feist, S.W. and Verner-Jeffreys, D.W. 2011. *Francisella* infections in fish and shellfish. *J Fish Dis* **34**: 173–87.

Bootland, L.M. and Leong, J.A.C. 2011. Infectious haematopoietic necrosis virus, in *Viral, Bacterial and Fungal Infections*, 2nd edn (eds P.T.K. Woo and D.W. Bruno). Wallingford, CAB, 66–109.

Buchanan, J.T., Stannard, J.A., Lauth, X., *et al.*, 2005. *Streptococcus iniae* phosphoglucomutase is a virulence factor and target for vaccine development. *Infect Immun* **73**: 6935–44.

Carrias, A.A., Terhune, J.S., Sayles, C.A. and Chappel, J.A. 2008. Effects of an extended hatchery phase and vaccination against enteric septicemia of catfish on the production of channel catfish, *Ictalurus punctatus*, fingerlings. *J World Aquac Soc* **39**: 259–66.

Cheng, S., Hu, Y., Zhang, M. and Sun, L. 2010. Analysis of the vaccine potential of a natural avirulent *Edwardsiella tarda* isolate. *Vaccine* **28**: 2716–21.

Clark, T.G. and Cassidy-Hanley, D. 2005. Recombinant subunit vaccines: potentials and constraints. *Dev Biol (Basel)* **121**: 153–63.

Cooper II,, R.K., Shotts Jr.,, E.B. and Nolan, L.K. 1996. Use of a mini-transposon to study chondroitinase activity associated with *Edwardsiella ictaluri*. *J Aquat Anim Health* **8**: 319–24.

Curtiss, III,, R. and Kelly, S.M. 1987. *Salmonella typhimurium* deletion mutants lacking adenylate cyclase and cyclic AMP receptor protein are avirulent and immunogentic. *Infect Immun* **55**: 3035–43.

Daly, J.G., Griffiths, S.G., Kew, A.K., *et al.*, 2001. Characterization of attenuated *Renibacterium salmoninarum* strains and their use as live vaccines. *Dis Aquat Org* **44**: 121–6.

De Kinkelin, P. and Béarzotti-Le Beer, M. 1981. Immunization of rainbow trout against viral haemorrhagic septicemia (VHS) with a thermoresistant variant of the virus. *Dev Biol Stand* **49**: 431–9.

Enzmann, P.-J., Fichtner, D., Schütze, H. and Walliser, G. 1998. Development of vaccines against VHS and IHN: oral application, molecular marker and discrimination of vaccinated fish from infected populations. *J Appl Ichthyol* **14**: 179–83.

Evans, J.J., Klesius, P.H. and Shoemaker, C.A. 2006. A modified live *Edwardsiella tarda* vaccine for aquatic animals. US Patent No. 7,067,122.
Fijan, N., Petrinec, Z., Štancl, Z., *et al.*, 1977. Vaccination of carp against spring viremia: comparison of intraperitoneal and peroral application of live virus to fish kept in ponds. *Bull Off Int Épizoot* **87**: 441–2.
Frey, J. 2007. Biological safety concepts of genetically modified live bacterial vaccines. *Vaccine* **25**: 5598–605.
Fujihara, M.P. and Nakatani, R.E. 1971. Antibody production and immune responses of rainbow trout and coho salmon to *Chondrococcus columnaris*. *J Fish Res Board Can* **28**: 1253–8.
Gantois, I., Ducatelle, R., Timbermount, L., *et al.*, 2006. Oral immunization of laying hens with live vaccine strains of TAD *Salmonella* vac® E and TAD *Salmonella* vac® T reduces internal egg contamination with *Salmonella enteritidis*. *Vaccine* **24**: 6250–55.
Godwin, U.B., Flores, M., Quiniou, S., *et al.*, 2000. MHC class II *A* genes in the channel catfish (*Ictalurus punctatus*). *Dev Comp Immunol* **24**: 609–22.
Gomez-Casado, E., Estepa, A. and Coll, J.M. 2011. A comparative review on European-farmed finfish RNA viruses and their vaccines. *Vaccine* **29**: 2657–71.
Griffiths, S.G., Melville, K.J. and Salonius, K. 1998. Reduction of *Renibacterium salmoninarum* culture activity in Atlantic salmon following vaccination with avirulent strains. *Fish Shellfish Immunol* **8**: 607–19.
Grove, S., Høie, S. and Evensen, Ø. 2003. Distribution and retention of antigens of *Aeromonas salmonicida* in Atlantic salmon (*Salmo salar* L.) vaccinated with a Δ*aro*A mutant or formalin-inactivated bacteria in oil-adjuvant. *Fish Shellfish Immunol* **15**: 349–58.
Hartman, J.X. and Noga, E.J. 1980. Channel catfish virus disease vaccine and method of preparation thereof and method of immunization therewith. US Patent No. 4,219,543.
Hernanz Moral, C., Flaño Del Castillo, E., López Fierro, P., *et al.*, 1998. Molecular characterization of the *Aeromonas hydrophila aro*A gene and potential use of an auxotrophic *aro*A mutant as a live attenuated vaccine. *Infect Immun* **66**: 1813–21.
Hoiseth, S.K. and Stocker, B.A.D. 1981. Aromatic dependent *Salmonella typhimurium* are non-virulent and effective as live vaccines. *Nature* **291**: 238–9.
Igarashi, A. and Iida, T. 2002. A vaccination trial using live cells of *Edwardsiella tarda* in tilapia. *Fish Pathol* **37**: 145–8.
Ishiguro, E.E., Kay, W.W., Ainsworth, T., *et al.*, 1981. Loss of virulence during culture of *Aeromonas salmonicida* at high temperature. *J Bacteriol* **148**: 333–40.
Itano, T., Kawakami, H., Kono, T. and Sakai, M. 2006. Live vaccine trials against nocardiosis in yellowtail *Seriola quinqueradiata*. *Aquaculture* **261**: 1175–80.
Karsi, A., Gülsoy, N., Corb, E., *et al.*, 2009. High-throughput bioluminescence-based mutant screening strategy for identification of bacterial virulence genes. *Appl Environ Microbiol* **75**: 2166–75.
Klesius, P.H. and Shoemaker, C.A. 1997. Heterologous isolates challenge of channel catfish, *Ictalurus punctatus*, immune to *Edwardsiella ictaluri*. *Aquaculture* **157**: 147–55.
Klesius, P.H. and Shoemaker, C.A. 1999. Development and use of modified live *Edwardsiella ictaluri* vaccine against enteric septicemia of catfish. *Adv Vet Med* **41**: 523–37.
Klesius, P.H., Shoemaker, C.A. and Evans, J.J. 2000. *In ovo* methods for utilizing live *Edwardsiella ictaluri* against enteric septicemia in channel catfish. US Patent No. 6,153,202.
Klesius, P.H., Evans, J.J. and Shoemaker, C.A. 2004. Warmwater fish vaccinology in catfish production. *Anim Health Res Rev* **5**: 305–11.
Klesius, P.H., Shoemaker, C.A. and Evans, J.J. 2011. Modified live *Aeromonas hydrophila* vaccine for aquatic animals. US Patent No. 7,988,977 B2.
Kölbl, O. 1989. *Process for producing an avirulent cold blood virus*. World Intellectual Property Organization, WO/1989/005154.
LaFrentz, B.R., LaPatra, S.E., Call, D.R. and Cain, K.D. 2008. Isolation of rifampicin resistant *Flavobacterium psychrophilum* strains and their potential as live attenuated vaccine candidates. *Vaccine* **26**: 5582–9.
LaFrentz, B.R., Welch, T.J., Shoemaker, C.A., *et al.*, 2011. Modified live *Edwardsiella ictaluri* vaccine, AQUAVAC-ESC, lacks multidrug resistance plasmids. *J Aquat Anim Health* **23**: 195–9.
Laing, K.J. and Hansen, J.D. 2011. Fish T-cells: recent advances through genomics. *Dev Comp Immunol* **35**: 1282–95.
Lawrence, M.L. and Banes, M.M. 2005. Tissue persistence and vaccine efficacy of an O polysaccharide mutant strain of *Edwardsiella ictaluri*. *J Aquat Anim Health* **17**: 228–32.
Lawrence, M.L., Cooper, R.K. and Thune, R.L. 1997. Attenuation, persistence, and vaccine potential of an *Edwardsiella ictaluri pur*A mutant. *Infect Immun* **65**: 4642–51.

Lawrence, M.L., Banes, M.M. and Williams, M.L. 2001. Phenotype and virulence of a transposon derived lipopolysaccharide O side-chain mutant strain of *Edwardsiella ictaluri*. *J Aquat Anim Health* **13**: 291–9.
Leung, K.Y., Wong, L.S., Low, K.W. and Sin, Y.M. 1997. Mini-Tn5 induced growth- and protease-deficient mutants of *Aeromonas hydrophila* as live vaccines for blue gourami, *Trichogaster trichopterus* (Pallas). *Aquaculture* **158**: 11–22.
Linde, K., Beer, J. and Bondarenko, V. 1990. Stable *Salmonella* live vaccine strains with two or more attenuating mutations and any desired level of attenuation. *Vaccine* **8**: 278–82.
Locke, J.B., Colvin, K.M., Datta, A.K., *et al.*, 2007. *Streptococcus iniae* capsule impairs phagocytic clearance and contributes to virulence in fish. *J Bacteriol* **189**: 1279–87.
Locke, J.B., Aziz, R.K., Vicknair, M.R., *et al.*, 2008. *Streptococcus iniae* M-like protein contributes to virulence in fish and is a target for live attenuated vaccine development. *PloS ONE* **3**: e2824.
Locke, J.B., Vicknair, M.R., Ostland, V.E., *et al.*, 2010. Evaluation of *Streptococcus iniae* killed bacterin and live attenuated vaccines in hybrid striped bass through injection and bath immersion. *Dis Aquat Org* **89**: 117–23.
Lorenzen, E., Brudeseth, B.E., Wiklund, T. and Lorenzen, N. 2010. Immersion exposure of rainbow trout (*Oncorhynchus mykiss*) fry to wildtype *Flavobacterium psychrophilum* induces no mortality, but protects against later intraperitoneal challenge. *Fish Shellfish Immunol* **28**: 440–44.
Marsden, M.J., Vaughan, L.M., Fitzpatrick, R.M., *et al.*, 1998. Potency testing of a live genetically attenuated vaccine for salmonids. *Vaccine* **16**: 1087–94.
Marsden, M.J., Vaughan, L.M., Foster, T.J. and Secombes, C.J. 1996. A live (Δ*aro*A) *Aeromonas salmonicida* vaccine for furunculosis preferentially stimulates T-cell responses relative to B-cell responses in rainbow trout (*Oncorhynchus mykiss*). *Infect Immun* **64**: 3863–9.
Mast, J. and Goddeeris, B.M. 1999. Development of immunocompetence of broiler chickens. *Vet Immunol Immunopathol* **70**: 245–56.
Milev-Milovanovic, I., Long, S., Wilson, M., *et al.*, 2006. Identification and expression analysis of interferon gamma genes in channel catfish. *Immunogenetics* **58**: 70–80.
Norqvist, A., Hagström, A. and Wolf-Watz, H. 1989. Protection of rainbow trout against vibriosis and furunculosis by the use of attenuated strains of *Vibrio anguillarum*. *Appl Environ Microbiol* **55**: 1400–5.
Novoa, B., Romero, A., Mulero, V., *et al.*, 2006. Zebrafish (*Danio rerio*) as a model for the study of vaccination against viral hemorrhagic septicemia virus (VHSV). *Vaccine* **24**: 5806–16.
Nusbaum, K.E. and Morrison, E.E. 1996. Entry of 35 S-labeled *Edwardsiella ictaluri* into channel catfish (*Ictalutus punctatus*). *J Aquat Anim Health* **8**: 146–9.
Panangala, V.S., Shoemaker, C.A., Klesius, P.H., *et al.*, 2009. Cross-protection elicited in channel catfish (*Ictalurus punctatus* Rafinesque) immunized with a low dose of virulent *Edwardsiella ictaluri* strains. *Aquacult Res* **40**: 915–26.
Peatman, E., Terhune, J., Baoprasertkul, P., *et al.*, 2008. Microarray analysis of gene expression in the blue catfish liver reveals early activation of the MHC class I pathway after infection with *Edwardsiella ictaluri*. *Mol Immunol* **45**: 553–66.
Perelberg, A., Ronen, A., Hutoran, M., *et al.*, 2005. Protection of cultured *Cyprinus carpio* against a lethal viral disease by an attenuated virus vaccine. *Vaccine* **23**: 3396–403.
Pridgeon, J.W. and Klesius, P.H. 2011a. Development and efficacy of a novobiocin-resistant *Streptococcus iniae* as novel vaccine in Nile tilapia (*Oreochromis niloticus*). *Vaccine* **29**: 5986–93.
Pridgeon, J.W. and Klesius, P.H. 2011b. Development of a novobiocin-resistant *Edwardsiella ictaluri* as a novel vaccine in channel catfish (*Ictalurus punctatus*). *Vaccine* **29**: 5631–7.
Pridgeon, J.W. and Klesius, P.H. 2011c. Development and efficacy of novobiocin and rifampicin resistant *Aeromonas hydrophila* as novel vaccines in channel catfish and Nile tilapia. *Vaccine* **29**: 7896–904.
Pridgeon, J.W., Yeh, H.-Y., Shoemaker, C.A., *et al.*, 2012. Global gene expression in channel catfish after vaccination with an attenuated *Edwardsiella ictaluri*. *Fish Shellfish Immunol* **32**: 524–33.
Romero, A., Figueras, A., Thoulouze, M.I., *et al.*, 2008. Infectious hematopoietic necrosis recombinant viruses induced protection for rainbow trout (*Oncorhynchus mykiss*). *Dis Aquat Org* **80**: 123–35.
Romero, A., Dios, S., Bremont, M., *et al.*, 2011. Interaction of the attenuated recombinant rIHNV-Gvhsv GFP virus with macrophages from rainbow trout (*Oncorhynchus mykiss*). *Vet Immunol Immunopathol* **140**: 119–29.
Ronen, A., Perleberg, A., Abramowitz, J., *et al.*, 2003. Efficient vaccine against the virus causing a lethal disease in cultured *Cyprinus carpio*. *Vaccine* **21**: 4677–84.

Russo, R., Shoemaker, C.A., Panangala, V.S. and Klesius, P.H. 2009. *In vitro* and *in vivo* interaction of macrophages from vaccinated and non-vaccinated channel catfish (*Ictalurus punctatus*) to *Edwardsiella ictaluri*. *Fish Shellfish Immunol* **26**: 543–52.

Sabin, A.B., Hennessen, W.A. and Winsser, J. 1954. Studies on variants of poliomyelitis virus I. Experimental segregation and properties of avirulent variants of three immunologic types. *J Exp Med* **99**: 551–76.

Salonius, K., Siderakis, C., MacKinnon, A.M. and Griffiths, S.G. 2005. Use of *Arthrobacter davidanieli* as a live vaccine against *Renibacterium salmoninarum* and *Piscirickettsia salmonis* in salmonids. *Dev Biol (Basel)* **121**: 189–97.

Santander, J., Mitra, A. and Curtiss, III,, R. 2011. Phenotype, virulence and immunogenicity of *Edwardsiella ictaluri* cyclic adenosine 3',5'-monophosphate receptor protein (Crp) mutants in catfish host. *Fish Shellfish Immunol* **31**: 1142–53.

Schnell, M.J., Mebatsion, T. and Conzelmann, K.K. 1994. Infectious rabies viruses from cloned cDNA. *EMBO J* **13**: 4195–203.

Schurig, G.G., Roop, II,, R.M., Bagchi, T., *et al.*, 1991. Biological properties of RB51; a stable rough strain of *Brucella abortus*. *Vet Microbiol* **28**: 171–88.

Seder, R.A. and Hill, A.V.S. 2000. Vaccines against intracellular infections requiring cellular immunity. *Nature* **406**: 793–8.

Shoemaker, C.A. and Klesius, P.H. 1997. Protective immunity against enteric septicemia in channel catfish, *Ictalurus punctatus* (Rafinesque), following controlled exposure to *Edwardsiella ictaluri*. *J Fish Dis* **20**: 361–8.

Shoemaker, C.A., Klesius, P.H. and Bricker, J.M. 1999. Efficacy of a modified live *Edwardsiella ictaluri* vaccine in channel catfish as young as seven days post hatch. *Aquaculture* **176**: 189–93.

Shoemaker, C.A., Klesius, P.H. and Evans, J.J. 2002. *In ovo* method for utilizing the modified live *Edwardsiella ictaluri* vaccine against enteric septicemia in channel catfish. *Aquaculture* **203**: 221–7.

Shoemaker, C.A., Klesius, P.H. and Evans, J.J. 2007. Immunization of eyed channel catfish, *Ictalurus punctatus*, eggs with monovalent *Flavobacterium columnare* vaccine and bivalent *F. columnare* and *Edwardsiella ictaluri* vaccine. *Vaccine* **25**: 1126–31.

Shoemaker, C.A., Klesius, P.H., Evans, J.J. and Arias, C.R. 2009. Use of modified live vaccines in aquaculture. *J World Aquac Soc* **40**: 573–85.

Shoemaker, C.A., Klesius, P.H., Drennan, J.D. and Evans, J.J. 2011. Efficacy of a modified live *Flavobacterium columnare* vaccine in fish. *Fish Shellfish Immunol* **30**: 304–8.

Smith, B.P., Reina-Guerra, M., Stocker, B.A., *et al.*, 1984. Aromatic-dependent *Salmonella dublin* as a parenteral modified live vaccine for calves. *Am J Vet Res* **45**: 2231–5.

Sommerset, I., Krossøy, B., Biering, E. and Frost, P. 2005. Vaccines for fish in aquaculture. *Exp Rev Vaccines* **4**: 89–101.

Soto, E., Wiles, J., Elzer, P., *et al.*, 2011. Attenuated *Francisella asiatica iglC* mutant induces protective immunity to francisellosis in tilapia. *Vaccine* **29**: 593–8.

Sun, Y., Liu, C.-S. and Sun, L. 2010. Isolation and analysis of the vaccine potential of an attenuated *Edwardsiella tarda* strain. *Vaccine* **28**: 6344–50.

Sundell, K., Högfors-Rönnholm, E. and Wiklund, T. 2014. Vaccination against diseases caused by *Flavobacteriaceae* species, in *Fish Vaccination* (eds R. Gudding, A. Lillehaug and Ø. Evensen). Oxford, John Wiley & Sons Ltd., 273–288.

Swain, P., Behera, T., Mohapatra, D., *et al.*, 2010. Derivation of rough attenuated variants from smooth virulent *Aeromonas hydrophila* and their immunogenicity in fish. *Vaccine* **28**: 4626–31.

Tan, Y.P., Lin, Q., Wang, X.H., *et al.*, 2002. Comparative proteomic analysis of extracellular proteins of *Edwardsiella tarda*. *Infect Immun* **70**: 6475–80.

Temprano, A., Riaño, J., Yugueros, J., *et al.*, 2005. Potential use of a *Yersinia ruckeri* O1 auxotrophic *aroA* mutant as a live attenuated vaccine. *J Fish Dis* **28**: 419–27.

Thornton, J.C., Garduño, R.A. and Kay, W.W. 1994. The development of live vaccines for furunculosis lacking the A-layer and O-antigen of *Aeromonas salmonicida*. *J Fish Dis* **17**: 195–204.

Thoulouze, M.I., Bouguyon, E., Carpentier, C. and Brémont, M. 2004. Essential role of the NV protein of *Novirhabdovirus* for pathogenicity in rainbow trout. *J Virol* **78**: 4098–107.

Thune, R.L., Collins, L.A. and Pena, M.P. 1997. A comparison of immersion, immersion/oral combination and injection methods for the vaccination of channel catfish *Ictalurus punctatus* against *Edwardsiella ictaluri*. *J World Aquac Soc* **28**: 193–201.

Thune, R.L., Fernandez, D.H. and Battista, J.R. 1999. An *aro*A mutant of *Edwardsiella ictaluri* is safe and efficacious as a live, attenuated vaccine. *J Aquat Anim Health* **11**: 358–72.
Tizard, I. 1999. Grease, anthraxgate, and kennel cough: a revisionist history of early veterinary vaccines. *Adv Vet Med* **41**: 7–24.
Vaughan, L.M., Smith, P.R. and Foster, T.J. 1993. An aromatic-dependent mutant of the fish pathogen *Aeromonas salmonicida* is attenuated in fish and is effective as a live vaccine against the salmonid disease furunculosis. *Infect Immun* **61**: 2172–81.
Vestergård-Jørgensen, P.E. 1982. Egtved virus: temperature dependent immune response of trout to infection with low virulence virus. *J Fish Dis* **5**: 47–55.
Vivas, J., Riaño, J., Carracedo, B., *et al.*, 2004. The auxotrophic *aroA* mutant of *Aeromonas hydrophila* as a live attenuated vaccine against *A. salmonicida* infections in rainbow trout (*Oncorhynchus mykiss*). *Fish Shellfish Immunol* **16**: 193–206.
Wang, Y., Wang, Q., Yang, W., *et al.*, 2013. Functional characterization of *Edwardsiella tarda* twin-arginine translocation system and its potential use as a biological containment in live attenuated vaccine of marine fish. *Appl Microbiol Biotechnol* **97**: 3545–557.
Wehrli, W., Knusel, P., Schmid, K. and Staehelin, M. 1968. Interaction of rifamycin with bacterial RNA polymerase. *Proc Natl Acad Sci* **61**: 667–73.
Wilcox, C.L., Crnic, L.S. and Pizer, L.I. 1992. Replication, latent infection, and reactivation in neuronal culture with a herpes simplex virus thymidine kinase-negative mutant. *Virology* **187**: 348–52.
Wise, D.J. and Terhune, J. 2001. The relationship between vaccine dose and efficacy in channel catfish *Ictalurus punctatus* vaccinated as fry with a live attenuated strain of *Edwardsiella ictaluri* (RE-33). *J World Aquac Soc* **32**: 177–83.
Wise, D.J., Klesius, P.H., Shoemaker, C.A. and Wolters, W.R. (2000) Vaccination of mixed and full-sib families of channel catfish *Ictalurus punctatus* against enteric septicemia of catfish with a live attenuated *Edwardsiella ictaluri* isolate (RE-33). *J World Aquac Soc* **31**: 206–12.
Yu, L.-P., Hu, Y.-H., Sun, B.-G. and Sun, L. 2012. C312M: an attenuated *Vibrio anguillarum* strain that induces immunoprotection as an oral and immersion vaccine. *Dis Aquat Org* **102**: 33–42.
Zhang, G.H. and Hanson, L.A. 1995. Deletion of thymidine kinase gene attenuates channel catfish herpesvirus while maintaining infectivity. *Virology* **209**: 658–63.
Zhang, Y., Arias, C.R., Shoemaker, C.A. and Klesius, P.H. 2006. Comparison of lipopolysaccharide and protein profiles between *Flavobacterium columnare* strains from different genomovars. *J Fish Dis* **29**: 657–63.
Zhu, K., Chi, Z., Li, J., *et al.*, 2006. The surface display of haemolysin from *Vibrio harveyi* on yeast cells and their potential applications as live vaccine in marine fish. *Vaccine* **24**: 6046–52.

5 DNA Vaccines

Eirik Biering[1] and Kira Salonius[2]

[1]Norwegian Veterinary Institute, Trondheim, Norway
[2]Independent Consultant, Prince Edward Island, Canada

ABSTRACT

DNA vaccination is genetic immunization that relies on the use of a gene or genes encoding protective antigens, instead of the antigens themselves. DNA vaccines are genetic constructs containing one or more genes derived from a pathogen, and they are designed to facilitate the transient production of protein from these genes in the vaccinee with the aim to elicit a protective immune response. DNA vaccines are usually in the form of a purified bacterial plasmid, a circular molecule of DNA able to replicate in bacterial hosts. The constructs will contain regulatory elements to ensure both replication of the plasmid in the bacterial host for production purposes, and expression of the vaccine genes in the vaccinated animal. In some cases the nomenclature NAV (nucleic acid vaccine) or genetic vaccine is used, and those terms also include vaccines that are based on other nucleic acids than DNA (including RNA).

5.1 INTRODUCTION

Most vaccines in aquaculture are inactivated products formulated with an adjuvant and delivered by injection, and they confer protection mainly by initiating production of protective antibodies. This technology works well for many bacterial diseases (Sommerset *et al.*, 2005) as neutralizing antibodies in many cases are sufficient to prevent or stop a bacterial infection. For viral diseases, however, it is often necessary to stimulate the cellular arms of the immune response in order to obtain sufficient protection (Biering *et al.*, 2005). The fact that most of the viral vaccines used in aquaculture today have limited efficacy (Gomez-Casado *et al.*, 2011) clearly illustrates that the approach with inactivated protein antigens is suboptimal for many viral diseases.

DNA vaccination is genetic immunization that relies upon the use of a gene or genes encoding protective antigens, instead of the antigens themselves. DNA vaccines are genetic

eirik.biering@vetinst.no

Fish Vaccination, First Edition. Edited by Roar Gudding, Atle Lillehaug and Øystein Evensen.

constructs containing one or more genes derived from a pathogen, and they are designed to facilitate the transient production of protein from these genes in the vaccinee with the aim to elicit a protective immune response. DNA vaccines are usually in the form of a purified bacterial plasmid, a circular molecule of DNA able to replicate in bacterial hosts. The constructs will contain regulatory elements to ensure both replication of the plasmid in the bacterial host for production purposes, and expression of the vaccine genes in the vaccinated animal (Figure 5.1). In some cases the nomenclature NAV (nucleic acid vaccine) or genetic vaccine is used, and those terms also include vaccines that are based on other nucleic acids than DNA (including RNA).

DNA vaccines are generally delivered by intramuscular injection without an adjuvant. The plasmids will transfect cells, mainly myocytes but also professional antigen-presenting cells like dendritic cells (Liu, 2011). The transfected cells produce protein from the plasmids and present this on MHC class I molecules, in this way mimicking a viral infection. This leads to stimulation of all three arms of the adaptive immune system; namely antibodies, helper T-cells and cytotoxic T lymphocytes (CTLs). The immune response toward DNA vaccines in fish has recently been reviewed (Kurath, 2008; Tonheim *et al.*, 2008) and it has been divided into three phases. The first is the early antiviral response (EAVR) that is non-specific but, at least for the rhabdovirus viral hemorrhagic septicemia virus (VHSV), is also able to provide heterologous protection against a virus not included in the vaccine (Sommerset *et al.*, 2003). The ensuing specific antiviral response (SAVR) is often characterized by the appearance of specific antibodies and increased protection that is followed by the long-term antiviral response (LAVR), where protection and antibody titers are reduced but still significant. A specific advantage of DNA vaccines is that because of the activation of the cellular arm of the immune system, they are effective in killing virus harbored intracellularly, which is a specific advantage over conventional inactivated vaccines to treat pre-existing disease. Accordingly, DNA vaccines are able to imitate a viral infection to a much greater extent than inactivated vaccines, and in some cases this results in a better protective immune response.

5.2 COMPARISON OF DNA VACCINES WITH CONVENTIONAL INACTIVATED PRODUCTS: ADVANTAGES AND DISADVANTAGES

5.2.1 Development of test vaccines

Bacterial vaccines can be quite uncomplicated to develop once the causative agent has been identified. The bacterium can then be grown, inactivated and formulated with or without adjuvant and tested in challenge experiments. This procedure is more difficult for viral vaccines. If the aim is an inactivated product based upon cell culture grown virus, it is necessary to have a receptive culture and optimized growth conditions before test vaccines are produced. If the aim is a recombinant subunit vaccine, it is necessary to identify the protective antigen(s), clone them into an expression system, recover the antigens in an active form and formulate test vaccines. Usually it is necessary to test several antigens and expression systems in order to achieve success. By comparison, DNA vaccines are much quicker to construct, the only prerequisite being detailed knowledge of the genomics of the pathogen. Today such sequence data are usually quite easy to obtain, especially for viruses, but information is available even

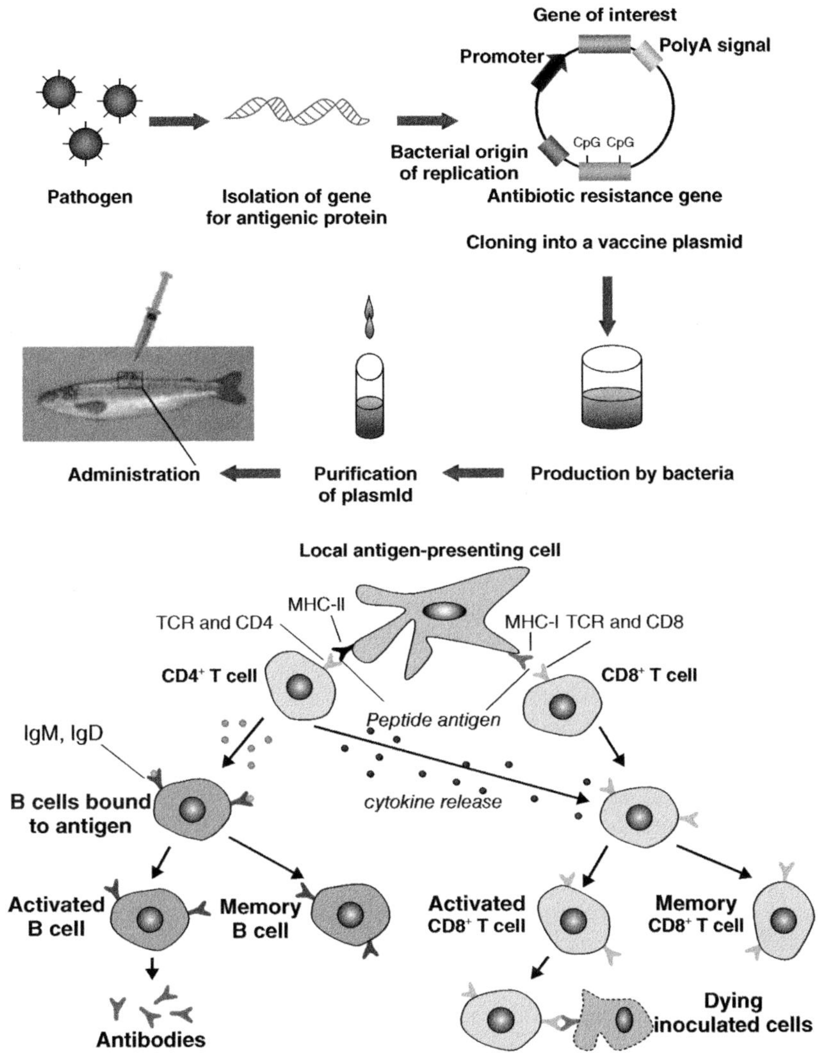

Fig. 5.1 A general and simplified overview of the adaptive immune response. DNA vaccines that have been taken up by, for example, muscle cells and processed may be completely degraded or may be expressed by the muscle cells. The transfected cells produce and release the plasmid encoding antigens that will be subjected to uptake in APCs (antigen presenting cells). APCs present peptides, being the breakdown products of the antigens, on MHC-I and II to CD8+ and CD4+ cells following uptake of endogenously and exogenously derived antigens, respectively. Activation of naïve CD4+ cells will initiate cellular and humoral adaptive responses such as activation of B cells to secrete antibodies specific to this antigen, whereas binding of the T-cell receptor of CD8+ cells to MHC-I presented peptides, with aid of cytokines produced by Th1 cells, will facilitate a cytotoxic T-cell response, eliminating virus-infected cells producing and expressing the virus antigen. One feature of the adaptive immune response is the generation of memory cells that need a short time to be activated during a later infection with the same pathogen. CD4, cluster of differentiation 4 co-receptors; CD8, cluster of differentiation 8 co-receptors; MHC-I, major histocompatibility complex class I protein; MHC-II, major histocompatibility complex class II protein; IgM, immunoglobulin M; IgD, immunoglobulin D; TCR, T-cell receptor; Th1, T helper 1. (Source: Adapted from Dufour 2001.)

for more complex organisms like the salmon louse (Skern-Mauritzen *et al.*, 2013). Selected sequences are then subcloned into a vaccine construct and test vaccines can be produced. This is a generic process that is quick to perform compared with cell culture of virus or heterologous expression. It also makes the process of culturing pathogens under containment superfluous, and it is easy to construct several test vaccines with different genes and combinations of genes. Even multivalent products can be made quite easily (Einer-Jensen *et al.*, 2009), and it is possible to use conserved genes that provide cross-protection towards several related viral strains (Ulmer *et al.*, 1993). In fact, vaccine discovery using nucleic acids – DNA, and potentially more recently RNA – has many advantages and it will be a standard method of choice for antigen selection in many cases. A more difficult matter than the design of a construct is ultimately realizing the efficacy of a DNA vaccine. In an animal model such as Atlantic salmon, it remains to be seen whether the difficulty in discovering highly efficacious DNA vaccines for many of the viral disease targets is due to inadequate construct design, transfection, protein production, or cell trafficking.

5.2.2 Production and storage

When a satisfactory test vaccine has been designed, the next step is production on a small scale for testing. It is relatively simple to produce most bacterial vaccines for fish. The microorganism in question is grown in a suspension culture, inactivated, processed and formulated with an adjuvant, or used without adjuvant for immersion vaccination. On the other hand, viral vaccines are more complicated to produce. Either it is necessary to grow the virus in a cell culture in order to obtain sufficient quantity of antigen, or one can clone the protective antigen in a heterologous expression system and produce the antigen recombinantly. Cell culture production of virus is generally expensive and complicated, and as new viruses appear, a susceptible cell line suitable for large-scale production is not always available. Heterologous expression also has its pitfalls. It can be difficult to produce the antigen in an immunologically active form, and yields are not always sufficient to secure an economic production. Compared with these types of production that must be optimized on a case-by-case basis, production of a DNA vaccine plasmid is relatively generic, even though yield can be affected by the size of the genes included. Large-scale production of plasmids in the bacterium *E. coli* is easily done on an industrial scale. However, as the purification process involves volumes of buffer that can be on a par with the volumes of fermentation processes to produce conventional bacterial antigens, there is no particular economy of scale. As specifications for acceptable quality and purity have not been established, the onus is on the manufacturer to prove a quality standard that is appropriate for safety and efficacy in the target animal. Plasmids are also relatively stable under various conditions, potentially making storage and transport easier compared with oil-adjuvanted vaccine emulsions that can be unstable and break down during storage if such conditions (such as room temperature storage) are proven in the documentation of the vaccine throughout the shelf life.

5.2.3 Formulation and delivery

Except for live vaccines and bacterial vaccines made for immersion, most fish vaccines today use an oil-adjuvant in order to obtain sufficient and prolonged protection. The vaccines are multivalent, conferring protection to several diseases of both bacterial and viral etiology (Sommerset *et al.*, 2005). These products are injected intraperitoneally (IP), and in the salmon industry this is usually done automatically. Adjuvants like Vaxfectin might be used in combination with DNA vaccines (Hartikka *et al.*, 2001; Sullivan *et al.*, 2010), and as recently reviewed, it is also possible to include sequences in the construct that may increase the potency (cytokines, co-stimulatory sequences and targeting molecules) in addition to improving delivery and uptake of the construct (Liu, 2011). Within aquaculture it is customary to formulate "naked" DNA vaccines in saline and deliver them by intramuscular (IM) injection. So far, IP injection of DNA vaccines has given little or reduced efficacy as compared with IM injection (Corbeil *et al.*, 2000; McLauchlan *et al.*, 2003). It thus follows that it is difficult to include DNA vaccines in the combination products used by the salmon industry today.

5.3 DNA VACCINES FOR VETERINARY USE

As reviewed before (Kutzler and Weiner, 2008; Liu, 2011), only three DNA vaccines are licensed today, and all are for veterinary use. Two of these are against viral diseases, namely the West Nile-Innovator® for horses against the West Nile virus (Davis *et al.*, 2001), and Apex-IHN® for salmon against *Infectious hematopoietic necrosis virus* IHNV (Salonius *et al.*, 2007). The technology can also be used to prevent non-infectious diseases such as cancer, and the third product, Oncept™, prevents melanoma in dogs (Bergman *et al.*, 2003). It is also possible to deliver biologically active molecules such as hormones without the aim of eliciting an immune response. This is demonstrated by a fourth registered DNA-plasmid product, LifeTide® SW 5, which increases litter survival in pigs (Khan *et al.*, 2010). As of today, no DNA vaccines are licensed for humans.

The original impetus for developing nucleic acid or DNA vaccines for fish was a desire to induce the potent cellular and humoral immune responses attainable by live organism-based vaccines with a simple, highly purified subunit plasmid DNA. The technology therefore is most applicable to the development of viral vaccines. DNA vaccines for the rhabdoviruses VHSV and IHNV are well described (Anderson *et al.*, 1996; Lorenzen *et al.*, 1998; Corbeil *et al.*, 1999). The disease model and the efficacy of vaccines based on constructs utilizing glycoproteins have resulted in opportunities regarding the dosing (Garver *et al.*, 2005), early innate immune responses (Kim *et al.*, 2000), heterology of protection across virus species (Lorenzen *et al.*, 1998) and the fate of DNA vaccines in farmed fish (Salonius *et al.*, 2007). In non-salmonid fish, a DNA vaccine against spring viremia of carp virus has been reported to give significant protection (relative percent survival or RPS: 48) in common carp (Kanellos *et al.*, 2006) and also in ornamental koi with a highly significant RPS of 50–80 under severe challenge at 28 days post-vaccination (Emmenegger and Kurath, 2008).

Outside of the family *Rhabdoviridae*, the reports of efficacy of DNA vaccines for other finfish disease models are somewhat less convincing. This could be related to differences in efficiency and form of assembly, presentation or trafficking of proteins in fish cells after DNA vaccination. Mikalsen and coworkers reported that a DNA vaccine expressing infectious salmon anemia virus (ISAV) haemagglutinin-esterase in Atlantic salmon demonstrated RPS of 39.5–60.5% (Mikalsen *et al.*, 2005). A plasmid construct encoding the open reading frame of the whole polyprotein of *Infectious pancreatic necrosis virus* (IPNV) showed good protection with 84% RPS against control mortality of 34% (Mikalsen *et al.*, 2004), but there are no further reports in the literature regarding work with IPNV or ISAV DNA vaccines.

Given the requirements to document a DNA vaccine and the uncertainty about acceptance in Europe, it is not surprising that the industry has pursued documentation for registration of only those DNA vaccines where there is strong evidence of superiority to conventional vaccines and where there is a serious animal welfare issue regarding the disease without an effective vaccine. More recently, there are two reports on evaluation of the efficacy of salmonid alphavirus (SAV) 3 subtype plasmid vaccines. Xu and coworkers (2012) compared the efficacy of plasmid DNA vaccines based on the E1 and E2 spike proteins, E1 and E2 subunit vaccines, and a conventional cell-culture-grown inactivated SAV vaccine. At 4 weeks post-challenge, a single injection of the conventional vaccine resulted in a 49-fold reduction in viral load over a control group vaccinated with plasmid blank. When compared with a series of prime-boost strategies where a primary vaccination was followed up at 6 weeks with a second vaccination, only one prime-boost strategy, 20 μg E1 DNA vaccine followed by 50 μg protein of an E1subunit vaccine, had a significant reduction in viral load (8.5-fold). In addition, a SAV nucleic acid vaccine (NAV) was evaluated based on the severity of pancreatic and heart tissue necrosis by histopathology and load of viral RNA as determined by R-qPCR (Simard *et al.*, 2009). Evaluation of protection levels at 10 weeks and 28 weeks post-vaccination revealed a strong and lasting protective response against infection with 10 and 20 ug doses. The reduction in viral load and disease in infected Atlantic salmon was compared with a commercially available inactivated oil-adjuvanted SAV vaccine. The NAV had superior efficacy at both 10 and 28 weeks post-vaccination. Given that there are still serious economic losses and animal welfare concerns regarding salmon pancreas disease in Northern Europe despite the use of SAV vaccines (Gomez-Casado *et al.*, 2011), this may be the first opportunity where there is impetus to pursue authorization of a nucleic acid vaccine for use in aquaculture in Europe.

5.4 BIOSECURITY AND REGULATORY CONSIDERATIONS

Safety considerations are central for the licensing of all pharmaceutical products, and for food-producing animals like fish that are reared in close contact with the environment, these are (i) safety to the animal, (ii) safety to the environment and (iii) safety to the user and consumer. Safety issues related to DNA vaccination of food-producing animals in general have been thoroughly reviewed by Holm (2004) and for fish also by Lorenzen and LaPatra (2005). It is apparent that, in many aspects, DNA vaccines are safer than comparable technologies. As no oil-adjuvant is used, post-vaccination peritonitis associated with traditional vaccines used in aquaculture is absent (Lillehaug *et al.*, 1992; Midtlyng *et al.*, 1996; Garver *et al.*, 2005; Kurath *et al.*, 2006). Recently it has also been shown that severe side-effects following vaccination with oil-adjuvanted vaccines may be linked to development of systemic autoimmunity in vaccinated salmon (Koppang *et al.*, 2008; Haugarvoll *et al.*, 2010) with potential for negative impact on fish health and welfare. With DNA vaccines there is no risk of reversion to virulence or incomplete inactivation, which may be issues related to live vaccines and inactivated vaccines respectively. As discussed by Holm (2004), issues regarding immunological tolerance or autoimmunity in the vaccinee have been mentioned, but risk potential appears minimal compared with the side-effects associated with traditional products. The main concerns are thus related to integration of the vaccine construct in the genome of the vaccinee and its possible spread to the environment, the offspring or the consumer. Even though chromosomal integration has been detected following electroporation delivery of plasmid DNA (Wang *et al.*, 2004), available data indicate that it is a very rare event (Holm, 2004; Tonheim *et al.*, 2008), and the risk of integration of one salmon DNA vaccine after IM injection has been estimated to be ~43-fold less than the risk for spontaneous mutation (Salonius *et al.*, 2007). It thus follows that germ line integration would be an even rarer event and, in all probability, risk to the consumer is negligible. These risks would certainly increase if the vaccine construct was designed to integrate, but risk assessment will always be done on a case-by-case basis with a thorough evaluation of the properties of the particular plasmid in question. It is important to keep in mind that the amount of remnant vaccine DNA in a fish fillet in any case will be infinitesimally small compared with the total amount of nucleic acids present in food. The safety considerations of DNA in food have been analysed and it was concluded that recombinant DNA in food will not represent new risks different from those already due to unmodified nucleic acids (Jonas *et al.*, 2001).

The regulation of DNA vaccines are described elsewhere in this volume; here we will only briefly discuss some problems related to the European legislation of genetically modified organisms (GMOs). In Europe there are some uncertainties as to whether the regulatory framework pertinent to GMOs (Directive 2001/18/EC) will apply to DNA vaccinated animals. A DNA vaccine itself consists only of genetic material and is not considered to be an organism (as per the definition of an organism in Article 2 of the directive) as it is not able, on its own, to replicate or transfer genetic material into the genome of the fish. Public consultation and GMO labelling are made compulsory under Directive 2001/18/EC, and the directive also requires a marketing authorization for GMO products, an environmental risk assessment, and surveillance after marketing. In Europe, the status of plasmid DNA vaccinated fish is still being assessed. The licensing procedure for a GMO in Europe is a complicated procedure, fully comparable with the similar process for licensing of a vaccine. However, as the responsibility for obtaining a license for a vaccine clearly lies with the producer of the medicine, so far it is unclear who should be the applicant for a license to market a DNA vaccinated fish if it is ultimately defined to be genetically modified. Furthermore, as Directive 2001/18/EEC is applicable to GMOs with stable and well-defined modifications that can be risk-assessed and detected for surveillance purposes, it is unclear how risk assessment and surveillance should be performed on DNA vaccinated fish. There is no defined genetic modification to assess or identify, only a risk that the vaccine could be integrated at any given place in the vaccinee's genome. However, the regulation (EC) 1829/2003 on genetically modified food and feed states in Article 16 that:

> Products obtained from animals fed with genetically modified feed or treated with genetically modified medicinal products will be subject neither to the authorisation requirements nor to the labelling requirements referred to in this Regulation.

It thus follows that if a DNA vaccine falls within the definition of a genetically modified medicinal product, the fish itself is not considered to be a GMO. This problem and possible solutions have been discussed in more detail by Foss and Rogne in two papers (Foss and Rogne, 2003, 2007). Clearly, as long as these regulatory issues are not resolved, vaccine producers will be reluctant to introduce DNA vaccines to the European market.

In conclusion, DNA vaccination appears to be an effective approach in some cases where traditional technology so far has failed to provide effective products. As development continues, new applications will appear, but DNA vaccination is not likely to be the universal solution to all product development within aquaculture. Most likely it has the potential to be an attractive supplement to traditional products. The use of vaccines has made the most progress in salmon farming, and Europe is the main salmon-producing region in the world and also a major market. For DNA vaccine technology to be able to prove its potential for fish, it is necessary therefore to have regulatory clarifications of a DNA vaccine within the EU.

REFERENCES

Anderson, E.D., Mourich, D.V., Fahrenkrug, S.C., *et al.*, 1996. Genetic immunization of rainbow trout (*Oncorhynchus mykiss*) against infectious hematopoietic necrosis virus. *Mol Mar Biol Biotechnol* **5**: 114–22.

Bergman, P.J., McKnight, J., Novosad, A., *et al.*, 2003. Long-term survival of dogs with advanced malignant melanoma after DNA vaccination with xenogeneic human tyrosinase: a phase I trial. *Clin Cancer Res* **9**: 1284–90.

Biering, E., Villoing, S., Sommerset, I. and Christie, K.E. 2005. Update on viral vaccines for fish. *Dev Biol (Basel)* **121**: 97–113.

Corbeil, S., LaPatra, S.E., Anderson, E.D., *et al.*, 1999. Evaluation of the protective immunogenicity of the N, P, M, NV and G proteins of infectious hematopoietic necrosis virus in rainbow trout *Oncorhynchus mykiss* using DNA vaccines. *Dis Aquat Org* **39**: 29–36.

Corbeil, S., Kurath, G. and LaPatra, S.E. 2000. Fish DNA vaccine against infectious hematopoietic necrosis virus: efficacy of various routes of immunisation. *Fish Shellfish Immunol* **10**: 711–23.

Davis, B.S., Chang, G.J., Cropp, B., *et al.*, 2001. West Nile virus recombinant DNA vaccine protects mouse and horse from virus challenge and expresses *in vitro* a noninfectious recombinant antigen that can be used in enzyme-linked immunosorbent assays. *J Virol* **75**: 4040–47.

Einer-Jensen, K., Delgado, L., Lorenzen, E., *et al.*, 2009. Dual DNA vaccination of rainbow trout (*Oncorhynchus mykiss*) against two different rhabdoviruses, VHSV and IHNV, induces specific divalent protection. *Vaccine* **27**: 1248–53.

Emmenegger, E.J. and Kurath, G. 2008. DNA vaccine protects ornamental koi (*Cyprinus carpio koi*) against North American spring viremia of carp virus. *Vaccine* **26**: 6415–21.

Foss, G.S. and Rogne, S. 2003. Gene medication or genetic modification? The devil is in the details. *Nat Biotechnol* **21**: 1280–81.

Foss, G.S. and Rogne, S. 2007. When gene medication is also genetic modification –regulating DNA treatment. *Vaccine* **25**: 5613–18.

Garver, K.A., Conway, C.M., Elliott, D.G. and Kurath, G. 2005. Analysis of DNA-vaccinated fish reveals viral antigen in muscle, kidney and thymus, and transient histopathologic changes. *Mar Biotechnol (NY)* **7**: 540–53.

Gomez-Casado, E., Estepa, A. and Coll, J.M. 2011. A comparative review on European-farmed finfish RNA viruses and their vaccines. *Vaccine* **29**: 2657–71.

Hartikka, J., Bozoukova, V., Ferrari, M., *et al.*, 2001. Vaxfectin enhances the humoral immune response to plasmid DNA-encoded antigens. *Vaccine* **19**: 1911–23.

Haugarvoll, E., Bjerkas, I., Szabo, N.J., *et al.*, 2010. Manifestations of systemic autoimmunity in vaccinated salmon. *Vaccine* **28**: 4961–9.

Holm A. 2004. *DNA-vaccines for food-producing animals. Technical review and discussion of safety issues.* Ministry of Food, Agriculture and Fisheries and the Danish Veterinary Institute, Copenhagen.

Jonas, D.A., Elmadfa, I., Engel, K.H., *et al.*, 2001. Safety considerations of DNA in food. *Ann Nutr Metab* **45**: 235–54.

Kanellos, T., Sylvester, I.D., D'Mello, F., *et al.*, 2006. DNA vaccination can protect *Cyprinus carpio* against spring viraemia of carp virus. *Vaccine* **24**: 4927–33.

Khan, A.S., Bodles-Brakhop, A.M., Fiorotto, M.L. and Draghia-Akli, R. 2010. Effects of maternal plasmid GHRH treatment on offspring growth. *Vaccine* **28**: 1905–10.

Kim, C.H., Johnson, M.C., Drennan, J.D., *et al.*, 2000. DNA vaccines encoding viral glycoproteins induce nonspecific immunity and Mx protein synthesis in fish. *J Virol* **74**: 7048–54.

Koppang, E.O., Bjerkås, I., Haugarvoll, E., *et al.*, 2008. Vaccination-induced systemic autoimmunity in farmed Atlantic salmon. *J Immunol* **181**: 4807–14.

Kurath, G. 2008. Biotechnology and DNA vaccines for aquatic animals. *Rev Sci Tech* **27**: 175–96.

Kurath, G., Garver, K.A., Corbeil, S., *et al.*, 2006. Protective immunity and lack of histopathological damage two years after DNA vaccination against infectious hematopoietic necrosis virus in trout. *Vaccine* **24**: 345–54.

Kutzler, M.A. and Weiner, D.B. 2008. DNA vaccines: ready for prime time? *Nat Rev Genet* **9**: 776–88.

Lillehaug, A., Lunder, T. and Poppe, T.T. 1992. Field testing of adjuvanted furunculosis vaccines in Atlantic salmon, *Salmo salar* L. *J Fish Dis* **15**: 485–96.

Liu, M.A. 2011. DNA vaccines: an historical perspective and view to the future. *Immunol Rev* **239**: 62–84.

Lorenzen, N. and LaPatra, S.E. 2005. DNA vaccines for aquacultured fish. *Rev Sci Tech* **24**: 201–13.

Lorenzen, N., Lorenzen, E., Einer-Jensen, K., *et al.*, 1998. Protective immunity to VHS in rainbow trout (*Oncorhynchus mykiss*, Walbaum) following DNA vaccination. *Fish Shellfish Immunol* **8**: 261–70.

McLauchlan, P.E., Collet, B., Ingerslev, E., *et al.*, 2003. DNA vaccination against viral haemorrhagic septicaemia (VHS) in rainbow trout: size, dose, route of injection and duration of protection-early protection correlates with Mx expression. *Fish Shellfish Immunol* **15**: 39–50.

Midtlyng, P.J., Reitan, L.J. and Speilberg, L. 1996. Experimental studies on the efficacy and side-effects of intraperitoneal vaccination of Atlantic salmon (*Salmo salar* L.) against furunculosis. *Fish Shellfish Immunol* **6**: 335–50.

Mikalsen, A.B., Torgersen, J., Aleström, P., *et al.*, 2004. Protection of Atlantic salmon *Salmo salar* against infectious pancreatic necrosis after DNA vaccination. *Dis Aquat Org* **60**: 11–20.

Mikalsen, A.B., Sindre, H., Torgersen, J. and Rimstad, E. 2005. Protective effects of a DNA vaccine expressing the infectious salmon anemia virus hemagglutinin-esterase in Atlantic salmon. *Vaccine* **23**: 4895–905.

Salonius, K., Simard, N., Harland, R. and Ulmer, J.B. 2007. The road to licensure of a DNA vaccine. *Curr Opin Investig Drugs* **8**: 635–41.

Simard, N.C., Hay, V., Aarflot, L., *et al.*, 2009. Evaluation of a DNA vaccine prototype for the control of salmon pancreas disease virus (SPDV) in Atlantic salmon, *Salmo salar*. Oral presentation and abstract, 14th EAFP International Conference, Prague.

Skern-Mauritzen R, Malde K, Besnier F, *et al.*, 2013. How does sequence variability affect *de novo* assembly quality? *J Nat Hist* **47**: 901–10.

Sommerset, I., Krossoy, B., Biering, E. and Frost, P. 2005. Vaccines for fish in aquaculture. *Exp Rev Vaccines* **4**: 89–101.

Sommerset, I., Lorenzen, E., Lorenzen, N., *et al.*, 2003. A DNA vaccine directed against a rainbow trout rhabdovirus induces early protection against a nodavirus challenge in turbot. *Vaccine* **21**: 4661–7.

Sullivan, S.M., Doukas, J., Hartikka, J., *et al.*, 2010. Vaxfectin: a versatile adjuvant for plasmid DNA- and protein-based vaccines. *Exp Opin Drug Deliv* **7**: 1433–46.

Tonheim, T.C., Bøgwald, J. and Dalmo, R.A. 2008. What happens to the DNA vaccine in fish? A review of current knowledge. *Fish Shellfish Immunol* **25**: 1–18.

Ulmer, J.B., Donnelly, J.J., Parker, S.E., *et al.*, 1993. Heterologous protection against influenza by injection of DNA encoding a viral protein. *Science* **259**: 1745–9.

Wang, Z., Troilo, P.J., Wang, X., *et al.*, 2004. Detection of integration of plasmid DNA into host genomic DNA following intramuscular injection and electroporation. *Gene Ther* **11**: 711–21.

Xu, C., Mutoloki, S. and Evensen, Ø. 2012. Superior protection conferred by inactivated whole virus vaccine over subunit and DNA vaccines against salmonid alphavirus infection in Atlantic salmon (*Salmo salar* L.). *Vaccine* **30**: 3918–28.

6 Mucosal Vaccination of Fish

Jan H.W.M. Rombout[1,2] and Viswanath Kiron[1]

[1]Faculty of Biosciences and Aquaculture, University of Nordland, Bodø, Norway
[2]Cell Biology and Immunology, Wageningen University, The Netherlands

ABSTRACT

For the continued development of aquaculture, fish disease prevention is essential and vaccination appears to be the most suitable method. The number of commercially applied vaccines is increasing, but many must be delivered by injection. This may be the most effective route, but is also labour-intensive, costly and unsuitable for small fish. As most pathogens enter the body via mucosal surfaces, protection at that level would also be highly desirable. In addition, oral vaccination via feed could solve some of the drawbacks associated with injection vaccination, particularly if the vaccine can be produced in a cost-effective way and when formulated with similar or lower quantities of vaccine than needed for immersion vaccination. From 1942, when the first oral vaccination was reported by Duff, until present times, many reports have indicated the promise of "mucosal" vaccines. However, in most cases they have never entered commercial production. In this chapter many vaccination approaches are reviewed with a focus on their uptake, immune stimulation, and where possible, their potential as future vaccines is discussed.

6.1 INTRODUCTION

Disease prevention by vaccination is the most appropriate method for pathogen control – economically, environmentally, and ethically. However, much research is necessary to improve existing suboptimal vaccines and to develop novel vaccines against viral and bacterial diseases. Efficacy, safety and vaccine delivery route deserve special attention. In addition, novel vaccination methods have to be cost-effective, easy to apply, and if possible less stressful to the animal.

Among the novel methods, mucosal vaccination seems to possess all the desired criteria. In this chapter state-of-the-art knowledge regarding this type of vaccination will be reviewed, and

jhwmrombout@gmail.com

Fish Vaccination, First Edition. Edited by Roar Gudding, Atle Lillehaug and Øystein Evensen.

the reasons why it is not yet extensively used will be discussed. Information on the mucosal immune system, suitable mucosal antigens and adjuvants and uptake mechanisms are included. Finally, attention will be paid to species-specific differences in mucosal anatomy and function in prominent farmed fish species.

6.2 HISTORY OF "MUCOSAL" VACCINATION

The history of mucosal vaccination started with the publication of a paper in the *Journal of Immunology* by Duff (1942) that revealed reduced mortality after a prolonged (>64 days) feeding with *Aeromonas salmonicida*-containing feed and a subsequent immersion challenge. A reduction in mortality from 75% in the control group to 25% in the orally vaccinated group was reported, and the protection appeared to correlate with antibody production. Thereafter, limited attention was given to fish vaccination in general as chemotherapeutic treatment became popular in the control of fish diseases. In 1976 the first *Yersinia ruckeri* vaccine was licensed in the US for oral administration, followed shortly by acceptance of a *Vibrio anguillarum/ordalii* vaccine for immersion application (Plant and LaPatra, 2011). However, the majority of vaccines developed since then have been based on intraperitoneal (IP) injection and immersion/bath vaccination. Immersion can be considered as mucosal vaccination as antigens are taken up by the mucosal epithelia of organs such as the skin, gills and gut, and possibly evoke local immune reactions in these organs. In most studies only mortality was monitored, and little, if any, attention was paid to the uptake mechanisms and subsequent local or systemic immune responses. For a more detailed historical overview one can refer to Van Muiswinkel (2008) and Plant and Lapatra (2011). In addition, Table 6.1 gives a comparison of injection and mucosal vaccination based on survival/mortality from a selection of studies performed during the period 1977–83.

Based upon the mortality values given in this table it can be concluded that while oral vaccination against *V. anguillarum* and *Y. ruckeri* confers protection in salmonids, injection and immersion vaccination are in general more effective. However, Johnson and Amend (1983a,b) also showed that intestinal vaccination might be promising if undegraded antigens can be

Table 6.1 Comparison of the efficacy of systemic (injection) and mucosal vaccination (immersion; oral/anal) of salmonids (Atlantic salmon or rainbow trout) against bacterial diseases in the late 1970s and early 1980s, based on mortality (%).

Reference/pathogen	**Modes of vaccination**				
	Control*	**Injection**	**Immersion**	**Oral**	**Anal**
Vibrio anguillarum					
Håstein *et al.* (1977)	46	19	42	76	–
Baudin-Laurencin and Tangtrongpiros (1980)	34	1.5	2	32	–
Evelyn and Ketchetson (1980)	42	1	2	18	–
Amend and Johnson (1981)	52	0	4	27	–
Horne *et al.* (1982)	100	7	53	94	–
Johnson and Amend (1983b)	55	–	–	15–45	0
Yersinia ruckeri					
Johnson and Amend (1983a,b)	65	–	18	24	3

*Control fish were not vaccinated, but challenged.

brought into the posterior part of the gut. Antigens must, therefore, be protected in a way such that they escape digestion in the foregut and reach the endgut, where they can be taken up and processed efficiently (Rombout *et al.*, 1985; Rombout and van den Berg, 1989) in a variety of fish species (Rombout *et al.*, 2011). Although it has been claimed that oral vaccination with (bio)encapsulated vaccines can be protective, successful commercial applications have not been reported, probably due to their low cost-effectiveness compared with injection or immersion vaccination.

6.3 MUCOSAL VERSUS SYSTEMIC IMMUNITY IN FISH

It is well documented in mammals that exposure of mucosal surfaces to antigen results in a local response, finally resulting in secretion of antigen-specific IgA at mucosal surfaces. Mammals have a common mucosal immune system, in which stimulation of one epithelium can also result in specific IgA responses in other mucosal organs (Brandtzaeg and Pabst, 2004). This phenomenon is in principle based upon the existence of so-called systemic and mucosal homing receptors on immune competent cells. Once immune cells are "educated" in a mucosal organ, they return specifically to only such tissues based on recognition of mucosal address molecules present on the endothelium of high endothelial venules. In this way, body surfaces can be protected by specific antibodies evoked at another mucosal surface. In principle, mucosal vaccination is a powerful tool to protect the organism at exposed sites, where most pathogens attempt to enter the body. It has to be stated that the number of mucosal vaccines in mammals is still very limited, which may be partly due to the fact that injection vaccines are cost-effective in medical and veterinary fields. Moreover, the affinity and memory formation in systemic responses is much better than that resulting from mucosal responses. In addition, nearly all vaccines contain adjuvants to reduce the amount of antigen necessary – a wide variety of systemic adjuvants are currently available and these are more effective than mucosal adjuvants.

Contrary to normal practice in mammals, mucosal vaccines may be more desirable in fish as they allow large-scale application and are less labour-intensive compared with injection application. Moreover, mucosal application is a relatively stress-free method that could be used even on young fish that are too small to inject. At present, immersion is the most widely used mucosal vaccination method, but as shown in Table 6.1, it is less effective than injection. Upon drinking, antigens can enter the skin, gills and even the gut, although the mechanisms have not been clearly demonstrated. These vaccines have been developed empirically based on their efficacy as determined by mortality studies. Little is known, however, about the type of response evoked or the responses that confer effective protection. In fish we have to be careful with stimulation of single mucosal surfaces, as the common mucosal immune system may not function as in mammals. There are no indications of specific homing of B- and T-cells in carp mucosae (Rombout, unpublished) or intraepithelial T-cells in the gut mucosa of trout (Bernard *et al.*, 2006). On the other hand, oral or anal immunization of carp resulted in the presence of detectable antibodies in the skin mucus, while they were absent in the serum following oral immunization of ayu (Kawai *et al.*, 1981) and carp (Rombout *et al.*, 1986). At present we have to avoid firm conclusions on this aspect, since we know from research on carp that mucosal antibodies can differ from serum antibodies (Rombout *et al.*, 1993). More recently a new type of immunoglobulin H chain was reported in carp (IgZ; Savan *et al.*, 2005a), rainbow trout

(IgT; Hansen *et al.*, 2005) and fugu (IgT; Savan *et al.*, 2005b), and this IgT- like molecule was suggested to have a mucosal function in trout (Zhang *et al.*, 2010). This function may also be partly retained in carp, as a chimeric form of the molecule (having both μ and ζ domains) was described, bearing a preference for mucosal tissues (Ryo *et al.*, 2010). In any case, this explains why in carp a monoclonal antibody against serum IgM (mAb: WCI12) could be used for detection of mucosal responses, which is not the case for the trout anti-IgM mAb (Zhang *et al.*, 2010). Therefore we must be careful in drawing firm conclusions for fish in general, due to species differences. The pIgR, an Ig binding molecule allowing transcytosis of Ig towards the mucus, has been found in a variety of fish species (Rombout *et al.*, 2011), and at least in trout this molecule also seems to bind IgT (Zhang *et al.*, 2010). While it appears that IgM, and IgT/IgZ transport to mucus takes place in polarized cells, such as enterocytes or hepatocytes, it is not logical to assume the same function for skin epithelial cells. Skin will also be protected well when immunoglobulins are bound to epithelial cells and not transported. Unpublished data on the pIgR of carp has shown that there is a single amino acid difference in the cleavage area of the molecule which seems to be organ-dependent. Although speculative, this difference may allow a different processing pathway for pIgR. As very little is known about this, more attention has to be paid to improve our understanding of mucosal immunity in fish, particularly of the prominent cultured species, to develop cost-effective vaccines that are capable of protecting the animals, both at the mucosal as well as the systemic level.

6.4 IMMERSION VACCINATION

According to the fish vaccination delivery review of Plant and LaPatra (2011), immersion is probably the simplest method of vaccination, but it is not suitable for all farming conditions. They classified the different methods of immersion vaccination as follows:

(1) *Direct immersion*, where the fish are transferred to water containing vaccine for a short period (around 30 seconds) and subsequently returned to the holding tank (Lillehaug, 2014). As this method is generally effective without any pre-treatment, based on protection values, it is at present the most widely used protocol. However, data presented in Table 6.1 show that the degree of protection attained through direct immersion does not always reach that obtained by injection.

(2) *Hyperosmotic infiltration*, in which the animals are initially placed in a hyperosmotic solution of sodium chloride for a few minutes prior to immersion in a vaccine solution. This method is considered stressful, although a paper of Huising *et al.* (2003) reported that increased cortisol levels and skin and gill damage were only registered over a short period. This temporary damage may have an adjuvant function as it results in better antigen uptake in skin and gills and increased immune responses. Plant and LaPatra (2011) reported conflicting results regarding the efficacy of this method. In carp it was shown that osmotic infiltration vaccination induced mucosal skin responses 6–8 weeks after vaccination with systemic responses detectable from week 4 (Huising *et al.*, 2003). This difference may be due to the longer transit time of mucosal Ig bound to the skin epithelial cells by the pIgR.

(3) *Spray vaccination*, originally developed for delivery of *V. anguillarum* to large fish (>20 g), is considered stressful (Ellis, 1988), and is therefore rarely used.

(4) *Ultrasound/immersion* is a relatively new approach, in which high-frequency sound (20 kHz) is used to enhance the permeability of cells. Levels of uptake and protection comparable to IP injection were observed (Plant and LaPatra, 2011). It has been used for viral hemorrhagic septicemia virus (VHSV) DNA vaccine delivery in rainbow trout, resulting in a relative percent survival of 50 (Fernandez-Alonso *et al.*, 2001). Although this procedure requires five times less antigen compared with normal immersion delivery, the amount of bacterial antigen or plasmid needed is very high and probably limits widespread application of this method in aquaculture.

(5) *Puncture/immersion* uses a multiple puncture instrument for creating small lesions in the skin of fish prior to immersion vaccination. Using this method, Nakanishi *et al.* (2002) obtained protection levels similar to those achieved with a *Streptococcus iniae* bacterin IP injection in rainbow trout.

Hyperosmotic immersion is in fact comparable to ultrasound and multiple puncture approaches. In principle, skin and gill damage breaches the protective barriers of fish, thereby enabling better antigen delivery, greater responses and increased protection. All the other techniques are impractical in normal aquaculture situations, most probably due to acute stress, a need for repeated application and increased equipment costs. However, the benefit of evoking a local/mucosal response has been long overlooked, as has the contribution of antigens presented in the gut following drinking.

6.5 ORAL VACCINATION

Oral vaccination is in theory the most appealing method due to its ease of administration, lack of stress induction and suitability for mass vaccination at all ages (Vandenberg, 2004; Rombout *et al.*, 2011, Plant and LaPatra, 2011). However, it also has disadvantages, including the amount of vaccine ingested per animal and the amount of undegraded vaccine reaching the so-called second segment of the hindgut, where antigen uptake occurs (Rombout *et al.*, 2011). Although already reported by Duff in 1942, oral vaccination has a history of being inconsistent in efficacy, which according to Plant and LaPatra (2011) may partly be explained by the limitations described above. Differences in the digestive tracts of cultured fish species also influence vaccine effectiveness. Gastric versus non-gastric species, short and long intestinal tracts, and even the absence of a second segment (Inami *et al.*, 2009), makes it difficult to promote oral vaccination strongly. We will summarize a variety of methods that are employed to deliver antigen safely to the hindgut, induce local or systemic immune responses, and, most importantly, induce immunological memory and achieve long-term protection.

6.5.1 Oral vaccination with unprotected antigens

Following studies with unprotected vaccines it became clear that protection levels were considerably lower than those obtained with injection or immersion (Table 6.1), even when daily administration was continued for a longer period. For instance, in the first oral vaccination study by Duff (1942), trout had to be fed for 64–70 days to achieve mortality reduction from 75% to 25%. The extended administration period, which is not cost-effective due to the very high amounts of vaccine needed, has not discouraged scientists from testing this repeated ingestion technique, probably to ensure that all animals ingested sufficient antigen.

On the other hand, repeated administration of protein antigens has been shown to induce immunosuppression and/or tolerance in mammals (Brandtzaeg and Pabst, 2004). Similar genetic-dependent suppression was reported for carp, and suggested for other species (Joosten *et al.*, 1997a). In order to improve the efficiency of this technique, antigen degradation in the stomach and foregut must be reduced, and the frequency of administration minimized.

6.5.2 Bioencapsulation

Many fish species are initially fed with live feed, such as rotifers, brine shrimp (*Artemia*) and water fleas (*Daphnia*). These organisms are filter feeders and can ingest particulate antigens like bacteria. As these live feeds can release antigens in the posterior part of the digestive tract of fish, they could be employed to bioencapsulate vaccines. Early attempts on ayu (Kawai *et al.*, 1989), carp and sea bream (Joosten *et al.*, 1995) were promising, as the young fish developed immunological memory. Lin *et al.* (2005) found good protection in zebrafish vaccinated using this method. Other positive side-effects were reported: European sea bass had better growth, improved feed conversion, and lower stress responses when vaccinated with *V. anguillarum* bioencapsulated in *Artemia* (Chair *et al.*, 1994). However, it also became clear that this vaccination procedure can only be applied when the immune system is relatively well developed. Too early vaccination can result in fish being confronted with antigens during the self/non-self recognition stage and thus leading to reduced responses. This phenomenon, termed neonatal tolerance in mammals, has also been demonstrated in carp 1–2 months post-fertilization (Joosten *et al.*, 1995).

Another approach based on bio-encapsulation is the use of microalgae. For instance *Chlamydomonas reinhardtii* has been used as an antigen delivery system in fish (Siripornadulsil *et al.*, 2007). The *Renibacterium salmoninarum* protein 57 was expressed in this microalgae and the transformed algae were administered by immersion or via feed. Although the two delivery modes led to specific antibody responses, specific antibodies in the skin mucus were detectable only following immersion.

6.5.3 Edible vaccines

Advances in scientific research have led to the development of genetically modified plants capable of producing relevant antigens in their leaves, fruits or bulbs (Richter and Kipp, 1999). These plant products can be cultured in large quantities and processed for direct incorporation in the fish feed. In this way it is possible to produce a bio-encapsulated vaccine that is protected against degradation in the foregut of fish. Although edible vaccines may be cost-effective, in most cases the amount of antigen produced by the plant is too low to obtain immune responses in vaccinated fish. Until now only Companjen *et al.* (2005, 2006) has reported the use of such a vaccine for carp. The G protein of the spring viremia of carp virus (SVCV) coupled to LTB (heat labile enterotoxin of *Escherichia coli*) or a green fluorescent protein (GFP) coupled to LTB were incorporated into a plasmid used for transfection of potato cells. The resultant LTB-GFP potato tubers produced an amount of GFP suitable for the study of uptake and immune responses in fish. Uptake of GFP coupled to LTB was much better than GFP alone, indicating that LTB is a suitable intestinal adjuvant for enhancing antigen uptake. Further, immunological memory against GFP was reported. Even though LTB and protein G form a very stable LTB-G construct in potato tubers, the amount of LTB-G present in the tubers is too low for oral immunization. This procedure might, however, be very useful when more LTB-G can be accumulated in the plant tubers or in another plant species suitable for incorporation in fish feeds.

6.5.4 Microbial biofilms

Biofilms are also used for oral immunization of fish. To develop biofilms, bacteria are cultured on minute particles of chitin, on which they aggregate. When these biofilms are fed to fish, the outer layer of the bacterial aggregate protects the inner bacteria from digestion. Chitin-based, heat-inactivated *Aeromonas hydrophila* biofilm delivered to catla, rohu and common carp via feed provided significant protection when challenged with *A. hydrophila*, as well as being taken up more efficiently and generating higher antibody responses than normally cultured bacterial cells (Azad *et al.*, 1999, 2000). Similar results were obtained for walking catfish (*Clarias batrachus*) using the same vaccine (Nayak *et al.*, 2004). To check the eventual contribution of mucosal immune responses, this biofilm vaccine was tested on common carp (40 g). Fish were orally vaccinated for 10 days, and blood and gut mucosa samples were obtained from each fish ($n = 5$ on each sample day) on 0, 10, 20 and 30 days post-vaccination (0 dpv = 10 days after the first oral vaccination). The ELISA results of anti-*A. hydrophila* responses are shown for serum in Figure 6.1A (left) and gut mucus samples in Figure 6.1B (right).

From Figure 6.1 it is clear that both systemic as well as mucosal responses were measurable following oral biofilm vaccination. The same vaccination protocol has been shown to result in protective responses in common carp (Azad *et al.*, 1999, 2000). In serum the antibody titers are clearly higher after 30 dpv and comparable with 21 dpi. In the gut mucus *Ah*-antibody levels rise gradually after 10 days of oral feeding to reach the highest level at 30 dpv. It has to be stated that an mAb against serum IgM (WCI12), which has lower affinity for mucus Ig, a chimeric molecule with μ and ζ domains (Ryo *et al.*, 2010), was used in this experiment and is probably not the most sensitive way to monitor mucosal responses. These are, however, the first available data on the different kinetics of systemic and mucosal responses in fish.

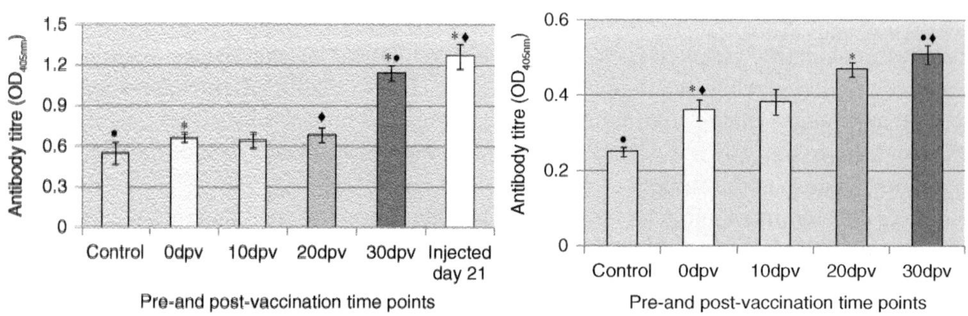

Fig. 6.1 (a) Serum *Ah*-antibody titers at OD 405 nm (mean ± SEM) in carp- from control, oral vaccinated and IP injected animals. ANOVA followed by Dunnett's multiple comparison test was employed to compare between 0 dpv and the other time points in the vaccination group. Unpaired t-test was used for the comparison between the control and vaccination group at 30 dpv as well as to compare the vaccination group (20 dpv) and injection group (21 days after IP injection). (b) Gut mucus *Ah*-antibody titers (OD at 405 nm (mean ± SEM) from control and vaccinated animals. Same symbols denote significant differences ($P < 0.05$) between the groups (Source: Rombout *et al.*, unpublished).

6.5.5 Microencapsulation

The potential of nano- and microparticles for oral antigen delivery has been studied in several fish species employing a variety of different polymers, both natural and synthetic. Antigens are generally encapsulated inside the particle, but may also be covalently linked to them. In general, particles used in these approaches are non-toxic, biodegradable and hence suitable for oral delivery. Most studies report good uptake in the endgut, increased specific antibody production and/or better protection using the following particles: alginate microparticles (Joosten *et al.*, 1997b; Romalde *et al.*, 2004; Rodrigues *et al.*, 2006; Tian *et al.*, 2008a), liposomes (Yasumoto *et al.*, 2006a,b), poly D,L-lactide-co-glycolic acid (PLGA) microparticles (O'Donnell *et al.*, 1996; Lavelle *et al.*, 1997; Ellis, 1998; Benoit *et al.*, 2001; Tian *et al.*, 2008b), and chitosan microparticles (Kumar *et al.*, 2008; Tian *et al.*, 2008c).

Alginate micro particles can be produced in a way that they are resistant to digestion in various fish species. For instance, different formulations of alginate particles were necessary for carp (a-gastric) and trout (gastric), to obtain systemic as well as mucosal responses (Joosten *et al.*, 1997b). In the aforementioned study, immunological memory was reported, but protection against vibriosis was not measured. More recently in Japanese flounder, alginate particles were used in combination with plasmid DNA expressing a major capsid protein of lymphocystis disease virus (LCDV). The expression of the viral protein and a reporter gene (GFP) in various tissues of fish indicated that it is also an effective strategy for oral DNA vaccination (Tian *et al.*, 2008a). On the other hand, less promising results were obtained by others using alginate microparticles (Maurice *et al.*, 2004 (goldfish); Altun *et al.*, 2010 (rainbow trout); Leal *et al.*, 2010 (Nile tilapia)). When an IPNV DNA-vaccine was administered orally (by pipette) to brown and rainbow trout, very good RPS values were obtained, validating the potential of this delivery system (de Las Heras *et al.*, 2010). As stated earlier by Joosten *et al.* (1997b), formulation of the alginate particles has to be adapted for each species to overcome degradation of the antigens in the foregut, while taking care that the particles are not too stable and are released within the appropriate gut segment. It is not yet clear whether the particles employed in these studies are the appropriate ones or not. It remains unclear whether these particles will be cost-effective in aquaculture.

PLGA and chitosan particles, claimed to be biodegradable mucoadhesive microspheres (Plant and LaPatra, 2011), are very suitable for encapsulation of pDNA vaccines (Tian *et al.*, 2008b,c). The report of Tian *et al.* (2008b) showed that PLGA particles loaded with plasmids can be transported by the gut, and when these plasmids are expressed in the body, specific antibodies are produced. Although the method seems suitable for oral DNA-vaccination, the exact transport mechanism by the gut epithelium is not yet completely clear and there is some doubt of its cost-effectiveness for use in aquaculture. Another recent study (Altun *et al.*, 2010) showed that PLGA particles are slightly more potent in providing protection than alginate particles.

The antigen delivery capacity of *chitosan* particles has been investigated in fish, and all reports (Ramos *et al.*, 2005; Kumar *et al.*, 2008; Tian *et al.*, 2008c) have validated their suitability. Kumar *et al.* (2008) reported partial protection against vibriosis (RPS = 46) when a plasmid DNA encoding the *V. anguillarum* outer membrane protein 38 was orally delivered to Asian sea bass.

Polyethylene glycol (PEG) has also been used for encapsulation, and when employed as a vaccine against VHSV in rainbow trout, RPS values above 60 were obtained (Adelmann *et al.*, 2008).

6.5.6 Alternative methods

Vaccines based on attenuated bacteria can also be delivered to fish, either by immersion or orally. When the outer membrane protein of *Vibrio harveyi* was transformed into the commensal bacterium *Pseudomonas fluorescens*, encapsulated in alginate microparticles and subsequently orally delivered to Japanese flounder, a RPS of 61 was recorded (Sun *et al.*, 2009).

A protective coating of feed pellets either with or without absorption enhancers like vitamin E or sodium lauryl sulfate appears to be effective. Oral vaccination against vibriosis with antigen incorporated in the aforementioned feed type generated similar antibody levels as obtained for IP injection in African catfish (Vervarcke *et al.*, 2004).

Anti-proteases and membrane permeability enhancers added to a potential salmonid vaccine helped in protecting the antigens from digestion. This oral adjuvant, patented as Oralject^{TM}, when applied in Nile tilapia against *Streptococcus iniae*, gave RPS values of 63, compared with 100 upon IP injection (Shoemaker *et al.*, 2006).

6.6 PERSPECTIVES

Among the mucosal vaccination techniques discussed above, microencapsulated oral vaccines hold potential for use in fish. Despite this, there are few oral vaccines on the market, possibly due to their poor stability in aquatic feeds, the limited protection achieved (Komar *et al.*, 2004), and most likely due to their poor cost-effectiveness. The development of "edible vaccines" may in fact be the solution for wider application of oral vaccination in aquaculture. For instance, the combination of viral trimeric G proteins with LTB produced in plants appears to be very stable and may function as both vaccine and mucosal adjuvant. Subsequent incorporation into fish feeds may result in useful oral vaccines. However, the amount of transgenic protein produced by the plants should be adequate to avoid further concentration steps prior to their use in feeds. Additional research on fish is needed to achieve optimal effect with small amounts of antigen. As in mammals, suitable intestinal adjuvants are needed to reach this goal.

Immersion may be more effective when combined with ultrasound or other controlled skin or gill damage, which enhances uptake and immune responses in fish. Although this approach may appear promising, further research should focus on both the effects of these methods and the welfare of the vaccinated fish.

The rather recent discovery of fish pIgR and a new Ig class (IgT or IgZ) may be very helpful in validating the mucosal responses of fish, especially its significance in protective mechanisms. Molecular biological approaches during the past decade have revealed an array of immune molecules in fish. Some of them are already considered as good adjuvant candidates (Secombes, 2011), boosting immune responses and eliciting appropriate protective responses.

Finally, mucosal vaccination of fish is a rather underutilized technique in aquaculture. The recent advances in the field of defense mechanisms in fish are bound to encourage researchers to attempt newer delivery modes and techniques to develop suitable mucosal vaccines for farmed fish.

REFERENCES

Adelmann, M., Köllner, B., Bergmann, S.M., *et al.*, 2008. Development of an oral vaccine for immunisation of rainbow trout (*Oncorhynchus mykiss*) against viral haemorrhagic septicaemia. *Vaccine* **26**: 837–44.

Altun, S., Kubilay, A., Ekici, S., *et al.*, 2010. Oral vaccination against lactococosis in rainbow trout (*Oncorhynchus mykiss*) using sodium alginate and poly (lactide-co-glycolide) carrier. *Kafkas Univ Vet Fak Derg* **16**: S211–17.

Amend, D.F. and Johnson, K.A. 1981. Current status and future need of *Vibrio anguillarum* bacterins. *Dev Biol Stand* **49**: 403–17.

Azad, I.S., Shankar, K.M., Mohan, C.V. and Kalita, B. 1999. Biofilm vaccine of *Aeromonas hydrophila* standardization of dose and duration for oral vaccination of carps. *Fish Shellfish Immunol* **9**: 519–28.

Azad, I.S., Shankar, K.M., Mohan, C.V. and Kalita, B. 2000. Uptake and processing of biofilm and free cell vaccines of *Aeromonas hydrophila* in Indian major carps and common carp following oral vaccination–antigen localization by a monoclonal antibody. *Dis Aquat Org* **43**: 103–8.

Baudin-Laurencin, F. and Tangtrongpiros, J. 1980. Some results of vaccination against vibriosis in Brittany, in *Fish Diseases* (ed. W. Ahne). Third COPRAQ Session. Berlin, Springer, 60–68.

Benoit, M.-E., Ribet, C., Distexhe, J., *et al.*, 2001. Studies on the potential of microparticles EnTropping pDNA-Poly(aminoacids) complexes as vaccine delivery systems. *J Drug Target* **9**: 253–66.

Bernard, D., Sox, A., Rigottier-Gois, L., *et al.*, 2006. Phenotypic and functional similarity of gut intraepithelial and systemic T cells in a teleost fish. *J Immunol* **176**: 3942–9.

Brandtzæg, P. and Pabst, R. 2004. Let's go mucosal: communication on slippery ground. *Trends Immunol* **25**: 570–77.

Chair, M., Gapasin, R.S.J., Dehasque, M. and Sorgeloos, P. 1994. Vaccination of European sea bass fry through bioencapsulation of *Artemia nauplii*. *Aquac Int* **2**: 254–61.

Companjen, A.R., Florack, D.E.A., Bastiaans, C.I., *et al.*, 2005. Development of a cost-effective oral vaccination method against viral diseases in fish. *Dev Biol (Basel)* **121**: 143–50.

Companjen, A.R., Florack, D.E.A., Slootweg, T., *et al.*, 2006. Improved uptake of plant derived LTB-linked proteins in carp gut and induction of specific humoral immune responses upon infeed delivery. *Fish Shellfish Immunol* **21**: 251–60.

De Las Heras, A.I., Saint-Jean, S.R. and Perez-Prieto, S.I. 2010. Immunogenic and protective effects of an oral DNA vaccine against infectious pancreatic necrosis virus in fish. *Fish Shellfish Immunol* **28**: 562–70.

Duff, D.C.B. 1942. The oral immunization of trout against *Bacterium salmonicida*. *J Immunol* **44**: 87–94.

Ellis, A.E. 1988. General principles of fish vaccination, in *Fish Vaccination* (ed. A.E. Ellis). London, Academic Press, 1–19.

Ellis, A.E. 1998. Meeting the requirements for delayed release of oral vaccines for fish. *J Appl Ichthyol* **14**: 149–52.

Evelyn, T.P.T. and Ketchetson, J.E. 1980. Laboratory and field observations on anti-vibriosis vaccines, in *Fish Diseases* (ed. W. Ahne). Third COPRAQ-Session. Berlin, Springer, 60–68.

Fernandez-Alonso, M., Rocha, A. and Coll, J.M. 2001. DNA vaccination by immersion and ultrasound to trout haemorrhagic septicaemia virus. *Vaccine* **19**: 3067–75.

Hansen, J.D., Landis, E.D. and Phillips, R.B. 2005. Discovery of a unique Ig heavy chain isotype (IgT) in rainbow trout: implications for a distinct B cell developmental pathway in teleost fish. *Proc Natl Acad Sci USA* **102**: 6919–24.

Håstein, T., Refsti, T. and Gjedrem, T. 1977. Preliminary results of vaccination trials against vibriosis in rainbow trout. *Bull Off Int Epizoot* **87**: 487–8.

Horne, M.T., Tatner, M., McDerment, S., *et al.*, 1982. Vaccination of rainbow trout, *Salmo gairdneri* Richardson, at low temperatures and the long persistence of protection. *J Fish Dis* **5**: 343–5.

Huising, M.O., Guichelaar, T., Hoek, C., *et al.*, 2003. Increased efficacy of immersion vaccination in fish with hyperosmotic pretreatment. *Vaccine* **21**: 4178–93.

Inami, M., Taverne-Thiele, A.J., Schrøder, M.B., *et al.*, 2009. Immunological differences in intestine and rectum of Atlantic cod (*Gadus morhua* L.). *Fish Shellfish Immunol* **26**: 751–9.

Johnson, K.A. and Amend, D.F. 1983a. Comparison of efficacy of several delivery methods using *Yersinia ruckeri* bacterin on rainbow trout, *Salmo gairdneri* Richardson. *J Fish Dis* **6**: 331–6.

Johnson, K.A. and Amend, D.F. 1983b. Efficacy of *Vibrio anguillarum* and *Yersinia ruckeri* bacterins applied by oral and anal intubation of salmonids. *J Fish Dis* **6**: 473–6.

Joosten, P.H.M., Avilés-Trigueros, M., Sorgeloos, P. and Rombout, J.H.W.M. 1995. Oral vaccination of juvenile carp (*Cyprinus carpio*) and gilthead seabream (*Sparus aurata*) with bioencapsulated *Vibrio anguillarum* bacterin. *Fish Shellfish Immunol* **5**: 289–99.

Joosten, P.H.M., Engelsma, M.Y., van der Zee, M.D. and Rombout, J.H.W.M. 1997a. Induction of oral tolerance in carp (*Cyprinus carpio* L.) after feeding protein antigens. *Vet Immunol Immunopathol* **60**: 187–96.

Joosten, P.H.M., Tiemersma, E., Threels, A., *et al.*, 1997b. Oral immunization of fish against *Vibrio anguillarum* using alginate microparticles. *Fish Shellfish Immunol* **7**: 471–85.

Kawai, K., Kusuda, R. and Itami, T. 1981. Mechanisms of protection in ayu orally vaccinated for vibriosis. *Fish Pathol* **15**: 257–62.

Kawai, K., Yamamoto, S. and Kusuda, R. 1989. Plankton-mediated oral delivery of *Vibrio anguillarum* vaccine to juvenile ayu. *Nippon Suisan Gakkaishi* **55**: 35–40.

Komar, C., Enright, W.J., Grisez, L. and Tan, Z. 2004. Understanding fish vaccination. *Aqua Culture Asia Pacific Magazine* **Nov/Dec**: 27–9.

Kumar, S.R., Ishaq Ahmed, V.P., Parameswaran, V., *et al.*, 2008. Potential use of chitosan nanoparticles for oral delivery of DNA vaccine in Asian sea bass (*Lates clacrifer*) to protect from *Vibrio (Listonella) anguillarum*. *Fish Shellfish Immunol* **25**: 47–56.

Lavelle, E.C., Jenkins, P.G. and Harris, J.E. 1997. Oral immunization of rainbow trout with antigen microencapsulated in poly(DL-lactide-co-glycolide) microparticles. *Vaccine* **15**: 1070–78.

Leal, C.A.G., Carvalho-Castro, G.A., Sacchetin, P.S.C., *et al.*, 2010. Oral and parental vaccines against *Flavobacterium columnare*: evaluation of humoral immune response by ELISA and *in vivo* efficiency in Nile tilapia (*Oreochromis niloticus*). *Aquac Int* **18**: 657–66.

Lillehaug, A. 2014. Vaccination strategies and procedures, in *Fish Vaccination* (eds R. Gudding, A. Lillehaug and Ø. Evensen). Oxford, John Wiley & Sons, Ltd., 140–152.

Lin, J.H., Yu, C.C., Lin, C.C. and Yang, H.L. 2005. An oral delivery system for recombinant subunit vaccine to fish. *Dev Biol (Basel)* **121**: 175–80.

Maurice S, Nussinovitch A, Jaffe N, *et al.*, 2004. Oral immunization of *Carassius auratus* with modified recombinant A-layer proteins entrapped in alginate beads. *Vaccine* **23**: 450–59.

Nakanishi, T., Kiryu, I. and Ototake, M. 2002. Development of a new vaccine delivery method for fish: percutaneous administration by immersion with application of a multiple puncture instrument. *Vaccine* **20**: 3764–9.

Nayak, D.K., Asha, A., Shankar, K.M. and Mohan, C. 2004. Evaluation of biofilm of *Aeromonas hydrophila* for oral vaccination of *Clarias batrachus* – a carnivore model. *Fish Shellfish Immunol* **16**: 613–19.

O'Donnell, G.B., Reilly, P., Davidson, G.A. and Ellis, A.E. 1996. The uptake of gamma globulin incorporated into poly (D,L-lactide-co-glycolide) microparticles following oral intubation in Atlantic salmon, *Salmo salar* L. *Fish Shellfish Immunol* **6**: 507–20.

Plant, K.P. and LaPatra, S.E. 2011. Advances in fish vaccine delivery. *Dev Comp Immunol* **35**: 1256–62.

Ramos, E.A., Relucio, J.L.V. and Torres-Villanueva, C.A.T. 2005. Gene expression in tilapia following oral delivery of chitosan-encapsulated plasmid DNA incorporated into fish feeds. *Mar Biotechnol (NY)* **7**: 89–94.

Richter, L. and Kipp, P.B. 1999. Transgenic plants as edible vaccines. *Curr Top Microbiol Immunol* **240**: 159–76.

Rodrigues, A.P., Hirsch, D., Figueiredo, H.C.P., *et al.*, 2006. Production and characterisation of alginate microparticles incorporating *Aeromonas hydrophila* designed for fish oral vaccination. *Process Biochem* **41**: 638–43.

Romalde, J.L., Luzardo-Alvárez, A., Ravelo, C., *et al.*, 2004. Oral immunization using alginate microparticles as a useful strategy for booster vaccination against lactococcosis. *Aquaculture* **236**: 119–29.

Rombout, J.H.W.M. and van den Berg, A.A. 1989. Immunological importance of the second gut segment of carp. I. Uptake and processing of antigens by epithelial cells and macrophages. *J Fish Biol* **35**: 13–22.

Rombout, J.H.W.M., Lamers, C.H.J., Helfrich, M.H., *et al.*, 1985. Uptake and transport of intact macromolecules in the intestinal epithelium of carp (*Cyprinus carpio* L.). *Cell Tiss Res* **239**: 519–30.

Rombout, J.H.W.M., Blok, L.J., Lamers, C.H.J. and Egberts, E. 1986. Immunization of carp (*Cyprinus carpio* L.) with a *Vibrio anguillarum* bacterin: indications for a common mucosal immune system. *Dev Comp Immunol* **10**: 341–51.

Rombout, J.H.W.M., Taverne. N., van de Kamp, M. and Taverne-Thiele, A.J. 1993. Differences in mucus and serum immunoglobulin of carp (*Cyprinus carpio* L.). *Dev Comp Immunol* **17**: 309–17.

Rombout, J.H.W.M., Abelli, L., Picchietti, S., *et al.*, 2011. Teleost intestinal immunology. *Fish Shellfish Immunol* **31**: 616–26.

Ryo, S., Wijdeven, R., Tyagi, A., *et al.*, 2010. Common carp have two subclasses of bony fish specific IgZ showing differential expression in response to infection. *Dev Comp Immunol* **34**: 1183–90.

Savan, R., Aman, A., Nakao, M., *et al.*, 2005a. Discovery of a novel immunoglobulin heavy chain gene chimera from common carp (*Cyprinus carpio* L.). *Immunogenetics* **57**: 458–63.

Savan, R., Aman, A., Sato, K., *et al.*, 2005b. Discovery of a new class of immunoglobulin heavy chain from fugu. *Eur J Immunol* **35**: 3320–31.

Secombes, C.J. 2011. Fish immunity: the potential impact on vaccine development and performance. *Aquac Res* **42** (suppl. 1): 90–92.

Shoemaker, C.A., Vandenberg, G.W., Desormeaux, A., *et al.*, 2006. Efficacy of *Streptococcus iniae* modified bacterin delivered using Oralject^{TM} technology in Nile tilapia (*Oreochromis niloticus*). *Aquaculture* **255**: 151–6.

Siripornadulsil, S., Dabrowski, K. and Sayre, R. 2007. Microalgal vaccines. *Adv Exp Med Biol* **616**: 122–8.

Sun, K., Zhang, W., Hou, J. and Sun, L. 2009. Immunoprotective analysis of VhhP2, a *Vibrio harveyi* vaccine candidate. *Vaccine* **27**: 2733–40.

Tian, J., Sun, X.Q., Chen, X., *et al.*, 2008a. Formation and oral administration of alginate microspheres loaded with pDNA codon for lymphocystis disease virus (LCDV) to Japanese flounder. *Fish Shellfish Immunol* **24**: 592–9.

Tian, J., Sun, X.Q., Chen, X., *et al.*, 2008b. The formulation and immunization of oral poly (DL-lactide-co-glycolide) microparticles containing a plasmid vaccine against lymphocystis disease virus in Japanese flounder (*Paralichthys olivaceus*). *Int Immunopharmacol* **8**: 900–908.

Tian, J., Yu, J. and Sun, X.Q. 2008c. Chitosan microspheres as candidate plasmid vaccine carrier for oral immunization of Japanese flounder (*Paralichthys olivaceus*). *Vet Immunol Immunopathol* **126**: 220–29.

Vandenberg, G.W. 2004. Oral vaccines for finfish: academic theory or commercial reality. *Annu Health Res Rev* **5**: 302–4.

Van Muiswinkel, W.B. 2008. A history of fish immunology and vaccination I. The early days. *Fish Shellfish Immunol* **25**: 397–408.

Vervarcke, S., Ollevier, F., Kinget, R. and Michoel A. 2004. Oral vaccination of African catfish with *Vibrio anguillarum* O2: effect on antigen uptake and immune response by absorption enhancers in lag time coated pellets. *Fish Shellfish Immunol* **16**: 407–14.

Yasumoto, S., Yoshimura, T. and Miyazaki, T. 2006a. Oral immunization of common carp with a liposome vaccine containing *Aeromonas hydrophila* antigen. *Fish Pathol* **41**: 45–9.

Yasumoto, S., Kuzuya, Y., Yasuda, M., *et al.*, 2006b. Oral immunization of common carp with a liposome vaccine fusing herpesvirus antigen. *Fish Pathol* **41**: 141–5

Zhang, Y.-A., Salinas, I., Li, J., *et al.*, 2010. IgT, a primitive immunoglobulin class specialized in mucosal immunity. *Nat Immunol* **11**: 827–35.

7 Adjuvants in Fish Vaccines

Carolina Tafalla[1], Jarl Bøgwald[2], Roy A. Dalmo[2],
Hetron Mweemba Munang'andu[3] and Øystein Evensen[3]

[1]Animal Health Research Center (CISA-INIA), Madrid, Spain
[2]Norwegian College of Fishery Science, UiT The Arctic University of Norway, Tromsø, Norway
[3]Norwegian School of Veterinary Science, Oslo, Norway

ABSTRACT

Vaccination is the preferred method to control infectious diseases in aquaculture industry worldwide. Unfortunately, vaccines are usually not able to confer protection on their own, especially those vaccines based on recombinant or inactivated antigens. Therefore, adjuvants are used to improve vaccine efficacy. Traditional adjuvants such as mineral and vegetable oils are routinely used in different commercial bacterial and viral vaccines for fish, but they can only be used for delivery by injection, and produce unwanted side-effects. Vaccines against intracellular pathogens of fish still have room for improvement, and some of the possible alternatives are discussed in this chapter. Oral vaccination is considered as the most desirable method of vaccine delivery to fish, but to date no specific oral adjuvants are commercialized. One can foresee that antigen-adjuvant combinations that direct immune responses are likely to come into use in the future, also combined with no or minor side-effects. In this review, we summarize the current status of vaccine adjuvants used in fish vaccines and discuss some of the most promising new-generation adjuvants that may help to overcome the limitations of fish vaccinology.

7.1 INTRODUCTION

Disease prevention by vaccination is, on economic, environmental and ethical grounds, the most appropriate method for pathogen control currently available to the aquaculture sector. Traditionally, vaccines comprise either live, attenuated, replicating or non-replicating pathogens, inactivated pathogens or their subunits. Inactivated vaccines based on either killed pathogens or isolated pathogen subunits are, in many cases, weakly immunogenic with low vaccine efficacies, while live vaccines are not licensed for use in aquaculture in many countries. Thus, adjuvants are required for present as well as the new-generation vaccines to be protective.

roy.dalmo@uit.no

Fish Vaccination, First Edition. Edited by Roar Gudding, Atle Lillehaug and Øystein Evensen.

In the past, fish vaccines were produced by a trial-and-error approach (conventional vaccine design) including pathogen identification and cultivation, followed by vaccine formulation containing whole cell preparation and oils. Luckily enough, these strategies were quite efficient, gaining huge reductions in mortality and a drastic reduction in antibiotic usage throughout the aquaculture industry. This was the case in Western "high-cost" aquaculture. Given the very high growth perspectives of aquaculture production, especially in Asian countries, the need for efficacious vaccines is still present. In addition, many of the economically disastrous diseases of today are due to intracellular pathogens, and for this type of pathogen the development of effective vaccines has not been easy going. The most promising future vaccines that induce protection against certain viruses are DNA vaccines. Intramuscular injection of DNA plasmids encoding an immunogenic antigen has proven to elicit protective immunity in fish for many viral pathogens. Because the fish cells produce the antigen themselves, it is exposed on the cell surface either directly, or processed and presented in the context of both major histocompatibility complex (MHC) class I and MHC class II, thus effectively triggering both humoral and cellular immune responses (Biering and Salonius, 2014). Therefore, fish vaccine approaches should be subjected to rational vaccine design wherein a combination of a tailored adjuvant system with the most appropriate antigen(s) is used to create vaccines that may provide more effective immune responses against specific pathogens with minimal side-effects.

Many aspects of fish immunology are in the discovery phase, and we are far from the recognition of which immune mechanisms may be the really protective ones for a given pathogen. Moreover, as we know of today, there are close to 22,000 different fish species, and most of them have their "immune peculiarities". Without a doubt, the innate defense system of fish is quite efficacious and may cope with many infectious pathogens, helping the fish to eradicate viruses, bacteria and even parasites. However, many infectious agents may escape innate defense mechanisms, and thus an adaptive immune response must come into play. The adaptive immune response provides the vertebrate immune system with the ability to recognize and remember specific pathogens, to be able to mount secondary responses each time this pathogen is encountered. In higher vertebrates, adaptive immunity to extracellular pathogens is generally mediated by humoral immune responses (antibodies), while immunity to intracellular pathogens (including viruses) often relies upon cellular immune responses, including cytotoxic T-cells. In fish, the regulation of these elements greatly differs between mammalian systems and even among different fish species. There is a tight, functional link between the innate and adaptive system, as revealed in mammalian immunology, that has not been much explored in fish immunology. This link, governed by several innate receptors and signaling molecules such as cytokines and transcription factors, may provide the key for the future rational design of vaccine adjuvants, since recent advances in immunology have shown that the magnitude and specificity of the signals perceived by the innate immune cells following vaccination shape the subsequent adaptive immune responses.

7.2 VACCINE FORMULATIONS

In general, a vaccine formulation is made up of two components, namely the specific moiety that stimulates the adaptive immune response, and a non-specific moiety that evokes innate immune responses. The specific moiety is made of the antigenic components of microorganisms used for vaccine production, while the non-specific moiety is made of adjuvants. The criterion for selecting a formulation is dependent upon the nature of the immune response to be evoked, avoidance of adverse side-effects and stability of the vaccine. Among the prime factors to be taken into account when choosing a vaccine formulation is the safety of the final product. The potential benefit of obtaining protective immunity has to be weighed against the possible side-effects caused by adjuvants used in the formulation. For practical reasons it is important that vaccine formulations are relatively easy to manufacture, cost-effective and that they should have a long shelf-life.

7.3 PRINCIPLES OF ADJUVANT ACTIONS

Adjuvants, as derived from the term *adjuvare* which means "to help", are helper substances that enhance the immune response to the immunogens. Adjuvants assist with an early onset of immunity, long duration of effector responses such as antibody formation or cytotoxic T-cell activity, and avoidance of booster immunizations (Singh and O'Hagan, 2003). The mechanisms of "adjuvanticity" are complex. They facilitate delivery of antigen (to the secondary lymphoid organs) for a sufficient period of time (Singh and O'Hagan, 2003). At present, the classification of adjuvants that distinguishes between "signal 1" and "signal 2" facilitators has been widely acknowledged (Schijns, 2001). According to this two-signal model, both the presentation of an antigen (signal 1) and the additional secondary signals (signal 2) are required for later activation of T and B lymphocytes (Ribeiro and Schijns, 2010). Signal 1 is dependent upon the fate (e.g., antigen degradation processes) of the vaccine antigen in time (e.g., depot effect of emulsions), place/injection site, and concentration, ultimately improving its availability to immune cells. The signal 1 modality is independent of receptors, while signal 2 facilitators are mostly acting upon innate immune receptors. Moreover, signal 2 adjuvants may lead to an increased innate response together with release of cytokines and DAMPS (danger-associated molecular pattern molecules) that may further modulate the succeeding immune receptor expression and response with respect to T-cell differentiation and activities, given that MHC-peptide complexes have been recognized by T-cell receptors (TCRs). When optimal, this may provide an adequate environment for a robust antigen-specific immune response. In summary, adjuvants will become more important in the way they guide the type of adaptive response against a specific pathogen. Therefore, adjuvants have now been defined as a group of heterogenous compounds able to modulate the intrinsic immunogenicity of an antigen (Guy, 2007). They can be classed according to their chemical nature or physical properties; however, since even related compounds can have very different immunomodulating activities, novel classifications have focused upon the immunological events they induce, even though for many of them the exact mechanism of action is currently unknown.

7.4 ANTIGENIC COMPONENT

The antigenic component constitutes the specific moiety of a vaccine that is responsible for the induction of a protective adaptive immune response in vaccinated fish. Antigens can be made of purified proteins, glycoproteins, carbohydrates or peptides that encode the immunogenic component of a microorganism. Optimization of the antigenic component in a vaccine formulation includes the selection of the most protective vaccine strain, designing genetically engineered immunogenic proteins as vaccine antigens, as well as finding the optimal dose that induces the production of a protective adaptive response in vaccinated fish.

7.5 ADJUVANTS

The various aspects of adjuvants include:

(1) enhancing the immune response to the antigen while at the same time prolonging the duration of immune responses;
(2) modulating the breadth, affinity and specificity of antibody responses;
(3) stimulating the expression of potent cellular-mediated immune responses;
(4) increasing immunogenicity for weak antigens and seroconversion for low responders;
(5) promoting induction of mucosal immunity;
(6) facilitating the reduction of antigen doses and reducing the need for booster vaccinations;
(7) reducing antigen competition in multivalent vaccines.

7.6 ANTIGEN DELIVERY SYSTEMS

Antigen delivery systems can be used to direct the pathway by which antigens are processed in the host. Antigens delivered into the intracellular compartments evoke a cellular immune response, while antigens deposited in extracellular compartments are neutralized by humoral responses. Therefore, the choice of delivery system can be used to evoke exclusively a cellular or humoral immune response. Thus far, delivery systems explored to channel antigens for fish vaccines into the intra- or extracellular compartments include the use of emulsion suspensions, biodegradable microparticles, and fusion of antigens with bacterial toxins.

7.7 DELIVERY VEHICLES

The main role of adjuvants as "delivery vehicles" is related to the signal 1 concept, including: (i) carrying the antigens and immunomodulators; (ii) enabling slow release of the antigens, thereby reducing the need for high frequency of booster vaccination; (iii) protecting the antigen during uptake; (iv) being biodegradable; and (v) serving as an immunostimulant that attracts antigen-presenting sites to the site of antigen deposition. Suffice to mention that while the role of delivering antigens can be separated from immune stimulation, most adjuvants are designed in such a way that the antigen delivery vehicle also serves as an immunostimulant. Consequently, increasingly more complex delivery systems are being developed, aimed at improving the efficiency of antigen delivery, while simultaneously trying to increase the potency of immune stimulation. For example, Fredriksen and Grip (2012) showed that poly-(lactide-co-glycolic acid) PLGA nanoparticles had the capacity to stimulate a strong innate response that could enhance the uptake of encapsulated antigens, and yet PLGA nanoparticles are also known to possess the characteristic of having a controlled release of antigens, which gives them the potential to serve as a single-dose vaccine, thereby eliminating the need for booster vaccinations. However, more work is required to elucidate the efficacy of these innovations in fish vaccinology.

7.8 EMULSION VACCINES

The term "emulsion" is used to describe a system in which an immiscible liquid is dispersed, what is referred to as the dispersed phase, in a second liquid known as the continuous phase. For fish vaccines, the most commonly used emulsion formulations are water-in-oil adjuvants in which the water phase carries the antigens in water globulets while the oil phase serves as a stabilizer. Generally, most emulsion vaccines are administered by injection and they deposit their antigens in extracellular compartments leading to humoral responses orchestrated by the MHC-II pathway, which is supported by the Th2 response. Emulsion formulations constitute the greater bulk of commercial vaccines currently used in aquaculture, where the oil-adjuvanted vaccines play a key role.

7.8.1 Oil-adjuvant vaccines

Vaccination of Atlantic salmon against furunculosis and vibriosis/cold-water vibriosis with oil-adjuvant vaccines results in the induction of long-lasting and protective immunity. In terms of level of protection, use of oil-adjuvant vaccines against furunculosis will not result in clinical disease outbreaks after transfer to seawater. However, the drawback is that oil-adjuvant vaccines result in the formation of visible injection-site lesions that persist through to harvest size (Midtlyng *et al.*, 1996). This may on some occasions result in downgrading of fish at slaughter or after processing. The intra-abdominal lesions are recognized grossly as melanization and adhesions between internal organs or between the organs and the peritoneal wall (Mutoloki *et al.*, 2004; Poppe and Koppang, 2014).

Retention of antigens at the injection site is believed to be a prerequisite for long-term protection, known as the depot effect. This characteristic is known for gel-type adjuvants, such as aluminum hydroxide, and emulsion-based adjuvants. An emulsion is defined as a dispersion of a liquid, called the dispersed phase, in a second liquid, called the continuous phase, with which the first one is not miscible. The antigens of a water-in-oil emulsion are located in the water droplets (mainly). Retention of lipopolysaccharide (LPS) and A-layer protein of *Aeromonas salmonicida* subsp. *salmonicida* (*A. salmonicida*) in head kidney and of LPS in spleen has been observed 16 weeks following intraperitoneal injection of mono- and trivalent killed vaccines with Al_2PO_4 adjuvant. Høie *et al.* (1996) demonstrated that *A. salmonicida* 16S rDNA can be detected by PCR 16 weeks after intraperitoneal injection of formalin-killed bacteria. It has also been shown that LPS of *A. salmonicida* is retained in the kidney as long as 18 months post-vaccination, as demonstrated by immunohistochemistry (Evensen *et al.*, 2005).

7.8.2 Particle-based/formulated vaccines

Particles can potentially improve the signal 1 cascades by a sustained depot effect (slow release), injection site localization and efficacious presentation of antigens. Microparticles offer a promising option to oil emulsions, and their beneficial use as carriers for vaccine delivery has been widely discussed (Sinyakov *et al.*, 2006). An association of antigen(s) with microparticles can be achieved by covalent linkage or physical entrapment. Compared with the latter technique, where the antigen is non-covalently, physically incorporated in the interior of the microparticle, covalent coupling offers distinct advantages: less antigen is required, processing and presentation by antigen-presenting cells is more efficient, a higher stability during storage is obtained, and any excess material can easily be regained. With the use of microparticles, a very low dose of encapsulated antigen may induce a robust humoral response. The structure and properties of microparticles may change markedly with slight alterations in production conditions, and nanoparticles can be prepared in a physico-chemically reproducible manner within narrow size limits. For this reason, adjuvants on the basis of these submicron polymeric particles were developed and have also been suggested for use as potent adjuvants in mammalian systems (Cui and Mumper, 2003). Strictly speaking, particulate vaccine carriers may themselves produce biological effects belonging to signal 2 facilitators, as pointed out by Oyewumi *et al.* (2010).

Encapsulation of vaccines in biocompatible and biodegradable PLGA polymers has been studied for over 20 years. Antigen is released from the microspheres by diffusion through matrix pores and by matrix degradation. Biodegradation rates can be regulated by alterations in polymer composition and molecular weights. So far, a few studies have been carried out on fish with regard to uptake and degradation of PLGA particles and the immune response obtained. For the most part these studies have been on oral administration (O'Donnell *et al.*, 1996; Lavelle *et al.*, 1997; Tian *et al.*, 2008; Altun *et al.*, 2010; Tian and Yu, 2011). A recent article appeared on parenteral immunization of Indian major carp, rohu (*Labeo rohita*), with PLGA-encapsulated antigen (Behera *et al.*, 2010). Outer membrane proteins (OMPs) of *A. hydrophila* were encapsulated in PLGA microparticles and mixed with Freund's incomplete adjuvant (FIA) in an emulsion, or administered alone by IP injection in rohu. At 21 and 42 days after immunization, the antibody titers were significantly higher in the PLGA-encapsulated antigen group containing FIA (Behera *et al.*, 2010).

A dose-dependent transient increase of antibody response following IP injection of PLGA particles containing human gamma globulin (HGG) has been shown by Fredriksen and Grip (2012), where microparticle carriers were superior compared with nanoparticles. Furthermore, when the formulation of PLGA-entrapped HGG was performed with ß-glucan or oil, it resulted in a continuous increase of antibodies over time (up to 120 days). A more recent study on the use of micro- and nanoparticle formulations, including inactivated antigens of infectious pancreatic necrosis virus, yielded less promising results (Munang'andu *et al.*, 2012), and particle-based vaccines were by far inferior to standard water-in-oil emulsions containing the same antigen.

Oral vaccines encapsulated in PLGA have been also used in Japanese flounder (Tian *et al.*, 2008; Tian and Yu, 2011), rainbow trout (Lavelle *et al.*, 1997; Altun *et al.*, 2010; Adomako *et al.*, 2012) and Atlantic salmon (O'Donnell *et al.*, 1996). In the case of Japanese flounder, a plasmid encoding the major capsid protein of lymphocystis disease virus (LCDV) was constructed and encapsulated in PLGA. Controls were naked plasmid vaccine and empty PLGA particles (Tian and Yu, 2011). The fish were orally intubated, and 28 days post-vaccination the fish were challenged by intramuscular injection with LCDV. Vaccine effects were evaluated by observing the presence and number of lymphocystis nodules. The cumulative percentage of Japanese flounder with nodules after challenge was greatly reduced in the group receiving the plasmid coding for the LCDV protein in PLGA particles in the period of 15 to 120 days post-immunization (Tian and Yu, 2011). In addition, the levels of antibody in sera of fish vaccinated with PLGA microcapsules increased for up to nine weeks, although from this point it started to decrease (Tian *et al.*, 2008).

In rainbow trout, oral vaccination against lactococcosis was attempted with antigens encapsulated in PLGA particles dispersed in feed (Altun *et al.*, 2010). Relative percent survival of the PLGA-vaccine amounted to 63%, and booster vaccination with oral administration of the

PLGA-vaccine gave a RPS of more than 60%, 120 days after the first vaccination. Also in rainbow trout, human gamma globulin (HGG) was microencapsulated in PLGA (Lavelle *et al.*, 1997). Specific antibodies were detected in the intestinal mucus of fish that were administered with the microencapsulated antigen after boosting with soluble HGG, but not in fish that were primed with the soluble antigen. Finally, feeding of rainbow trout with feed containing plasmid DNA encoding IHNV G protein microencapsulated in PLGA induced slightly higher amounts of neutralizing antibodies against IHNV, although there was no increased survival after experimental challenge with IHNV (Adomako *et al.*, 2012).

7.9 BIODEGRADABLE PARTICULATE DELIVERY SYSTEMS

This delivery system is attained by either encapsulating or covalently linking the antigens to biodegradable carrier particles. Particulate delivery systems explored for fish vaccines thus far include liposomes, chitosans, alginate microspheres and PLGA nanoparticles. The advantages of a particulate delivery system are that they:

(1) protect the antigen against degradation during uptake;
(2) concomitantly deliver the antigens and costimulatory components to the same antigen-presenting cells (APCs);
(3) induce prolonged release of antigens;
(4) have the possibility of delivering antigens using the mucosal route; and
(5) particulate antigens released in the phagosomes have the ability to enter either the MHC-I or MHC-II pathways (Burgdorf and Kurts, 2008).

Antigens encapsulated in particles of the order of 100 nm in diameter are easily taken up by APCs while those ≥ 0.5 μm are internalized by phagocytosis (De Temmerman *et al.*, 2011). Although particulate vaccines have shown the ability to evoke humoral responses in fish, their ability to induce cellular responses in fish is yet to be elucidated in detail. Much as particulate vaccines have attracted a lot of interest for mucosal and parenteral delivery of antigens, a lot of research is currently ongoing to optimize the performance of these vaccines before they are commercialized.

7.10 FUSION PROTEIN DELIVERY SYSTEM

The channeling of antigens into the cytosol has mainly been a phenomenon of live and DNA vaccines, and as such only these types of vaccines have been linked to MHC-I responses. However, new approaches are being sought to deliver non-replicative antigens into the cytosol in order to evoke the classical MHC-I pathway. One efficient strategy is the binding of antigens to bacteria toxin receptors that translocate the antigens into the cytosol, which has been referred to as the express ticket to the MHC-I pathway by some scientists (Smith *et al.*, 2002). The rationale behind this principle is that many bacteria species have the ability to translocate their toxins across cell membranes, and as such, fusing heterologous antigens to competent bacteria toxin receptors could serve as a delivery strategy for translocating antigens into the cytosol. Once an antigen is fused with the bacteria toxin, the toxin–antigen complex is internalized into the cell via the receptor-mediated endocytosis, and when the endosome is acidified, the antigen is transported to the cytosol by retrograde translocation. Once in the cytosol, antigens are then processed to produce peptides that are presented to the MHC-I molecules. Although several bacteria toxins have been exploited for the delivery of different antigens into the endoplasmic reticulum (ER) in mammalia (Smith *et al.*, 2002), only a few bacteria toxins have been explored for this delivery system in fish vaccinology (Munang'andu *et al.*, 2012).

7.11 IMMUNOMODULATORS

The immunomodulator facilitates signal 2 effects. This includes activating relevant cytokines and upregulation of costimulatory molecules that attract different cell types, such as macrophages and dendritic cells, to the sites of antigen deposition for the uptake and onward processing of antigens for presentation to B- or T-cells in order to evoke a strong priming of the adaptive immune system. These modulators are often referred to as signal 2 facilitating adjuvants. The choice of immunomodulator is influenced by the type of adaptive immune response to be induced, avoidance of adverse side-effects, and the ability of the immunomodulator to improve the potency of the antigen used in the vaccines. Table 7.1 shows some of the immunomodulators explored for fish vaccines. These substances activate and

Table 7.1 Examples of adjuvants used for inactivated fish vaccines.

Category	Adjuvant
Gel-type	Aluminum hydroxide
	Potassium aluminum phosphate
Microbial components	CpG
	Bacterial polysaccharides (LPS)
	Tetanus and measles virus
	Mycobacterium butyricum
	Mycobacterium bovis
	Mycobacterium chelonae
	Mycobacteria cell walls
	Flagellin
Oil-emulsion and emulsifiers	Freund's complete adjuvant (FCA)
	Freund's incomplete adjuvant (FIA)
	Mineral oil and sorbitan sesquioleate
	Montanide ISA
Biodegradable particulates	Alginates
	Liposomes
	Biodegradable microspheres
	Saponins
	PLGA nanoparticles
	Chitosans
	Beta-glucans
Cytokines and chemokines	Interleukins
	Chemokines
Vitamins and other chemical compounds	Levamisole
	Vitamin C
	Vitamin E

facilitate the maturation of macrophages and dendritic cells into effective antigen presenting cells (APCs). However, the paradigm in vaccine formulation is to find immunomodulators that skew the adaptive immune response towards a humoral or cellular mediated immune response. Although it is a common phenomenon that inactivated vaccines induce humoral responses, research has shown that immunomodulators can be designed to evoke cellular responses for non-replicative antigens. As such, immunomodulators serve as an extra incentive to antigen delivery by evoking cellular mediated immune responses that non-replicative antigens on their own might not evoke. Examples of immunomodulators or signal 2 facilitating adjuvants are given below.

An important characteristic of signal 2 adjuvants is their resemblance to conserved microbial molecular patterns, designated as pathogen-associated microbial patterns (PAMPs) by pathogen recognition receptors (PRRs) that include toll-like receptors (TLRs), NOD-like receptors, dectin-1 or RIG-like helicases, which are predominantly found on cells of the innate immune system. Nowadays, this first recognition is considered critical in signal 2 induction and downstream activation of distinct T helper cell subsets. Recent work on adjuvants has especially focused on different PRR ligands including different PAMPs, as well as other endogenous TLR ligands (DAMPs) such as heat-shock proteins (hsp), studying their ability to induce targeted Th responses. Once there is a production and expression of IL-2 (T-cell growth factor) and its alpha subunit of the IL-2 receptors (CD25) during, for example, activation of naïve Th cells into Th0 cells, proliferation of Th cells begins. Th0 cells will differentiate into Th1 or Th2 cells depending on the cytokine environment, wherein IFN-γ drives Th1 cells while IL-4 induces Th2 cell production/differentiation (Steinman, 2007). Additionally, after many cell generations the Th cell progenitors differentiate into effector Th cells, memory Th cells, and regulatory Th cells. The vaccine adjuvants that are in use in veterinary and human medicine aid differentiation of Th cells into several T cell lineages, such as Th1, Th2, Th9 and Th17 (Dong, 2008; Chen *et al.*, 2011).

7.11.1 Aluminum-containing adjuvants

The adjuvant property of aluminum salts was discovered in 1926 (Glenny *et al.*, 1926). Aluminum compounds, especially aluminum phosphate and aluminum hydroxide, are some of the few adjuvants that have been allowed and considered safe to use in human vaccines. Aluminum adjuvants have been shown to induce Th2 responses almost exclusively, thus they have been used as adjuvants with great success, being particularly effective at promoting protective humoral immunity. It was believed that alum activated the NLRP3 inflammasome, thus inducing necrotic cell death that released the danger signal uric acid (Coffman *et al.*, 2010). However, very recently, it has been discovered that being a crystal, alum binds dendritic cell plasma membrane lipids with substantial force, independent of inflammasome and membrane proteins (Flach *et al.*, 2011). The subsequent lipid reassembling activates an abortive phagocytic response that leads to antigen uptake. Such activated dendritic cells, without further association with alum, show high affinity and stable binding to $CD4^+$ T-cells via the adhesion molecules intercellular adhesion molecule-1 (ICAM-1) and lymphocyte function-associated antigen-1 (LFA-1).

Only a few studies have been performed with aluminum adjuvants in the optimization of fish vaccines. A vaccine against *A. salmonicida* mixed with potassium aluminum sulfate (alum) as an adjuvant was tested in Atlantic salmon 15 years ago (Mulvey *et al.*, 1995). Alum appeared to increase the protection against challenge, but the results were not statistically significant.

In another study, an *Escherichia coli* mutant was used for vaccination against *Edwardsiella ictaluri*-induced enteric septicaemia of catfish (*Ictalurus punctatus*) (Tyler and Klesius, 1994). Killed *E. coli* bacteria with or without alum were administered IP to catfish and the fish were challenged with virulent *E. ictaluri* bacteria. Fish given *E. coli* in alum showed an enhanced survival (92%) compared with the fish for which *E. coli* was administered alone (54%) or fish given saline (56%). Quite recently, an aluminum hydroxide adjuvanted *E. tarda* vaccine was prepared and injected IP in Japanese flounder. The RPS was found to be 69% (Jiao *et al.*, 2010a), while immunization with the antigen alone followed by an experimental challenge gave a RPS of 34%; however, the FIA-coupled vaccine showed a RPS of 81%. More recently, an experiment has been carried out by Fan *et al.* (2012) in which formalin-inactivated reddish body iridovirus (TRBIV) was mixed with alum and either injected or bath-administered twice in turbot. The resulting relative survival rates were 83.3% and 90.5%, respectively.

7.11.2 Saponins

Saponins are natural glycosides of steroid or triterpene that have been widely explored as adjuvants in different mammalian systems due to their capacity to stimulate simultaneous Th1 and Th2 responses (Sun *et al.*, 2009). The most widely used saponins are Quil A (also used in immune stimulating complexes (ISCOMs)) and their derivatives; however, due to their high cell cytotoxicity and instability in the aqueous phase, different kinds of saponins are being explored. In Japanese flounder, formalin-killed *E. tarda* cells were administered to fish by feeding in the absence or presence of curdlan or curdlan together with Quil A saponin. Although the addition of curdlan alone gave higher survival rates, the group in which the vaccine was administered with both curdlan and Quil A showed significantly better survival (Ashida *et al.*, 1999).

7.11.3 ß-glucans

ß-glucans are known to stimulate the non-specific immune response of both mammals and fish where dectin-1 may be involved (Robertsen *et al.*, 1999, Dalmo and Bøgwald, 2008). The binding to dectin-1 may induce an adaptive Th1/Th17 cell activation (Carvalho *et al.*, 2012). Whether a similar T-cell differentiation process also occurs in fish is not yet known. To obtain protective effects against diseases the glucan is usually injected IP, and it is suggested that the effects of glucans are both dose-dependent and short-lived. The immunostimulant or adjuvant effect of ß-glucans has been reported in many past publications (Nikl *et al.*, 1991; Chen and Ainsworth, 1992; Rørstad *et al.*, 1993; DeBaulney *et al.*, 1996; Midtlyng *et al.*, 1996; Figueras *et al.*, 1998; Ashida *et al.*, 1999; Selvaraj *et al.*, 2005; Kamilya *et al.*, 2006). In general, the use of glucans may result in elevated antibody responses, higher cell-mediated activities (innate) and to some degree protection. This has already been reviewed by Bricknell and Dalmo (2005); however, to our knowledge there are hardly any recent publications on the adjuvant activity of glucans in fish.

7.11.4 TLR ligands

A number of so-called toll-like receptor (TLR) ligands (agonists) may induce strong innate responses that may be decisive for the outcome of adaptive responses. Teleost fish species may possess close to twice the number of different TLRs compared with mammalian species, and one may think about how diverse the immune response may be with respect to fish TLR-induced signaling. A review article on immune-relevant genes including TLR-like receptors in fish has recently been published by Zhu *et al.* (2013). In general, those TLRs that, after ligand binding, induce the production of IL-12 favor a Th1 response (TLR 3, 4, 5, 7, 8, 9 and 11), and in addition the activation of these TLRs may induce cross-presentation of antigens facilitating a cytotoxic T-cell response under certain conditions (Manicassamy and Pulendran, 2009). It should be mentioned that ligand binding to TLRs 3 and 4, 7 and 9 may also induce type I IFN responses via interferon regulating factors.

7.11.5 Flagellin

The structural protein of gram-negative flagella is called flagellin and is a potent activator of a broad range of cell types within the innate and adaptive immune system. Several studies have demonstrated the ability of flagellin and its fusion construct (antigen) to act as an adjuvant (Mizel and Bates, 2010). Flagellin is known to induce immune responses via TLR5 signaling, resulting in a mixed Th1 and Th2 response. It has also been reported that inflammasomes containing NLRC4/IPAF may bind cytosolically-located flagellin inducing IFN-γ expression (Coffman *et al.*, 2010). During the last decade, the adjuvant effect of flagellin has widely been studied in vertebrates, and during the last couple of years also in fish (Wilhelm *et al.*, 2006; Jiao *et al.*, 2009, 2010b).

Jiao and coworkers studied different vaccine concepts against *E. tarda* in the Japanese flounder to obtain effective protective formulations, based on both recombinant proteins and DNA vaccine constructs encoding flagellin (Jiao *et al.*, 2009, 2010b). The best performing vaccine concept was the one consisting of a chimeric DNA vaccine coding for the *E. tarda* proteins Eta6 fused in-frame to FliC, the flagellin for *E. tarda*. Although they found that *E. tarda* FliC induced low protective immunity by itself, it could function as a molecular adjuvant and potentiate the specific immune response induced by the *E. tarda* antigen Eta6. Upregulation of immune genes following immunization with flagellin has been described by Hynes *et al.* (2011), where TNF-α, IL-6, IL-8 and IL-1ß were significantly upregulated compared with non-adjuvanted controls. In this study, however, there was no induction of specific antibody response against flagellin or the model antigen *Limulus polyhemus* hemolymph (LPH) in the Atlantic salmon.

Piscirickettsiosis is a severe disease reported in salmonids that has caused especially great problems for the Chilean aquaculture industry. A recombinant subunit vaccine was developed in order to control the disease due to poor responses after treatment by antibiotics. Three experimental formulations were prepared containing two or three recombinant proteins of the bacterium, and the formulations were emulsified with FIA (Wilhelm *et al.*, 2006). The highest protective response was obtained with a vaccine formulation containing the subunit of the flagellum and chaperonins Hsp60 and Hsp70 of *P. salmonis*, suggesting that the use of more than one recombinant protein antigen is needed to obtain a good protective effect against this disease.

7.11.6 Poly I:C

Polyinosinic polycytidylic acid (poly I:C) is a double-stranded polyribonucleotide mimicking a viral infection, binds to TLR3, and therefore has been widely used to induce a type I IFN in many species including fish (Eaton, 1990; Jensen *et al.*, 2002, Plant *et al.*, 2005). IFNs are cytokines with a major role in the innate defense against viral infections. This non-specific antiviral activity of poly I:C has recently been tested in rainbow trout infected with *Infectious hematopoietic necrosis virus* (IHNV) (Kim *et al.*, 2009). Fish pre-injected with poly I:C were protected against IHNV challenge 2 days later, and IHNV-specific antibodies were detected in survivors. The survivors showed a 100% survival rate following re-challenge with IHNV both 21 and 49 days after the primary IHNV challenge (Kim *et al.*, 2009), demonstrating that the fish were in an antiviral state during the virus exposure. The use of poly I:C gave the fish an important advantage for posterior specific antibody production. A similar study was performed in the sevenband grouper *Epinephelus septemfasciatus* in which fish were immunized against the nodavirus *Red-spotted grouper nervous necrosis virus* (RGNNV) (Nishizawa *et al.*, 2009). Fish injected with 50 mg poly I:C per fish or more intramuscularly (IM) and challenged IM with RGNNV 2 days post-injection showed more than 90% survival. When surviving fish were re-challenged with RGNNV 3 weeks after the primary challenge, no mortalities were detected in the group that had been previously exposed to Poly I:C, since upon RGNNV challenge the antibodies against RGNNV were higher in these fish. All survivors that were re-challenged with RGNNV showed even higher levels of specific antibodies (Nishizawa *et al.*, 2009). Following up this work, the same research group performed a field trial exploring the vaccine efficacy of a RGNNV vaccine followed by poly I:C injection. The poly I:C-adjuvanted vaccine showed reasonably high efficacy, but a one-shot poly I:C injection in sevenband grouper 20 days after a natural RGNNV outbreak also induced significant protection (93.7%) compared with non-treated fish (9.8%) (Oh *et al.*, 2012).

A prophylactic strategy using poly I:C was also used by Takami and coworkers in Japanese flounder experimentally infected with *Viral hemorrhagic septicemia virus* (VHSV) (Takami *et al.*, 2010). The survival rate in Japanese flounder after VHSV challenge following poly I:C administration was 100%, while all untreated fish died within 9 days. Survival rates of the fish given a secondary challenge of VHSV were 100% in the poly I:C-VHSV group (Poly I:C-VHSV-VHSV group), while non-immunized fish showed 0% survival.

7.11.7 CpG ODN

Bacterial DNA and synthetic oligodeoxynucleotides (ODNs) expressing unmethylated CpG motifs trigger an immunostimulatory cascade that culminates in the maturation, differentiation and proliferation of multiple immune cells, including B and T lymphocytes, NK cells, monocytes, macrophages and dendritic cells. CpG motifs are approximately 20 times less common in mammalian than microbial DNA, and therefore are recognized as a danger signal by cells that express TLR9. In mammals, it has been widely demonstrated that CpG ODNs function as adjuvants when co-administered with vaccines, being able to both accelerate and magnify the immune response (Bode *et al.*, 2011). Although many studies have been carried out on the immunomodulatory effects of CpGs in fish (Carrington and Secombes, 2007; Liu *et al.*, 2010a,b), only a few studies have focused on the adjuvant effect of these molecules.

Chinook salmon (*O. tshawytscha*) reared in the Pacific Northwest of the US often suffer from infection with *Renibacterium salmoninarum*, the causative agent of bacterial kidney disease (BKD). The result from a study where whole-cell vaccines with or without CpG ODN adjuvants were used was that CpG ODN did not significantly increase the vaccine efficacy compared with a whole-cell based vaccine (Rhodes *et al.*, 2004).

In a study of rainbow trout, four groups were IM injected with a commercially available, non-adjuvanted aqueous vaccine against furunculosis containing inactivated cultures of *A. salmonicida* (Aquavac Furovac 5) alone, or together with CpG ODN 1982, CpG ODN 2133 or ODN 2143. The fish were challenged with IP injection of a pathogenic strain of *A.*

salmonicida seven weeks after injection, and the only group that showed a significantly lower mortality compared with those injected with Furovac alone (mortality of 52%) was the group injected with Furovac and the CpG ODN 2143, where only 21% of the fish died (Carrington and Secombes, 2007).

The protective effect of CpG motifs was also studied by Liu and coworkers (2010a,b) in turbot and Japanese flounder; 16 CpG ODNs were synthesized and examined for the ability to inhibit bacterial dissemination in Japanese flounder blood. Four ODNs with the strongest inhibitory effects were selected and a plasmid pCN6 was constructed containing the sequences of the four selected ODNs. Japanese flounder were injected IM with plasmids pCN6 and pCN3 (control) and PBS. Four weeks post-vaccination the fish were challenged with *A. hydrophila* and mortality was monitored over a period of 20 days. Accumulated mortalities were 30%, 66.7% and 63.3% in pCN6-, pCN3-, and PBS-immunized flounder, respectively (Liu *et al.*, 2010b). Fish were also vaccinated as above and challenged with *E. tarda* 4 weeks after vaccination, and the mortalities were 53.3%, 90%, and 93.3% respectively. Therefore, the pCN6 plasmid provided a non-specific protection against both *A. hydrophila* and *E. tarda* infections – even at four weeks post-injection. This non-specific protective effect has also been observed in fish parasitic infections, since certain CpGs (e.g., CpG-ODN 1668 and CpG-ODN 2359) have also been shown to have protective effects against *Miamiensis avidus* (Kang *et al.*, 2012). Following on, a salmonid alphavirus (SAV) vaccine containing antigen plus CpG and poly I:C as adjuvants induced a significant production of neutralizing antibodies and conferred some level of protection, as evaluated by the proportion of SAV-positive fish compared with controls (Thim *et al.*, 2012). The authors reported that the adjuvanted vaccines induced prominent IFN type I expression.

To analyze the adjuvant effect of CpGs in turbot, fish were vaccinated with a *Vibrio harveyi* recombinant subunit vaccine, DegQ, in combination with a CpG that had been shown to provide antibacterial effects in the host species after injection. Fish were vaccinated by IP injection including all the appropriate controls, and 28 days after vaccination the fish were challenged by a virulent strain of *V. harvey*, and accumulated mortalities were recorded (Liu *et al.*, 2010a). The only vaccine formulation that induced a significant protection was DegQ + pCN5 CpG. The duration of the adjuvant effect was found to last at least 50 days.

One of the unique features of DNA vaccines is the ability to stimulate both cellular and humoral immune responses through the administration of a bacterial plasmid coding for a protective antigen (Weiner and Kennedy, 1999; Biering and Salonius, 2014). Thus, these DNA vaccines possess intrinsic immunostimulatory capacity due to the presence of CpG motifs in the bacterial plasmid backbone. Therefore, the inclusion of additional CpG motifs in the vaccine plasmid would provide us with an intrinsic adjuvant within the same construct, being an easy method to increase the immunogenicity. A recent work by Martinez-Alonso *et al.* (2011) explored the possibility of increasing the immunogenicity of a VHSV DNA vaccine though the introduction of several copies (either two or four) of a fragment containing multiple CpG sequences of known immunostimulatory effects into the DNA vaccine. The addition of these CpG motifs significantly increased the titer of neutralizing antibodies in serum and increased the levels of transcription of several immune genes such as Mx or MHC-I, demonstrating for the first time that additional CpG motifs may also be used to increase the immunogenicity of these DNA vaccines.

7.12 STABILIZERS

Stabilizers and preservatives are substances that ensure that vaccines have a stable shelf-life and that they maintain their immunogenic properties during adsorption when administered in fish. For example, emulsifiers as such surfactants, which are chemical compounds containing a hydrophobic and non-hydrophilic polar group made of fatty acid chains, are added to vaccines to stabilize their polarity. The hydrophilic:lipophilic balance (HLB) of emulsifiers determines whether the vaccine product is polarized towards the aqueous phase as a water-in-oil (w/o) emulsion, or polarized towards the oily phase constituted as an oil-in-water (o/w) emulsion. A low HLB ratio is indicative of a high affinity for an aqueous w/o emulsion, while a high HLB ratio has a propensity for a high affinity linked to o/w emulsion. Similarly, an intermediate HLB ratio is indicative of w/o/w emulsion. Overall, the coalescence of the dispersed phase in the continuous phase has an impact on storage, but with careful selection of appropriate emulsifiers and HLB ratios, formulations with a long shelf-life can be obtained. Other stabilizers used in formulations include amino acids and sugars that protect vaccines from adverse conditions like the freeze-drying process.

7.13 CONCLUDING REMARKS AND PERSPECTIVES

A future development of efficacious vaccines for use in aquaculture should be undertaken by utilising highly antigenic proteins together with adjuvants in a formulation that provides signal 1 and 2. Such adjuvants would have to balance the ability to trigger a specific immunological response targeted at, for example, viral pathogens, against the reactogenic potential that these ligands possess. New, rationally designed vaccines will have the advantage of oil adjuvants that induce strong and durable immune responses. Thus, the search for real molecular correlates of protection should be pursued vigorously.

7.14 ACKNOWLEDGEMENTS

This work was supported by Starting Grant 2011 (Project No. 280469) from the European Research Council and project AGL2011-29676 from the Spanish Ministerio de Economia y Competitividad (Plan Nacional AGL2011-29676). Financial support was also received under the Grant Agreement 311993 TARGETFISH. Furthermore, The Research Council of Norway (contract no. 183204/S40) and the Tromsø Research Foundation are acknowledged for their support.

REFERENCES

Adomako, M., St-Hilaire, S., Zheng, Y., *et al.*, 2012. Oral DNA vaccination of rainbow trout, *Oncorhynchus mykiss* (Walbaum), against infectious haematopoietic necrosis virus using PLGA [poly(D,L-lactic-co-glycolic acid)] nanoparticles. *J Fish Dis* **35**: 203–14.

Altun, S., Kubilay, A., Ekici, S., *et al.*, 2010. Oral vaccination against lactococcosis in rainbow trout (*Oncorhynchus mykiss*) using sodium alginate and poly (lactide-co-glycolide) carrier. *Kafkas Univ Vet Fak Derg* **16**: S211–17.

Ashida, T., Okimasu, E., Ui, M., *et al.*, 1999. Protection of Japanese flounder *Paralichthys olivaceus* against experimental edwardsiellosis by formalin-killed *Edwardsiella tarda* in combination with oral administration of immunostimulants. *Fish Sci* **65**: 527–30.

Behera, T., Nanda, P.K., Mohanty, C., *et al.*, 2010. Parenteral immunization of fish, *Labeo rohita* with Poly D,L-lactide-co-glycolic acid (PLGA) encapsulated antigen microparticles promotes innate and adaptive immune responses. *Fish Shellfish Immunol* **28**: 320–25.

Biering, E. and Salonius, K. 2014. DNA vaccines, in *Fish Vaccination* (eds R. Gudding, A. Lillehaug and Ø. Evensen). Oxford, John Wiley & Sons, Ltd., 47–55.

Bode, C., Zhao, G., Steinhagen, F., *et al.*, 2011. CpG DNA as a vaccine adjuvant. *Exp Rev Vaccines* **10**: 499–511.

Bricknell, I. and Dalmo, R.A. 2005. The use of immunostimulants in fish larval aquaculture. *Fish Shellfish Immunol* **19**: 457–72.

Burgdorf, S. and Kurts, C. 2008. Endocytosis mechanisms and the cell biology of antigen presentation. *Curr Opinion Immunol* **20**: 89–95.

Carrington, A.C. and Secombes, C.J. 2007. CpG oligodeoxynucleotides up-regulate antibacterial systems and induce protection against bacterial challenge in rainbow trout (*Oncorhynchus mykiss*). *Fish Shellfish Immunol* **23**: 781–92.

Carvalho, A., Giovannini, G., De Luca, A., *et al.*, 2012. Dectin-1 isoforms contribute to distinct Th1/Th17 cell activation in mucosal candidiasis. *Cell Mol Immunol* **9**: 276–86.

Chen, D. and Ainsworth, A.J. 1992. Glucan administration potentiates immune defence mechanisms of channel catfish, *Ictalurus punctatus* Rafinesque. *J Fish Dis* **15**: 295–304.

Chen, Z., Lin, F., Gao, Y., *et al.*, 2011. FOXP3 and RORγt: transcription regulation of Treg and Th17. *Int Immunopharmacol* **11**: 536–42.

Coffman, R.L., Sher, A. and Seder, R.A. 2010. Vaccine adjuvants: putting innate immunity to work. *Immunity* **33**: 492–503.

Cui, Z. and Mumper, R.J. 2003. Microparticles and nanoparticles as delivery systems for DNA vaccines. *Crit Rev Ther Drug Carrier Syst* **20**: 103–37.

Dalmo, R.A. and Bøgwald, J. 2008. ß-glucans as conductors of immune symphonies. *Fish Shellfish Immunol* **25**: 384–96.

DeBaulny MO, Quentel C, Fournier V, *et al.*, 1996. Effect of long-term oral administration of ß-glucan as an immunostimulant or an adjuvant on some non-specific parameters of the immune response of turbot *Scophthalmus maximus*. *Dis Aquatic Org* **26**: 139–47.

De Temmerman, M.L., Rejman, J., Demeester, J., *et al.*, 2011. Particulate vaccines: on the quest for optimal delivery and immune response. *Drug Discov Today* **16**: 569–82.

Dong, C. 2008. T_H17 cells in development: an updated view of their molecular identity and genetic programming. *Nat Rev Immunol* **8**: 337–48.

Eaton, W.D. 1990. Antiviral activity in four species of salmonids following exposure to poly inosinic:cytidylic acid. *Dis Aquat Org* **9**: 193–8.

Evensen, Ø., Brudeseth, B. and Mutoloki, S. 2005. The vaccine formulation and its role in inflammatory processes in fish – effects and adverse reactions. *Dev Biol (Basel)* **121**: 117–25.

Fan, T.J., Hu, X.Z., Wang, L.Y., *et al.*, 2012. Development of an inactivated iridovirus vaccine against turbot viral reddish body syndrome. *J Ocean Univ China* **11**: 65–9.

Figueras, A., Santarem, M.M. and Novoa, B. 1998. Influence of the sequence of administration of ß-glucans and a *Vibrio damsela* vaccine on the immune response of turbot (*Scophthalmus maximus* L.). *Vet Immunol Immunopathol* **64**: 59–68.

Flach, T.L., Ng, G., Hari, A., *et al.*, 2011. Alum interaction with dendritic cell membrane lipids is essential for its adjuvanticity. *Nat Med* **17**: 479–87.

Fredriksen, B.N. and Grip, J. 2012. PLGA/PLA micro- and nanoparticle formulations serve as antigen depots and induce elevated humoral responses after immunization of Atlantic salmon (*Salmo salar* L.). *Vaccine* **30**: 656–67.

Glenny, A.T., Pope, C.G., Waddington, H. and Wallace, U. 1926. Immunological notes. XXIII. The antigenic value of toxoid precipitated by potassium alum. *J Pathol Bacteriol* **29**: 31–40.

Guy, B. 2007. The perfect mix: recent progress in adjuvant research. *Nat Microbiol* **5**: 505–17.

Høie, S.H., Heum, M. and Thoresen, O.F. 1996. Detection of *Aeromonas salmonicida* by polymerase chain reaction in Atlantic salmon vaccinated against furunculosis. *Fish Shellfish Immunol* **6**: 199–206

Hynes, N.A., Furnes, C., Fredriksen, B.N., *et al.*, 2011. Immune response of Atlantic salmon to recombinant flagellin. *Vaccine* **29**: 7678–87.

Jensen, I., Albuquerque, A., Sommer, A.I. and Robertsen, B. 2002. Effect of poly I:C on the expression of Mx proteins and resistance against infection by infectious salmon anaemia virus in Atlantic salmon. *Fish Shellfish Immunol* **13**: 311–26.

Jiao, X.D., Zhang, M., Hu, Y.H. and Sun, L. 2009. Construction and evaluation of DNA vaccines encoding *Edwardsiella tarda* antigens. *Vaccine* **27**: 5195–202.

Jiao, X.D., Cheng, S., Hu, Y.H. and Sun, L. 2010a. Comparative study of the effects of aluminum adjuvants and Freund's incomplete adjuvant on the immune response to an *Edwardsiella tarda* major antigen. *Vaccine* **28**: 1832–7.

Jiao, X.D., Hu, Y.H. and Sun, L. 2010b. Dissection and localization of the immunostimulating domain of *Edwardsiella tarda* FliC. *Vaccine* **28**: 5635–40.

Kamilya, D., Maiti, T.K., Joardar, S.N. and Mal, B.C. 2006. Adjuvant effect of mushroom glucan and bovine lactoferrin upon *Aeromonas hydrophila* vaccination in catla, *Catla catla* (Hamilton). *J Fish Dis* **29**: 331–7.

Kang, Y.J. and Kim, K.H. 2012. Effect of CpG-ODNs belonging to different classes on resistance of olive flounder (*Paralichthys olivaceus*) against viral hemorrhagic septicemia virus (VHSV) and *Miamiensis avidus* (Ciliata; Scuticociliata) infections. *Aquaculture* **324**: 39–43.

Kim, H.J., Oseko, N., Nishizawa, T. and Yoshimizu, M. 2009. Protection of rainbow trout from infectious hematopoietic necrosis (IHN) by injection of infectious pancreatic necrosis virus (IPNV) or Poly(I:C). *Dis Aquat Org* **83**: 105–13.

Lavelle, E.C., Jenkins, P.G. and Harris, J.E. 1997. Oral immunization of rainbow trout with antigen microencapsulated in poly(DL-lactide-co-glycolide) microparticles. *Vaccine* **15**: 1070–78.

Liu, C.S., Sun, Y., Hu, Y.H. and Sun, L. 2010a. Identification and analysis of a CpG motif that protects turbot (*Scophthalmus maximus*) against bacterial challenge and enhances vaccine-induced specific immunity. *Vaccine* **28**: 4153–61.

Liu, C.S., Sun, Y., Hu, Y.H. and Sun, L. 2010b. Identification and analysis of the immune effects of CpG motifs that protect Japanese flounder (*Paralichthys olivaceus*) against bacterial infection. *Fish Shellfish Immunol* **29**: 279–85.

Manicassamy, S. and Pulendran, B. 2009. Modulation of adaptive immunity with Toll-like receptors. *Semin Immunol* **21**: 185–93.

Martinez-Alonso, S., Martinez-Lopez, A., Estepa, A., *et al.*, 2011. The introduction of multi-copy CpG motifs into an antiviral DNA vaccine strongly upregulates its immunogenicity in fish. *Vaccine* **29**: 1289–96.

Midtlyng, P.J., Reitan, L.J. and Speilberg, L. 1996. Experimental studies on the efficacy and side-effects of intraperitoneal vaccination of Atlantic salmon (*Salmo salar* L.) against furunculosis. *Fish Shellfish Immunol* **6**: 335–50.

Mizel, S.B. and Bates, J.T. 2010. Flagellin as an adjuvant: cellular mechanisms and potential. *J Immunol* **185**: 5677–82.

Mulvey, B., Landolt, M.L. and Busch, R.A. 1995. Effects of potassium aluminium sulphate (alum) used in an *Aeromonas salmonicida* bacterin in Atlantic salmon, *Salmo salar* L. *J Fish Dis* **18**: 495–506.

Munang'andu, H.M., Fredriksen, B.N., Mutoloki, S., *et al.*, 2012. Comparison of vaccine efficacy for different antigen delivery systems for infectious pancreatic necrosis virus vaccines in Atlantic salmon (*Salmo salar* L.) in a cohabitation challenge model. *Vaccine* **30**: 4007–16.

Mutoloki, S., Alexandersen, S. and Evensen Ø. 2004. Sequential study of antigen persistence and concomitant inflammatory reactions relative to side-effects and growth of Atlantic salmon (*Salmo salar* L.) following intraperitoneal injection with oil-adjuvanted vaccines. Fish Shellfish Immunol **16**: 633–44.

Nikl, L., Albright, L.J. and Evelyn, T.P.T. 1991. Influence of seven immunostimulants on the immune response of coho salmon to *Aeromonas salmonicida*. *Dis Aquat Org* **12**: 7–12.

Nishizawa, T., Takami, I., Kokawa, Y. and Yoshimizu, M. 2009. Fish immunization using a synthetic double-stranded RNA Poly(I:C), an interferon inducer, offers protection against RGNNV, a fish nodavirus. *Dis Aquat Org* **83**: 115–22.

O'Donnell, G.B., Reilly, P., Davidson, G.A. and Ellis, A.E. 1996. The uptake of human gamma globulin incorporated into poly (D,L-lactide-co-glycolide) microparticles following oral intubation in Atlantic salmon, *Salmo salar* L. *Fish Shellfish Immunol* **6**: 507–20.

Oh, M.J., Takami, I., Nishizawa, T., *et al.*, 2012. Field tests of Poly I:C immunization with nervous necrosis virus (NNV) in sevenband grouper, *Epinephelus septemfasciatus* (Thunberg). *J Fish Dis* **35**: 187–91.

Oyewumi, M.O., Kumar, A. and Cui, Z. 2010. Nano-microparticulates as immune adjuvants: correlating particle sizes and the resultant immune responses. *Exp Rev Vaccines* **9**: 1095–107.
Plant, K.P., Harbottle, H. and Thune, R.L. 2005. Poly I:C induces an antiviral state against ictalurid herpesvirus 1 and Mx1 transcription in the channel catfish (*Ictalurus punctatus*). *Dev Comp Immunol* **29**: 627–35.
Poppe, T. and Koppang, E.O. 2014. Side effects of vaccination, in *Fish Vaccination* (eds R. Gudding, A. Lillehaug and Ø. Evensen). Oxford, John Wiley & Sons, Ltd., 153–61.
Ribeiro, C.M.S. and Schijns, V.E.J.C. 2010. Immunology of vaccine adjuvants. *Methods Mol Biol* **626**: 1–14.
Rhodes, L.D., Rathbone, C.K., Corbett, S.C., *et al.*, 2004. Efficacy of cellular vaccines and genetic adjuvants against bacterial kidney disease in Chinook salmon (*Oncorhynchus tshawytscha*). *Fish Shellfish Immunol* **16**: 461–74.
Robertsen, B. 1999. Modulation of the non-specific defence of fish by structurally conserved microbial polymers. *Fish Shellfish Immunol* **9**: 269–90.
Rørstad, G., Aasjord, P.M. and Robertsen, B. 1993. Adjuvant effect of a yeast glucan in vaccines against furunculosis in Atlantic salmon (*Salmo salar* L.). *Fish Shellfish Immunol* **3**: 179–90.
Schijns, V.E.J.C. 2001. Induction and direction of immune responses by vaccine adjuvants. *Crit Rev Immunol* **21**: 456–63.
Selvaraj, V., Sampath, K. and Sekar, V. 2005. Administration of yeast glucan enhances survival and some non-specific and specific immune parameters in carp (*Cyprinus carpio*) infected with *Aeromonas hydrophila*. *Fish Shellfish Immunol* **19**: 293–306.
Singh, M. and O'Hagan, D.T. 2003. Recent advances in veterinary vaccine adjuvants. *Int J Parasitol* **33**: 469–78.
Sinyakov, M.S., Dror, M., Lublin-Tennenbaum, T., *et al.*, 2006. Nano- and microparticles as adjuvants in vaccine design: success and failure is related to host natural antibodies. *Vaccine* **24**: 6534–41.
Smith, D.C., Lord, J.M., Roberts, L.M., *et al.*, 2002. 1st class ticket to class I: protein toxins as pathfinders for antigen presentation. *Traffic* **3**: 697–704.
Steinman, L. 2007. A brief history of T(H)17, the first major revision in the T(H)1/T(H)2hypothesis of T cell-mediated tissue damage. *Nat Med* **13**: 139–45.
Sun, H.X., Xie, Y. and Ye, Y.P. 2009. Advances in saponin-based adjuvants. *Vaccine* **27**: 1787–96.
Takami, I., Kwon, S.R., Nishizawa, T. and Yoshimizu, M. 2010. Protection of Japanese flounder *Paralichthys olivaceus* from viral hemorrhagic septicemia (VHS) by Poly(I:C) immunization. *Dis Aquat Org* **89**: 109–15.
Thim, H.L., Iliev, D.B., Christie, K.E., *et al.*, 2012. Immunoprotective activity of a salmonid alphavirus vaccine: comparison of the immune responses induced by inactivated whole virus antigen formulations based on CpG class B oligonucleotides and poly I:C alone or combined with an oil adjuvant. *Vaccine* **30**: 4828–34.
Tian, J., Sun, X., Chen, X., *et al.*, 2008. The formulation and immunisation of oral poly(DL-lactide-co-glycolide) microcapsules containing a plasmid vaccine against lymphocystis disease virus in Japanese flounder (*Paralichthys olivaceus*). *Int Immunopharmacol* **8**: 900–908.
Tian, J. and Yu, J. 2011. Poly(lactic-co-glycolic acid) nanoparticles as candidate DNA vaccine carrier for oral immunization of Japanese flounder (*Paralichthys olivaceus*) against lymphocystis disease virus. *Fish Shellfish Immunol* **30**: 109–17.
Tyler, J.W. and Klesius, P.H. 1994. Protection against enteric septicemia of catfish (*Ictalurus punctatus*) by immunization with the R-mutant, *Escherichia coli* (J5). *Am J Vet Res* **55**: 1256–60.
Weiner, D.B. and Kennedy, R.C. 1999. Genetic vaccines. *Sci Am* **281**: 50–57.
Wilhelm, V., Miquel, A., Burzio, L.O., *et al.*, 2006. A vaccine against the salmonid pathogen *Piscirickettsia salmonis* based on recombinant proteins. *Vaccine* **24**: 5083–91.
Zhu, L.-Y., Nie, L., Zhu, G., *et al.*, 2013. Advances in research of fish immune-relevant genes: A comparative overview of innate and adaptive immunity in teleosts. *Dev Comp Immunol* **39**: 39–62.

8 The Innate Immune Response in Fish

Jorunn B. Jørgensen

Norwegian College of Fishery Science, UiT The Arctic University of Norway, Tromsø, Norway

ABSTRACT

Investigations aimed at unraveling the breadth of innate immunity in bony fish have uncovered both phylogenetically conserved as well as novel mechanisms absent in higher vertebrates. By homology cloning and utilization of genomic and transcriptomic data available for several teleost species, many "innate" genes have been identified, including pattern recognition receptors like the toll-like receptors and a variety of cytokines. Progress has also been made related to the bioactivity of many of these molecules but, in many aspects, studies of their functional activity are still in their infancy. Fish possess important innate cells including macrophages, neutrophils, and several non-specific cytotoxic cell types, but discrimination between different leukocyte subsets according to the mammalian CD nomenclature is difficult, partly due to the lack of tools like CD-specific antibodies. In this chapter we discuss recent advances in the understanding of innate immunity in fish.

8.1 INTRODUCTION

The innate immunity system is the first line of defense against infection and is immediately available to combat threats. It exists both in invertebrates and vertebrates and provides broad-spectrum host defense against a wide range of pathogens. Innate immunity constitutes the only mechanisms of defense for organisms "below" the jawless fishes. Approximately 450 million years ago, antigen-specific, adaptive immunity is thought to have emerged with the introduction of recombination-activating genes (RAGs) into the germline of ancestral jawed cartilaginous fish (Agrawal *et al.*, 1998). The RAG-dependent genomic rearrangements were the basis for the development of immunoglobulins (Igs) and T-cell receptors now associated with B- and T-cells, respectively (Flajnik and Kasahara, 2010). Recent evidence has also shown that the small group of extant jawless fishes possesses the facility to generate antigen-specific immunity (Pancer *et al.*, 2004; Deng *et al.*, 2010). For the jawed fishes and

jorunn.jorgensen@uit.no

Fish Vaccination, First Edition. Edited by Roar Gudding, Atle Lillehaug and Øystein Evensen.

the higher vertebrates, the innate immunity serves a dual role: controlling and destroying pathogens and, additionally, triggering a comprehensive immune response needed for development of a proper adaptive immune response.

8.2 INNATE IMMUNITY: A *SENSING* AND AN *EFFECTOR* ARM

Innate immunity can broadly be divided into a sensing arm and an effector arm. The former deals with how all multicellular organisms, including fish, recognize infection, and the latter with how cellular responses are involved in combating infections. Each arm of innate immunity may further be divided into cellular and humoral components, and Figure 8.1 gives an outline of some of these components found in fish. All four topics will be discussed here, and we will start by describing different cell types important for innate immunity in fish, followed by descriptions of cell-based innate immune sensing and different humoral effectors including cytokines and complement components (Figure 8.1).

8.3 PROFESSIONAL PHAGOCYTES: THE MACROPHAGES AND THE NEUTROPHILIC GRANULOCYTES

In vertebrates, innate immunity is largely dependent upon myeloid cells – professional phagocytes that engulf and destroy pathogens. Myeloid cells include mononuclear and polymorphonuclear phagocytes. The mononuclear phagocytes are the macrophages, derived from monocytes, and the closely related myeloid dendritic cells (DCs), also of monocyte origin, which are highly efficient at presenting antigens to T-cells of the adaptive immune system. The macrophages were among the first leukocytes to be isolated and studied in fish (Braun-Nesje *et al.*, 1981), and as in mammals, there is a diversity of macrophage phenotypes as documented in two recent reviews (Hanington *et al.*, 2009; Forlenza *et al.*, 2011).

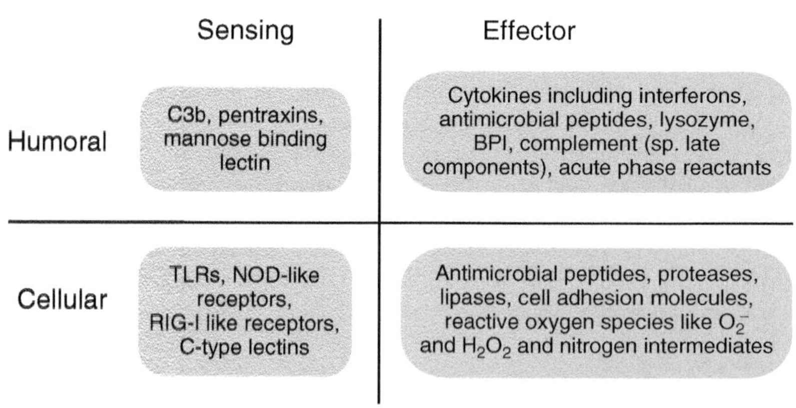

Fig. 8.1 The *sensing* and *effector* arms of the innate immune system in fish have cellular and humoral components.

Neutrophilic granulocytes or neutrophils are the main polymorphonuclear type of phagocytes described in fish (Ellis, 2001). Teleosts do not have a bone marrow and lymph nodes. In these species the monocytopoeisis, in general, occurs in the head kidney (pronehros); additionally, the head kidney functions as an organ for antigen-trapping (Zapata and Cooper, 1990).

Both macrophages and granulocytes are important inflammatory cells in fish and are mobilized upon infection or tissue injury. Macrophages represent the resident phagocytic cells in the peritoneal cavity, while neutrophilic granulocytes appear during inflammatory response. The principal characteristics used to identify fish macrophages include their morphology (bean-shaped nucleus and high cytoplasmic-to-nuclear ration), the presence of non-specific esterase and endogenous peroxidase activities, and their pinocytic and phagocytic abilities (Ellis, 2001; Lieschke *et al.*, 2001; Traver *et al.*, 2003). No monocyte-macrophage-specific "cluster of differentiation" (CD) antigens are defined in fish; however, with several fish genomes being sequenced, there is an increasing list of candidate genes with homology to mammalian antigens that can be tested. Of note, the lipopolysaccharide (LPS)-sensing system, consisting of MD2, CD14 and TLR4, which is a prominent characteristic of mammalian macrophages, is incompletely represented in fish (Iliev *et al.*, 2005). Of these molecules, only TLR4 homologs are detected in some, but not in all, of the fish genomes sequenced so far (Jault *et al.*, 2004). Neutrophils are also efficient phagocytes in fish, and these cells can be distinguished from the macrophages due to their morphology (smaller size compared with macrophages, and lobed nucleus) (Lieschke *et al.*, 2001). A unique cell type in fish is the melanomacrophages. They contain varying amounts of melanin particles and can be found in the head kidney and spleen, but also in inflamed tissues of most species. These cells are thought to be a part of the antigen-presenting cell system (Agius and Roberts, 2003; Koppang *et al.*, 2003).

Phagocytosis and intracellular killing are main tasks for the phagocytes, and microorganisms are engulfed by these cells into membrane-delimited compartments known as phagosomes. The phagosomes fuse with granules to produce a phagolysosome, in which the microorganisms are exposed to antimicrobial peptides (AMPs), enzymes and reactive oxygen species (ROS). These components synergize and effectively kill microorganisms. Many studies, mainly using head kidney-derived monocytes/macrophages and also neutrophils, have demonstrated inducible antimicrobial responses in these cells (Neumann *et al.*, 2001; Rodriguez *et al.*, 2003; Plouffe *et al.*, 2005). This includes respiratory burst and subsequent production of reactive oxygen species (ROS) (Jørgensen and Robertsen, 1995; Rodriguez *et al.*, 2003) and inducible nitric oxide synthetase (iNOS) producing nitrogen intermediates with antimicrobial effect (Laing *et al.*, 1999; Stafford *et al.*, 2002; Forlenza *et al.*, 2008). There is also increasing evidence that fish possess AMPs such as defensins, natural resistance-associated macrophage protein (Nramp), NK-lysin and hepcidin (Falco *et al.*, 2008; Casadei *et al.*, 2009; Nam *et al.*, 2010), which are also important components of the phagocyte killing machinery. Further description of AMPs can be found in a recent review by (Zhu *et al.*, 2013). In addition to their ability to eliminate pathogens by phagocytosis and antimicrobial secretions, it has been shown that neutrophils can trap and kill microorganisms by the release of extracellular structures composed of DNA and antimicrobial proteins called neutrophil extracellular traps (NETs) (Brinkmann and Zychlinsky, 2007). By techniques like confocal and light microscopy, the presence of such NETs has been demonstrated for activated fish neutrophils (Palic *et al.*, 2007).

Beside the directly antimicrobial role of the mononuclear fish phagocytes, these cells express MHC class II (Iliev *et al.*, 2010), and they have the molecular machinery necessary for antigen processing and presentation (Vallejo *et al.*, 1991a,b; Wittamer *et al.*, 2011; Mutoloki *et al.*, 2014).

8.4 NATURAL KILLER (NK)-LIKE CELLS

NK cells are a lineage of cells related to lymphocytes that recognize infected and/or stressed cells and respond by directly killing these cells and by secreting inflammatory cytokines. NK cells in mammals have an important role in antiviral defense, both by directly killing virus-infected cells, but also as major producers of IFN-γ which is a cytokine mediating antiviral activity. In contrast to cytotoxic T-lymphocytes, the NK-like cells kill cells in a non-MHC restricted manner and without need for prior sensitization. Evidence that fish possess NK-like cells has come from both *in vivo* and *in vitro* studies. For example, it has been shown that fish leukocytes can spontaneously kill a variety of xenogeneic cells without the need for prior immunization (Fischer *et al.*, 1998; Somamoto *et al.*, 2000). Two different non-specific cytotoxic cells termed NK-like cells and non-specific cytoxic cells (NCC) have been extensively studied in channel catfish reviewed by Shen *et al.* (2002). Both cell types are able to kill classical targets of mammalian NK cells like xenogeneic and allogeneic cells. Similar to the mammalian NK cells, the channel catfish NK-like cells are large, granular cells isolated from peripheral blood (Shen *et al.*, 2004), while the NCC cells are small, agranular lymphocytes found in lymphoid tissues (Evans *et al.*, 1984a,b,c). The NCC cells express a 34 kDa protein named the NCC-receptor protein 1 (Jaso-Friedmann *et al.*, 1997a,b, 2001). This receptor is believed to recognize a single, highly conserved target antigen suggested to be expressed on potential targets. NCC cells are postulated to represent an evolutionary precursor of mammalian NK cells and they have been reported in a number of other fish species reviewed in Plouffe *et al.* (2005). Other NK-like cytotoxic leukocytes are found in several fish species, and there are ongoing studies to identify receptors that share sequence and structural relationships with mammalian NK cell receptors (Fischer *et al.*, 2006; Yoder and Litman, 2011). Progress in identifying receptors that regulate NK-like cell cytotoxicity in fish will be indispensable for further characterization of cellular cytotoxicity in fish. How the piscine cytotoxic cells are triggered, and how their receptors distinguish infected from uninfected cells, are important issues to be addressed to widen the knowledge about cellular cytotoxic responses in teleosts.

8.5 THE SENSING ARM OF INNATE IMMUNITY

The innate immune system is available immediately to combat infectious agents, and unlike the adaptive immune system, it is not dependent upon complex mechanisms for selection and expansion of cell clones that react to foreign substances. Instead, the innate system responds to common structures shared by certain groups of microbes or other potentially pathogenic agents. These common structures are called pathogen-associated molecular patterns, or PAMPS. Detection of PAMPS by the host occurs via soluble and cell-associated germline-encoded pathogen recognition receptors (PRRs; Figure 8.2). In the last 10 years there has been huge progress in the studies of the innate immune receptors that sense viruses and bacteria in fish, and most PRR families found in mammals have also been identified in

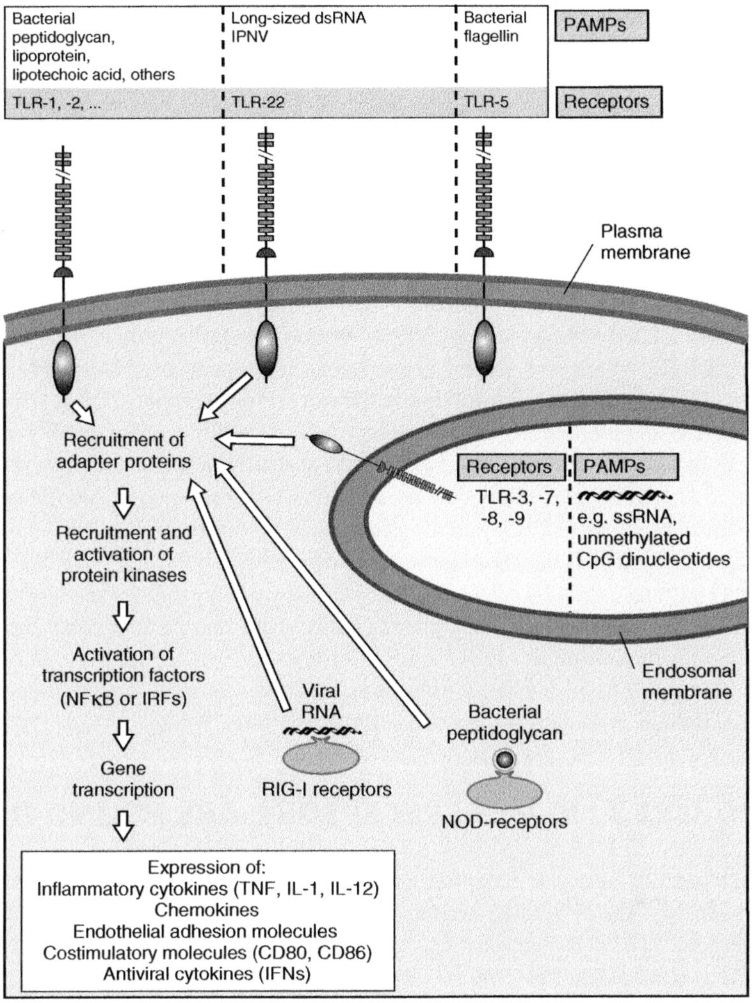

Fig. 8.2 Specificities and functions of pathogen recognition receptors (PRRs). Different PRRs respond to different microbial molecules, including lipoprotein and nucleic acids. Most PRRs activate similar signaling mechanisms, resulting in cellular responses that are central to innate immunity responses.

piscine species, which so far include the toll-like receptors (TLRs), RIG-I-like receptors, NOD-like receptors, C-type lectins and complement components (Zhu *et al.*, 2013). However, characterization of their interactions with specific PAMPS and deciphering the signaling pathways induced upon receptor ligation are incomplete in most piscine species.

8.6 TLRS ARE THE BEST STUDIED PRRS IN FISH

Among the best-studied PRRs are the toll-like receptors (TLRs), of which 17 types have been described in different fish species so far (Palti, 2011). In humans, two major subtypes of TLRs are identified based on their cellular localization; TLR1, 2, 4, 5, 6 and 10 (type I) are found on the cell surface and recognize microbial lipids and sugars derived from different bacteria and fungi, while TLR3, 7, 8 and 9 (type II) reside within the endosomal compartments and primarily respond to nucleic acids such as double-stranded (ds) or single stranded (ss)-RNA and CpG DNA, derived from viruses and bacteria. Representatives from both of these subtypes are identified in fish (Rebl *et al.*, 2010; Palti, 2011). However, the fish TLRs have a much greater diversity compared with mammals, and additionally six non-mammalian TLRs are identified in fish. These include TLR14, which shares sequence and structural similarities with TLR1 and 2 (Oshiumi *et al.*, 2003; Jault *et al.*, 2004; Meijer *et al.*, 2004; Hwang *et al.*, 2011; Star *et al.*, 2011), and the fish-specific TLR-branch including TLR 19, 20, 21 22 and 23 (Oshiumi *et al.*, 2003; Meijer *et al.*, 2004). Within the latter group, the one studied in detail is fugu TLR22, which was shown to recognize long-sized dsRNA on the cell surface (Matsuo *et al.*, 2008). Fish TLRs exhibit distinct features; for example, TLR5, which in mammals is a membrane-bound receptor that recognizes the flagellin component of bacterial flagella, is found both as a membrane-bound (TLR5M) and soluble (TLR5s) protein in rainbow trout (Tsujita *et al.*, 2004) and other species as well (Oshiumi *et al.*, 2003; Hwang *et al.*, 2010). The membrane-bound TLR5 signaling in trout in response to flagellin, as measured by NFκB activation, is amplified through interaction with the soluble form (TLR5s) in a positive feedback loop (Tsujita *et al.*, 2004). Atlantic cod TLRs are unique due to the absence of several TLRs that recognize bacterial surface antigens (TLR1, TLR2 and TLR5), while the families of TLRs that recognize nucleic acids (TLR7, TLR8, TLR9 and TLR22) are expanded (Star *et al.*, 2011). These data point to an increased importance of the recognition of pathogens through the nucleic acid detection system for the cod immune defense.

8.7 NOD-LIKE AND RIG-I RECEPTORS ARE FOUND IN FISH

Two additional families of innate receptors have been described in fish that join the TLRs as key pathogen sensors: the NOD-like receptors (NLRs) (Laing *et al.*, 2008) and the retinoic acid-inducible gene I (RIG-I)-like receptors (RLRs). Both of them are intracellular cytosolic receptors, mainly involved in bacterial or viral defense, respectively. The NLR family members are best known for their ability to signal NFκB activation (NOD1 and NOD2) or secretion of the pro-inflammatory cytokines IL-1β and IL-18 (NALPs) (Chen *et al.*, 2009). In mammals, NLRs are primarily expressed in immune cells (lymphocytes and APCs such as macrophages and DCs), but they are also expressed in non-immune cells such as epithelial cells (Chen *et al.*, 2009). The teleost NLR-family genes were firstly identified in the zebrafish genome, and consist of three different subfamilies of NLRs, including one unique subfamily (Laing *et al.*, 2008). NLR genes have also been identified in a number of other fish species including channel catfish (Sha *et al.*, 2009; Rajendran *et al.*, 2012a), flounder (Park *et al.*, 2012), grass carp (Chen *et al.*, 2010) and rainbow trout (Chang *et al.*, 2011b), and in general the genes are widely expressed in various tissues and leukocyte cell-lines. One of the catfish NLR genes, named NOD1, was induced after challenge with the intracellular bacteria *Edwardsiella ictaluri*, while the others appeared to be constitutively expressed (Sha *et al.*, 2009). This may suggest the catfish NOD1 is involved in immunity against intracellular pathogens. Overexpression of trout NOD2 effector domains resulted in increased expression of several pro-inflammatory genes, type I and type II IFNs, and also a variety of caspases. These results suggest that fish NOD2 are involved in inflammation, and might regulate apoptosis and trigger antibacterial and antiviral defense (Chang *et al.*, 2011b).

The RLRs comprise three members: RIG-I, MDA-5 and LGP2. All of them are RNA helicases responsible for detection of cytoplasmic viral RNA (Kumar *et al.*, 2011). RIG-I has been cloned in grass carp (Yang *et al.*, 2011) and channel catfish (Rajendran *et al.*, 2012b), and LGP2 and MDA5 in rainbow trout (Chang *et al.*, 2011a) and grass carp (Wang *et al.*, 2012). In rainbow trout both MDA5 and LPG2 possess high binding affinity for poly I:C (Chang *et al.*, 2011a). Furthermore, MDA5 derived from rainbow trout (Chang *et al.*, 2011a), Japanese flounder (Ohtani *et al.*, 2011) and grass carp (Wang *et al.*, 2012), and rainbow trout LGP2, exhibit antiviral functions (Chang *et al.*, 2011a), thus demonstrating that fish RLRs, like their mammalian homologs, have roles in host surveillance against viral infections. There are several recent reviews about innate recognition in fish, where a more detailed description about the genomics and biology of piscine PRRs can be found (Zhang and Gui, 2012; Zhu *et al.*, 2013).

8.8 LECTINS ARE MULTIFUNCTIONAL SENSOR MOLECULES FOR CARBOHYDRATE LIGANDS

Lectins are a group of sugar-binding proteins that can specifically bind to carbohydrate structures from viruses, bacteria, fungi and animals, and in turn agglutinate various cells to exert their biological functions. In animals, lectins are important components of the innate immune response by inducing phagocytosis, activating platelets, initiating the complement cascade and enhancing natural killer cell activity (Vasta *et al.*, 2004). Lectins are also regulators of the adaptive immunity by mediating the recognition of bacterial and viral components by DCs. Many studies in higher vertebrates have demonstrated that binding of antigen by lectins results in its internalization into lysosomal compartments and loading of MHC class II molecules with antigenic peptides for CD4 T-cell presentation (van Vliet *et al.*, 2007).

C-type lectins (CTLs) are members of the PRR family. The CTLs are named after their ability to interact with carbohydrate residues of glycoproteins through the C-type carbohydrate recognition domain (CRD) or C-type lectin domain. CTLs are further classified into several groups comprising the collectins, selectins, and the mannose-macrophage receptors, which are directly involved in immune functions (Vasta *et al.*, 2011). The collectins include the mannose-binding lectin (MBL), which upon association with the serine protease MASP leads to the activation of the complements system (see further details below). Several members of the C-type lectin family have been discovered in fish, including rainbow trout, common carp, turbot, and zebrafish (Vasta *et al.*, 2011). All these C-type lectins are significantly induced by bacterial invasion and show different functions of agglutination and inhibition with various pathogens.

Another lectin identified in fish is the DC-specific ICAM-3 grabbing nonintegrin (DC-SIGN), also known as CD209, which is a type II transmembrane protein. Furthermore, DC-SIGN is an important adhesion receptor known to mediate DC maturation, migration and T-cell activation. The first fish DC-SIGN was identified in zebrafish and was shown to share characteristic features with mammalian DC-SIGN family members, including a typical CRD in the extracellular domain (Lin *et al.*, 2009). Functional assays showed that *in vivo* T-cell activation and antibody production induced by exogenous keyhole limpet hemocyanin antigen could be significantly blocked by anti-DC-SIGN antibody treatment. Phagocytosis measurements sustained that the DC-SIGN protein is not directly involved in antigen uptake by APCs, but might have a role in APC migration and aggregation, followed by downstream T-cell activation (Lin *et al.*, 2009). Since fish DCs have also been discovered in recent years, an interesting question is whether DC-SIGN is a functional molecule in fish DC that participate in fish adaptive responses.

8.9 PRRs AND THE INDUCTION OF IMMUNITY

Upon binding to their PAMPs, most TLRs, NLRs and RLRs lead to activation of different signaling pathways that regulate the activation of different transcription factors, such as NFκB and interferon regulatory factors (IRFs) (Kumar *et al.*, 2011). NFκB activation results in enhanced inflammatory cytokine responses, induction of DC maturation (CD80, CD83, CD86), chemokines and chemokine receptors (Janeway and Medzhitov, 2002). As a result, PRR triggering, in particular activation of TLRs, switches the immature DC phenotype to an inflammatory phenotype that is capable of inducing adaptive immune responses, instructing both antigen-specific CD4 and CD8 T-cell responses and humoral responses. IRF activation primarily results in IFN induction, which in addition to its direct antiviral activity also has a broader role in shaping up the host immune response (Kumar *et al.*, 2011). There are numerous studies in different fish species, including *in vitro* stimulation of leukocytes or *in vivo* treatments using PRRs agonists, demonstrating that such treatments result in enhanced cytokine and chemokine production, upregulation of co-stimulatory molecules and also protection against infections (Jørgensen *et al.*, 2001a,b; Jensen *et al.*, 2002b; Jensen and Robertsen, 2002; Pedersen *et al.*, 2006; Purcell *et al.*, 2006b; Strandskog *et al.*, 2007, 2008a; Kileng *et al.*, 2008). Well-studied PRR agonists in both mammals and fish are synthetic nucleic acids including CpG-oligonucleotides and poly I:C, which have been shown to induce robust type I IFN responses and have, consequently, augmented the antiviral response against infections with IPNV, ISAV and SPDV in Atlantic salmon (Jensen *et al.*, 2002a; Jørgensen *et al.*, 2003; Strandskog *et al.*, 2011). It is also clear that the interplay between innate signals is necessary for shaping up the immune responses and, for example, the activation of multiple TLRs can result in complementary or synergistic effects (Strandskog *et al.*, 2008b, 2011; Thim *et al.*, 2012).

8.10 CYTOKINES IN INNATE IMMUNITY

Cytokines are small cell-signaling protein molecules that encompass a large and diverse family. They consist of immunomodulating agents such as interleukins and IFNs. About 35 interleukins are currently described in mammals, and homologs to most of these molecules are found in bony fish (Secombes *et al.*, 2011). Although many piscine cytokine genes have been identified, there is still limited information about their biological function. In this chapter we will focus on the cytokines IL-1β, TNF-α and type I IFNs, which are important cytokines released from innate immune cells and are among the best characterized fish cytokines so far.

8.10.1 The pro-inflammatory cytokines IL-1β and TNF-α

Virtually all nucleated cells, especially endo-/epithelial cells and macrophages, are potent producers of IL-1 and TNF-α. Both cytokines belong to multigene families with members involved in diverse immunological and developmental pathways.

The IL-1 family has a central role in the regulation of immune and, most notably, inflammatory responses, and it includes 11 members, of which mammalian IL-1α, IL-1β and IL-18 have been extensively characterized (Barksby *et al.*, 2007). To date only homologs to IL-1β and IL-18 have been discovered in fish (Secombes *et al.*, 2011). IL-1β genes have been cloned from many species of teleost fish, including salmon (Ingerslev *et al.*, 2006), trout (Zou *et al.*, 1999), cod (Seppola *et al.*, 2008), and carp (Engelsma *et al.*, 2003). In most species, more than one IL-1β gene is present and, for example, salmonids possess three different IL-1β genes, named IL-1β1, 2, and 3 (Husain *et al.*, 2012). Expression analysis of IL-1β in different tissues in healthy fish has revealed a ubiquitous expression pattern, but the highest basal levels are found in immunological organs like the spleen, head kidney and gills (Ingerslev *et al.*, 2006; Husain *et al.*, 2012).

Human IL-1β is synthesized as an inactive 31-kDa precursor (pro-IL-1β), which requires processing to produce the secreted, bioactive 17-kDa mature protein. Processing occurs mainly through the action of the cysteine protease, caspase1 (Thornberry *et al.*, 1992). Prior to its ability to process IL-1β, caspase 1 itself is activated in response to PAMPs in a multiprotein complex known as the inflammasome (Martinon *et al.*, 2002). By sequence analysis of piscine IL-1β genes, no obvious caspase 1 cleaving site has been found (Secombes *et al.*, 2011). Despite this, there is indirect evidence that IL-1β is processed by potential caspases in fish owing to studies showing bioactivity of truncated recombinant trout IL-1β (Hong *et al.*, 2004) or demonstrating processed forms of IL-1β in fish cell cultures (Pelegrin *et al.*, 2004). A more definitive proof was recently given, when a fully processed form (about 18 kDa) of IL-1β was detected in zebrafish primary leukocytes infected by the intracellular pathogen *Francisella noatunensis* (Vojtech *et al.*, 2012). When these cells were preincubated by caspase inhibitors, the processing was partly inhibited. In the same study two putative zebrafish inflammatory caspase orthologs were shown to cleave IL-1β with different specificities. This work suggests that the inflammasome platform of immune activation might exist in fish.

In higher vertebrates, IL-1β has been shown to mediate a wide range of inflammatory effects, including the acute phase-response, activation of macrophages and subsequent secretion of cytokines such TNF and IL-6, and activation of T, B and NK cells. In fish leukocytes, IL-1β is transcriptionally upregulated during infection (Husain *et al.*, 2012; Wang *et al.*, 2009) and proinflammatory stimuli (Strandskog *et al.*, 2008b; Wang *et al.*, 2009; Husain *et al.*, 2012); also, recombinant Il-1β affects cell proliferation and immune gene expression (Peddie *et al.*, 2001, 2002; Buonocore *et al.*, 2005).

Like IL-1, TNF-α is a pleiotropic cytokine and a major regulator of leukocyte trafficking and inflammation (Ware, 2003). TNF-α belongs to the TNF ligand superfamily, which includes structurally related proteins involved in a number of cellular signaling pathways, and the reader is also referred to an excellent publication describing this superfamily in teleosts (Wiens and Glenney, 2011). TNF-α gene homologs have been identified in different fish species (Laing *et al.*, 2001; Saeij *et al.*, 2003; Zou *et al.*, 2003b), and similar to IL-1β, the number of genes (1–3) varies between the species (Zou *et al.*, 2002; Haugland *et al.*, 2007; Saeij *et al.*, 2003; Savan *et al.*, 2005). This is presumably a result of the fish specific gene/genome duplication (Meyer and Van de Peer, 2005).

TNF-α is a type II transmembrane glycoprotein, with an extracellular C-terminal domain and a cytoplasmic tail, and it can be found both as a membrane-bound and a soluble molecule. The soluble form exists as a trimer, composed of three identical TNF-α subunits that bind to the receptor. Expression studies have revealed that TNF-α is constitutively expressed in head kidney and gill tissues, and it is also LPS-inducible in isolated head kidney leukocytes (Laing *et al.*, 2001). There are species-specific differences between fish TNF-α molecules related to their ability to activate phagocytes directly. For example, in rainbow trout, carp and goldfish, recombinant TNF-α protein stimulates phagocytic activity *in vitro*, albeit at different concentrations (Zou *et al.*, 2003a; Grayfer *et al.*, 2008; Forlenza *et al.*, 2009). Opposite results are found in sea bream; in this species, TNF-α is a potent activator of endothelial cells, but it does not activate phagocytes directly (Roca *et al.*, 2008). Supernatants from sea bream endothelial cells treated with TNF-α were shown to promote the adhesion, migration and activation of leukocytes. This is analogous to the functions of mammalian TNF, where stimulation of endothelial cells with TNF-α increases the expression of adhesion molecules and the synthesis of chemotactic mediators such as IL-8. Thereby, TNF-α promotes leukocyte recruitment and activation and contributes to the inflammatory process. Like in mammals, the induction of the two cytokines TNF-α and IL-1β are mediated through the activation of the mitogen-activated protein kinase p38 (Hansen and Jørgensen, 2007).

8.11 INTERFERONS

During viral infections, some of the most important defense molecules to be produced are the IFNs, named for their ability to interfere with viral replication. Therefore, induction of IFN is a key event during viral infections, and their regulation is controlled at many different levels. Most viruses make dsRNA or ssRNA that act as PAMPs which are recognized by PRRs and cause activation of transcription factors, followed by expression of type I IFNs as described earlier. This innate response establishes an antiviral state in the infected cell and its neighbors and alerts immune cells to danger (Figure 8.3). In mammals, the IFNs are classified into three types according to their biological and structural properties: type I IFN (including IFN-α and IFN-β), type II IFN (IFN-γ) and type III (IFN-λ).

In fish, the induction of secreted molecules with IFN properties was described about 40 years ago (de Kinkelin and Dorson, 1973), but it was not until 2003 that the first fish type I IFNs were cloned in three fish species: zebrafish (Altmann *et al.*, 2003), Atlantic salmon (Robertsen *et al.*, 2003), and pufferfish (Lutfalla *et al.*, 2003). Like in mammals, fish possess multiple copies of the IFN-genes (Zou and Secombes, 2011) and Atlantic salmon, for example, possess at least 11 IFN genes, divided into 3 subtypes (Sun *et al.*, 2009), and recent studies have revealed distinct roles for the different salmon subtypes (Svingerud *et al.*, 2012). The IFNs signal through the JAK/STAT pathway and in mammals they upregulate the expression of several hundred IFN-stimulated genes (ISGs), which establish the "antiviral" state (Figure 8.3). Many of these ISGs have direct antiviral function, and a direct antiviral activity against pathogenic viruses has been demonstrated for Mx, ISG15 and PKR in Atlantic salmon and Japanese flounder (Caipang *et al.*, 2003; Larsen *et al.*, 2004; Zhu *et al.*, 2008). Still, the functions of most fish ISGs remain unknown.

Homologs to IFN-γ have been found in several fish species (Zou *et al.*, 2005; Igawa *et al.*, 2006; Milev-Milovanovic *et al.*, 2006; Stolte *et al.*, 2008; Furnes *et al.*, 2009). Zou *et al.* (2005)

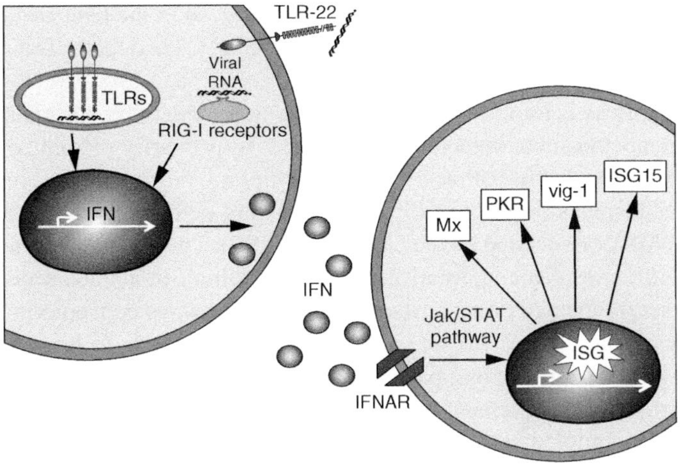

Fig. 8.3 Fish virus induced genes and IFN type I signaling. Following virus entry in the cell, viral nucleic acids bind different sensors as RLRs and TLRs. Additionally fish possess TLR-22, a unique cell-surface receptor, which binds dsRNA. Activation of these sensors leads to the induction and secretion of IFNs. IFNs have auto- and paracrine activity mediated through interactions with a transmembrane receptor (IFNAR) that activates the JAK/STAT pathway. It then leads to the induction of interferon-stimulated genes (ISGs) such as Mx, ISG15, and vig/viperin.

demonstrated that trout IFN-γ has functional properties in common with its mammalian counterpart, including the ability to activate macrophages, and studies in other species including goldfish have confirmed this (Grayfer *et al.*, 2010). Both type I IFNs and IFN-γ derived from different fish species have been produced as recombinant proteins and tested for their bioactivity (Zou *et al.*, 2007; Ohta *et al.*, 2011; Sun *et al.*, 2011). Fish IFN-γ induces gene expression of many ISGs that also respond to type I IFNs, suggesting there is cross-activation of the innate response by type I and type II IFNs; however, the ISG-inducing potential of IFN-γ is much weaker compared with that of type I IFNs, and a relatively high dose of IFN-γ is required to confer virus resistance (Sun *et al.*, 2011). In addition, fish IFN-γ has been proven to induce TLR8 and TLR9 expression in salmon (Skjæveland *et al.*, 2008, 2009).

Many highly pathogenic viruses have evolved mechanisms to evade an IFN response, and the balance between the robustness of host immune response and viral antagonistic mechanisms determines whether or not the virus is cleared. Several viruses infecting salmonids, including ISAV and IPNV, have been shown to interfere with IFN responses (Garcia-Rosado *et al.*, 2008; Skjesol *et al.*, 2009). By identifying IFN-antagonizing virus proteins, it will be possible to make attenuated viruses where such proteins are crippled or absent and these can be used as vaccine candidates to trigger more pronounced innate responses.

8.12 THE COMPLEMENT SYSTEM

The complement system, as we know it from well-studied mammalian species, is composed of about 30 distinct plasma proteins and membrane-associated proteins, and plays a pivotal role in innate immunity. The three different routes of complement activation (classical, alternative and lectin pathway) involve several proteins that are produced in the liver by hepatocytes and secreted in plasma. Additionally, there are proteins like C1q, C7 and factor D that are produced mainly in extra-hepatic tissue.

The classical pathway is initiated by the C1q recognition unit, which is mainly synthesized by cells of the monocyte–macrophage lineage. The C1q primarily recognizes antibodies in immune complexes. The lectin pathway is activated upon binding of the serum lectin MBL or ficolin to sugar residues on the surface of the invading pathogen, leading to complement activation via the MBL-associated serine protease (MASP). The spontaneous activation of C3 is the basis for initiation of the alternative pathway, resulting in abundant deposition of C3 cleavage fragments on the activating surface. All three pathways converge in the generation of C3 convertase whihc cleaves C3 into C3a and C3b. C3b binds to hydroxylic groups of carbohydrates or proteins of invading pathogens or self-structures.

The main function of complement is the opsonization of microbes with C3b, which then can be recognized by complement receptors (CR1 and CR3) expressed on phagocytes. Another function is its cytolytic activity, where target-bound C3b forms a protease complex to activate C5 into C5a and C5b, which becomes a scaffold for the formation of the membrane-attack complex (MAC) by C6-C9. MAC can induce osmotic lysis of cells including microbes. The small peptide fragments C3a, C4a and C5a are chemotactic for leukocytes, stimulate the release of inflammatory mediators, and act on endothelial cells to enhance movement of leukocytes and plasma proteins into tissues.

As shown by trout, carp and zebrafish data, it is now evident that almost all the homologs of mammalian complements components are also present in bony fish and can be activated through all three complement activation pathways. For further information there are several comprehensive reviews on the complement system in teleost fish (Boshra *et al.*, 2006; Nakao *et al.*, 2011). An interesting feature of the teleost complement system is the isotypic diversity of several components such as C3, C4, C5, C7 and MBL, factor B, and factor I, generated by gene duplication (Nakao *et al.*, 2006). The C3 isoforms in trout and carp are the most extensively studied at both protein and cDNA levels. The C3 isoforms differ structurally in some functional sites, particularly in the thioester-catalytic site defining the binding specificity of the thioester site to either hydroxyl groups or amino groups. These isoforms are shown to differ in hemolytic activity and in binding specificity to targets such as sheep and rabbit erythrocytes, bacteria, and yeast. The functional elements that are responsible for the different binding preferences of the C3 isoforms are still unknown. It is, though, suggested that the C3 diversification might represent an evolutionary strategy to expand or enhance immune recognition and effector function of teleost complement (Nakao *et al.*, 2006). In fish, the mRNA expression of complement components is not only restricted to the liver, and these are found in other organs like head kidney, renal kidney, intestine, gill, skin, brain and gonads (Gonzalez *et al.*, 2007a,b; Løvoll *et al.*, 2007a; Encinas *et al.*, 2010). Furthermore, upon treatment with immunostimulants, trout C3 isoforms showed differential expression between different organs (Løvoll *et al.*, 2007b).

Complement-mediated phagocytosis is demonstrated in fish, and C3b has been reported as a mediator of this opsonic activity in several teleost species (Schraml *et al.*, 2006; Jenkins and Ourth, 1993). However, the specific receptors involved in this process are still sparsely described (Nakao *et al.*, 2011). Chemo-attractive activity of teleost C3a and C5a has been demonstrated in trout and carp (Kato *et al.*, 2004; Rotllant *et al.*, 2004).

8.13 CONCLUDING REMARKS AND PERSPECTIVES

As described above, homology-hunting of "innate" genes in the immune system of bony fish have identified a wide range of important molecules including pathogen recognition receptors, complement components and a variety of cytokines. These studies have been followed up by analyses of their expression profiles under different conditions such as infections, immunostimulation and vaccination, and in some cases comprehensive analysis by microarray has been used for global gene expression profiling (Purcell *et al.*, 2006a; Krasnov *et al.*, 2011). Progress has also been made related to the bioactivity of many of these molecules, but in many aspects, studies of their functional activity are still in their infancy. To further elucidate the role of innate immunity, the research focus must shift towards the proteins and cellular effector functions. APCs, like DCs and macrophages, have key roles in translating information from the innate response into a language understood by the cells of the adaptive immune system, and further characterization of these cell types and their link to adaptive immunity is of particular interest for future studies in bony fish.

REFERENCES

Agius, C. and Roberts, R.J. 2003. Melano-macrophage centres and their role in fish pathology. *J Fish Dis* **26**: 499–509.

Agrawal, A., Eastman, Q.M. and Schatz, D.G. 1998. Transposition mediated by RAG1 and RAG2 and its implications for the evolution of the immune system. *Nature* **394**: 744–51.

Altmann, S.M., Mellon, M.T., Distel, D.L. and Kim, C.H. 2003. Molecular and functional analysis of an interferon gene from the zebrafish, *Danio rerio*. *J Virol* **77**: 1992–2002.

Barksby, H.E., Lea, S.R., Preshaw, P.M. and Taylor, J.J. 2007. The expanding family of interleukin-1 cytokines and their role in destructive inflammatory disorders. *Clin Exp Immunol* **149**: 217–25.

Boshra, H., Li, J. and Sunyer, J.O. 2006. Recent advances on the complement system of teleost fish. *Fish Shellfish Immunol* **20**: 239–62.

Braun-Nesje, R., Bertheussen, K., Kaplan, G. and Seljelid, R. 1981. Salmonid macrophages: separation, *in vitro* culture and characterization. *J Fish Dis* **4**: 141–51.

Brinkmann, V. and Zychlinsky, A. 2007. Beneficial suicide: why neutrophils die to make NETs. *Nat Rev Microbiol* **5**: 577–82.

Buonocore F, Forlenza M, Randelli E, *et al.*, 2005. Biological activity of sea bass (*Dicentrarchus labrax* L.) recombinant interleukin-1ß. *Mar Biotechnol* **7**: 609–17.

Caipang, C.M.A., Hirono, I. and Aoki, T. 2003. *In vitro* inhibition of fish rhabdoviruses by Japanese flounder, *Paralichthys olivaceus* Mx. *Virology* **317**: 373–82.

Casadei, E., Wang, T., Zou, J., *et al.*, 2009. Characterization of three novel ß-defensin antimicrobial peptides in rainbow trout (*Oncorhynchus mykiss*). *Mol Immunol* **46**: 3358–66.

Chang, M., Collet, B., Nie, P., *et al.*, 2011a. Expression and functional characterization of the RIG-I-like receptors MDA5 and LGP2 in rainbow trout (*Oncorhynchus mykiss*). *J Virol* **85**: 8403–12.

Chang, M., Wang, T., Nie, P., *et al.*, 2011b. Cloning of two rainbow trout nucleotide-binding oligomerization domain containing 2 (NOD2) splice variants and functional characterization of the NOD2 effector domains. *Fish Shellfish Immunol* **30**: 118–27.

Chen, G., Shaw, M.H., Kim, Y.G. and Nunez, G. 2009. NOD-like receptors: role in innate immunity and inflammatory disease. *Annu Rev Pathol* **4**: 365–98.

Chen, W.Q., Xu, Q.Q., Chang, M.X., *et al.*, 2010. Molecular characterization and expression analysis of nuclear oligomerization domain proteins NOD1 and NOD2 in grass carp *Ctenopharyngodon idella*. *Fish Shellfish Immunol* **28**: 18–29.

de Kinkelin, P. and Dorson, M. 1973. Interferon production in rainbow trout (*Salmo gairdneri*) experimentally infected with Egtvedt virus. *J Gen Virol* **19**: 125–7.

Deng, L., Velikovsky, C.A., Xu, G., *et al.*, 2010. A structural basis for antigen recognition by the T cell-like lymphocytes of sea lamprey. *Proc Natl Acad Sci USA* **107**: 13408–13.

Ellis, A.E. 2001. The immunology of teleosts, in *Fish Pathology* (ed. R.J. Roberts). London, W.B. Saunders, 133.

Encinas, P., Rodriguez-Milla, M.A., Novoa, B., *et al.*, 2010. Zebrafish fin immune responses during high mortality infections with viral haemorrhagic septicemia rhabdovirus. A proteomic and transcriptomic approach. *BMC Genomics* **11**: 518.

Engelsma, M.Y., Stet, R.J., Saeij, J.P. and Verburg-van Kemenade, B.M. 2003. Differential expression and haplotypic variation of two interleukin-1ß genes in the common carp (*Cyprinus carpio* L.). *Cytokine* **22**: 21–32.

Evans, D.L., Carlson, R.L., Graves, S.S. and Hogan, K.T. 1984a. Nonspecific cytotoxic cells in fish (*Ictalurus punctatus*). IV. Target cell binding and recycling capacity. *Dev Comp Immunol* **8**: 823–33.

Evans, D.L., Graves, S.S., Cobb, D. and Dawe, D.L. 1984b. Nonspecific cytotoxic cells in fish (*Ictalurus punctatus*). II. Parameters of target cell lysis and specificity. *Dev Comp Immunol* **8**: 303–12.

Evans, D.L., Hogan, K.T., Graves, S.S., *et al.*, 1984c. Nonspecific cytotoxic cells in fish (*Ictalurus punctatus*). III. Biophysical and biochemical properties affecting cytolysis. *Dev Comp Immunol* **8**: 599–610.

Falco, A., Chico, V., Marroqui, L., *et al.*, 2008. Expression and antiviral activity of a ß-defensin-like peptide identified in the rainbow trout (*Oncorhynchus mykiss*) EST sequences. *Mol Immunol* **45**: 757–65.

Fischer, U., Ototake, M. and Nakanishi, T. 1998. *In vitro* cell-mediated cytotoxicity against allogeneic erythrocytes in ginbuna crucian carp and goldfish using a non-radioactive assay. *Dev Comp Immunol* **22**: 195–206.

Fischer, U., Utke, K., Somamoto, T., *et al.*, 2006. Cytotoxic activities of fish leucocytes. *Fish Shellfish Immunol* **20**: 209–26.

Flajnik, M.F. and Kasahara, M. 2010. Origin and evolution of the adaptive immune system: genetic events and selective pressures. *Nat Rev Genet* **11**: 47–59.

Forlenza, M., Scharsack, J.P., Kachamakova, N.M., *et al.*, 2008. Differential contribution of neutrophilic granulocytes and macrophages to nitrosative stress in a host-parasite animal model. *Mol Immunol* **45**: 3178–89.

Forlenza, M., Magez, S., Scharsack, J.P., *et al.*, 2009. Receptor-mediated and lectin-like activities of carp (*Cyprinus carpio*) TNF-α. *J Immunol* **183**: 5319–32.

Forlenza, M., Fink, I.R., Raes, G. and Wiegertjes, G.F. 2011. Heterogeneity of macrophage activation in fish. *Dev Comp Immunol* **35**: 1246–55.

Furnes, C., Seppola, M. and Robertsen, B. 2009. Molecular characterisation and expression analysis of interferon gamma in Atlantic cod (*Gadus morhua*). *Fish Shellfish Immunol* **26**: 285–92.

Garcia-Rosado, E., Markussen, T., Kileng, O., *et al.*, 2008. Molecular and functional characterization of two infectious salmon anaemia virus (ISAV) proteins with type I interferon antagonizing activity. *Virus Res* **133**: 228–38.

Gonzalez, S.F., Buchmann, K. and Nielsen, M.E. 2007a. Complement expression in common carp (*Cyprinus carpio* L.) during infection with *Ichthyophthirius multifiliis*. *Dev Comp Immunol* **31**: 576–86.

Gonzalez, S.F., Chatziandreou, N., Nielsen, M.E., *et al.*, 2007b. Cutaneous immune responses in the common carp detected using transcript analysis. *Mol Immunol* **44**: 1664–79.

Grayfer, L., Walsh, J.G. and Belosevic, M. 2008. Characterization and functional analysis of goldfish (*Carassius auratus* L.) tumor necrosis factor-alpha. *Dev Comp Immunol* **32**: 532–43.

Grayfer, L., Garcia, E.G. and Belosevic, M. 2010. Comparison of macrophage antimicrobial responses induced by type II interferons of the goldfish (*Carassius auratus* L.). *J Biol Chem* **285**: 23537–47.

Hanington, P.C., Tam, J., Katzenback, B.A., *et al.*, 2009. Development of macrophages of cyprinid fish. *Dev Comp Immunol* **33**: 411–29.

Hansen, T.E. and Jørgensen, J.B. 2007. Cloning and characterisation of p38 MAP kinase from Atlantic salmon: A kinase important for regulating salmon TNF-2 and IL-1ß expression. *Mol Immunol* **44**: 3137–46.

Haugland, Ø., Mercy, I.S., Romøren, K., *et al.*, 2007. Differential expression profiles and gene structure of two tumor necrosis factor-α variants in Atlantic salmon (*Salmo salar* L.). *Mol Immunol* **44**: 1652–63.

Hong, S., Zou, J., Collet, B., *et al.*, 2004. Analysis and characterisation of IL-1 ß processing in rainbow trout, *Oncorhynchus mykiss*. *Fish Shellfish Immunol* **16**: 453–9.

Husain, M., Bird, S., Zwieten, R.V., *et al.*, 2012. Cloning of the IL-1ß3 gene and IL-1ß4 pseudogene in salmonids uncovers a second type of IL-1ß gene in teleost fish. *Dev Comp Immunol* **38**: 431–46.

Hwang, S.D., Asahi, T., Kondo, H., *et al.*, 2010. Molecular cloning and expression study on Toll-like receptor 5 paralogs in Japanese flounder, *Paralichthys olivaceus*. *Fish Shellfish Immunol* **29**: 630–38.

Hwang, S.D., Kondo, H., Hirono, I. and Aoki, T. 2011. Molecular cloning and characterization of Toll-like receptor 14 in Japanese flounder, *Paralichthys olivaceus*. *Fish Shellfish Immunol* **30**: 425–9.

Igawa, D., Sakai, M. and Savan, R. 2006. An unexpected discovery of two interferon gamma-like genes along with interleukin (IL)-22 and −26 from teleost: IL-22 and −26 genes have been described for the first time outside mammals. *Mol Immunol* **43**: 999–1009.

Iliev, D.B., Jørgensen, S., Rode, M., Krasnov, A., Harneshaug, I., Jørgensen, J.B., 2010. CpG-induced secretion of MHCIIb from salmon (*Salmo salar*) APCs. *Dev Comp Immunol* **34**: 29–41.

Iliev, D.B., Roach, J.C., Mackenzie, S., *et al.*, 2005. Endotoxin recognition: in fish or not in fish? *FEBS Lett* **579**: 6519–28.

Ingerslev, H.C., Cunningham, C. and Wergeland, H.I. 2006. Cloning and expression of TNF-α, IL-1ß and COX-2 in an anadromous and landlocked strain of Atlantic salmon (*Salmo salar* L.) during the smolting period. *Fish Shellfish Immunol* **20**: 450–61.

Janeway, C.A., Jr., and Medzhitov, R. 2002. Innate immune recognition. *Annu Rev Immunol* **20**: 197–216.

Jaso-Friedmann, L., Leary, J.H. III, and Evans, D.L. 1997a. NCCRP-1: a novel receptor protein sequenced from teleost nonspecific cytotoxic cells. *Mol Immunol* **34**: 955–65.

Jaso-Friedmann, L., Leary, J.H. III,, Warren, J., *et al.*, 1997b. Molecular characterization of a protozoan parasite target antigen recognized by nonspecific cytotoxic cells. *Cell Immunol* **176**: 93–102.

Jaso-Friedmann, L., Leary, J.H. III, and Evans, D.L. 2001. The non-specific cytotoxic cell receptor (NCCRP-1): molecular organization and signaling properties. *Dev Comp Immunol* **25**: 701–11.

Jault, C., Pichon, L. and Chluba, J. 2004. Toll-like receptor gene family and TIR-domain adapters in *Danio rerio*. *Mol Immunol* **40**: 759–71.

Jenkins, J.A. and Ourth, D.D. 1993. Opsonic effect of the alternative complement pathway on channel catfish peripheral blood phagocytes. *Vet Immunol Immunopathol* **39**: 447–59.

Jensen, I. and Robertsen, B. 2002. Effect of double-stranded RNA and interferon on the antiviral activity of Atlantic salmon cells against infectious salmon anemia virus and infectious pancreatic necrosis virus. *Fish Shellfish Immunol* **13**: 221–41.

Jensen, I., Albuquerque, A., Sommer, A.I. and Robertsen, B. 2002a. Effect of poly I:C on the expression of Mx proteins and resistance against infection by infectious salmon anaemia virus in Atlantic salmon. *Fish Shellfish Immunol* **13**: 311–26.

Jensen, I., Larsen, R. and Robertsen, B. 2002b. An antiviral state induced in Chinook salmon embryo cells (CHSE-214) by transfection with the double-stranded RNA poly I:C. *Fish Shellfish Immunol* **13**: 367–78.

Jørgensen, J.B. and Robertsen, B. 1995. Yeast ß-glucan stimulates respiratory burst activity of Atlantic salmon (*Salmo salar* L.) macrophages. *Dev Comp Immunol* **19**: 43–57.

Jørgensen, J.B., Johansen, A., Stenersen, B. and Sommer, A.I. 2001a. CpG oligodeoxynucleotides and plasmid DNA stimulate Atlantic salmon (*Salmo salar* L.) leucocytes to produce supernatants with antiviral activity. *Dev Comp Immunol* **25**: 313–21.

Jørgensen, J.B., Zou, J., Johansen, A. and Secombes, C.J. 2001b. Immunostimulatory CpG oligodeoxynucleotides stimulate expression of IL-1ß and interferon-like cytokines in rainbow trout macrophages via a chloroquine-sensitive mechanism. *Fish Shellfish Immunol* **11**: 673–82.

Jørgensen, J.B., Johansen, L.H., Steiro, K. and Johansen, A. 2003. CpG DNA induces protective antiviral immune responses in Atlantic salmon (Salmo salar L.). *J Virol* **77**: 11471–9.

Kato, Y., Nakao, M., Shimizu, M., *et al.*, 2004. Purification and functional assessment of C3a, C4a and C5a of the common carp (*Cyprinus carpio*) complement. *Dev Comp Immunol* **28**: 901–10.

Kileng, O., Albuquerque, A. and Robertsen, B. 2008. Induction of interferon system genes in Atlantic salmon by the imidazoquinoline S-27609, a ligand for Toll-like receptor 7. *Fish Shellfish Immunol* **24**: 514–22.

Koppang, E.O., Hordvik, I., Bjerkås, I., *et al.*, 2003. Production of rabbit antisera against recombinant MHC class II ß chain and identification of immunoreactive cells in Atlantic salmon (*Salmo salar*). *Fish Shellfish Immunol* **14**: 115–32.

Krasnov, A., Timmerhaus, G., Schiotz, B.L., *et al.*, 2011. Genomic survey of early responses to viruses in Atlantic salmon, *Salmo salar* L. *Mol Immunol* **49**: 163–74.

Kumar, H., Kawai, T. and Akira, S. 2011. Pathogen recognition by the innate immune system. *Int Rev Immunol* **30**: 16–34.

Laing, K.J., Hardie, L.J., Aartsen, W., *et al.*, 1999. Expression of an inducible nitric oxide synthase gene in rainbow trout *Oncorhynchus mykiss*. *Dev Comp Immunol* **23**: 71–85.

Laing, K.J., Wang, T., Zou, J., *et al.*, 2001. Cloning and expression analysis of rainbow trout *Oncorhynchus mykiss* tumour necrosis factor-α. *Eur J Biochem* **268**: 1315–22.

Laing, K.J., Purcell, M.K., Winton, J.R. and Hansen, J.D. 2008. A genomic view of the NOD-like receptor family in teleost fish: identification of a novel NLR subfamily in zebrafish. *BMC Evol Biol* **8**: 42.

Larsen, R., Røkenes, T.P. and Robertsen, B. 2004. Inhibition of infectious pancreatic necrosis virus replication by Atlantic salmon Mx1 protein. *J Virol* **78**: 7938–44.

Lieschke, G.J., Oates, A.C., Crowhurst, M.O., *et al.*, 2001. Morphologic and functional characterization of granulocytes and macrophages in embryonic and adult zebrafish. *Blood* **98**: 3087–96.

Lin, A.F., Xiang, L.X., Wang, Q.L., *et al.*, 2009. The DC-SIGN of zebrafish: insights into the existence of a CD209 homologue in a lower vertebrate and its involvement in adaptive immunity. *J Immunol* **183**: 7398–410.

Lutfalla, G., Crollius, H.R., Stange-thomann, N., *et al.*, 2003. Comparative genomic analysis reveals independent expansion of a lineage-specific genefamily in vertebrates: The class II cytokine receptors and their ligands in mammals and fish. *BMC Genomics* **4**: 29.

Løvoll, M., Dalmo, R.A. and Bøgwald, J. 2007a. Extrahepatic synthesis of complement components in the rainbow trout (*Oncorhynchus mykiss*). *Fish Shellfish Immunol* **23**: 721–31.

Løvoll, M., Fischer, U., Mathisen, G.S., *et al.*, 2007b. The C3 subtypes are differentially regulated after immunostimulation in rainbow trout, but head kidney macrophages do not contribute to C3 transcription. *Vet Immunol Immunopathol* **117**: 284–95.

Martinon, F., Burns, K. and Tschopp, J. 2002. The inflammasome: a molecular platform triggering activation of inflammatory caspases and processing of proIL-ß. *Mol Cell* **10**: 417–26.

Matsuo, A., Oshiumi, H., Tsujita, T., *et al.*, 2008. Teleost TLR22 recognizes RNA duplex to induce IFN and protect cells from birnaviruses. *J Immunol* **181**: 3474–85.

Meijer, A.H., Gabby Krens, S.F., Medina Rodriguez, I.A., *et al.*, 2004. Expression analysis of the Toll-like receptor and TIR domain adaptor families of zebrafish. *Mol Immunol* **40**: 773–83.

Meyer, A. and Van de Peer, Y. 2005. From 2R to 3R: evidence for a fish-specific genome duplication (FSGD). *Bioessays* **27**: 937–45.

Milev-Milovanovic, I., Long, S., Wilson, M., 2006. Identification and expression analysis of interferon gamma genes in channel catfish. *Immunogenetics* **58**: 70–80.

Mutoloki, S., Jørgensen, J.B. and Evensen, Ø. 2014. The adaptive immune response in fish, in *Fish Vaccination* (eds R. Gudding, A. Lillehaug and Ø. Evensen). Oxford, John Wiley & Sons, Ltd., 104–115.

Nakao, M., Kato-Unoki, Y., Nakahara, M., *et al.*, 2006. Diversified components of the bony fish complement system: more genes for robuster innate defense? *Adv Exp Med Biol* **586**: 121–38.

Nakao, M., Tsujikura, M., Ichiki, S., *et al.*, 2011. The complement system in teleost fish: progress of post-homolog-hunting researches. *Dev Comp Immunol* **35**: 1296–308.

Nam, B.H., Moon, J.Y., Kim, Y.O., *et al.*, 2010. Multiple ß-defensin isoforms identified in early developmental stages of the teleost *Paralichthys olivaceus*. *Fish Shellfish Immunol* **28**: 267–74.

Neumann, N.F., Stafford, J.L., Barreda, D., *et al.*, 2001. Antimicrobial mechanisms of fish phagocytes and their role in host defense. *Dev Comp Immunol* **25**: 807–25.

Ohta, T., Ueda, Y., Ito, K., *et al.*, 2011. Anti-viral effects of interferon administration on sevenband grouper, *Epinephelus septemfasciatus*. *Fish Shellfish Immunol* **30**: 1064–71.

Ohtani, M., Hikima, J., Kondo, H., *et al.*, 2011. Characterization and antiviral function of a cytosolic sensor gene, MDA5, in Japanese flounder, *Paralichthys olivaceus*. *Dev Comp Immunol* **35**: 554–62.

Oshiumi, H., Tsujita, T., Shida, K., *et al.*, 2003. Prediction of the prototype of the human Toll-like receptor gene family from the pufferfish, *Fugu rubripes*, genome. *Immunogenetics* **54**: 791–800.

Palic, D., Ostojic, J., Andreasen, C.B. and Roth, J.A. 2007. Fish cast NETs: neutrophil extracellular traps are released from fish neutrophils. *Dev Comp Immunol* **31**: 805–16.

Palti, Y. 2011. Toll-like receptors in bony fish: from genomics to function. *Dev Comp Immunol* **35**: 1263–72.

Pancer, Z., Amemiya, C.T., Ehrhardt, G.R., *et al.*, 2004. Somatic diversification of variable lymphocyte receptors in the agnathan sea lamprey. *Nature* **430**: 174–80.

Park, S.B., Hikima, J., Suzuki, Y., *et al.*, 2012. Molecular cloning and functional analysis of nucleotide-binding oligomerization domain 1 (NOD1) in olive flounder, *Paralichthys olivaceus*. *Dev Comp Immunol* **36**: 680–87.

Peddie, S., Zou, J., Cunningham, C. and Secombes, C.J. 2001. Rainbow trout (*Oncorhynchus mykiss*) recombinant IL-1ß and derived peptides induce migration of head-kidney leucocytes *in vitro*. *Fish Shellfish Immunol* **11**: 697–709.

Peddie, S., Zou, J. and Secombes, C.J. 2002. A biologically active IL-1ß derived peptide stimulates phagocytosis and bactericidal activity in rainbow trout, *Oncorhynchus mykiss* (Walbaum), head kidney leucocytes *in vitro*. *J Fish Dis* **25**: 351–60.

Pedersen, G.M., Johansen, A., Olsen, R.L. and Jørgensen, J.B. 2006. Stimulation of type I IFN activity in Atlantic salmon (*Salmo salar* L.) leukocytes: synergistic effects of cationic proteins and CpG ODN. *Fish Shellfish Immunol* **20**: 503–18.

Pelegrin, P., Chaves-Pozo, E., Mulero, V. and Meseguer, J. 2004. Production and mechanism of secretion of interleukin-1ß from the marine fish gilthead seabream. *Dev Comp Immunol* **28**: 229–37.

Plouffe, D.A., Hanington, P.C., Walsh, J.G., *et al.*, 2005. Comparison of select innate immune mechanisms of fish and mammals. *Xenotransplantation* **12**: 266–77.

Purcell, M.K., Nichols, K.M., Winton, J.R., *et al.*, 2006a. Comprehensive gene expression profiling following DNA vaccination of rainbow trout against infectious hematopoietic necrosis virus. *Mol Immunol* **43**: 2089–106.

Purcell, M.K., Smith, K.D., Aderem, A., *et al.*, 2006b. Conservation of Toll-like receptor signaling pathways in teleost fish. *Comp Biochem Physiol Part D - Genomics Proteomics* **1**: 77–88.

Rajendran, K.V., Zhang, J., Liu, S., *et al.*, 2012a. Pathogen recognition receptors in channel catfish: I. Identification, phylogeny and expression of NOD-like receptors. *Dev Comp Immunol* **37**: 77–86.

Rajendran, K.V., Zhang, J., Liu, S., *et al.*, 2012b. Pathogen recognition receptors in channel catfish: II. Identification, phylogeny and expression of retinoic acid-inducible gene I (RIG-I)-like receptors (RLRs). *Dev Comp Immunol* **37**: 381–9.

Rebl, A., Goldammer, T. and Seyfert, H.-M. 2010. Toll-like receptor signaling in bony fish. *Vet Immunol Immunopathol* **134**: 139–50.

Robertsen, B., Bergan, V., Røkenes, T., *et al.*, 2003. Atlantic salmon interferon genes: cloning, sequence analysis, expression, and biological activity. *J Interferon Cytokine Res* **23**: 601–12.

Roca, F.J., Mulero, I., Lopez-Munoz, A., *et al.*, 2008. Evolution of the inflammatory response in vertebrates: fish TNF-α is a powerful activator of endothelial cells but hardly activates phagocytes. *J Immunol* **181**: 5071–81.

Rodriguez, A., Esteban, M.A. and Meseguer, J. 2003. Phagocytosis and peroxidase release by seabream (*Sparus aurata* L.) leucocytes in response to yeast cells. *Anat Rec A Discov Mol Cell Evol Biol* **272**: 415–23.

Rotllant, J., Parra, D., Peters, R., *et al.*, 2004. Generation, purification and functional characterization of three C3a anaphylatoxins in rainbow trout: role in leukocyte chemotaxis and respiratory burst. *Dev Comp Immunol* **28**: 815–28.

Saeij, J.P., Stet, R.J., de Vries, B.J., *et al.*, 2003. Molecular and functional characterization of carp TNF: a link between TNF polymorphism and trypanotolerance? *Dev Comp Immunol* **27**: 29–41.

Savan, R., Kono, T., Igawa, D. and Sakai, M. 2005. A novel tumor necrosis factor (TNF) gene present in tandem with theTNF-α gene on the same chromosome in teleosts. *Immunogenetics* **57**: 140–50.

Schraml, B., Baker, M.A. and Reilly, B.D. 2006. A complement receptor for opsonized immune complexes on erythrocytes from *Oncorhynchus mykiss* but not *Ictalarus punctatus*. *Mol Immunol* **43**: 1595–603.

Secombes, C.J., Wang, T. and Bird, S. 2011. The interleukins of fish. *Dev Comp Immunol* **35**: 1336–45.

Seppola, M., Larsen, A.N., Steiro, K., *et al.*, 2008. Characterisation and expression analysis of the interleukin genes, IL-1ß, IL-8 and IL-10, in Atlantic cod (*Gadus morhua* L.). *Mol Immunol* **45**: 887–97.

Sha, Z., Abernathy, J.W., Wang, S., *et al.*, 2009. NOD-like subfamily of the nucleotide-binding domain and leucine-rich repeat containing family receptors and their expression in channel catfish. *Dev Comp Immunol* **33**: 991–9.

Shen, L., Stuge, T.B., Zhou, H., *et al.*, 2002. Channel catfish cytotoxic cells: a mini-review. *Dev Comp Immunol* **26**: 141–9.

Shen, L., Stuge, T.B., Bengten, E., *et al.*, 2004. Identification and characterization of clonal NK-like cells from channel catfish (*Ictalurus punctatus*). *Dev Comp Immunol* **28**: 139–52.

Skjæveland, I., Iliev, D.B., Strandskog, G. and Jørgensen, J.B. 2009. Identification and characterization of TLR8 and MyD88 homologs in Atlantic salmon (*Salmo salar*). *Dev Comp Immunol* **33**: 1011–17.

Skjæveland, I., Iliev, D.B., Zou, J., *et al.*, 2008. A TLR9 homolog that is up-regulated by IFN-γ in Atlantic salmon (*Salmo salar*). *Dev Comp Immunol* **32**: 603–7.

Skjesol, A., Aamo, T., Hegseth, M.N., *et al.*, 2009. The interplay between infectious pancreatic necrosis virus (IPNV) and the IFN system: IFN signaling is inhibited by IPNV infection. *Virus Res* **143**: 53–60.

Somamoto, T., Nakanishi, T. and Okamoto, N. 2000. Specific cell-mediated cytotoxicity against a virus-infected syngeneic cell line in isogeneic ginbuna crucian carp. *Dev Comp Immunol* **24**: 633–40.

Stafford, J.L., Galvez, F., Goss, G.G. and Belosevic, M. 2002. Induction of nitric oxide and respiratory burst response in activated goldfish macrophages requires potassium channel activity. *Dev Comp Immunol* **26**: 445–59.

Star, B., Nederbragt, A.J., Jentoft, S., *et al.*, 2011. The genome sequence of Atlantic cod reveals a unique immune system. *Nature* **477**: 207–10.

Stolte, E.H., Savelkoul, H.F., Wiegertjes, G., *et al.*, 2008. Differential expression of two interferon-γ genes in common carp (*Cyprinus carpio* L.). *Dev Comp Immunol* **32**: 1467–81.

Strandskog, G., Ellingsen, T. and Jørgensen, J.B. 2007. Characterization of three distinct CpG oligonucleotide classes which differ in ability to induce IFN α/ß activity and cell proliferation in Atlantic salmon (*Salmo salar* L.) leukocytes. *Dev Comp Immunol* **31**: 39–51.

Strandskog, G., Skjæveland, I., Ellingsen, T. and Jørgensen, J.B. 2008a. Double-stranded RNA- and CpG DNA-induced immune responses in Atlantic salmon: comparison and synergies. *Vaccine* **26**: 4704–15.

Strandskog, G., Skjæveland, I., Ellingsen, T. and Jørgensen, J.B. 2008b. Double-stranded RNA- and CpG DNA-induced immune responses in Atlantic salmon: Comparison and synergies. *Vaccine* **26**: 4704–15.

Strandskog, G., Villoing, S., Iliev, D.B., *et al.*, 2011. Formulations combining CpG containing oliogonucleotides and poly I:C enhance the magnitude of immune responses and protection against pancreas disease in Atlantic salmon. *Dev Comp Immunol* **35**: 1116–27.

Sun, B., Robertsen, B., Wang, Z. and Liu, B. 2009. Identification of an Atlantic salmon IFN multigene cluster encoding three IFN subtypes with very different expression properties. *Dev Comp Immunol* **33**: 547–58.

Sun, B., Skjæveland, I., Svingerud, T., *et al.*, 2011. Antiviral activity of salmonid gamma interferon against infectious pancreatic necrosis virus and salmonid alphavirus and its dependency on type I interferon. *J Virol* **85**: 9188–98.

Svingerud, T., Solstad, T., Sun, B., *et al.*, 2012. Atlantic salmon type I IFN subtypes show differences in antiviral activity and cell-dependent expression: evidence for high IFNb/IFNc-producing cells in fish lymphoid tissues. *J Immunol* **189**: 5912–23.

Thim, H.L., Iliev, D.B., Christie, K.E., *et al.*, 2012. Immunoprotective activity of a salmonid alphavirus vaccine: comparison of the immune responses induced by inactivated whole virus antigen formulations based on CpG class B oligonucleotides and poly I:C alone or combined with an oil adjuvant. *Vaccine* **30**: 4828–34.

Thornberry, N.A., Bull, H.G., Calaycay, J.R., *et al.*, 1992. A novel heterodimeric cysteine protease is required for interleukin-1ß processing in monocytes. *Nature* **356**: 768–74.

Traver, D., Paw, B.H., Poss, K.D., *et al.*, 2003. Transplantation and *in vivo* imaging of multilineage engraftment in zebrafish bloodless mutants. *Nat Immunol* **4**: 1238–46.

Tsujita, T., Tsukada, H., Nakao, M., *et al.*, 2004. Sensing bacterial flagellin by membrane and soluble orthologs of Toll-like receptor 5 in rainbow trout (*Onchorhynchus mykiss*). *J Biol Chem* **279**: 48588–97.

Vallejo, A.N., Miller, N.W. and Clem, L.W. 1991a. Phylogeny of immune recognition: processing and presentation of structurally defined proteins in channel catfish immune responses. *Dev Immunol* **1**: 137–48.

Vallejo, A.N., Miller, N.W. and Clem, L.W. 1991b. Phylogeny of immune recognition: role of alloantigens in antigen presentation in channel catfish immune responses. *Immunology* **74**: 165–8.

van Vliet, S.J., den Dunnen, J., Gringhuis, S.I., *et al.*, 2007. Innate signaling and regulation of dendritic cell immunity. *Curr Opin Immunol* **19**: 435–40.

Vasta, G.R., Ahmed, H. and Odom, E.W. 2004. Structural and functional diversity of lectin repertoires in invertebrates, protochordates and ectothermic vertebrates. *Curr Opin Struct Biol* **14**: 617–30.

Vasta, G.R., Nita-Lazar, M., Giomarelli, B., *et al.*, 2011. Structural and functional diversity of the lectin repertoire in teleost fish: relevance to innate and adaptive immunity. *Dev Comp Immunol* **35**: 1388–99.

Vojtech, L.N., Scharping, N., Woodson, J.C. and Hansen, J.D. 2012. Roles of inflammatory caspases during processing of Zebrafish interleukin-1ß in *Francisella noatunensis* infection. *Infect Immun* **80**: 2878–85.

Wang, T., Bird, S., Koussounadis, A., *et al.*, 2009. Identification of a novel IL-1 cytokine family member in teleost fish. *J Immunol* **183**: 962–74.

Wang, L., Su, J., Yang, C., *et al.*, 2012. Genomic organization, promoter activity of grass carp MDA5 and the association of its polymorphisms with susceptibility/resistance to grass carp reovirus. *Mol Immunol* **50**: 236–43.

Ware, C.F. 2003.The TNF superfamily. *Cytokine Growth Factor Rev* **14**: 181–4.

Wiens, G.D. and Glenney, G.W. 2011. Origin and evolution of TNF and TNF receptor superfamilies. *Dev Comp Immunol* **35**: 1324–35.

Wittamer, V., Bertrand, J.Y., Gutschow, P.W. and Traver, D. 2011. Characterization of the mononuclear phagocyte system in zebrafish. *Blood* **117**: 7126–35.

Yang, C., Su, J., Huang, T., *et al.*, 2011. Identification of a retinoic acid-inducible gene I from grass carp (*Ctenopharyngodon idella*) and expression analysis *in vivo* and *in vitro*. *Fish Shellfish Immunol* **30**: 936–43.
Yoder, J.A. and Litman, G.W. 2011. The phylogenetic origins of natural killer receptors and recognition: relationships, possibilities, and realities. *Immunogenetics* **63**: 123–41.
Zapata, A.G. and Cooper, E.L. 1990. *The Immune System*. Chichester, John Wiley & Sons, Ltd.
Zhang, Y.B. and Gui, J.F. 2012. Molecular regulation of interferon antiviral response in fish. *Dev Comp Immunol* **38**: 193–202.
Zhu, L.Y., Nie, L., Zhu, G., *et al.*, 2013. Advances in research of fish immune-relevant genes: A comparative overview of innate and adaptive immunity in teleosts. *Dev Comp Immunol* **39**: 39–62.
Zhu, R., Zhang, Y.-B., Zhang, Q.-Y. and Gui, J.-F. 2008. Functional domains and the antiviral effect of the double-stranded RNA-dependent protein kinase PKR from *Paralichthys olivaceus*. *J Virol* **82**: 6889–901.
Zou, J., Grabowski, P.S., Cunningham, C. and Secombes, C.J. 1999. Molecular cloning of interleukin 1beta from rainbow trout *Oncorhynchus mykiss* reveals no evidence of an ice cut site. *Cytokine* **11**: 552–60.
Zou, J., Wang, T., Hirono, I., *et al.*, 2002. Differential expression of two tumor necrosis factor genes in rainbow trout, *Oncorhynchus mykiss*. *Dev Comp Immunol* **26**: 161–72.
Zou, J., Peddie, S., Scapigliati, G., *et al.*, 2003a. Functional characterisation of the recombinant tumor necrosis factors in rainbow trout, *Oncorhynchus mykiss*. *Dev Comp Immunol* **27**: 813–22.
Zou, J., Secombes, C.J., Long, S., *et al.*, 2003b. Molecular identification and expression analysis of tumor necrosis factor in channel catfish (*Ictalurus punctatus*). *Dev Comp Immunol* **27**: 845–58.
Zou, J., Carrington, A., Collet, B., *et al.*, 2005. Identification and bioactivities of IFN-γ in rainbow trout Oncorhynchus mykiss: the first Th1-type cytokine characterized functionally in fish. *J Immunol* **175**: 2484–94.
Zou, J., Tafalla, C., Truckle, J. and Secombes, C.J. 2007. Identification of a second group of type I IFNs in fish sheds light on IFN evolution in vertebrates. *J Immunol* **179**: 3859–71.
Zou, J. and Secombes, C.J. 2011. Teleost fish interferons and their role in immunity. *Dev Comp Immunol* **35**: 1376–87.

9 The Adaptive Immune Response in Fish

Stephen Mutoloki[1], Jorunn B. Jørgensen[2] and Øystein Evensen[1]

[1]Norwegian School of Veterinary Science, Oslo, Norway
[2]Norwegian College of Fishery Science, UiT The Arctic University of Norway, Tromsø, Norway

ABSTRACT

The adaptive immune system is a system by which an animal acquires protection against pathogens following an encounter. As the term suggests, the response is "adapted" to the particular pathogen and is thus specific. Key features are that it is slow to develop, taking several days to weeks, but gets refined with time and is quick and effective upon subsequent encounters with the same pathogen, and thus it is characterized by anamnesis. Dendritic cells are specialized for antigen capture, migration and T stimulation. Recent advances have been made in identifying these cells in fish, and these studies have laid the foundation for future work aimed at understanding antigen presentation in bony fish. Central to the adaptive response are the lymphocytes, cell types responsible for the diversity of antigen recognition, specificity and memory. The cells can broadly be divided into B-cells responsible for antibody production, and T-cells that mediate cell-mediated immunity. T-cells are subdivided into cytotoxicity T-cells that directly kill infected and abnormal cells, and helper T-cells that modulate other immune cells through cytokine production. Helper T-cells are classified into several groups depending on the cytokine profile they produce. Teleost fish have been demonstrated to possess the necessary prerequisites of a functional adaptive system similar to that of mammals, although important differences exist. Firstly, the adaptive immune response of fish is temperature-dependent, and on average takes longer to develop compared with mammalian counterparts. There are fewer antibody isotypes (IgM, IgD and IgT), with only two being shown to respond to antigen stimulation. There is no class switching of antibodies; instead, specific antibody isotypes are produced by specific subsets of B-cells. The IgM isotype is dominant systemically, while IgT is predominant in the gut mucosa and possibly the skin. Studies done so far indicate that, for the most part, the cell-mediated response is conserved in teleost. However, additional studies are still required to gain a better understanding of the functions of the adaptive immune system, especially where the T-cell response is concerned. Finally,

oystein.evensen@nmbu.no

Fish Vaccination, First Edition. Edited by Roar Gudding, Atle Lillehaug and Øystein Evensen.

orthologs of most proteins taking part in the adaptive immune response, while conserved, seem to exist as more than one copy in teleost fish. There is a need to examine the contribution of the additional genes not least from a comparative point of view, but also from a functional perspective.

9.1 INTRODUCTION

In the previous chapter on innate immunity, its role as the first line of defense and the mechanisms affected to eliminate the pathogens with the goal of protecting the individual were described. Not all insults are resolved following activation of the innate immune system, as some pathogens have evolved sophisticated mechanisms by which they can evade it and establish infection. When this happens, some of the cells involved in the innate immune response such as macrophages and dendritic cells trigger the onset of the adaptive immune response (also referred to as specific or acquired immunity). The adaptive immune system is believed to have emerged early in vertebrate evolution, about 450 million years ago, between the divergence of the cyclostomes and cartilaginous fish, and is found in all jawed vertebrates. It has a greater capacity to respond to infections than the innate system. The main features of the adaptive immune system and how it differs from the innate system are summarized in Table 9.1.

The adaptive response takes time to develop, but also improves as it progresses. Unlike the innate immune system, it relies upon gene recombination to generate structures that are used for the recognition of antigens. This system has exquisite specificity and offers more diversity for antigen recognition. Furthermore, it is "smart" in the sense that it "learns" from encounters with the pathogen and is able to "remember" the invaders, so that on subsequent invasion it can respond rapidly and more effectively. This is the property that serves as the basis for vaccine design against pathogens.

Being a diverse group with more than 20,000 members, the parameters and competences of fish adaptive immune systems vary greatly even between closely related species. What is known so far about how they respond to infection is mainly from studies in teleost fish, therefore the rest of the chapter will be mainly restricted to teleost species. In general, the existence of lymphocytes in fish has been known for many years. Their identification was initially based

Table 9.1 Differences between mammalian innate and adaptive immune systems.

	Innate immunity	Adaptive immunity
Antigen recognition structures	Germ-line encoded	Generated by gene re-assortment
Specificity of antigen recognition	General classes of pathogens (e.g. bacteria, viruses, fungi) but can make fine distinctions	Very high
Response	Immediate	Takes time to develop
Cell types	Phagocytes, dendritic cells, NK cells	B and T lymphocytes
Memory	None, reacts with equal potency with repeated exposure	Yes, memory cells remember specific pathogen and the response more effective on second exposure

on morphology, and their staining characteristics in IgM-based assays. Using such assay, it was possible to sort the cells, by panning or flow cytometry and subjecting them to functional tests (e.g., allograft rejection and response), to known B- and T-cell mitogens (lipopolysaccharides and concanavalin A (Con A)). Recently, more tools have become available for the identification of subpopulations of these cells, owing to advances in molecular biology and genetics.

9.2 LYMPHOCYTES ARE THE KEY CELLS OF THE ADAPTIVE IMMUNE SYSTEM

The key cell type of the adaptive immune system is the lymphocyte. These cells are responsible for the diversity and specificity of antigen recognition as well as memory. Two distinct types are recognized, and these are the B- and T-cells. In mammals, lymphocytes originate from the bone marrow, and in contrast with the cells of the innate system that have a myeloid lineage, lymphocytes have a lymphoid lineage. B lymphocytes mature within the bone marrow (or bursa of Fabricius in birds), while T lymphocytes migrate to the thymus where they undergo positive selection and maturation prior to seeding the secondary lymphoid organs.

Fish lack bone marrow, so both B- and T-cells are believed to originate from the head kidney, a bone marrow equivalent. The maturation of B-cells occurs within the head kidney, while the thymus is important for the maturation of T lymphocytes (Ellis *et al.*, 1988; Clem *et al.*, 1991; Salinas *et al.*, 2011). Lymphoid structures like germinal centers, B-cell follicles, lymph nodes and mucosa associated lymphoid tissues (MALTs) that are found in mammals are absent in fish, although MALTs are believed to be represented by a primitive gut associated lymphoid tissue (GALT) found as diffuse subepithelial lymphoid aggregates (Zapata and Amemiya, 2000). More recently, the interbranchial lymphoid organ has been discovered in the gill area of salmon, and this has been suggested to be an important site for T-cell aggregation (Koppang *et al.*, 2010). Its function is, however, yet to be elucidated in more detail.

9.3 ANTIGEN TRAPPING AND ACTIVATION OF THE LYMPHOCYTES

Head kidneys and spleen are the main organs of antigen trapping in teleost fish (Press and Evensen, 1999). Lymphocyte recirculation through distinct tissues of the head kidney in plaice was shown to occur, while antigen stimulation of lymphocytes followed by the formation of spherical aggregates of pyroninophilic cells and plasma cells in carp were also demonstrated. The pyroninophilic stage is thought to be the proliferative stage of B-cells. The spleen, on the other hand, is more highly organized in advanced species, although not to the extent of that in higher vertebrates. This organ has ellipsoid structures known to be involved in trapping of immune complexes (Press and Evensen, 1999). Following antigen stimulation, lymphocytes undergo similar kinetics to that in head kidney to differentiate into plasma cells. Melano-macrophage centers (MMC), found in close proximity with structures of antigen trapping in both head kidney and spleen as well as other tissues undergoing chronic inflammation, are believed to be primitive analogs of the germinal centers of higher vertebrates. Indeed, small lymphocytes were reported to migrate to these areas, and given that the MMC are also areas of antigen retention, it has been suggested that they are sites for immune processing. Despite all these insights, clarity in how antigen presentation occurs and activation of lymphocytes is still lacking.

9.4 ANTIGEN PRESENTING CELLS (APCS) OF MYELOID ORIGIN

Besides the directly antimicrobial role of the mononuclear fish phagocytes described in the chapter on innate immunity (Jørgensen, 2014), these cells express MHC class II (Iliev *et al.*, 2010) and they have the molecular machinery necessary for antigen processing and presentation (Vallejo *et al.*, 1991; Wittamer *et al.*, 2011). However, there is sparse knowledge about antigen presentation in fish. For example, basic questions such as where antigen presentation takes place and which cell types are responsible for stimulating clonal T-cell proliferation are still unanswered. The seminal studies of APC function in fish were conducted in channel catfish, where it was shown that peripheral blood leukocyte (PBL)-derived monocytes were required as accessory cells in mixed leukocyte reactions with Ig-negative cell (most likely T-cells) (Sizemore *et al.*, 1984). In mammals, dendritic cells (DCs) are widely regarded as the most potent and versatile APCs of the immune system, due to their superior capacity to stimulate naïve T-cell responses. DCs have diverse morphology depending on their ontogeny and, more specifically, stage of differentiation (Geissmann *et al.*, 2010). The name of this heterogenous cell group was first proposed by Steinman *et al.* (1979) who had observed that certain adherent splenocytes develop a characteristic stellate morphology *in vitro*. Now, DCs have been defined as a system of APCs united by certain molecular cell-surface phenotypes and functions (Steinman, 2007). Immature DCs are present in the periphery where they sample the environment for foreign antigens. Upon activation, they migrate toward the T-cell areas of secondary lymphoid organs (Figure 9.1). During this migration, they lose their ability to internalize antigen and they acquire the capacity to present antigens to naïve T-cells, a process referred to as DC maturation (Randolph *et al.*, 2005a,b).

Recent studies in zebrafish (Lugo-Villarino *et al.*, 2010) and rainbow trout (Bassity and Clark, 2012) have identified APCs with features resembling mammalian DCs, including high expression of surface MHCII and co-stimulatory factors like CD80 and CD86. In zebrafish these cells were enriched by their affinity to the lectin peanut agglutinin, and electron-microscopy studies revealed that these cells had morphological characteristics different from other myeloid cells (Lugo-Villarino *et al.*, 2010). Furthermore, functional assays revealed that these cells showed antigen-specific recall responses. In rainbow trout, the DC-like cells expressed high levels of surface MHC-II and showed a stronger ability to stimulate mixed leukocyte reactions compared with other professional APCs like macrophages and B-cells (Lugo-Villarino *et al.*, 2010). The trout dendritic cells could be directly isolated from the spleen; additionally, large numbers could be derived from head kidney and PBLs *in vitro* (Bassity and Clark, 2012). In Atlantic salmon head kidney, three distinct populations of MHC-II expressing cells were detected by flow cytometry analysis (Iliev *et al.*, 2010). One of them is Ig^+ cells (presumably B-cells) (<10%), while the majority are Ig-negative and express high levels of surface MHC-II. The high percentage of myeloid cells expressing high levels of MHC-II underscores the importance of the head kidney as a source for APCs in fish, and also suggests that this might be an important site where antigen presentation takes place.

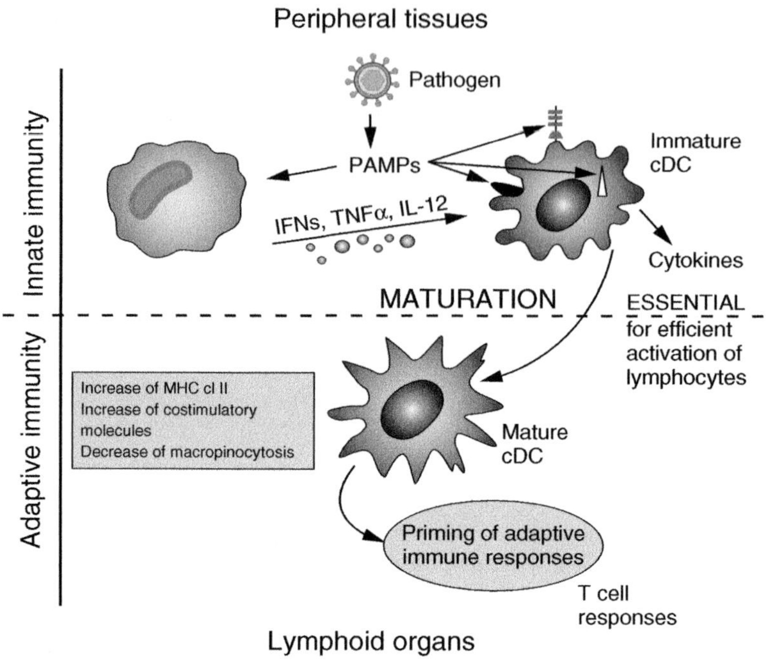

Fig. 9.1 Activation and maturation of dendritic cells (DCs). Immature DCs in the periphery respond to pathogen PAMPs and internalize the pathogen. Additionally other innate cells including monocytes/macrophages, also activated by PAMPs, secrete cytokines like type I IFNs and TNFα and subsequent activate the DCs. This results in maturation of DCs, and these cells will increase their expression of MHC-II and co-stimulatory molecules, migrate to lymphoid organs and present antigens to naïve T-cells.

Beside the morphological characterization of fish APCs, it has also been demonstrated that these cells can be efficiently activated by TLR ligands (Iliev *et al.*, 2010; Bassity and Clark, 2012) or by co-stimulatory molecules like CD40L (Lagos *et al.*, 2012), and upon stimulation these cells switch from an immature phenotype to an inflammatory phenotype, with high expression of surface MHC-II and with a reduced capacity to internalize antigen (Iliev *et al.*, 2010). The latter features are characteristic of mature DCs (Randolph *et al.*, 2005a,b).

9.5 IMMUNOGLOBULINS AND B LYMPHOCYTES

Three classes of immunoglobulin isotypes have so far been identified in teleost fish. The most abundant in systemic circulation is IgM. The main producers of this antibody isotype are plasma cells and plasmablasts located in the head kidney (Bromage *et al.*, 2004; Zwollo *et al.*, 2005). This isotype shows functional heterogeneity with monomeric, dimeric and tetrameric forms. Class-switching does not occur in teleosts, and in addition there is poor affinity maturation of IgM responses. Nevertheless, this antibody isotype has been used as a marker for protection against several extracellular bacterial diseases such as furunculosis and vibriosis, consistent with humoral immunity in higher vertebrates. It has also been linked to the protection against viral diseases in Atlantic salmon such as infectious pancreatic necrosis (Munang'andu *et al.*, 2013) and pancreas disease (Xu *et al.*, 2012). Interestingly, for infectious pancreatic necrosis, high antibody titers post-vaccination (at the start of the challenge) and not during the challenge were associated with protection. Antibodies appeared to be consumed during the course of the challenge, with mortality setting in early in the groups with low or without any antibody titers. No correlation was observed with antibodies generated against the challenge virus (e.g. in non-vaccinated controls), suggesting that pre-challenge antibodies play a significant role in limiting infection and its outcomes, probably by neutralizing the virus in circulation (Munang'andu *et al.*, 2013). These results add impetus to the role of IgM in teleosts in controlling intracellular pathogens. Whether vaccination in fish followed by infection induces memory recall reminiscent of mammals is one question that remains to be answered.

Passive immunization trials where serum antibodies from vaccinated fish were transferred to non-vaccinated fish have been shown to induce protection. For example, some workers showed that unvaccinated Nile tilapia (*Oreochromis niloticus*) were protected by serum antibodies passively transferred from fish that were immunized against *Streptococcus iniae* (LaFrentz *et al.*, 2011). In another study, Bercovier and others showed reduced infection in tilapia protected by passively transferred antibodies from vaccinated fish that had high antibody titers against *Streptococcus difficile* (Bercovier *et al.*, 1997). These studies clearly demonstrate the role of antibodies in the protection of unvaccinated fish.

The second antibody isotype, IgD, has only been characterized in channel catfish (*Ictalurus punctatus*) at protein level (Edholm *et al.*, 2010), although it has been cloned in several teleost species. In the channel catfish, the protein form was shown to be a monomer and the secreted one lacks the variable region, so consequently its function remains unclear. The Fc region of the antibody has, however, been suggested to function as a pattern recognition molecule, and furthermore, these fish (catfish) have been shown to contain IgD-armed granulocytes.

The third isotype, IgT, is expressed in several teleost fish species with the exception of channel catfish. This antibody is predominantly found in the gut mucosa where it is present in multimeric forms, suggesting that it is an equivalent of IgA. A monomeric form has also been observed in the serum. As with IgM, IgT is induced by pathogens affecting the gut (Zhang *et al.*, 2011). This antibody isotype, however, remains poorly understood with only a few studies having been carried out in fish (Salinas *et al.*, 2011). The location of the secreting cells is unknown, and so are the mechanisms by which the antibodies are transported to the mucosal surfaces.

In common with the immunoglobulin isotypes, B-cell subsets producing these antibodies have also been demonstrated. The catfish is one of the best studied teleost fish species when it comes to B lymphocytes, and in this species three subsets have been described, namely IgM^{+}/IgD^{-} (IgM), IgM^{+}/IgD^{+} and IgM^{-}/IgD^{+}(IgD) on the basis of B-cell receptors (BCRs) (Edholm *et al.*, 2010). In other species like rainbow trout, however, only two subsets, $IgM^{+}/IgD^{+}/IgT^{-}$ and $IgM^{-}/IgD^{-}/IgT^{+}$, have been reported. B-cells that express IgT do not express IgM and vice versa, suggesting that IgM- and IgT-producing cells exist as mutually exclusive B-cell lineages. The absence of isotype class-switching suggests that teleosts have a different mechanism of generating B-cell isotype diversity compared with tetrapods (Zhang *et al.*, 2011). IgM^{+} B-cells are the major B-cell population in systemic circulation, while IgT^+ B-cells comprise a minor subpopulation. However, the latter is dominant in the gut mucosa and has also been found in the mucus of the trout skin, igniting speculation that IgT is specialized for mucosal immunity (Sunyer, 2012). Both IgM^+ and IgT^+ B-cells have been shown to have potent phagocytic and microbial capabilities (Li *et al.*, 2006).

9.6 T LYMPHOCYTES

T lymphocytes are the subtypes that orchestrate cell-mediated immune responses. In mammals, these cells can be separated into αβ or γδ T-cells, depending on whether their T-cell receptors (receptors by which they bind antigens, abbreviated TCR) contain TCR-α with a -β chain or TCR-γ or -δ chain. αβ-T-cells are more abundant in circulation and in lymphoid organs, and are considered the "conventional T-cells", while the γδ-T-cells are found more in mucosal and epithelial tissues, do not seem to require antigen processing and presentation through MHC molecules to recognize pathogens, and are thus considered to belong to cells of the innate system. For the rest of the chapter, reference will only be made to αβ-T-cells, unless otherwise stated.

Mature T lymphocytes share certain common traits like TCR, CD3, CD28, and CD45 that are either surface molecules or are involved in pathogen recognition and signaling. As with BCR on B lymphocytes, the diversity of TCR is attained by gene re-assortment. T-cells only recognize antigens in association with MHC molecules, and this means that antigens must be on surfaces of other cells in order to be recognized by these cells.

T-cells can further be separated into two functional groups depending on whether they are cytotoxic or helpers. Cytotoxic T lymphocytes (CTLs) are involved in the direct killing of infected or abnormal cells by releasing molecules to induce apoptosis. The target cells are identified because they display fragments of pathogens or abnormal proteins in association with the MHC-I molecules on their surfaces. In this way, the host is able to protect itself against intracellular pathogens that are not easily accessible. T helper (T_H) cells, on the other hand, act indirectly by secreting cytokines that activate other immune cells to respond to a given threat.

In teleost, T lymphocytes constitute a minor population in circulation, although they are believed to be present in greater numbers in mucosal areas. Studies of their functions are an area that has lagged behind owing to the lack of reagents or tools. In the last two decades, however, most laboratories have taken advantage of the availability of expressed sequence tag (EST) databases and rapidly growing fish genomes coupled with homology cloning strategies to characterize these cells. As an example, T-cell clonal expansion and repertoire diversity in rainbow trout were characterized by immunoscope spectratyping (Boudinot *et al.*, 2001), while TCR genes were described in several species and shown to contain both conserved and novel characteristics (reviewed by Laing and Hansen, 2011). CD3 chains, CD28 and other T-cell co-stimulatory and co-inhibitory molecules were also demonstrated in several species (Araki *et al.*, 2005; Bernard *et al.*, 2006, 2007; Liu *et al.*, 2008). Many of the surface markers used to differentiate between naïve, memory and effector T-cells, for example CC chemokine receptor 7 and CD44, CD45RA were demonstrated (Laing and Hansen, 2011). However, the functional aspects of putative responses of different T-cell subsets remain poorly understood.

9.7 CYTOTOXIC T-CELLS

Cytotoxic T lymphocytes (CTLs) are the effector cells of the cytotoxic responses. They express CD8 molecules, TCR co-receptors involved in the cell's MHC-I interaction. Indeed antibodies against these molecules have been used to identify and sort out the cell population in several species (Araki *et al.*, 2008; Hetland *et al.*, 2010; Shibasaki *et al.*, 2010).

The first fish species in which specific CTLs were demonstrated was the channel catfish (Miller *et al.*, 1986). Thereafter, both alloantigen- and virus-specific cytotoxicity were demonstrated in ginburna crucian carp and rainbow trout systems (Nakanishi *et al.*, 2002; Fischer *et al.*, 2006; Castro *et al.*, 2011). Peripheral blood from fish immunized against *Viral hemorrhagic septicemia virus* (VHSV) using a DNA vaccine encoding VHSV G protein efficiently lysed VHSV-infected but not *Infectious hematopoietic necrosis virus* (IHNV)-infected histocompatible cells (Utke *et al.*, 2008).

Genetic sequences for molecules released by CTLs to induce apoptosis, such as granzymes, perforins and FasL (CD95), have been identified in several fish species. In fact, for FasL, mammalian antibodies have been shown to cross-react with sea bream leukocytes and catfish T-cell lines (Cuesta *et al.*, 2003; Long *et al.*, 2004), demonstrating conservation of these molecules. Recombinant perforin has been produced and shown to be lytic in the presence of calcium ions (Laing and Hansen, 2011). Genetic sequences of CD107 molecules used to measure degranulation of CTL have been identified in several species.

9.8 HELPER T-CELLS

As mentioned above, helper T-cells (T_H) produce cytokines that are critical in the cell- and humoral-mediated immune responses. A common feature of all T_H cells is the expression of a surface glycoprotein CD4 which is responsible for the specificity in the cellular interaction with MHC-II proteins. A structurally conserved ortholog of mammalian CD4 as well as additional CD4-like genes have been demonstrated in many teleost fish (reviewed in Laing and Hansen, 2011). These molecules have also been used as targets for anti-CD4 monoclonal antibodies in ginbuna crucian carp (Shibasaki *et al.*, 2010). In mammals, they are classified into several effector and regulatory subsets depending upon the type of cytokine profile that they produce (Figure 9.2). T_H1 cells are important in cell-mediated responses; T_H2 cells in humoral responses; T_H17 cells enhance responses to extracellular bacteria; while regulatory T-cells (Tregs) are involved in the regulation or suppression of immune responses in order to prevent immune-mediated damage. Recently, other T_H phenotypes have been discovered including T_H22, T_H9 and Tfh (reviewed by Dong, 2006; Reiner, 2007).

In teleost fish, many orthologs representing different helper T-cell subsets and their transcription factors have been demonstrated either at genetic or functional level (Laing and Hansen, 2011). IFN-γ (IFN-γ 2), a hallmark T_H1 cytokine, and another closely related molecule with little sequence homology to the mammalian IFN-γ (fish IFN-γ 1) have been sequenced in many fish species (Zou and Secombes, 2011). In zebrafish, trout and goldfish, recombinant IFN-γ has been shown to induce antiviral and inflammatory genes, and in common with the mammalian counterpart, the main producers of this cytokine in fish are T-cells and NK cells, although fish macrophages and B-cells are also capable of producing IFN-γ. T-bet, the hallmark transcription factor of T_H1 cells, has also been sequenced in fish

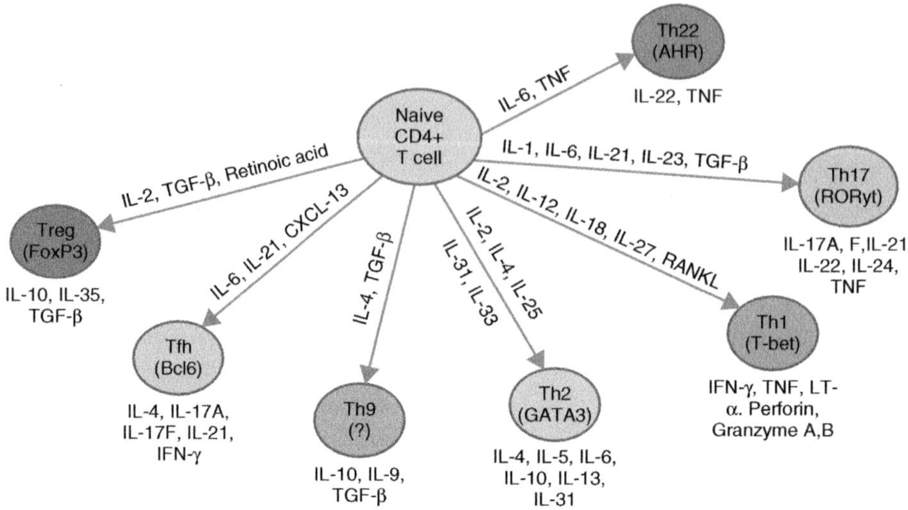

Fig. 9.2 CD4+ T-cell differentiation. Each T-cell subset has a characteristic cytokine signature that favors its differentiation (on arrow) and that it produces (below). The transcription factors are given in brackets. Th1 are activated in response to intracellular microbes, organ-specific autoimmune disorders and chronic inflammation; Th2: extracellular parasites and allergic disorders; Th9: role not clear; Th22: skin homeostasis and pathology; Tfh: help follicular B-cells. Bcl6 = B cell leukemia/lymphoma-6; RANKL = Receptor activator of nuclear factor kappa-B ligand.

and shown to be differentially regulated during experimental infection against viruses in grass carp (Wang *et al.*, 2013).

Classical T_H2 cytokines have not been functionally characterized in fish thus far. At genetic level, IL-4/13A and IL-4/13B are found as two paralogs related to a common ancestor of IL-4 and IL-13 (Li *et al.*, 2007), while GATA-3, the master transcription factor, is conserved in teleost fish in terms of sequence and developmental functions relative to mammals.

T_H17 cells secrete cytokines that are members of a multigene family IL-17A to F in mammals. In addition, these cells also secrete IL-22. Three forms are found in teleost fish. Whilst gene expression studies involving IL-17A have been undertaken (Mutoloki *et al.*, 2010), functional characterization is still required. Another T-cell subset recently demonstrated to secrete IL-22 is T_H22. However, unlike T_H17 cells, these cells are incapable of producing IL-17 (Eyerich *et al.*, 2010). T_H22 cells, although described in teleosts, are not yet well characterized, and more work is required to ascertain their existence. Other subsets include Tfh, T_H9 and Tregs. Tfh cells have a specialized role in helping follicular B-cells to become long-lived plasma cells. In mammals they secrete IL-21. They are also able to secrete IL-10- suggesting that they play a suppressive role. IL-21 has been discovered in the pufferfish genome and at a functional level in salmonids, although the cells producing it have not been definitively proven. It remains to be seen whether this cytokine in fish performs the functions akin with its mammalian counterpart, namely induction of antibody production. The transcription factor, B-cell leukemia/lymphoma-6 (Bcl-6), is uniquely required and has been identified in bony fish although not yet reported in teleost fish. There are no reports of T_H9 in fish so far ,while as for Tregs, the transcription factor Foxp3 has been demonstrated in many species. It is most highly expressed in T-cell associated tissues such as thymus and spleen, and its expression is reciprocal to that of IL-17 in zebra fish embryo, consistent with its known role of inhibiting T_H17 cells.

REFERENCES

Araki, K., Suetake, H., Kikuchi, K. and Suzuki, Y. 2005. Characterization and expression analysis of CD3varepsilon and CD3gamma/delta in fugu, *Takifugu rubripes*. *Immunogenetics* **57**: 158–63.

Araki, K., Akatsu, K., Suetake, H., *et al.*, 2008. Characterization of CD8+ leukocytes in fugu (*Takifugu rubripes*) with antiserum against fugu CD8α. Dev Comp Immunol **32**: 850–58.

Bassity, E. and Clark, T.G. 2012. Functional identification of dendritic cells in the teleost model, rainbow trout (*Oncorhynchus mykiss*). *PLoS One* **7**: e33196.

Bercovier, H., Ghittino, C. and Eldar, A. 1997. Immunization with bacterial antigens: infections with streptococci and related organisms. *Dev Biol Stand* **90**: 153–60.

Bernard, D., Riteau, B., Hansen, J.D., *et al.*, 2006. Costimulatory receptors in a teleost fish: typical CD28, elusive CTLA4. *J Immunol* **176**: 4191–200.

Bernard, D., Hansen, J.D., Du Pasquier, L., *et al.*, 2007. Costimulatory receptors in jawed vertebrates: conserved CD28, odd CTLA4 and multiple BTLAs. *Dev Comp Immunol* **31**: 255–71.

Boudinot, P., Boubekeur, S. and Benmansour, A. 2001. Rhabdovirus infection induces public and private T cell responses in teleost fish. *J Immunol* **167**: 6202–9.

Bromage, E.S., Kaattari, I.M., Zwollo, P. and Kaattari, S.L. 2004. Plasmablast and plasma cell production and distribution in trout immune tissues. *J Immunol* **173**: 7317–23.

Castro, R., Bernard, D., Lefranc, M.P., *et al.*, 2011. T cell diversity and TcR repertoires in teleost fish. *Fish Shellfish Immunol* **31**: 644–54.

Clem, L.W., Miller, N.W. and Bly, J.E. 1991. Evolution of lymphocyte subpopulations, their interactions and temperature sensitivities, in *Phylogenesis of Immune Functions* (eds G.W. Warr and N. Cohen). Boca Raton, FL, CRC Press, 191–213.

Cuesta, A., Esteban, M.A. and Meseguer, J. 2003. Identification of a FasL-like molecule in leucocytes of the teleost fish gilthead seabream (*Sparus aurata* L.). *Dev Comp Immunol* **27**: 21–7.

Dong, C. 2006. Diversification of T-helper-cell lineages: finding the family root of IL-17-producing cells. *Nat Rev Immunol* **6**: 329–33.

Edholm, E.S., Bengten, E., Stafford, J.L., *et al.*, 2010. Identification of two IgD+ B cell populations in channel catfish, *Ictalurus punctatus*. *J Immunol* **185**: 4082–94.

Ellis, A.E., Stapleton, K.J. and Hastings, T.S. 1988. The humoral immune response of rainbow trout (*Salmo gairdneri*) immunised by various regimes and preparations of *Aeromonas salmonicida* antigens. *Vet Immunol Immunopathol* **19**: 153–64.

Eyerich, S., Eyerich, K., Cavani, A. and Schmidt-Weber, C. 2010. IL-17 and IL-22: siblings, not twins. *Trends Immunol* **31**: 354–61.

Fischer, U., Utke, K., Somamoto, T., *et al.*, 2006. Cytotoxic activities of fish leucocytes. *Fish Shellfish Immunol* **20**: 209–26.

Geissmann, F., Manz, M.G., Jung, S., *et al.*, 2010. Development of monocytes, macrophages, and dendritic cells. *Science* **327**: 656–61.

Hetland, D.L., Jørgensen, S.M., Skjødt, K., *et al.*, 2010. *In situ* localisation of major histocompatibility complex class I and class II and CD8 positive cells in infectious salmon anaemia virus (ISAV)-infected Atlantic salmon. *Fish Shellfish Immunol* **28**: 30–39.

Iliev, D.B., Jørgensen, S.M., Rode, M., *et al.*, 2010. CpG-induced secretion of MHCIIß and exosomes from salmon (*Salmo salar*) APCs. *Dev Comp Immunol* **34**: 29–41.

Jørgensen, J.B. 2014. The innate immune response in fish, in *Fish Vaccination* (eds R. Gudding, A. Lillehaug and Ø. Evensen). Oxford, John Wiley & Sons, Ltd., 85–103.

Koppang, E.O., Fischer, U., Moore, L., *et al.*, 2010. Salmonid T cells assemble in the thymus, spleen and in novel interbranchial lymphoid tissue. *J Anat* **217**: 728–39.

LaFrentz, B.R., Shoemaker, C.A. and Klesius, P.H. 2011. Immunoproteomic analysis of the antibody response obtained in Nile tilapia following vaccination with a *Streptococcus iniae* vaccine. *Vet Microbiol* **152**: 346–52.

Lagos, L.X., Iliev, D.B., Helland, R., *et al.*, 2012. CD40L – a costimulatory molecule involved in the maturation of antigen presenting cells in Atlantic salmon (*Salmo salar*). *Dev Comp Immunol* **38**: 416–30.

Laing, K.J. and Hansen, J.D. 2011. Fish T cells: recent advances through genomics. *Dev Comp Immunol* **35**: 1282–95.

Li, J., Barreda, D.R., Zhang, Y.A., *et al.*, 2006. B lymphocytes from early vertebrates have potent phagocytic and microbicidal abilities. *Nat Immunol* **7**: 1116–24.

Li, J.H., Shao, J.Z., Xiang, L.X. and Wen, Y. 2007. Cloning, characterization and expression analysis of pufferfish interleukin-4 cDNA: the first evidence of Th2-type cytokine in fish. *Mol Immunol* **44**: 2078–86.

Liu, Y., Moore, L., Koppang, E.O. and Hordvik, I. 2008. Characterization of the CD3ζ, CD3γδ and CD3ε subunits of the T cell receptor complex in Atlantic salmon. *Dev Comp Immunol* **32**: 26–35.

Long, S., Wilson, M., Bengten, E., *et al.*, 2004. Identification of a cDNA encoding channel catfish interferon. *Dev Comp Immunol* **28**: 97–111.

Lugo-Villarino, G., Balla, K.M., Stachura, D.L., *et al.*, 2010. Identification of dendritic antigen-presenting cells in the zebrafish. *Proc Natl Acad Sci USA* **107**: 15850–55.

Miller, N.W., Deuter, A. and Clem, L.W. 1986. Phylogeny of lymphocyte heterogeneity: the cellular requirements for the mixed leucocyte reaction with channel catfish. *Immunology* **59**: 123–8.

Munang'andu, H.M., Fredriksen, B.N., Mutoloki, S., *et al.*, 2013. Antigen dose and humoral immune response correspond with protection for inactivated infectious pancreatic necrosis virus vaccines in Atlantic salmon (*Salmo salar* L). *Vet Res* **44**: 7.

Mutoloki, S., Cooper, G.A., Marjara, I.S., *et al.*, 2010. High gene expression of inflammatory markers and IL-17A correlates with severity of injection site reactions of Atlantic salmon vaccinated with oil-adjuvanted vaccines. *BMC Genomics* **11**: 336.

Nakanishi, T., Fischer, U., Dijkstra, J.M., *et al.*, 2002. Cytotoxic T cell function in fish. *Dev Comp Immunol* **26**: 131–9.

Press, C.McL. and Evensen, Ø. 1999. The morphology of the immune system in teleost fish. *Fish Shellfish Immunol* **9**: 309–18.

Randolph, G.J., Angeli, V. and Swartz, M.A. 2005a. Dendritic-cell trafficking to lymph nodes through lymphatic vessels. *Nat Rev Immunol* **5**: 617–28.

Randolph, G.J., Sanchez-Schmitz, G. and Angeli, V. 2005b. Factors and signals that govern the migration of dendritic cells via lymphatics: recent advances. *Springer Semin Immunopathol* **26**: 273–87.

Reiner, S.L. 2007. Development in motion: helper T cells at work. *Cell* **129**: 33–6.

Salinas, I., Zhang, Y.A. and Sunyer, J.O. 2011. Mucosal immunoglobulins and B cells of teleost fish. *Dev Comp Immunol* **35**: 1346–65.

Shibasaki, Y., Toda, H., Kobayashi, I., *et al.*, 2010. Kinetics of CD4+ and CD8α+ T-cell subsets in graft-versus-host reaction (GVHR) in ginbuna crucian carp *Carassius auratus langsdorfii*. *Dev Comp Immunol* **34**: 1075–81.

Sizemore, R.C., Miller, N.W., Cuchens, M.A., *et al.*, 1984. Phylogeny of lymphocyte heterogeneity: the cellular requirements for *in vitro* mitogenic responses of channel catfish leukocytes. *J Immunol* **133**: 2920–24.

Steinman, R.M. 2007. Dendritic cells: understanding immunogenicity. *Eur J Immunol* **37**: S53–60.

Steinman, R.M., Kaplan, G., Witmer, M.D. and Cohn, Z.A. 1979. Identification of a novel cell type in peripheral lymphoid organs of mice. V. Purification of spleen dendritic cells, new surface markers, and maintenance *in vitro*. *J Exp Med* **149**: 1–16.

Sunyer, J.O. 2012. Evolutionary and functional relationships of B cells from fish and mammals: insights into their novel roles in phagocytosis and presentation of particulate antigen. *Infect Disord Drug Targets* **12**: 200–212.

Utke, K., Kock, H., Schuetze, H., *et al.*, 2008. Cell-mediated immune responses in rainbow trout after DNA immunization against the viral hemorrhagic septicemia virus. *Dev Comp Immunol* **32**: 239–52.

Vallejo, A.N., Miller, N.W. and Clem, L.W. 1991. Phylogeny of immune recognition: processing and presentation of structurally defined proteins in channel catfish immune responses. *Dev Immunol* **1**: 137–48.

Wang, L., Shang, N., Feng, H., *et al.*, 2013. Molecular cloning of grass carp (*Ctenopharyngodon idellus*) T-bet and GATA-3, and their expression profiles with IFN-γ in response to grass carp reovirus (GCRV) infection. *Fish Physiol Biochem* **39**: 793–805.

Wittamer, V., Bertrand, J.Y., Gutschow, P.W. and Traver, D. 2011. Characterization of the mononuclear phagocyte system in zebrafish. *Blood* **117**: 7126–35.

Xu, C., Mutoloki, S. and Evensen, Ø. 2012. Superior protection conferred by inactivated whole virus vaccine over subunit and DNA vaccines against salmonid alphavirus infection in Atlantic salmon (*Salmo salar* L.). *Vaccine* **30**: 3918–28.

Zapata, A. and Amemiya, C.T. 2000. Phylogeny of lower vertebrates and their immunological structures. *Curr Top Microbiol Immunol* **248**: 67–107.

Zhang, Y.A., Salinas, I. and Oriol, S.J. 2011. Recent findings on the structure and function of teleost IgT. *Fish Shellfish Immunol* **31**: 627–34.

Zou, J. and Secombes, C.J. 2011. Teleost fish interferons and their role in immunity. *Dev Comp Immunol* **35**: 1376–87.

Zwollo, P., Cole, S., Bromage, E. and Kaattari, S. 2005. B cell heterogeneity in the teleost kidney: evidence for a maturation gradient from anterior to posterior kidney. *J Immunol* **174**: 6608–16.

10 Development, Production and Control of Fish Vaccines

Dag Knappskog[1], Joseph Koumans[2], Inger Kvitvang[3], Arne Marius Fiskum[3] and Rune Wiulsrød[4]

[1]MSD Animal Health, Bergen, Norway
[2]MSD Animal Health, Boxmeer, The Netherlands
[3]Pharmaq, Overhalla, Norway
[4]Pharmaq, Oslo, Norway

ABSTRACT

In global fish farming, the demand for safe and effective vaccines targeting different industrialized finfish species apply to both mature and emerging markets. In a few decades, production of biologicals for fish has developed from local manufacturers with an entrepreneurial basis to specialized industrial companies. As a prophylactic measure against identified pathogens, a wide range of different vaccines and combinations are commonly in use. Fish vaccines are basically divided into three categories: inactivated vaccines, live vaccines or DNA vaccines. As biologicals administered to food-producing animals, all process steps including development at the R&D stage, transfer and upscaling in production, purification, filling, packaging, labeling and testing of the final product are controlled by strict regulatory requirements set by national and international laws and guidelines.

10.1 INTRODUCTION

The vaccine industry has gone through a major development over the last decades. From traditional production in premises that combined science and practical knowledge, it is now a highly sophisticated, automated high-technology industry with advanced steering and quality systems. Scientists with biotechnology knowledge and personnel with practical expertise are now working together with engineers and system controllers.

From being local companies with an entrepreneurial basis, vaccine production is now dominated by large international industrial companies with interests going far beyond local needs. The complexity of the processes from the first idea via production to sales has made it necessary for the vaccine companies to improve their financial basis. As a result of this, companies have merged or been bought by larger companies.

dag.knappskog@merck.com

Fish Vaccination, First Edition. Edited by Roar Gudding, Atle Lillehaug and Øystein Evensen.

The existing fish vaccine companies are specialized enterprises or specialized departments of larger pharmaceutical companies, not only producing fish vaccines, but also developing and producing pharmaceutical products to cover demands in the fish farming industry, for products to combat sea lice and fungal infections to products for anesthesia and hormones.

Vaccines for the aquaculture industry consist of the active ingredient (antigen) dissolved in water (water-based) or in an emulsion of water and oil (oil-based). Vaccines may contain different forms of immune-enhancing agents or adjuvants, oil (e.g., mineral oil) being one of them. Different forms of oil-based vaccines exist – water in oil (wo), oil in water (ow) and water in oil in water (wow) – each form having different benefits and challenges. Addition of emulsifiers are needed to maintain the physical stability of the vaccine. The antigens can be localized in the water phase, in the oil phase, or in both. The vaccine may contain several antigens, both bacterial and viral, hence providing protection against several diseases. Oil-based vaccines are purely for intraperitoneal injection, while water-based vaccines can be intended for immersion or injection intraperitoneally, or intramuscularly in the case of DNA vaccines.

The development, production and control of vaccines for fish is regulated by national and international laws, regulations and guidelines (Holm *et al.*, 2014).

10.2 MANUFACTURING LICENSE

Production and control of vaccines are complicated processes that have high demands on premises, equipment and personnel. All commercial vaccine producers need approval from the authorities in the production country for production of vaccines. Such an approval is based upon comprehensive documentation of all relevant factors that may have an impact on the quality of the final product. Premises and equipment must have a satisfactory standard (see Figure 10.1), all processes must be validated, and the personnel must have the necessary competence.

Routines for internal controls must be in place, based on the modern principles for quality control (QC); these must be thoroughly described in standard operating procedures (SOPs). Hence, the production and control must be performed according to the principles of Good Manufacturing Practice (GMP).

In the EU/EEA the requirements include compliance with GMP directive 91/412/EEC, which covers manufacture of veterinary medicines. This is a critical requirement and is assessed by GMP audits of the site by the regulatory authorities.

10.2.1 Dossier

Detailed information with respect to development, safety, efficacy, production and control of a vaccine is gathered in a file called a dossier. There are certain requirements for the contents of a dossier for a vaccine. Within the European Economic Area (EEA) the common demands can be found in Commission Directive 2009/9/EC amending Directive 2001/82/EC, and these demands are further described in guidelines that are valid for the whole EEA.

A vaccine dossier describes the product and the producer. The product is described in a summary of the knowledge about the product: active ingredients, indication, user's manual, contra-indications, and so on. The description of the producer will give information about the organization, premises, product portfolio, and personnel. A copy of the production license will be included, and the producer will state that the principles of GMP are followed.

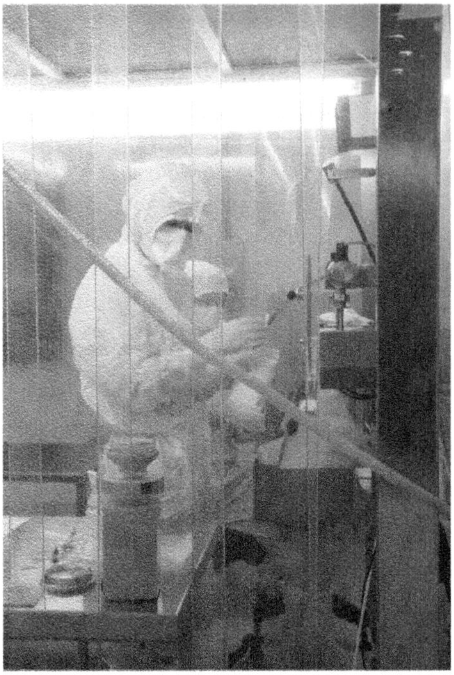

Fig. 10.1 Aseptic filling of vaccines. (Source: Reproduced with permission of Pharmaq.)

Description of the production process will be very detailed, including control tests of the finished product. In a vaccine the antigens are essential, and the dossier will contain all relevant information about origin, characterization, production and control of starting materials (with particular emphasis on materials from animal origin), storage and control.

The description will include details about the fermentation of the microorganisms, constitution of the growth media, and the downstream processing after harvest of the antigens. In this description there will also be information about the control tests performed during production. Samples will be taken at all stages of the production process, and these are to be examined following a plan and with specified methods. The methods used in the laboratory or during field trials should be quality assured and validated, following Good Manufacturing Practice (GMP) or Good Clinical Practice (GCP) (see Figure 10.2).

10.2.2 Quality systems

In order to be allowed to produce medicinal products, an effective quality system should be documented. A key principle is to have good systems in place, ensuring that the product is manufactured the same way every time it is produced. Principles and guidelines of Good Manufacturing Practice for veterinary medicinal products are laid down in Commission Directive 91/412/EEC and Eudralex, volume 4.

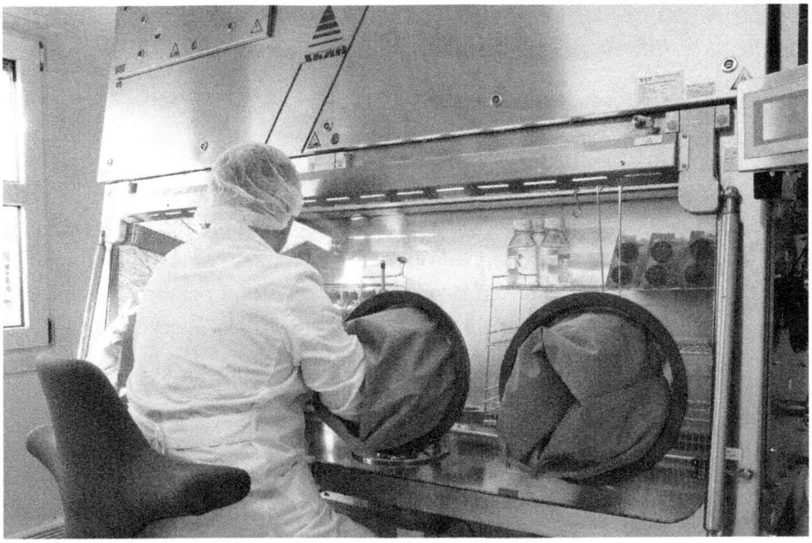

Fig. 10.2 Isolator for sterility testing. (Source: Reproduced with permission of Pharmaq.)

10.2.3 Quality management

Quality management (QM) covers all matters that individually or collectively influence the quality of a product. The system of QM appropriate for the manufacture of medicinal products should ensure that they are developed in a way that takes account of the requirements of Good Manufacturing Practice and Good Laboratory Practice. All systems and routines should be clearly described in standard operating procedures (SOPs). Quality management is the sum of all systems and routines required to fulfil the requirements set by the authorities. This includes systems that define responsibilities, quality documentation, training, control of manufacturing and test equipment, raw material specifications, laboratory testing and control, quality requirements in laboratory and field trials, preventive maintenance, risk management, deviation handling,

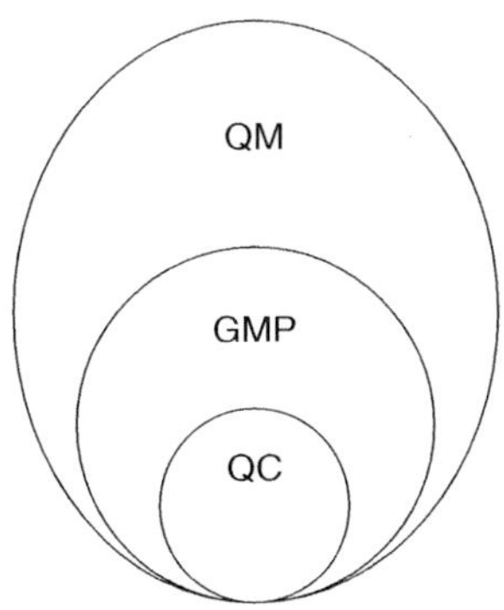

change of management, customer complaints and recalls, pharmacovigilance, approval of contract manufacturers/laboratories/suppliers and internal/external audits.

10.2.4 Good Manufacturing Practice

Good Manufacturing Practice (GMP) is the part of quality management that ensures that products are consistently produced and controlled to the quality standard appropriate to their intended use. GMP requires full traceability throughout the value chain. All activities from purchase of raw materials from approved suppliers through manufacturing and quality control are documented. All critical steps should be verified by a second person (four-eye principle). The quality of the product is dependent upon several things. The facility and the equipment must be fit for its purpose and satisfactorily qualified. Procedures and protocols have already been mentioned as important tools, in addition to a robust and well-defined process. The competence and attitude of personnel are key success factors. A lot of effort is put into training and documentation of each employee's competence.

10.2.5 Quality control

Quality control (QC) covers the part of GMP related to specifications, sampling, testing, document review and release of the product. Quality control is a tool used to verify that the product satisfies the defined specification – every time. Traditionally, the focus was on testing of the final product. This is now replaced by the philosophy that the quality is built into the whole process, and that samples should be taken throughout the process in order to verify the quality of the product. An effective quality system ensures the right quality each time. Quality control verifies that the product meets the specifications, rather than checking if the specifications are met.

Quality control is used for confirmation of the quality of the product, as set in the product specification. In addition, every batch of the product is also tested to verify safety and potency.

Classical bacterial/viral vaccines are usually inactivated by the use of formaldehyde. It is imperative to test that the formaldehyde has inactivated the live suspension. Samples are drawn at a minimum of two stages after inactivation to document that the material is inactivated. The inactivation process must be validated, that is, it must be shown that the inactivation process used is efficient for inactivation of the actual organism within two-thirds of the total inactivation period. Inactivation kinetics are also performed to show the speed and level of the inactivation effect that the formaldehyde has on the actual microorganism. The intermediate and final product must also be tested for purity/sterility.

For production of viral antigen, both the cell seed bank and the virus seed bank used for manufacture must be tested according to the requirements laid down in the European Pharmacopoeia (Ph.Eur). This testing is both complex and time-consuming, and includes extensive virus and sterility testing.

Ideally, all QC tests should be *in vitro*, but for vaccines it might be difficult to document safety and efficacy without the use of the target animal. Safety is tested by the use of an overdose of vaccine, to show that the vaccine itself is not harmful to the target animal. In general, a double dose is used for safety testing of inactivated vaccines, while ten times the normal dose is used to verify the safety of a live vaccine. The animals are frequently observed during the study, which normally lasts for three weeks. Any abnormal reactions are recorded.

Potency testing is important to document consistency of production. The test can be count of microorganisms (if it is a live vaccine), serological tests or quantification of antibody levels. For fish vaccines, potency is still usually performed *in vivo* on the target animal, where the mortality of the vaccinated group is compared with a group of unvaccinated fish. The potency is presented as RPS (relative percent survival), provided the mortality of the control group is at a satisfactory level. A reference vaccine may be used as a positive control.

10.3 VACCINE DEVELOPMENT

Once the relationship between a pathogen and a disease has been established, the development of a vaccine can start. The ideal vaccine is safe and efficacious, fast to develop and register, easy to supply in a sufficient number of doses at low cost, and easy to administer. Vaccines for aquatic animal health are particularly challenging to develop as they have to comply with many constraints (e.g., combination of many components in a single small injection volume) which differ with the intended target species. The choice of the antigen and the production system is dictated by the specific vaccine(s) it is intended for. Sometimes compromises can be made (you can't get what you want, but this is what we can deliver). In general we can discriminate between live, inactivated and DNA vaccines/antigens. Within these classifications we can make subdivisions.

10.3.1 Replicating vaccines

A classical live antigen can be a live attenuated strain obtained by serial passaging in a system that is different from the normal situation (e.g., other temperatures, cells from another species, medium lacking a specific component, etc.) (Shoemaker and Klesius, 2014). These antigens often take a long time to develop and hundreds of passages might be needed. However, in general they are considered to be very efficacious. Because the antigen can still replicate in the target animal they can be given at a low dose (a factor 1000-fold lower than an inactivated vaccine), and if well adapted to their culture system they can still be produced at a relatively high yield.

A live antigen based on targeted mutagenesis needs extensive knowledge of the molecular biology of the pathogen and a system in which specific mutations/truncations can be introduced in its genome (e.g., reversed genetics). Although sometimes obvious candidate genes for manipulation exist, these can also have large effects on their ability to mount an effective immune response and/or on the production characteristics of the pathogen. This can make them less suited for vaccine production, unless this effect can be counteracted by the culture conditions. These antigens are genetically modified organisms (GMOs), which means that they are treated as such with respect to the registration path they have to follow.

Special versions of live vaccines are vectors into which protective antigens of other pathogens are added. This has several advantages: it is a modular system that simplifies the production aspects, but it raises extra safety concerns with respect to new, previously non-existent characteristics, such as altered species specificity or tropism, which are introduced with the adding of the transgenes. This can be counteracted by making the vector replication defective (so-called single round of infection particles), but it is obvious that the large-scale production of such a vector is not easy to achieve.

Another advantage of live antigens in general is that they are efficacious on their own, without the need for an adjuvant. This has advantages with respect to their application method (oil-adjuvanted vaccines can in general only be administered by injection) and their safety profile with respect to local reactions. Live vaccines can be administered orally or by immersion, which enable vaccines of this type to be used on small fish (marine species), including relatively inexpensive fish species. Disadvantages can be their inability to combine with other inactivated antigens and their need for specific conditions (frozen or lyophilized) to maintain their efficacy during storage.

10.3.2 Non-replicating vaccines

Non-replicating (inactivated) vaccines can be based on either whole inactivated pathogens or recombinant subunits (Munang'andu *et al.*, 2014). Recombinant subunits are produced with the aid of an expression system, which can be bacteria, yeasts, plants, vertebrate cells, recombinant vertebrate or viral vectors infecting vertebrate cells. The type of expression system depends upon the level of post-translational processing (e.g., glycosylation) that is needed to produce an efficacious antigen. The choice of a subunit system can be made based upon safety aspects, even if the inactivated product is safe. Technical issues must be considered; it may simply not be possible to grow the pathogen in a production system, and molecular knowledge is needed of what component of the pathogen induces protection. Finally, the cost aspect needs evaluation because some salmonid viruses and their cell substrate grow very slowly, which can impact production cost and capacity.

In general, these types of vaccines need a high dose, or even repeated doses in combination with an adjuvant. They demand large-scale production systems with high yields at low costs. As the protection of subunit vaccines is only built upon the presence of a single antigen with few epitopes, field strain variation can have an effect on the level of protection that can be obtained with this type of vaccine. The same applies to vector vaccines which also contain transgenes that code for subunits of the pathogen they are produced to protect against.

Finally, while every type of vaccine demands specific types of antigens, the choice of a suitable production system for each specific type of vaccine also plays an important role.

10.3.3 DNA vaccines

DNA vaccination is genetic immunization that relies upon the use of a gene or genes encoding protective antigens, instead of the antigens themselves. DNA vaccines are genetic constructs containing one or more genes derived from a pathogen, and they are designed to facilitate the transient production of proteins from these genes in the vaccine with the aim of eliciting a protective immune response (Biering and Salonius, 2014). DNA vaccines are usually in the form of a purified bacterial plasmid, a circular molecule of DNA able to replicate in bacterial hosts. The constructs will contain regulatory elements to ensure both replication of the plasmid in the bacterial host for production purposes, and expression of the vaccine genes in the vaccinated animal. In some cases the nomenclature NAV (nucleic acid vaccine) or genetic vaccine is used, and those terms also include vaccines that are based upon other nucleic acids (including RNA).

10.4 DEVELOPMENT OF TESTS

Tests are developed to ensure the safety and efficacy of the product and to minimize costs and lost time in production because of early proof of deviations in the process. Tests are performed on the raw materials, the equipment and the infrastructure (e.g., environmental monitoring), the antigens, and the final product. Many of the tests are compulsory (e.g., batch safety test, batch efficacy test, inactivation control tests for an inactivated product, sterility tests, etc.). Some of the tests are internal tests intended to monitor the production process allowing for better control (e.g., glucose levels in a bioreactor in case of a batch-fed process). In all cases, test results are compared to specifications, after which predefined actions are taken. In some situations this could also mean that materials or antigens or even a vaccine is rejected. At all times, recall of a batch that has been released and is already with the customers has to be prevented.

The design of the test has to fulfil a number of constraints. Preferably tests are fast (results are obtained "live" and not retrospectively), objective (independent of the person performing the test), accurate (otherwise safety, efficacy and economics of the product could be compromised), and do not increase the cost–price of the product substantially.

10.5 TRANSFERS

One of the major challenges encountered during the transfer from research and development (R&D) to production is scaling up to the volumes that are actually used in production. Just imagine the freezing/thawing of a vial with 1 ml of antigen compared with freezing/thawing the contents of a 2000 l bioreactor (Figure 10.3). If not properly managed, the adaptations needed to ensure large-scale production could mean that authorities would consider the R&D batches and the large-scale production batches to be completely different products. Authorities therefore demand the registration batches to be at a minimum percentage of the actual scale of production.

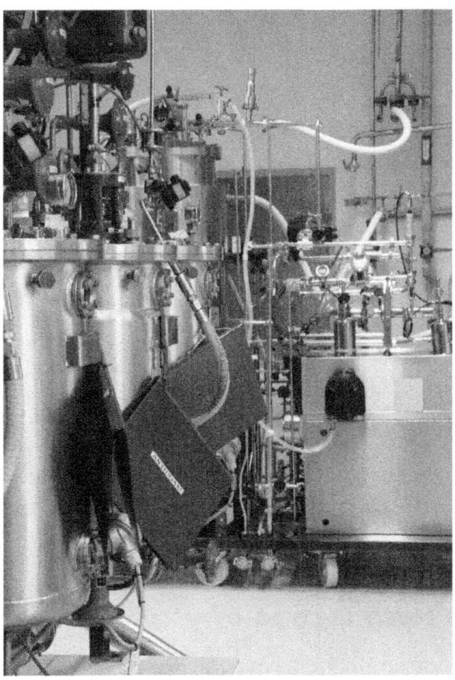

Fig. 10.3 Fermentor for production of bacterial antigens. (Source: Reproduced with permission of Pharmaq.)

The production process is documented in master manufacturing instructions (MMI), which are independent of the site of production, and the so-called batch manufacturing instructions, which are dedicated to a specific site of production. These instructions cover all the different stages of production.

Process development is a very specialized area, and is therefore often performed by so-called process development or technology support groups. These groups need to be involved early in the development of a new product to ensure that all registration experiments are performed with material equivalent to the actual product. They are often also involved in the production of batches at pilot scale and can help with the transfer of full-scale batches to production. Transfer of a product from one production site to another is also considered to be a transfer, and the process has to be validated and documented. Before transfer to production can take place, all necessary QC tests also have to be validated and transferred to the QC department. Tests performed on intermediate product during the production process, so-called in-process control (IPC) tests, are mostly performed at the site of production to avoid problems related to the transport of samples from one site to another.

10.6 MANUFACTURING

Vaccine manufacturing is a branch of the pharmaceutical industry, and a GMP-approved facility is a necessary basis for the production. Premises and equipment have to be validated for the purpose. Validation is also needed for processes, tests performed during production, and quality control tests. All these items have to be documented and approved. The concept is to prove quality and consistency of the product. Validation and training programs are important building stones in vaccine production.

10.6.1 Premises

A vaccine production plant has to be designed, planned, and constructed according to strict requirements and specifications. The aseptic area of the plant is the most critical for the product. To keep the product non-contaminated, several utility systems need to be in place, and entrances for people and materials have to be separated. Surfaces have to be without pores where contamination can build up. Air supply and ventilation have to be treated by HEPA-filters and often also moisture-treated to gain the optimum relative humidity. Clothing has to be made for the purpose of protecting the product as well as the operator. Charts for personal and material flow are important parts of GMP.

10.6.2 Production systems

In general, there are two types of production systems: adherent and in suspension. Most bacteria can grow in suspension, while most cell substrates for virus production grow adherent.

10.6.3 Production of bacterial antigens and subunits based on recombinant technology

Bacterial antigens are common components in animal and fish vaccines. Classical fermentation is often the basis for producing bacterial antigens. The antigen can be the bacteria itself or selected parts of it, or subunits (e.g., toxins). The starting point for production of a bacterial antigen is a master seed lot system where the master seed is the "mother" for all future antigens of a specific type.

Master seed (MS) can be grown on both solid and liquid growth media. The seed are stored freeze-dried/lyophilized or in stabilizing liquids and stored in ultra-freezers or in liquid nitrogen. Working seed (WS) is a further passage from the MS and is used for start-culture fermentation. The start culture could be the origin for several 1000 liters of bacteria.

The fermenter itself is traditionally a stainless steel tank where several parameters are controlled: stirring speed, dissolved oxygen, and pH. To reduce operating costs and validation work, disposable fermenters are developed; after being used once the fermenter is discharged. To reduce the contamination risk, a fermenter system is a closed system: that means no exposure to environment from inoculation to final product.

Fermentation is also the most common method when subunit antigens based on recombinant technology are produced. By genetic engineering the bacteria are modified to produce the specific protein serving as the antigen in the final vaccine. Once the production system is established, this method makes it possible to produce large amounts of antigen in a cost-effective way.

10.6.4 Virus cultivation

Since viruses are host-dependent, it is not possible to cultivate them solely in the presence of organic or inorganic nutrient medium. They can be grown only if living cells and tissues are used as culture medium. These tissues and cells act as the host for the virus under laboratory or production conditions. For this purpose, the relevant cells or tissues must be cultivated first.

There are three methods employed for virus cultivation that enable production of sufficient amounts of virus particles. Viruses can be cultivated through inoculation into animals, or in embryonated eggs. However, the standard method is production in cell cultures.

Cell cultures for virus production grow adherently. The standard production system for adherent cells is roller bottles, but lately more and more alternatives are available to allow for less open handling and better control of the culture conditions (e.g., cell factories, cell cubes and fixed bed bioreactors). An older alternative is the use of microcarriers, which allow adherent cells to be grown in conventional bioreactors. However, this system poses constraints on the volume of the bioreactors that can be used (typically 250–400 l, while suspension cells can be grown at 1000 l scale or even higher). New developments are the use of "closed systems" (e.g., tube welding) and the use of disposable systems (e.g., single-use bioreactors or SUBs). Closed systems greatly reduce the chances of contamination, while disposable systems have a positive effect on the down-time between different production runs and are less demanding on the infrastructure of the factory, which increases flexibility.

10.6.5 Inactivation

Inactivation is an essential part of the manufacturing process producing vaccines based on microorganisms. The method can impact both efficacy and safety of the vaccine. Inactivated vaccines require strict quality control to ensure that killed organisms are fully inactivated, and in this regard a validated inactivation process is required. Different methods are used: chemical, temperature and radiation methods are among these. Several parameters including concentration, temperature and duration of inactivation are central elements. Chemical agents such as formalin are commonly used, as they often maintain the structure of proteins or other biological molecular antigens that are important in developing an immune response.

10.6.6 Purification

Downstream processing includes all the purification steps required to recover or separate either bacterial or viral antigens from the culture broth. Lysis (cell disruption), homogenization (cell disruption), microfiltration (0.2–0.45 μm), ultrafiltration (<0.2 μm), diafiltration (buffer exchange), centrifugation and chromatographic purification are some of most common purification methods. A vaccine purification scheme might include one or more of these steps, depending upon the quality requirements for each specific antigen or vaccine.

Depending on the antigen, either inactivated bacterin or specific antigens, purification schemes might include simple steps such as microfiltration, centrifugation and ultrafiltration. However, if higher purity is required to reduce side-effects, further processing such as diafiltration and chromatographic purification might be included in the purification scheme.

For viral antigens released to the culture broth, either microfiltration or centrifugation might be sufficient for purification. However, if some of the media components such as fetal bovine serum or egg proteins trigger negative side-effects, further processing such as microfiltration or ultrafiltration might be required. If the viral antigen is contained within the cells, a cell disruption step (lysis or homogenization) will be included in the purification scheme. In general, downstream processing contributes to achieving a vaccine with better quality, improved stability and reduced risk of side-effects.

10.6.7 Filling, labelling and packing

For oil-based vaccines intended for injection, the product may be filled into plastic bottles or plastic type IV bags, usually containing 250–500 ml of product, or 5–10,000 single doses per unit, each single dose being 0.05 to 0.1 ml per individual fish.

Water-based injectable nucleic acid vaccines may be delivered in 250 ml plastic type IV bags or 5000 single doses per unit, each single dose being 0.05 ml per individual fish.

Immersion vaccines are water-based and typically filled into 1000 ml plastic bottles, each bottle typically sufficient for the vaccination of 20–100 kg of fish.

The bottle or bag specifications form part of the dossier information and cannot be changed without approval from the licensing authorities/medicines agency.

Each unit of vaccine will be labeled with an approved label containing information about the product and the producer, including batch number, storing conditions, shelf life, dose and fish size, and then packed into an outer container which is also labelled in accordance with the approved dossier. Any change in the label must be approved by the licensing authority.

10.6.8 Quality control and release

Throughout the production process and when the production is finalized, tests are performed to confirm compliance with the requirements of GMP. The final product is tested to confirm that the chemical and physical parameters are within the specification described in the dossier, and that the product meets the claims for potency and safety. Provided the product meets all requirements, a batch release certificate will be issued by the Qualified Person (Directives 2001/82 EC and 2001/83 EC). This is necessary to allow the sale and use of the product as indicated.

A batch release certificate will contain all details about the manufacture of the antigens, inactivation details, blending and formulation data and final product testing.

Final product testing for an oil-based injection vaccine may include, but not be restricted to:

(1) Inactivation, to ensure that the antigens are fully inactivated unless the product is designed as a live or attenuated vaccine.
(2) Safety, to ensure that there are no abnormal local or systemic reactions directly attributed to the vaccine.
(3) Appearance of the final product.
(4) Fill volume.
(5) Sterility, to ensure that there is no extraneous bacteria and/or fungi.
(6) Potency for each antigen in the vaccine to show consistent production.
(7) Residual formaldehyde, to show that rest concentration is below the level to be considered safe (<0.05%).
(8) Viscosity for the final product measured as cP.
(9) Particle size for the final product measured in μm.
(10) Miscibility to confirm that the product has formed a water-in-oil emulsion.

REFERENCES

Biering, E. and Salonius, K. 2014. DNA vaccines, in *Fish Vaccination* (eds R. Gudding, A. Lillehaug and Ø. Evensen). Oxford, John Wiley & Sons, Ltd., 47–55.

Commission Directive 91/412/EEC of 23 July 1991 laying down the principles and guidelines of good manufacturing practice for veterinary medicinal products. *Official Journal L* **228**, 17/8/1991, p. 70–73.

EU Directive 2001/82/EC, as amended (Veterinary Medicines).

European Pharmacopoeia. Available at http://www.edqm.eu/en/european-pharmacopoeia-publications-1401.html [accessed 10 April 2013].

GMP Guidelines, Eudralex vol. 4. Available at http://ec.europa.eu/health/documents/eudralex/vol-4/index_en.htm [accessed 10 April 2013].

Holm, A., Rippke, B. and Noda, K. 2014. Legal requirements and authorisation of fish vaccines, in *Fish Vaccination* (eds R. Gudding, A. Lillehaug and Ø. Evensen). Oxford, John Wiley & Sons, Ltd., 128–139.

Munang'andu, H., Mutoloki, S. and Evensen, Ø. 2014. Non-replicating vaccines, in *Fish Vaccination* (eds R. Gudding, A. Lillehaug and Ø. Evensen). Oxford, John Wiley & Sons, Ltd., 22–32.

Shoemaker, C.A. and Klesius, P.H. 2014. Replicating vaccines, in *Fish Vaccination* (eds R. Gudding, A. Lillehaug and Ø. Evensen). Oxford, John Wiley & Sons, Ltd., 33–46.

11 Legal Requirements and Authorization of Fish Vaccines

Anja Holm[1], Byron E. Rippke[2] and Ken Noda[3]

[1]Danish Health and Medicines Authority, Copenhagen, Denmark
[2]Center for Veterinary Biologics, USDA, Ames, Iowa, USA
[3]Food Safety and Consumer Affairs Bureau, Ministry of Agriculture, Forestry and Fisheries, Tokyo, Japan

ABSTRACT

A vaccine for fish must have an authorization from the competent authority of the country or region where it is to be used. The legislation, requirements and involved regulatory bodies for authorization and use may vary, and the precise rules and advice for a specific country should be sought from the relevant competent authority prior to any use or trade.

11.1 INTRODUCTION

Vaccines for humans and animals are defined as medicinal products, and they must go through a similar procedure for marketing authorization as therapeutic medicines. Vaccination may interfere with health programs for eradication and control of specific infectious diseases, and hence there may be rules governing the use of a vaccine in countries where a disease is absent or subject to control measures. Vaccines are normally used on prescription from a veterinarian or another qualified and authorized person, such as a fish health biologist in Norway. Vaccines are traded internationally, and in some regions, such as Europe, the requirements have been harmonized for many years by common legal directives. The central elements are the procedures for applications for marketing authorization and the system for inspection and authorization of manufacturers. An application for a marketing authorization consists of detailed descriptions of the production and control of the product and full documentation of relevant studies to evaluate the safety and efficacy of the vaccine.

11.2 MANUFACTURER AUTHORIZATION

A vaccine manufacturer must have a valid authorization for production, which is issued by the competent authority of the country where it is located. This requires detailed documentation of

anh@dkma.dk

Fish Vaccination, First Edition. Edited by Roar Gudding, Atle Lillehaug and Øystein Evensen.

the production process and – in the EU – that the international standard Good Manufacturing Practice (GMP) is followed (GMP Guidelines, Eudralex Vol. 4). The authorization must be renewed periodically. Inspections of the factory and all connected sites and processes may be performed by the competent authority at regular intervals or on request from other authorities. The inspection authorities from several regions of the world collaborate formally and exchange inspection reports and results.

11.2.1 Considerations for design of studies

(*Examples adapted from Guideline on the design of studies to evaluate the safety and efficacy of fish vaccines, EMA/CVMP/IWP/314550/2010*)

The legal basis for the guideline is EU Directive 2001/82/EC, as amended, and in particular Annex I thereof, Directive 2010/63/EC (regarding the protection of animals used for scientific purposes) and the relevant European Pharmacopoeia (Ph. Eur.) monographs (e.g., Ph. Eur. 0062, 5.2.6 and 5.2.7). Guidance on quality requirements for fish vaccines is outlined in the general guideline EMA/CVMP/IWP/206555/2010: *Requirements for the production and control of immunological veterinary medicinal products.*

In principle the results of all studies should be applicable, irrespective of where they are carried out; however, the applicant should take into account the various conditions (e.g., climatic, disease situation, water temperature, and salinity) as these may influence the outcome of the studies. The range of species, ages, sizes, weights and physiological status (e.g., smoltification, sexual maturation) of fish used in the studies must be representative of those to which the vaccine will be administered in the field for commercial purposes. For laboratory studies, fish of the minimum recommended vaccination age or size should be used, as this will eventually be expressed in the product information. Fish used in studies should preferably be derived from stock which will be used commercially.

The number of fish in the vaccinated and control groups should be sufficient to obtain statistically significant and clinically reliable results. However, for vaccination-challenge studies, the possibility of reducing the number of control non-vaccinated fish should be investigated as these fish will suffer disease and associated distress. If a pharmacopoiea monograph exists for the type of vaccine, these requirements must also be considered and complied with, as appropriate. The allocation of fish to vaccinated and control groups should be done randomly, using an appropriate method. In all tests, the vaccine and control should be administered in the same manner, and control fish should be handled identically to vaccinated fish.

If vaccinated and control fish are not housed in the same tank, to overcome tank effects that may be experienced between groups of fish which are kept under identical conditions but in different tanks, measures should be taken; for example, a minimum of two tanks could be used for each of the vaccinated and control groups. Effects of stocking density on the parameters to be determined should be taken into consideration.

Water quality parameters, such as temperature and salinity (e.g., freshwater versus seawater), used in each laboratory study during vaccination should be relevant to the environment under which the vaccine will be used for commercial purposes. Some studies may need to be performed at both high and low temperatures for the relevant fish species/disease distribution. Similarly, some studies may need to be performed following the main production practices for the species.

The vaccine formulation to be administered in the safety and efficacy studies should be the final formulation proposed for marketing, and the use of formulations that differ must be thoroughly justified. Dose, administration route and amount must represent the intended commercial use. The parameters evaluated should be appropriate to the proposed indications (including onset and duration of immunity claims, if relevant to the study design) and should be predetermined prior to conducting the studies.

The challenge model used in each study must be justified by the investigator and the relevance to the natural disease situation should be discussed. Items to be considered include: the relevance of the challenge organism(s) to the disease(s) against which protection is claimed; the method of administration of the challenge organism (e.g., cohabitant, injection, etc.); the water temperature; and the timings of (i) the challenge and (ii) the recording of the evaluation parameters.

To account for the fish being poikilothermic animals and taking into account the fact that immunity in fish is temperature-dependent and that the frequency and intensity of injection site reactions increases with higher water temperatures, comparative data from safety and efficacy laboratory studies involving fish should be based on "degree-days". Degree-days is the multiplication of water temperature in Celsius and number of days: 10°C for 5 days = 50 degree-days.

It is important to take into account the possible adverse effects of vaccine administration on development over the life-span of the target fish species. This is particularly important in the case of parenteral vaccines, as adhesions may have a negative effect on spawning, and adhesions/pigmentation/lesions may result in rejection or downgrading of fish at slaughter (Evensen *et al.*, 2005).

Data from well-controlled laboratory studies are preferred wherever relevant models are available, and field studies should serve to confirm the findings from the controlled studies. However, it is recognized that for some disease situations in fish, no (or only poor) challenge models exist. In such situations, with appropriate justification, more emphasis may be placed upon field studies conducted under conditions that reflect the disease situation in the field. The scope of the field studies is to ensure that the vaccine is efficacious and safe in the diversified conditions for aquaculture found in member states for the relevant fish species.

Records on the source of fish and the disease history in different pens or tanks must be kept. Previous medication, use of chemicals and vaccines should be known. Daily records of outbreaks of disease, mortality and medication are required, as well as known and stable management practice concerning, for example. hygiene, feeding, handling and use of feed additives and chemicals. Normally, data from both laboratory and full-scale field studies will be required. Where appropriate, the applicant should justify the lack of relevant data.

Development and testing of a new fish vaccine requires many experiments and trials. The number of fish used in laboratory and field studies for development of a vaccine and for later batch release of the vaccine is high, although the fish used in field studies would be vaccinated anyway. According to a report from the Norwegian Veterinary Institute, the number of fish may be reduced significantly (Ellingsen and Gudding, 2011). This can be done by combining experiments or substituting some of the experiments with *in vitro* tests, for example by measuring antigens responsible for protective immunity by an ELISA test (Romstad *et al.*, 2012), or by selecting the statistical methods carefully. Many authorities and guiding or governing bodies, including the European Pharmacopoeia, the International Cooperation on Harmonisation of Technical Requirements for Registration of Veterinary Medicinal Products (VICH) and the European Center for the Validation of Alternative Methods (ECVAM) encourage Three Rs approaches (Midtlyng *et al.*, 2011), but such methods must be properly validated to ensure the intended accuracy of information.

In the EU, directive 2010/63/EEC on the protection of animals used for scientific purposes will soon enter into force and make considerations on Three Rs obligatory.

11.3 FOOD SAFETY – MAXIMUM RESIDUE LIMITS

Vaccination of production animals may also have an influence on the quality of the food products derived from these animals. In some regions there are rules about product quality from agricultural or fishery authorities. Vaccines with adjuvants that give severe injection site reactions may cause reduced quality of the meat, potentially leading to downgrading at slaughter (Aunsmo *et al.*, 2008). For all veterinary medicines, including vaccines, administered to food-producing animals, the amount of residues remaining in edible tissues of the animal at slaughter must be below a set limit to ensure that there will be no harmful effect to the consumer. Such maximum residue limits (MRLs) are set for all pharmacologically active substances and excipients, but immunological antigens are exempted. For vaccines it would typically be excipients, adjuvants or preservatives present in the final product that would require that MRLs are set, or there is an evaluation concluding that no MRL is needed for consumer protection. In the EU, MRLs are set by the European Medicines Agency (EMA). Procedures for establishing worldwide agreed MRLs are led by the Codex Alimentarius. Internationally agreed MRLs are important to avoid trade barriers based upon differences in the acceptable residue levels in foodstuffs.

Most vaccines have no withdrawal period, that is, the withdrawal period is set to 0 days, because they present no risk for the consumer. The need for withdrawal periods is, however, evaluated by the competent authority for each individual product, and withdrawal periods > 0 days may be set for specific vaccines.

11.4 GENETICALLY MODIFIED ORGANISMS

Some vaccines contain genetically modified organisms (GMOs). In the EU such vaccines must be authorized for the entire European Union via the European Medicines Agency, and cannot be authorized by a national competent authority (see Figure 11.1). National competent authorities may, however, grant permission for clinical trials of such vaccines. There are several veterinary GMO vaccines authorized and marketed in EU, for example against influenza in horses and leukemia in cats. The authorization procedure involves the environmental agencies of the EU and EEA in accordance with Directive 2001/18/EEC (deliberate release of GMOs) in combination with the usual assessment of quality, safety and efficacy of the vaccine. The main aim of this directive is to make the procedure for granting consent for the deliberate release and placing on the market of GMOs more efficient and more transparent, to limit such consent to a period of ten years (renewable), and to introduce compulsory monitoring after GMOs have been placed on the market. It also provides for a common methodology to assess case-by-case the risks for the environment associated with the release of GMOs. Public consultation and GMO labeling are made compulsory under this directive. The objective of an environmental risk assessment is to identify and evaluate potential adverse effects of the GMO, either direct or indirect, immediate or delayed, upon human health and the environment, which the deliberate release or the placing on the market of GMOs may have.

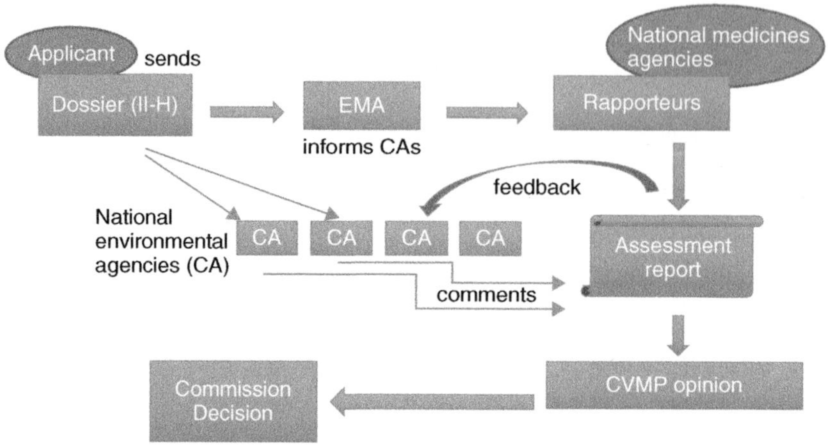

Fig. 11.1 The EU procedure for the environmental assessment of a vaccine containing a genetically modified organism (GMO).

11.5 DNA VACCINES

DNA vaccines, where bacterial plasmid DNA encoding for a relevant antigen is injected into an animal, are not defined as GMOs, but go through an ordinary authorization process. There are, however, several technical and safety-related issues, where DNA vaccines need special consideration compared with conventional vaccines (Holm, 2004). Moreover, in some regions a discussion is ongoing as to whether DNA-vaccinated animals must be classified as GMOs. There is an urgent need to define whether certain requirements must be fulfilled during the authorization process of the DNA vaccine, in order to avoid the vaccinated animal being considered to be a GMO and thereby falling under the above-mentioned directive (2001/18/EEC).

For fish, a DNA vaccine has been authorized in Canada against infectious hematopoietic necrosis virus (IHNV) (Canadian Food Inspection Agency, 2005; Salonius *et al.*, 2007).

11.6 PROHIBITION OF USE OF CERTAIN VACCINES

Many regions have control and surveillance programs for diseases that are absent or eradicated from their territory. In fish, bacterial kidney disease (BKD) and infectious pancreatic necrosis (IPN) are regulated in several countries. If a control program is installed, vaccination against the disease will also be strictly regulated by the competent authority. This means that even if a vaccine has a marketing authorization in a specific country, certain restrictions on the use of the vaccine – or a prohibition of use – may apply (e.g., Directive 2001/82, art. 71). Always consult the competent authority prior to the start of a new vaccination scheme.

11.7 USE OF VACCINES THAT ARE NOT AUTHORIZED

If there is a need to use a vaccine to control a disease and there is no authorized vaccine against this disease in the country, many regions and/or countries have special rules for exemption, or license under certain conditions. Many smaller markets may experience a lack of available products to control the diseases in the fish farms. It is very important that a flexible system is in place, so disease outbreaks can be avoided for the benefit of animal welfare and production. Normally, the responsible veterinarian must apply to the competent authority and submit the reasons for the requests and information about the intended vaccine to be used.

11.8 AUTOGENOUS VACCINES

Autogenous vaccines may be defined as inactivated immunological veterinary medicinal products that are manufactured from pathogens and antigens obtained from an animal or animals from a holding, and used for the treatment of that animal or the animals of that holding in the same locality. In the EU these are regulated under national law (i.e., not European law), and permission to produce or use such autogenous vaccines must be obtained from the national competent authority. In fish, immunization with bacterial antigens has been used against a number of infections, for example, streptococci and related organisms (Bercovier *et al.*, 1997).

11.9 REGIONAL RULES AND COMPETENT AUTHORITIES

Each region of the world has its own rules, procedures and authorities. The regulatory structure and guidelines are normally openly available at the websites of the national or regional authority. VICH and its outreach initiative are seeking to harmonize the requirements for authorization of medicines. VICH is a trilateral (EU–Japan–US) program aimed at harmonizing technical requirements for veterinary product registration, with Australia, Canada and New Zealand participating as observers. Its full title is the International Cooperation on Harmonisation of Technical Requirements for Registration of Veterinary Medicinal Products. VICH was officially launched in April 1996, and in 2011 the Outreach Initiative was adopted, where VICH encourages the wider harmonization of registration requirements and efficient use of resources in regions/countries that are not members of VICH.

VICH guidelines provide harmonized guidance that describes the data to be provided in an application dossier for a marketing authorization for a veterinary medicinal product. VICH also establishes guidelines on pharmacovigilance for veterinary medicinal products, that is, monitoring of their post-marketing safety and continued efficacy. However, VICH does not normally develop guidance on how to carry out the assessment of the data or on the assessment approach. Assessments are done by the regulatory authorities of the VICH countries and regions. When a VICH guideline is finally adopted, it supersedes the existing regional guidelines.

11.10 THE EUROPEAN UNION AND CONNECTED EEA COUNTRIES

The European Network consists of the European Medicines Agency (EMA) and National Competent Authorities (NCAs) from all 27 member states and three EEA countries (Norway, Iceland and Leichtenstein).

The EMA is in charge of the centralized procedures, the referral procedures and the MRL evaluations, and houses the central scientific committee, CVMP (Committee for Medicinal Products for Veterinary Use) with its working parties. The NCAs are responsible for their national market, and provides experts for the work of EMA and all the authorization procedures. In many NCAs both human and veterinary medicines are handled, and often both pharmaceutical and immunological products. However, there are also countries where human and veterinary medicines have separate authorities, and countries where the responsibility for pharmaceutical medicines and immunological products is split.

11.10.1 Procedures

The centralized procedure leads to an authorization that is valid in all member states and EEA countries (Figure 11.2). The marketing application is sent to EMA, which coordinates the scientific evaluation performed by CVMP. CVMP consists of one member per EU (+EEA) member state, and some additional elected members with special expertise. Each CVMP member coordinates with national experts on the specific field. The scientific opinion from CVMP is sent to the European Commission, which formally issues the marketing authorization in the EU. It is, however, possible subsequently to prohibit the use of a vaccine in a country, if a documented surveillance and control program for the relevant disease is in place.

The *decentralized procedure* (DCP) is used for new vaccines, where the manufacturer cannot or will not use the centralized procedure, and is valid only in those countries that are included in the procedure (two to all countries). One country acts as reference member state and performs the primary assessment, while other concerned member states may ask additional questions or conditions.

The *mutual recognition procedure* (MRP) is based upon an existing authorization for a vaccine in one member state (reference member state/RMS) within the EU/EEA. The concerned member states (one to all countries) are asked to accept the assessment and authorization of the RMS and issue similar authorizations for the product. For both DCP and MRP, the member states usually manage to find an agreement on the authorization application, so indications, proposed use and conditions can be accepted for the product and harmonized authorizations can be issued in the countries. If no agreement can be reached, the application is referred to

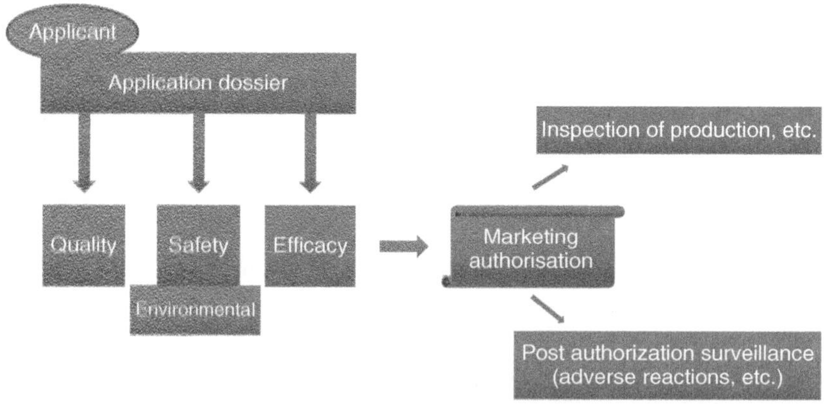

Fig. 11.2 Authorization of vaccines.

CVMP, which issues a scientific opinion on the issues of dispute. The European Commission and member states adopt a legally binding decision based upon the CVMP opinion, and all member states must comply with this.

A national procedure in only one country is also possible, and is handled and issued by the relevant NCA.

11.10.2 The European pharmacopoeia

The European Pharmacopoeia (Ph. Eur.) is an organization under the European Council with more than 50 participating countries. Its primary task is harmonization of the rules for production and control of medicines. Ph. Eur. issues monographs for many different vaccines, including many against serious animal diseases. Monographs exist only for some vaccines against fish diseases. In the EU, compliance with relevant Ph. Eur. monographs is part of the legal requirements for authorization.

The requirement for target animal batch safety tests has been deleted by the Ph. Eur in 2012 (coming into effect in 2013), although submission of such data is still a requirement for the regions participating in the VICH. Target animal batch safety tests may otherwise be waived by the regulatory authority when a sufficient number of consecutive production batches have been produced and found to comply with the test, thus demonstrating consistency of the manufacturing process (VICH GL50, draft 2011). It is expected that the regional requirements will be amended in the coming years.

11.10.3 Scientific advice

EMA/CVMP has established a veterinary Scientific Advice Working Party (SAWP-v), which gives advice to manufacturers and marketing authorization to applicants on specific requests related to the development of vaccines. The advice typically relates to the design of studies on scientific areas where no guidance is issued, or where existing guidance seems not relevant or unclear for the particular product. Applicants may contact EMA for further information on the procedures, fees, and special conditions for small- and medium-sized enterprises.

11.10.4 Minor use and minor species (MUMS)

CVMP has developed a specific guideline for vaccines for "Minor Use and Minor Species" (MUMS), or so called limited markets (EMA/CVMP/IWP/123243/2006). For most fish species and diseases, vaccines are needed, but the market potential may be so small that companies may have difficulties getting return on their investment. For such products, requirements may be relaxed or some of the scientific data can be submitted following the introduction of the product to the market. There may also be a possibility to get free scientific advice (Quigley, 2012). EMA's website displays useful documents in this respect, such as the latest list of MUMS designations and a gap analysis for diseases/species for which a vaccine is needed.

11.11 UNITED STATES OF AMERICA

In the US, the regulatory authority for veterinary vaccines is the US Department of Agriculture's (USDA) Center for Veterinary Biologics (CVB). CVB draws its authorities from the

Virus, Serum, Toxin Act (VSTA), which was originally passed and signed into law in March 1913. It regulated the sale and distribution of veterinary biological products moving in interstate commerce. In 1985, the VSTA was amended, bringing the sale and distribution of all veterinary biologics produced in the US under the authority of the CVB and establishing a single national regulatory framework. It is important to note that in the US, veterinary biological products fall under the regulatory authority of the USDA, and veterinary pharmaceutical products are regulated by the Food and Drug Administration.

11.11.1 Procedures

The Virus, Serum, Toxin Act makes it unlawful to sell or distribute, either within or from the US, veterinary biological products that are considered to be worthless, dangerous, contaminated, or harmful. Additionally, it requires that products that are sold or distributed must be prepared in a USDA-licensed facility, and in compliance with all USDA requirements. These requirements are documented in the Title 9 Code of Federal Regulations, Veterinary Services Memoranda, and Veterinary Biologics Notices. These regulations and documents work in concert to ensure that products produced and sold in or from the US are pure, safe, potent, and effective.

Once an application and the supporting material are received by the CVB, requirements for veterinary vaccines include multiple evaluations of various aspects of the product pre-licensing. This involves a series of steps that satisfactorily demonstrate the purity, safety, potency, and efficacy of the product. In general terms, this involves the following:

- A demonstration of the purity and identity of the seed and cell line used in producing the immunogen.
- Development of a consistent, well-controlled vaccine production process.
- Demonstration of efficacy, where efficacy generally reflects the prevention or mitigation of clinical disease in the host animal, supporting all intended label claims.
- Determination of adjuvant safety (if applicable) and withdrawal time requirements (for food animals).
- Demonstration of safety in the host animal in a full-scale field trial setting at multiple locations and under a variety of animal husbandry conditions.
- Validation of a potency assay that measures the potency of serials of vaccine.
- Successful production of commercial-scale serials of vaccine (Pre-licensing Serials).
- The licensing of aquaculture vaccines follows this same basic framework.
- After all of these requirements have been successfully completed, the manufacturer is granted a Biological Product license.

11.11.2 Types of product licenses/permits

The CVB grants several different licenses or permits for products, and they all are useful in meeting a variety of animal health needs.

Full biological product license. Products granted this type of license are licensed either with or without restrictions in distribution, and have met all applicable USDA requirements for purity, safety, potency and efficacy.

Conditional license. Products granted this type of license are licensed, often with some distribution restrictions, and have met all requirements for safety and purity, and have demonstrated an "expectation of efficacy". These products are generally licensed with the intent that they will achieve full licensure. What constitutes an expectation of efficacy is dependent upon the organism used in the product. This type of license is useful for responding to emerging disease situations, niche needs, or special circumstances within the marketplace.

Autogenous license. This type of license is granted for inactivated products intended for use in the herd, flock, or group of origin. They are intended to be used under the direction of a veterinarian or a person of appropriate expertise.

Biological product permit. This type of permit is issued to products produced outside of the US and imported for sale and distribution. They meet all of the USDA requirements for licensure, and have been deemed not to pose a risk to US animal health. The permit is issued to a responsible official located within the US at a quarantine facility, and not directly to the foreign manufacturer.

11.12 JAPAN

In Japan, medicinal products for human and veterinary use are under the regulation of Pharmaceutical Affairs Law (Law No. 145, 1960). The law is intended to provide regulations required to ensure the quality, efficacy and safety of drugs, quasi-drugs, cosmetics and medical devices at each stage of development, manufacturing, importing, marketing, retailing and usage. Subsequent Ministerial Ordinances specifically applied for veterinary medical products (VMPs) have been established by the Minister of Agriculture, Forestry and Fisheries (MAFF), and relating regulations and guidelines are also provided in accordance with the Ordinances. A person who is intending to distribute VMPs shall obtain marketing approval for each product from MAFF. The Animal Products Safety Division, Food Safety and Consumer Affairs Bureau, is responsible for establishment/amendment of the Ministerial Ordinances and relating Notifications. The National Veterinary Assay Laboratory (NVAL) is responsible for reviewing the application dossier for approval and establishment of guidelines for the applicants.

An application for approval of a new VMP undergoes an investigation by a committee of the Pharmaceutical Affairs Sub-Council (PASC), specialized in the category of the product (biologicals, antibiotics, general medicine, etc.). Ususally, fish-related VMPs are subject to the Committee on Aquaculture Products. VMPs intended for use in food-producing animals are also investigated for their residue in food by the Committee on Residue of Veterinary Drugs. The application is further subjected to a deliberation by the executive committee of the PASC. Additionally, VMPs for food-producing animals shall be assessed for safety to human health by the Food Safety Commission and, when required, maximum residue limits must be established for the concerned tissues by the Minister of Health, Labour and Welfare, prior to the approval.

The data required for approval of fish vaccines vary depending on the status of the products. For example, in the case of products containing new active ingredients, the applicant is required to submit a full dossier including: origin and history of development; physical, chemical and biological properties; manufacturing process; indications, effects, and potency; administration and dosage; stability; target animal safety; pharmacological action; and clinical trials. In the case of adjuvant-containing vaccines, a residue depletion study may also be required. Data for target animal safety shall meet the requirements of Ministerial Ordinance of Good Laboratory Practice (GLP) (Ordinance No. 74, 1997), and data for clinical trial are recommended to meet the requirements of Ministerial Ordinance of Good Clinical Practice (GCP) (Ordinance No.

75, 1997). Furthermore, it shall be confirmed that the manufacturing control and the quality control in a process complies with Good Manufacturing Practice (GMP) standards specified by the Ministerial Ordinance (Ordinance No. 18, 1994).

11.13 OTHER RELEVANT ORGANIZATIONS: OIE, FAO, WHO

In addition to the rules given by competent authorities, other relevant organizations have recommendations or rules for use and registration of vaccines.

The World Organization for Animal Health (OIE), with more than 170 member countries, works for global control of animal diseases. The OIE plays a very important role in the international harmonization of rules for veterinary work, eradication programs for serious animal diseases, reference laboratories, and authorization and use of veterinary medicines. OIE has issued the *OIE Aquatic Animal Health Code, 2011*, and the *Manual for Diagnostic Tests for Aquatic Animals*, which can be accessed online.

The Food and Agriculture Organization (FAO) is involved in vaccination programs against animal diseases, especially in developing countries.

The World Health Organization (WHO) is engaged in combating zoonoses, for example in relation to the development of avian influenza vaccines. The WHO also cooperates with the International Association of Biological Standardization, which mainly works with human vaccines, although they have organized international conferences on fish vaccination in Oslo in 1996 and Bergen in 2003.

REFERENCES

Aunsmo, A., Guttvik, A., Midtlyng, P.J., *et al.*, 2008. Association of spinal deformity and vaccine-induced abdominal lesions in harvest-sized Atlantic salmon, *Salmo salar* L. *J Fish Dis* **31**: 515–24.

Bercovier, H., Ghittino, C. and Eldar, A. 1997. Immunization with bacterial antigens: infections with streptococci and related organisms. *Dev Biol (Basel)* **90**: 153–60.

Canadian Food Inspection Agency. 2005. *DNA vaccine*. Available at http://epe.lac-bac.gc.ca/100/206/301/cfia-acia/2011-09-21/www.inspection.gc.ca/english/anima/vetbio/eaee/vbeaihnve.shtml [accessed 22 May 2013].

Codex alimentarius. Available at http://www.codexalimentarius.net/web/index_en.jsp [accessed 22 May 2013].

Ellingsen, K. and Gudding, R. 2011. The potential to increase use of the 3Rs in the development and validation of fish vaccines. Available at http://www.norecopa.no/norecopa/vedlegg/Rapporten---final.pdf

European Medicines Agency. http://www.ema.europa.eu/ema/ [accessed 22 May 2013].

EU Directive 2001/18/EC (Genetically Modified Organisms), EU Directive 2001/82/EC, as amended (Veterinary Medicines), EU Directive 2004/28/EC (Veterinary Medicines), EU Directive 2009/9/EC (technical requirements, = Amended annex 1 of Directive 2001/82/EC), and EU Directive 2010/63/EC (protection of test animals). Available at http://ec.europa.eu/health/documents/eudralex/vol-5/index_en.htm [accessed 22 May 2013].

European Pharmacopoeia. http://www.edqm.eu/en/european-pharmacopoeia-publications-1401.html [accessed 22 May 2013].

Evensen, Ø., Brudeseth, B. and Mutoloki, S. 2005. The vaccine formulation and its role in inflammatory processes in fish – effects and adverse effects. *Dev Biol (Basel)* **121**: 117–25.

EudraLex, Vol. 4: Good manufacturing practice (GMP) guidelines. Available at http://ec.europa.eu/health/documents/eudralex/vol-4/index_en.htm [accessed 22 May 2013].

EMA Guideline on the design of studies to evaluate the safety and efficacy of fish vaccines (EMA/CVMP/IWP/314550/2010). Available at http://www.ema.europa.eu/ema/pages/includes/document/open_document.jsp?webContentId=WC500118226 [accessed 22 May 2013].

Food and Agriculture Organization. http://www.fao.org/fishery/en [accessed 22 May 2013].

Guideline on requirements for the production and control of immunological veterinary medicinal products (EMA/CVMP/IWP/206555/2010, consultation). Available at http://www.ema.europa.eu/ema/pages/includes/document/open_document.jsp?webContentId=WC500104492 [accessed 22 May 2013].

Holm, A. 2004. *DNA-vaccines for food-producing animals. Technical review and discussion of safety issues.* Available at http://www.dfvf.dk/Admin/Public/Download.aspx?file=Files%2FFiler%2FPublikationer%2FDNA-vaccines_report_-_Final1.doc [accessed 22 May 2013].

Japanese authorisation procedures: *Outline of Regulation System of Veterinary Drugs in Japan.* Available at http://www.maff.go.jp/nval/english/ [accessed 22 May 2013].

Midtlyng, P.J., Hendriksen, C., Balks, E., *et al.*, 2011. Three Rs approaches in the production and quality control of fish vaccines. *Biologicals* **39**: 117–28.

OIE (World Organization for Animal Health). http://www.oie.int/international-standard-setting/terrestrial-manual/access-online/ [accessed 22 May 2013].

Quigley, K. 2012. Veterinary medicines: what is the MUMS/limited markets policy? *Regulatory Rapporteur* **9**: 8–9.

Romstad, A.B., Reitan, L.J., Midtlyng, P., *et al.*, 2012. Development of an antibody ELISA for potency testing of furunculosis (*Aeromonas salmonicida* subsp *salmonicida*) vaccines in Atlantic salmon (*Salmo salar* L). *Biologicals* **40**: 67–71.

Salonius, K., Simard, N., Harland, R. and Ulmer, J.B. 2007. The road to licensure of a DNA vaccine. *Curr Opin Invest Drugs* **8**: 635–41.

VICH website and guidelines. Available at http://www.vichsec.org/ [accessed 22 May 2013].

World Health Organization. http://www.who.int/about/en/ [accessed 22 May 2013].

12 Vaccination Strategies and Procedures

Atle Lillehaug

Norwegian Veterinary Institute, Oslo, Norway

ABSTRACT

Successful vaccination depends upon both the development of protective vaccines and their correct use. In addition to deciding which diseases to vaccinate against, the choice of vaccination method, the timing of vaccination, and the use of revaccination must be considered. For optimal protection, vaccination should be carried out some time before exposure to the actual pathogen, in order to give immunity sufficient time to develop. On the other hand, vaccination should not be carried out too early, as the degree of immunity declines with time. Water temperature may be an important factor when deciding when to vaccinate, as well as the size of fish, being the major parameter regulating the development of immuno-competence.

The overall aim of vaccination in aquaculture is to increase economic output by reducing losses due to disease, including expenses for medication and other costs, weighed up against the costs of vaccination. In general, vaccination by injection is most expensive, due to the extensive amount of work involved. However, the method gives superior protection. Vaccines can also be administered successfully by immersion, but due to the resulting lower levels of immunity, the outcome may be poorer, and the need for a booster vaccination may be greater when such a method is used. As regards vaccines with adjuvants, administration by injection is the only option.

If costs of vaccines, vaccination labour and side-effects are balanced against potential losses due to the actual disease in question, only a minor reduction in mortality in vaccinated fish will weigh up for the vaccination expenses. In fact, higher costs of vaccine and vaccination procedures, providing higher levels of protection against disease, may often be economically profitable when employed in valuable fish species.

atle.lillehaug@vetinst.no

Fish Vaccination, First Edition. Edited by Roar Gudding, Atle Lillehaug and Øystein Evensen.

12.1 INTRODUCTION

Optimal vaccination requires both the development of effective vaccines and their correct use. The term "vaccination strategy" includes the decision as to which diseases to vaccinate against, as well as the choice of vaccination procedure (Lillehaug, 1997). Vaccination procedure covers the choice of vaccine type and vaccination method, the timing of vaccination in relation to production cycle, water temperature and fish size, as well as the use of revaccination. These parameters are closely linked, and one cannot be settled without account being taken of the others.

An optimal vaccination strategy aims at protecting the fish against specific infections that are causing problems in the farm or the region in question. The level of protective immunity achieved should be adequate to overcome the infectious pressure, and should be highest when the risk of disease outbreak is greatest. Protection should last throughout the entire period of risk. In addition, the vaccination strategy should take into account the costs related to vaccination and the risk of side-effects. Overall, the vaccination strategy should aim at achieving a favorable solution, economically for the fish-farming industry, as well as from an animal welfare point of view.

12.2 TIMING OF VACCINATION

In order to achieve a protective immune response, the fish has to be immunocompetent at the time of vaccination. After vaccination, the curve for development of immunity follows a typical pattern, some time being taken before immunity reaches the level needed for protection, and before maximum protection is reached. The level of immunity then starts to decline after some time, and eventually drops below the limit for protection. The time needed for immunity to develop, the maximum level of protection, and duration of immunity will depend upon various factors, including water temperature, as well as the vaccination procedure used and characteristics of the vaccine product (i.e., inactivated or attenuated, use of adjuvant, etc.).

The vaccination strategy chosen must also be compatible with the production cycle of the fish species, ideally being done in due time before potential exposure to the actual pathogenic microorganism. Intensive aquaculture production systems are often split into two distinct phases. The first, including hatching, start-feeding and the first growth period, takes place under controlled conditions in tank systems with limited use of water, which makes it possible to control the introduction of pathogens (i.e., disinfection systems). Vaccination should be carried out during this period, prior to the following phase, grow-out in ponds or net-pens. For anadromous species, like salmonids, vaccination against pathogens in the marine environment should be carried out during the freshwater phase (Press and Lillehaug, 1995).

For some aquaculture productions, polyvalent vaccines against several infections constitute the dominant option for vaccination strategy, aiming at protecting the fish against several diseases after only a single operation of vaccination. Effective Atlantic salmon production is based on the use of oil-adjuvanted vaccines against several infectious agents, which allow the vaccination procedure to be limited to one injection only during the freshwater phase. This sole operation induces high levels of protection that last throughout the entire growth period in seawater. For the Norwegian market, all such vaccines contain *Vibrio anguillarum* serovars O1 and O2, *Vibrio salmonicida* and *Aeromonas salmonicida*, and they may also include *Moritella viscosa* and *Infectious pancreatic necrosis virus* (IPNV).

12.3 WATER TEMPERATURE

It is well known that the environment, including water temperature, influences the function of the immune system and the immune response of fish (Bowden, 2008). Previously, it was recommended to vaccinate fish, including salmonids, at relatively high temperatures, in order to avoid the potentially impaired immune response at low environmental temperatures (Bly and Clem, 1992). However, when relating to cold-water anadromous fish species, like salmonids, ambient water temperature may rise only very shortly before the time of sea transfer in the spring, and smoltification may have started when temperatures are going up. During this phase, the fish are vulnerable to handling (Eggset *et al.*, 1999), and the response to vaccination may be adversely affected (Maule *et al.*, 1987). Due to this conflict, clinical studies were carried out with Atlantic salmon on the relationship between water temperature, immune response, timing of vaccination, and protection achieved. Fingerlings were vaccinated against cold-water vibriosis at various water temperatures from 2–10°C, and challenged at different time intervals after vaccination (Lillehaug *et al.*, 1993). The results demonstrated that vaccination of Atlantic salmon against cold-water vibriosis may be performed at low water temperatures; there were even tendencies towards higher levels of protection in groups of fish vaccinated at lower temperatures, 2–6°C, both for dip- and injection-vaccinated fish.

Experiments reported by Lorenzen *et al.* (2011) with a DNA vaccine against viral hemorrhagic septicemia (VHS) in rainbow trout also confirmed that groups of fish vaccinated at 5°C, 10°C or 15°C, respectively, were all protected against virulent challenge, although the kinetics of the immune response was slower at the lowest water temperature. Another study with Atlantic salmon vaccinated with oil-containing, polyvalent vaccine at different temperatures from 2–8°C, and later kept at the respective temperatures until challenge, concluded that all temperature groups were protected against cold-water vibriosis, confirming the previously mentioned results. However, fish that were vaccinated and kept at 2°C were not protected against furunculosis, and fish in the 4°C group were only moderately protected, while there was a good effect in the 8°C group (Sevatdal and Dalen, 1997). The response to the antigens from *A. salmonicida* seemed to be delayed. However, the fish will develop protective immunity at a later stage, when the environmental water temperature rises, at least when oil-containing vaccines are used. With the warm-water species channel catfish, Martins *et al.* (2011) reported contrasting results when groups of fish were immunised with live theronts of *Ichthyophthirius multifiliis* and later exposed to virulent challenge; fish vaccinated at 15°C experienced higher mortality and impaired antibody response compared with groups vaccinated at higher temperatures, up to 30°C.

Altogether, one can conclude that the final level of protection does not seem to be notably affected by ambient temperature when fish are vaccinated, at least when being within "normal" variation for existence for the species in question. The effects of temperature may vary between fish species (warm water vs. cold water), and in relation to different types of antigens. The vaccine companies do, in general, only rarely indicate water temperature for vaccination, but Merck Animal Health recommend an interval from 21–29°C for their channel catfish vaccines.

12.4 SIZE OF FISH

Data concerning age or size of fish when the immune system has been fully developed have only been published for a few fish species. Commercially important species like carp and rainbow trout have been demonstrated to be able to mount a full immune response at approximately 2–3 months (Zapata *et al.*, 2006), and salmonids should not be vaccinated before they are immunologically mature at a weight of approximately 5 grams (Hart *et al.*, 1988). For manual handling purposes, salmonids are recommended to be 20 g before they are vaccinated by injection, and this suggestion will probably also be applicable for other fish species. The immune system of the cod also seems to be fully developed at approximately two months of age (Schrøder *et al.*, 1998), while the Atlantic halibut needs close to one month more to be immunologically mature (Øvergård *et al.*, 2011). On the other hand, the subtropical freshwater species channel catfish seems to give full response when vaccinated with a live *Edwardsiella ictaluri* vaccine only seven days post-hatch (Shoemaker *et al.*, 1999), illustrating the great variation in this subject area between fish species, and possibly between different antigens.

12.5 VACCINATION METHODS

Vaccine may be administered to fish by three basically different routes: parenterally by injection, or by immersion (delivering the antigens to the fish surface by dipping or bathing the fish in a vaccine solution, or spraying the vaccine onto the fish), or orally by incorporating the vaccine into the feed.

12.5.1 Injection vaccination

Vaccination by injection is the delivery method generally resulting in best protection, and is the only choice for adjuvanted products. Disadvantages of the method are the labour effort and highly specialized technical equipment required, and being unsuitable for use in small fish (i.e., <10 g) (Evensen, 2009).

Vaccination by the injection method is normally done via the intraperitoneal (IP) route. However, intramuscular injection may also be applied, which is the case for DNA-based products, including Apex-IHN (Novartis Animal Health), licensed in Canada for use in salmonids against infectious hematopoietic necrosis. Due to the local reactions induced in the abdominal cavity by adjuvanted vaccines after IP deposition, injection into the dorsal median sinus, the adipose tissue under the dorsal fin, has been tested in salmon brood fish in order to avoid problems with stripping of eggs, and still keeping the muscle filet unaffected by inflammatory reactions caused by the vaccine (Treasurer and Cox, 2008). Vaccines for injection are mostly inactivated products; however, the live *Arthrobacter* vaccine Renogen (Novartis Animal Health), used for prevention of salmonids against bacterial kidney disease, is to be injected IP.

The vaccination process starts with netting the fish, followed by lowering them into an anesthetic solution. The anesthetic benzocaine is mostly used for salmonids, while metacain is more applicable for marine fish like the cod (Karlsson *et al.*, 2012). The solution should be oxygenized, and it should be changed at intervals. Time for anesthetizing should be in the order of one minute, with water temperature affecting the time needed. When the fish has stopped wriggling and is lying still, they are netted further to a vaccination table. This is typically a steel surface with a brim or sideboard to keep fish and water on the table; the fish should stay wet during the whole process, and water should be running on the table. The operators grip single fish and inject the vaccine dose into the abdomen, before it is dropped into a pipe with running water to be transported back to a holding tank to wake up again.

Injection is made by use of an automatic repeating syringe connected to a vaccine bottle with a tube. The bottle must be well shaken prior to vaccination, and shaking should be repeated during the operation if needed, to avoid sedimentation of antigen and/or separation of water/oil emulsion. Vaccine dose varies with vaccine product. For oil-adjuvanted polyvalent vaccines in Atlantic salmon, the dose was originally 0.2 ml when they were introduced on the marked. However, due to problems with side-effects (intraperitoneal reactions), the doses have been reduced to 0.1 ml, and for some products even to 0.05 ml.

In salmonids, the injection site is recommended in the mid-line of the abdomen, approximately one fin length anterior to the pelvic fin base (Figure 12.1). The injection needle should have a diameter of 0.5–0.7 mm, and should only just penetrate the abdominal wall, a length of 3–5 mm usually being adequate (Figure 12.2). The needle should be changed regularly, when it is blunt; this also limits the risk of spreading infectious material between individuals.

Professional teams often carry out injection vaccination, with one person operating anesthesia and continuously supplying the vaccine table with an optimal number of fish. The staff of four to five injectors should be kept busy, avoiding individual fish lying too long on the table (Figure 12.3). The waking up of fish after vaccination must be surveyed, to assure an appropriate time and concentration of anesthetics. If waking up takes too long, the fish may pile up on the bottom, resulting in lack of oxygen and subsequent suffocation. In general, each step should be optimized to limit the time needed for the entire process.

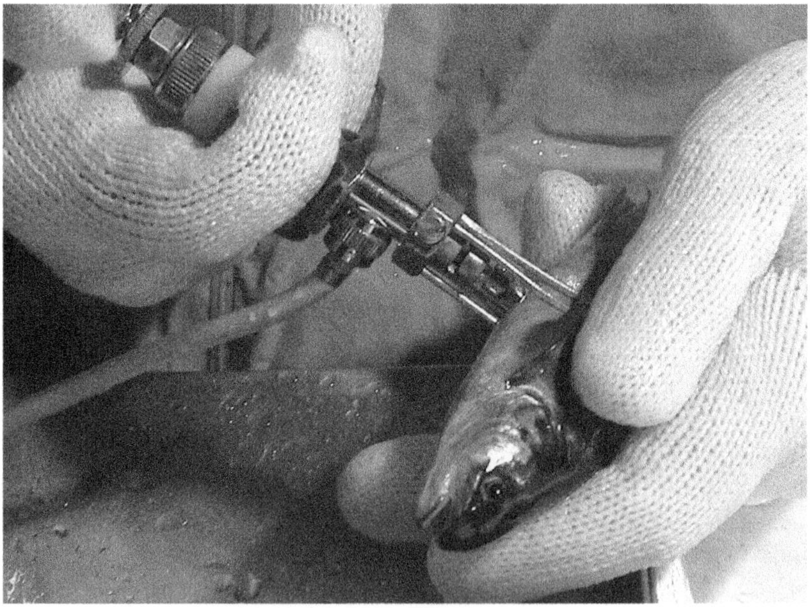

Fig. 12.1 Vaccination by intraperitoneal injection of Atlantic salmon smolt. The injection site is in the mid-line, approximately one fin length anterior to the pelvic fin base. Observe the metal loops on each side of the injection gun, guiding the needle to the injection site, and preventing self-injection of the vaccinator. (Source: Reproduced with permission of Pharmaq.)

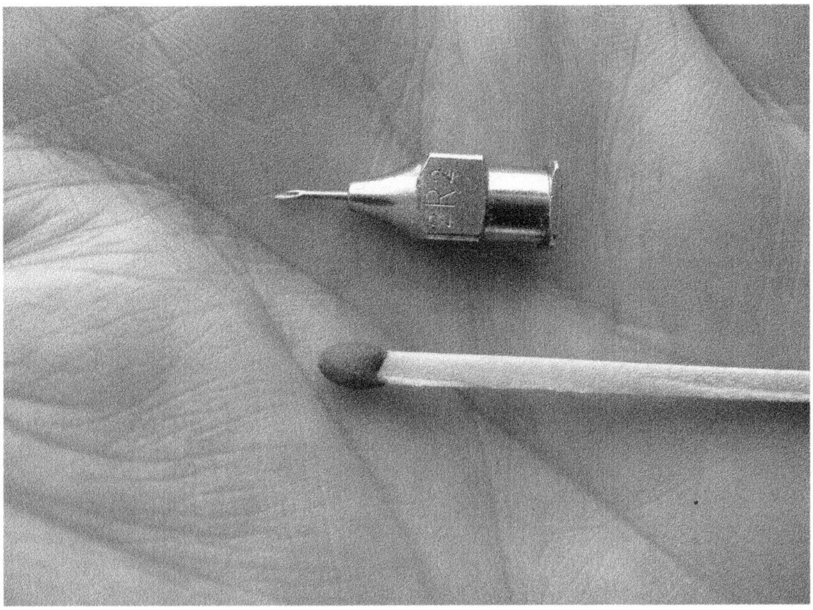

Fig. 12.2 The injection needle should be short, usually a length of 3–5 mm is adequate to penetrate the abdominal wall, and have a diameter of 0.5–0.7 mm. (Source: Reproduced with permission from Trygve T. Poppe.)

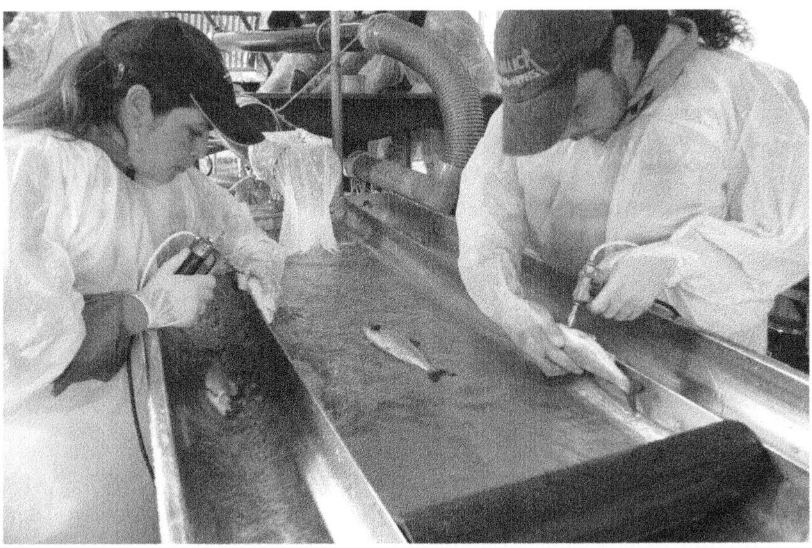

Fig. 12.3 Usually, mass injection vaccination of fish is done by professional teams. Observe the low number of fish transported in at a time, and the flowing water on the table and in the side pipes, in order to ensure a gentle handling process of a short time period. (Source: Reproduced with permission of Pharmaq.)

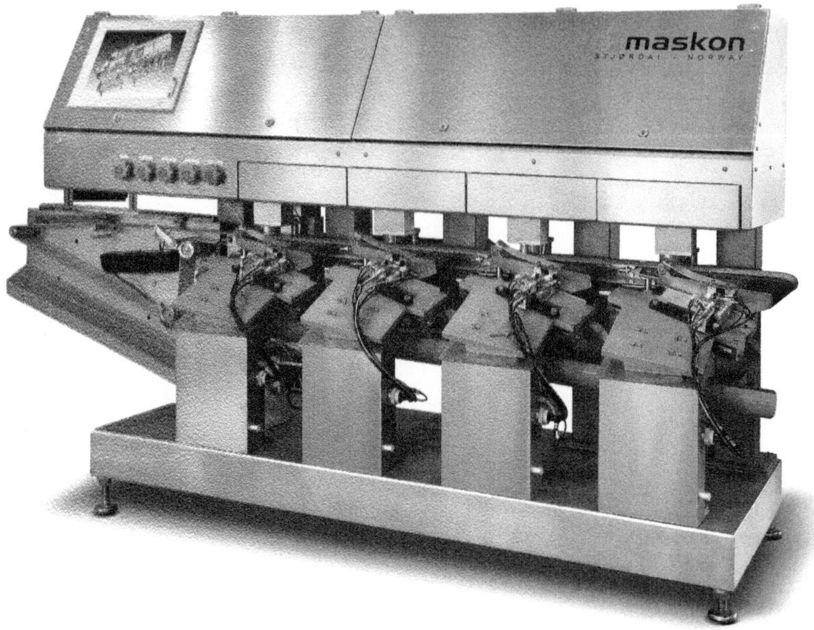

Fig. 12.4 Maskon machine for fully automatic high-speed injection vaccination of fish. (Source: Reproduced with permission of Skala Maskon.)

Self-injection of vaccine intended for fish may cause severe reactions in operators and must be avoided (Leira and Baalsrud, 1997). Protective gloves of metal string should be used, together with a double metal loop on the injection gun fitting around the fish body, guiding the needle to the injection site (Figure 12.1). Moreover, rubber gloves should be used when anesthetics are handled, due to human health and safety concerns.

Injection vaccination of fish has been subject to automation, and different equipment has been developed, from automatic injectors that have to be hand-fed, to fully automated machinery doing high-speed vaccination of the order of 10,000 fish per hour (see Figures 12.4 and 12.5).

12.5.2 Immersion/dip vaccination

When applying immersion vaccination methods, the surfaces of the fish (gills, skin, alimentary tract) are exposed to a dilution of the vaccine. The antigen uptake is considered to take place via the gills, the skin and the lateral line, and possibly also via the intestine (Nakanishi and Ototake, 1997). The fish may be dipped for a short period (30 seconds to one minute) in a relatively concentrated vaccine solution, or may swim for a prolonged time period in an extensively diluted mixture. The vaccine solution may also be sprayed onto the fish. Immersion vaccination is particularly convenient for small fish, fry and fingerlings, which are impractical to handle for injection. Vaccine consumption per individual is low for small fish, but increases proportionally with fish size (i.e., with total biomass of fish).

Dip vaccination is widely used with vaccines like formalin-inactivated cultures of vibrio-bacteria and *Yersinia ruckeri*, holding particulate antigens. Protection achieved is

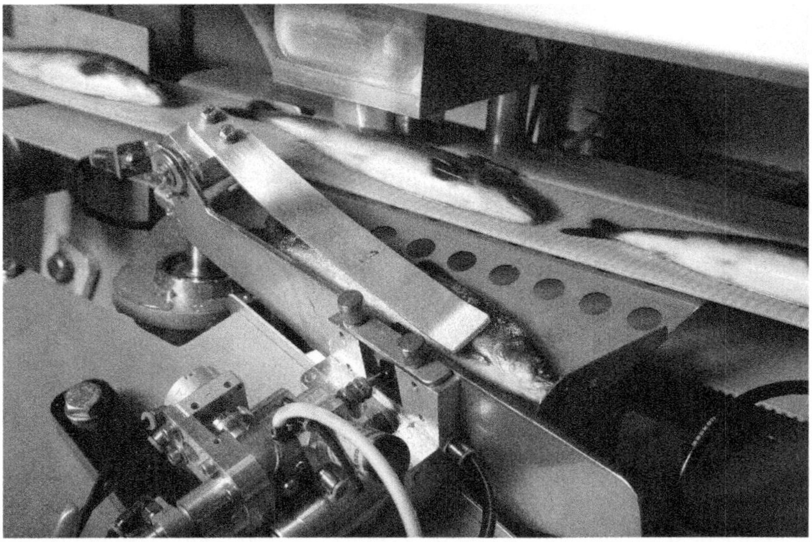

Fig. 12.5 Detail from injection unit, automatic injection vaccination of fish. (Source: Reproduced with permission of Skala Maskon.)

usually somewhat lower compared with use of the injection method with such vaccines. However, immersion is particularly applicable for live attenuated vaccines (Evensen, 2009). The *Flavobacterium columnare* vaccine Aquavac-Col, as well as the *E. ictaluri* vaccine Aquavac-Esc (both MSD Animal Health), are both avirulent live bacterial cultures to be administered by immersion in catfish fry one week post-hatch.

The usual procedure for dip vaccination includes the dilution of the vaccine in hatchery water, typically 1:10, in a container. At each dip, a quantity of fish should be netted in a big, slack net and immersed for a given time period (~30 seconds) in the vaccine solution. The container should have a volume scale engraved on the inner side, to make it possible to keep control of the biomass of fish being vaccinated. Alternatively, the tank should be placed on a weighing machine and read for each dip. Usually, a maximum of 100 kg should be vaccinated per litre of vaccine stock solution.

Bath vaccination is a modified procedure carried out without moving the fish from the holding tank; the water inlet is closed, and the water volume is lowered to increase fish density before vaccine is added to a concentration of typically 1:1000. The water supply is locked for one hour, and extra oxygen is added during vaccination. The same quantity of fish biomass may be vaccinated as with regular dipping, but the method generally gives a lower level of protection (Håstein and Refsti, 1986).

Several factors have been shown to affect the uptake of antigen from a vaccine solution during immersion, and thereby also the level of protection achieved after vaccination. Of greatest importance is the concentration of antigen, but also length of immersion time, as well as the nature of the antigen (particulate or soluble) causing the resulting immunity (Nakanishi and Ototake, 1997). Characteristics of the actual fish, like fish size and level of inflicted stress, do also influence the protective response. Different procedures have been tested with the aim of increasing antigen uptake during immersion. Experiments with immersion of the fish in a hypertonic salt solution prior to the vaccine bath have been carried out recurrently, first reported by Croy and Amend (1977). More recently, Huising *et al.* (2003) reported that a hyperosmotic bath increased the following uptake of a soluble antigen when common carp were vaccinated against *A. salmonicida*, resulting in improved protection. Ultrasound treatment prior to immersion has been reported to result in improved uptake of model antigens and enhanced antibody response in goldfish and carp (Navot *et al.*, 2005). Nakanishi *et al.* (2002) used an instrument with multiple needles to puncture the skin of juvenile rainbow trout before they were vaccinated against *Streptococcus iniae*, achieving increased protection against challenge. However, these procedures all include an extra handling step, making them less practical, and stressful manipulation of the fish is considered undesirable. So far such modifications of the immersion method have not come into practice in commercial aquaculture.

12.5.3 Oral vaccination

Since vaccines were first demonstrated to be effective to protect fish in aquaculture against disease, the idea of simply feeding vaccine to the huge, unmanageable and stress-sensitive fish populations has been an appealing idea. Numerous experiments have been reported, but the protective effect of oral vaccines is in general uncertain. Overall, oral delivery has not gained any ground in practical vaccination, due to poor protection and high consumption of antigen. There are reports of significant effects of oral vaccination as a booster after primary immersion vaccination (Thinh *et al.*, 2009), and there are today a few licensed products on the market. Aquavac ERM Oral vet. from MSD Animal Health is intended for revaccination of rainbow trout, which have earlier been vaccinated by immersion against enteric redmouth disease (*Y. ruckeri*), and Centrovet in Chile delivers oral products against infectious salmon anemia and salmon rickettsial syndrome, both as monovalent products and as a divalent vaccine.

Various methods have been tried out to protect the vaccine antigens against digestive degradation when passing the stomach and anterior intestine, to guide adequate amounts of antigens to the immune cells in the wall of the hindgut, which is supposed to be the important site for an immune response. Acid-resistant coatings, slow-release particles like alginate microparticles, and other principles of micro- and nanoparticles have been investigated (Plant and LaPatra, 2011). Vaccine antigens have also been incorporated into feed organisms like *Artemia*, by first feeding the vaccine antigen to the copepod. Other similar experiments have been made with water fleas and rotifers, and recently fly larvae have been used both as genetically engineered antigen producers, and as vehicles for vaccine delivery, by feeding the larvae to the fish. However, none of these experiments have led to a breakthrough regarding the applicability of oral vaccines under practical conditions, concerning acceptable antigen doses and protective immunity.

12.6 TIME FOR PROTECTION TO DEVELOP – DURATION OF PROTECTION

The time period from vaccination to potential exposure to the actual pathogen should be optimized in such a way that maximum protection coincides with the time of greatest risk of disease outbreak; if the fish are vaccinated too late, immunity will not have time to develop, and if they are vaccinated too early, immunity levels may have declined by the time they are exposed to the disease agent. Vaccine companies producing oil-adjuvanted vaccines for salmonids recommend a time period of at least 500 degree-days from vaccination to sea transfer, while the live *E. ictaluri* vaccine for channel catfish should be given at least two weeks prior to exposure at water temperatures between 21°C and 29°C, that is, 300–400 degree-days. Even for other non-adjuvanted products, both for immersion and injection, the recommended time periods prior to disease exposure are of this order.

Marine aquaculture of salmonids includes a grow-out phase in seawater of approximately one and a half years, and field experiences support the assumption that injectable vaccines with oil-adjuvants confer protective immunity during the entire period. Midtlyng *et al.* (1996) demonstrated an increase in specific antibody titers against *A. salmonicida*, as well as in level of protection measured as relative percent survival (RPS) in furunculosis challenge trials, from three to six months post-vaccination. Protection even in the second year in seawater was demonstrated in field experiments with vaccines in Atlantic salmon, both with a non-adjuvanted bacterin against cold-water vibriosis given twice by immersion (Lillehaug, 1991), as well as with vaccines against furunculosis adjuvanted with aluminum salts given by injection (Lillehaug *et al.*, 1992). However, the levels of protection were reduced during the second year in seawater compared with the first year.

Injection of non-adjuvanted experimental vaccines against *Streptococcus agalactiae* in Nile tilapia (Pasnik *et al.*, 2005) and against *A. salmonicida* in Atlantic salmon (Bricknell *et al.*, 1999) have demonstrated protection in challenge trials six and nine months post-vaccination, respectively, although there were tendencies towards a decline in levels of protection at these time points. Experimental DNA vaccines administered intramuscularly to rainbow trout against *Viral hemorrhagic septicemia virus* (McLauchlan *et al.*, 2003) and *Infectious hematopoetic necrosis virus* (Kurath *et al.*, 2006) gave significant protection against virulent challenges up to 9 and 25 months post-vaccination, respectively. Supplement of adjuvants to a vaccine can both improve the resulting level of protective immunity, as well as duration of protection, as shown by Ravelo *et al.* (2006), by adding different adjuvant products to a bacterin of *Lactococcus garvieae* used in rainbow trout.

12.7 BOOSTER VACCINATION

The use of a booster will increase the level of protection after vaccination (Tatner and Horne, 1985), and may be employed when vaccination once does not give adequate protection as a result, or when first vaccination has to be carried out in small fish that are not fully immunocompetent. In such cases, revaccination will typically be carried out a few weeks after primary immunization. Immersion vaccination will usually be the method of choice both for the primary and secondary vaccination in small fish, for instance as described by Angelidis *et al.* (2006) in sea bass juveniles.

A booster may also be utilized to restore protection at a time when susceptibility of fish to disease is increasing again, some months after the first vaccination. In such cases, vaccination typically has to be carried out in relatively large fish. Being practically difficult to handle for injection vaccination, and needing vast amounts of vaccine for immersion, such setups call for procedures of oral immunization. The vaccine Aquavac ERM Oral vet. (MSD Animal Health) is recommended for oral use in rainbow trout four to six months after primary vaccination by immersion.

12.8 VACCINATION ECONOMY

The implementation of a vaccination strategy should aim at achieving an economically favorable solution for the fish-farming industry. Disease and disease outbreaks caused by specific infectious agents generate expenses and economic losses, including reduced production due to direct losses of fish, and increased expenses for medication and extra work. In order to be able to estimate expenses of vaccination and disease, respectively, a model was developed, and it was applied to calculate the point of break-even between costs of vaccination and losses due to disease (Lillehaug, 1989). In addition to the vaccine itself, vaccination costs include labour costs of the actual vaccination method, as well as losses due to side-effects. The levels of protection achieved by the respective methods were taken into account, by including RPS into the formula. It was estimated that a reduction in disease losses by less than one percentage point due to vibriosis in Atlantic salmon, in the actual example, would pay for costs of vaccination, both for injection and immersion vaccination. Due to the superior RPS of injection, this method was shown to be economically beneficial if the disease caused significant mortalities in non-vaccinated fish.

The economic model was further developed by Thorarinsson and Powell (2006) and employed to evaluate the impact of disease risk, vaccine efficacy, and market price of fish products on the economic effects of vaccination against furunculosis in Atlantic salmon and vibriosis in sea bass production, respectively. They estimated net savings per kilo of produced fish of 0.42€ in Atlantic salmon, and 0.52€ in sea bass, respectively, for disease levels of 20% mortality in non-vaccinated fish during the entire production cycle. When deciding which vaccine product should be used, the product giving best protection under field conditions should be chosen, even if the price per dose is higher, due to a great impact of vaccine efficacy on the economic outcome.

REFERENCES

Angelides, P., Karagiannis, D. and Crump, E.M. 2006. Efficacy of a *Listonella anguillarum* (syn. *Vibrio anguillarum*) vaccine for juvenile sea bass *Dicentrarchus labrax* L. *Dis Aquat Org* **71**: 19–24.

Bly, J.E. and Clem, L.W. 1992. Temperature and teleost immune functions. *Fish Shellfish Immunol* **2**: 159–71.

Bowden, T.J. 2008. Modulation of the immune system of fish by their environment. *Fish Shellfish Immunol* **25**: 373–83.

Bricknell, I.R., King, J.A., Bowden, T.J, and Ellis, A.E. 1999. Duration of protective antibodies, and the correlation with protection in Atlantic salmon (*Salmo salar* L.), following vaccination with an *Aeromonas salmonicida* vaccine containing iron-regulated outer membrane proteins and secretory polysaccharide. *Fish Shellfish Immunol* **9**: 139–51.

Croy, T.R. and Amend, D.F. 1977. Immunization of sockeye salmon (*Oncorhynchus nerka*) against vibriosis using hyperosmotic infiltration. *Aquaculture* **12**: 317–25.

Eggset, G., Mortensen, A. and Løken, S. 1999. Vaccination of Atlantic salmon (*Salmo salar* L.) before and during smoltification; effects on smoltification and immunological protection. *Aquaculture* **170**: 101–12.

Evensen, Ø. 2009. Development in fish vaccinology with focus on delivery methodologies, adjuvants and formulations. *Op Méditerr Series A* **86**: 177–86.

Hart, S., Wrathmell, A.B., Harris, J.E. and Grayson, T.H. 1988. Gut immunology in fish: a review. *Dev Comp Immunol* **12**: 453–80.

Håstein, T. and Refsti, T. 1986. Vaccination of rainbow trout against vibriosis by injection, dip and bath. *Bull Eur Assoc Fish Pathol* **6**: 45–9.

Huising, M.O., Guichelaar, T., Hoek, C., *et al.*, 2003. Increased efficacy of immersion vaccination in fish with hyperosmotic pretreatment. *Vaccine* **21**: 4178–93.

Karlsson, A., Rosseland, B.O., Massabuau, J.C. and Kiessling, A. 2012. Pre-anaesthetic metomidate sedation delays the stress response after caudal artery cannulation in Atlantic cod (*Gadus morhua*). *Fish Physiol Biochem* **38**: 401–11.

Kurath, G., Garver, K.A., Corbeil, S., *et al.*, 2006. Protective immunity and lack of histopathological damage two years after DNA vaccination against infectious hematopoietic necrosis virus in trout. *Vaccine* **24**: 345–54.

Leira, H.L. and Baalsrud, K.J. 1997. Operator safety during injection vaccination of fish. *Dev Biol Stand* **90**: 383–7.

Lillehaug, A. 1989. A cost-effectiveness study of three different methods of vaccination against vibriosis in salmonids. *Aquaculture* **83**: 227–36.

Lillehaug, A. 1991. Vaccination of Atlantic salmon (*Salmo salar* L.) against cold-water vibriosis – duration of protection and effect on growth rate. *Aquaculture* **92**: 99–107.

Lillehaug, A. 1997. Vaccination strategies in seawater cage culture of salmonids. *Dev Biol Stand* **90**: 401–8.

Lillehaug, A., Lunder, T. and Poppe, T.T. 1992. Field testing of adjuvanted furunculosis vaccines in Atlantic salmon, *Salmo salar* L. *J Fish Dis* **15**: 485–96.

Lillehaug, A., Ramstad, A., Bækken, K. and Reitan, L.J. 1993. Protective immunity in Atlantic salmon (*Salmo salar* L.) vaccinated at different water temperatures. *Fish Shellfish Immunol* **3**: 143–56.

Lorenzen, E., Einer-Jensen, K., Rasmussen, J.S., *et al.*, 2011. The protective mechanisms induced by a DNA vaccine in fish depend on temperature. *Scand J Immunol* **73**: 392.

Martins, M.L., Xu, D.H., Shoemaker, C.A. and Klesius, P.H. 2011. Temperature effects on immune response and hematological parameters of channel catfish *Ictalurus punctatus* vaccinated with live theronts of *Ichthyophthirius multifiliis*. *Fish Shellfish Immunol* **31**: 774–80.

Maule, A.G., Schreck, C.B. and Kaattari, S.L. 1987. Changes in the immune system of coho salmon (*Oncorhynchus kisutch*) during the parr-to-smolt transformation and after implantation of cortisol. *Can J Fish Aquat Sci* **44**: 161–6.

McLauchlan, P.E., Collet, B., Ingerslev, E., *et al.*, 2003. DNA vaccination against viral haemorrhagic septicaemia (VHS) in rainbow trout: size, dose, route of injection and duration of protection – early protection correlates with Mx expression. *Fish Shellfish Immunol* **15**: 39–50.

Midtlyng, P.J., Reitan, L.J. and Speilberg, L. 1996. Experimental studies on the efficacy and side-effects of intraperitoneal vaccination of Atlantic salmon (*Salmo salar* L.) against furunculosis. *Fish Shellfish Immunol* **6**: 335–50.

Nakanishi, T. and Ototake, M. 1997. Antigen uptake and immune responses after immersion vaccination. *Dev Biol Stand* **90**: 59–68.

Nakanishi, T., Kiryu, I. and Ototake, M. 2002. Development of a new vaccine delivery method for fish: percutaneous administration by immersion with application of a multiple puncture instrument. *Vaccine* **20**: 3764–9.

Navot, N., Kimmel, E. and Avtalion, R.R. 2005. Immunisation of fish by bath immersion using ultrasound. *Dev Biol (Basel)* **121**: 135–42.

Øvergård, A.-C., Fiksdal, I.U., Nerland, A.H. and Patel, S. 2011. Expression of T-cell markers during Atlantic halibut (*Hippoglossus hippoglossus* L.) ontogenesis. *Dev Comp Immunol* **36**: 203–13.

Pasnik, D.J., Evans, J.J. and Klesius, P.H. 2005. Duration of protective antibodies and correlation with survival in Nile tilapia *Oreochromis niloticus* following *Streptococcus agalactiae* vaccination. *Dis Aquat Org* **66**: 129–34.

Plant, K.P. and LaPatra, S.E. 2011. Advances in fish vaccine delivery. *Dev Comp Immunol* **35**: 1256–62.

Press, C.McL. and Lillehaug, A. 1995. Vaccination in European salmonid aquaculture: a review of practices and prospects. *Br Vet J* **151**: 45–69.

Ravelo, C., Magarinos, B., Herrero, M.C., *et al.*, 2006. Use of adjuvanted vaccines to lengthen the protection against lactococcosis in rainbow trout (*Oncorhynchus mykiss*). *Aquaculture* **251**: 153–8.

Schrøder, M.B., Villena, A.J. and Jørgensen, T.Ø. 1998. Ontogeny of lymphoid organs and immunoglobulin producing cells in Atlantic cod (*Gadus morhua* L.). *Dev Comp Immunol* **22**: 507–17.

Sevatdal, S. and Dalen, V. 1997. Immunization of Atlantic salmon (*Salmo salar* L.) against furunculosis and cold water vibriosis at low temperatures. *Dev Biol Stand* **90**: 472.

Shoemaker, C.A., Klesius, P.H. and Bricker, J.M. 1999. Efficacy of a modified live *Edwardsiella ictaluri* vaccine in channel catfish as young as seven days post hatch. *Aquaculture* **176**: 189–93.

Tatner, M.F. and Horne, M.T. 1985. The effects of vaccine dilution, length of immersion time, and booster vaccinations on the protection levels induced by direct immersion vaccination of brown trout, *Salmo trutta*, with *Yersinia ruckeri* (ERM) vaccine. *Aquaculture* **46**: 11–18.

Thinh, N.H., Kuo, T.Y., Hung, L.T., *et al.*, 2009. Combined immersion and oral vaccination of Vietnamese catfish (*Pangasianodon hypophthalmus*) confers protection against mortality caused by *Edwardsiella ictaluri*. *Fish Shellfish Immunol* **27**: 773–6.

Thorarinsson, R. and Powell, D.B. 2006. Effects of disease risk, vaccine efficacy, and market price on the economics of fish vaccination. *Aquaculture* **256**: 42–9.

Treasurer, J. and Cox, C. 2008. Intraperitoneal and dorsal median sinus vaccination effects on growth, immune response, and reproductive potential in farmed Atlantic salmon *Salmo salar*. *Aquaculture* **275**: 51–7.

Zapata, A., Diez, B., Cejalvo, T., *et al.*, 2006. Ontogeny of the immune system of fish. *Fish Shellfish Immunol* **20**: 126–36.

13 Side-Effects of Vaccination

Trygve T. Poppe and Erling O. Koppang
Norwegian School of Veterinary Science, Oslo, Norway

ABSTRACT

Vaccination interferes with biological functions of the fish and may therefore cause some side-effects with consequences for economy and fish welfare. Although all delivery methods may cause side-effects, most of them are of minor significance. The most important are those associated with the use of injectable adjuvanted vaccines that may cause intra-abdominal lesions. These may compromise growth, health and fillet quality, and may also reach an extent and severity that exceeds what should be considered acceptable from an animal welfare point of view. Many farmed species may be affected, but the majority of side-effects following intraperitoneal administration are reported in Atlantic salmon.

13.1 INTRODUCTION

Vaccination is today common practice in large-scale salmon farming, and to some extent in other species as well. The vaccines are, in most countries, multivalent oil-adjuvanted vaccines. These vaccines have been very effective in reducing losses caused by furunculosis and other bacterial diseases, and modern large-scale farming of salmonids and some other species would not be sustainable without effective vaccination programs.

Most administration forms may cause acute or prolonged side-effects, but those caused by intraperitoneal injection of oil-adjuvanted vaccines in salmon are by far the most severe and will therefore constitute the main bulk of information in this chapter. Both immersion and bath vaccination may cause loss of appetite for a shorter or longer time with resultant growth retardation, but these side-effects are minor compared with the vast benefits of vaccination.

With the exception of Tasmania, virtually all salt-water farmed salmonids are vaccinated with oil-adjuvanted vaccines. The composition of the vaccines used may vary depending upon the zoosanitary situation in the area. Most vaccines used are multivalent, that is, they contain antigens from several different bacteria and viruses. In order to enhance and prolong the effect

trygve.poppe@nmbu.no

Fish Vaccination, First Edition. Edited by Roar Gudding, Atle Lillehaug and Øystein Evensen.

of the vaccine, an adjuvant is mixed with the antigens. Most adjuvants may cause side-effects of variable degree and severity. Over the years, several types of adjuvants have been tested, including aluminum salts (Lillehaug *et al.*, 1992), potassium aluminum sulfate (alum) (Horne *et al.*, 1984; Mulvey *et al.*, 1995), and hydrocarbon oils. The vaccines most widely used in salmonid aquaculture today usually contain some form of hydrocarbon oil (Haugarvoll *et al.*, 2010). Salmonid fish are immunized prior to smoltification and seawater transfer. After a few days of starvation, the fish are anesthetized and the vaccine is given intraperitoneally either by vaccination teams or by automated vaccination machines with a capacity of up to 20,000 fish per hour. The injection site is in the ventral midline, 1.5 fin lengths cranial to the base of the pelvic fins. Injection volume is usually 0.05 to 0.1 ml. In contrast to mammals, where an initial immunization is normally followed by a booster injection, salmonids are only injected once.

Since the very beginning, side-effects following injection vaccination were of great concern due to the intra-abdominal lesions that often occur. Worldwide, these lesions are first of all a problem in Atlantic salmon, while rainbow trout develop fewer and more moderate lesions. This may be due to the fact that vaccines for rainbow trout contain fewer antigens than those used in the salmon industry. Furthermore, some of the vaccines used for rainbow trout are non-adjuvanted and therefore less irritating. The concerns are partly associated with the animal welfare aspects and partly with quality issues like melanization and fibrous adhesions that may lead to retarded growth, downgrading and rejects (Midtlyng and Lillehaug, 1998).

Today, more than 20 years after the introduction of oil-adjuvanted vaccines in the salmon farming industry, side-effects still occur and may sometimes reach an extent and severity that exceeds what should be considered as acceptable from an animal welfare point of view. This is a surprising fact, given the enormous efforts that have been invested in optimization of the vaccines and the increased concern for the welfare of the animals. With increasing focus on fish welfare, there can be little doubt that even more effort should be invested in order to reduce/minimize the negative effects of this otherwise excellent preventive measure.

13.2 ACUTE SIDE-EFFECTS

The acute side-effects may grossly be divided into those resulting from poor handling, anesthesia, contamination of the vaccine, and genuine side-effects caused by the vaccine itself (Lillehaug, 1989). Inadequate routines, misproportioned equipment and anesthesia may all contribute to acute problems and mortality during or shortly after vaccination.

Poor water quality, contaminated vaccine or unhygienic vaccination procedures may cause the introduction of bacteria into the abdominal cavity concurrently with the vaccine. This may result in acute septicemia with extensive hemorrhage in the vent area, at the base of the pectoral and pelvic fins and ventral parts of the body a few days after vaccination. Olsen *et al.* (2006) described systemic post-vaccination infection focused within the peritoneal cavity with *Rhodococcus erythropolis* in Scotland and Norway. Internal lesions included ascites and petechiae on the peritoneal surface, liver and pyloric ceca. Histopathology revealed gram-positive rod-shaped bacteria in peritoneal lesions, subepicardially and in skeletal muscle. Interestingly, disease could not be reproduced by challenge with the isolated bacterium alone, while concurrent injection of the oil-adjuvanted vaccine resulted in 100% mortality. This indicates some type of physical or nutrition-related protection from the immune system of the fish. The source of the infection was never identified, but may have been the result of poor hygiene during immunization. Other bacteria frequently isolated from such cases include *Pseudomonas* spp. and *Aeromonas* spp.

Bjørge *et al.* (2011) showed experimentally that vaccinated salmon showed less interest in food and had decreased swimming activity compared with control fish in the first hours after vaccination. The severity of lesions also correlated with the latency to eat and activity during feeding. This reaction is similar to that of other species where pain has been produced experimentally by injection of acetic acid and points towards a general pain response to the injected material. Practical experience shows that latency to eat and altered behavior may last from a few days to a few weeks, depending on size of the fish, water temperature and other factors. Similarly, a short-term negative effect on growth has been demonstrated in rainbow trout (Rønsholdt and McLean, 1999), arctic char (Pylkkö *et al.*, 2000), whitefish (*Coregonus* sp.) (Koskela *et al.*, 2004), wolfish and halibut (Ingilæ *et al.*, 2000). Reaction to the vaccine will cause pain, restrict normal gut function and cause energy-demanding immune responses, with resultant loss of weight gain and poor animal welfare (Sørum and Damsgaard, 2004).

High post-vaccination mortality has been described in Atlantic salmon resulting from the use of misproportioned equipment and/or techniques resulting in vaccine being delivered into internal organs (liver, spleen, intestine, swim bladder) or vessels. Affected fish had pale gills, particularly near the tip of the filaments. Histopathology revealed oil droplets within the vessels of the filaments and in capillaries of the lamellae (Skrudland *et al.*, 2002). These embolic lesions subsequently resulted in necrosis of the distal parts of the filaments.

13.3 CHRONIC SIDE-EFFECTS

All vaccine deliveries to fish may cause some chronic effects, including dip vaccination, which is considered to be the most gentle delivery form (Lillehaug, 1991). Growth retardation may be the result of handling, anesthesia and other factors that may be difficult to explain. Fish with retarded growth after vaccination may show compensatory growth later in production (Berg *et al.*, 2006).

13.4 INJECTION SITE REACTIONS

The most common type of reaction seen in vaccinated fish is a rather localized fibrinous peritonitis in the area adjacent to the injection site. This is usually in the ventral midline and caudally to the pyloric ceca. Fibrinous strands typically form adhesions between the ventral body wall, spleen and pyloric ceca (Figure 13.1). The strands are usually easy to tear apart, cause minimal damage to the fillets and are probably of little concern to the fish.

Histologically, early lesions in salmon are characterized by neutrophilic infiltration followed by an increasing macrophage and lymphocyte response (Mutoloki *et al.*, 2006a,b). Mast cells commonly occur, in particular in proximity to the negative imprint of round oil droplets centrally in the lesions. Variable numbers of melanomacrophages may be present throughout the lesions. Fibrous tissue infiltrated with inflammatory cells forming long strands become progressively more common after some months. Mild and moderate lesions may be found between the walls of the pyloric ceca and pancreatic/adipose tissue, even in cases where macroscopic lesions are absent or scarce. In order to obtain a standardized scoring

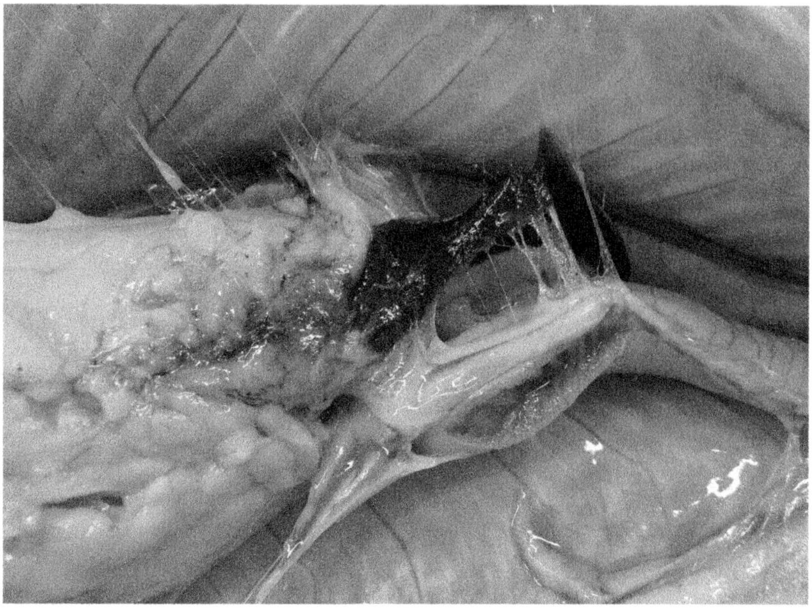

Fig. 13.1 Moderate injection-site adhesions with fibrinous strands between spleen, posterior gut and the body wall. Note melanization cranial to the spleen. (Source: Trygve T. Poppe.)

system for vaccine adhesions, the so-called "Speilberg scoring system" was introduced by Midtlyng *et al.* (1996). A score of zero implies unvaccinated fish or fish with no visible lesions, while score of six implies severe and widespread lesions throughout the abdominal cavity. In general, a Speilberg score up to 2.0 or 2.5 is considered acceptable from both an ethical and consumer-focused point of view.

13.5 EXTENSIVE ABDOMINAL LESIONS

Severe and widespread lesions sometimes occur, particularly in Atlantic salmon (Poppe and Breck, 1997). The extent and type of lesions may be highly variable and may compromise function, animal welfare and product quality. The occurrence of such lesions is rather unpredictable and has occurred at irregular intervals since the introduction of oil-adjuvanted vaccines. Some cases have been attributed to misinjections where the vaccine has been injected into abdominal organs (pyloric ceca, stomach wall, liver) causing extensive granulomatous inflammation and fusion of organs. Other cases have been characterized by extensive granulomatous adhesions in the dorsocranial part of the abdominal cavity, near the septum transversum, oesophagus, gonads, larger vessels and nerves (Figure 13.2). Lesions in this area may severely compromise normal gonad development and function of several organ systems. Clear, empty spaces are often present in the granulomatous tissue; these are the negative images of the oil droplets in the vaccine (Figure 13.3). Microscopically, such lesions are typically characterized by extensive granulomatous inflammation of considerable thickness and extent. Fibrous tissue, macrophages, lymphocytes and mast cells form large concentric structures around the

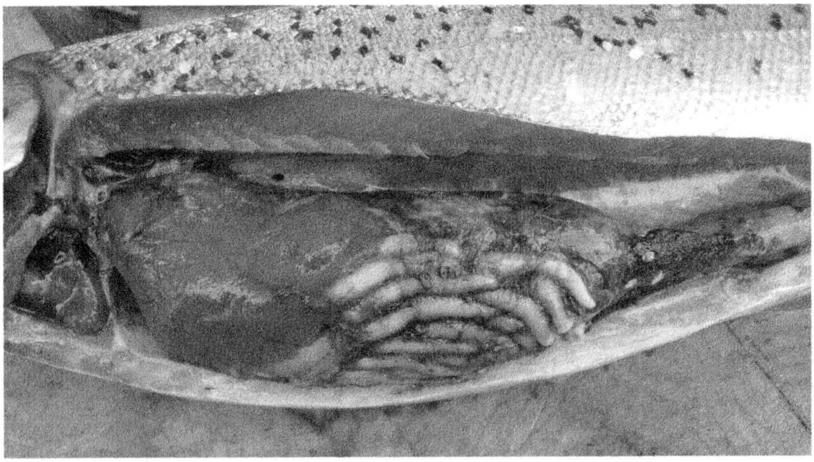

Fig. 13.2 Severe side-effects with granulomatous inflammation between pyloric ceca. Note extensive melanization of the lesion. (Source: Trygve T. Poppe.)

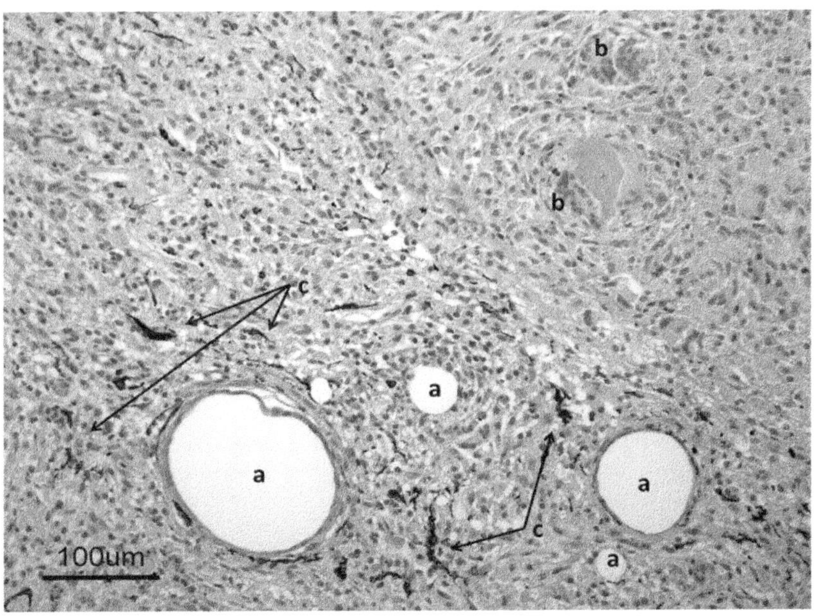

Fig. 13.3 Section showing granulomatous inflammation between ceca and the gut wall. (a) Negative imprint of oil droplets; (b) multinucleated giant cells; and (c) melanin is seen in a matrix of granulomatous tissue. H&E stain. (Source: Trygve T. Poppe.)

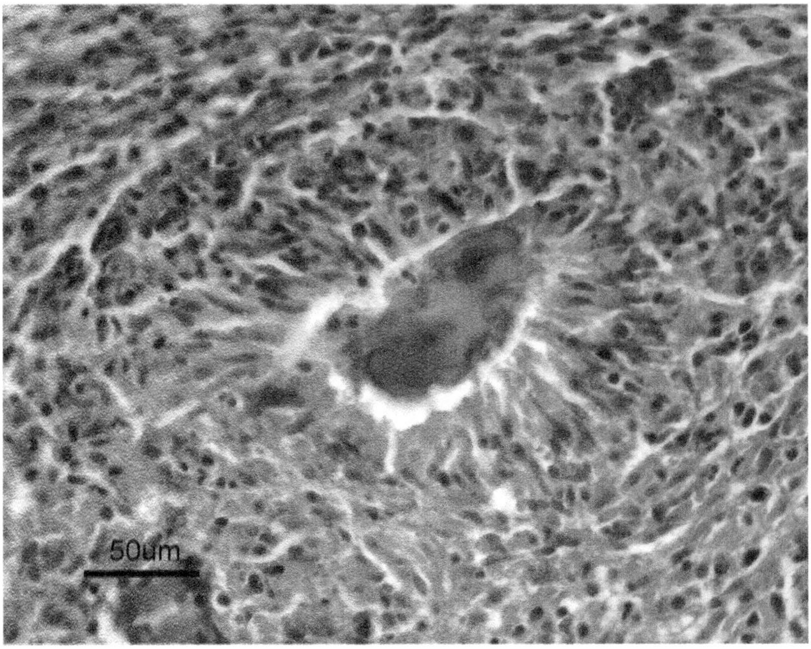

Fig. 13.4 Splendore-Hoeppli reaction in injection-site granulomatous tissue. Martius Scarlet Blue stain. (Source: Trygve T. Poppe.)

negative imprints of oil droplets. Multinuclear giant cells, Splendore-Hoeppli-like reactions, neovascularization and melanomacrophages may further add to this rather jumbled lesion (Figure 13.4). Cases with extensive melanization of both lesions and the peritoneal lining do also occur sporadically.

The etiology behind such lesions is partly unknown and certainly controversial. Concurrent disease like IPN or *Pseudomonas* infection has experimentally been shown to aggravate the severity of lesions and has been suspected in many field cases (Colquhoun *et al.*, 1998). The widespread occurrence of *Paranucleospora thereidon/Desmozoon salmonis* in and around salmon farms in Norway has prompted speculation about its possible contribution to the development of some lesions, but this has never been confirmed.

13.6 LESIONS IN OTHER ORGANS

Such lesions include muscle, the uveal tract and the kidney. Koppang *et al.* (2005) demonstrated severe intra-abdominal lesions and muscle necrosis with black pigmentation of fillets in salmon with gross lesions. Histology revealed negative imprints of oil droplets and made differentiation from other cases of black spots in the fillets easy. Inflammation in the eyes had been recorded as a systemic side-effect of vaccination (Koppang *et al.*, 2004), as has a generalized inflammatory response affecting most visceral organs including the spine (reviewed in Haugarvoll *et al.*, 2010). Here, cells with a spherical shape and flattened nuclei occurring in the inflammatory lesions were classified as Mott cells, which are dysfunctional

B cells. It has been noted previously that such cells tend to occur in vaccinated fish, and they have thus been called "vaccine cells" in routine diagnostic practice.

13.7 SKELETAL LESIONS

Skeletal malformations (platyspondyly) sometimes occur in farmed fish and have been shown to be of multifactorial etiology. Small fish, fast growth, time of vaccination, high incubation temperature and low phosphorus availability have all been shown to be associated with skeletal lesions. Furthermore, smolts transferred to seawater in the autumn develop more side-effects, including skeletal lesions, than smolts transferred to seawater in the spring (Fjelldal *et al.*, 2012). Affected areas of the vertebral column may comprise the anterior part ("humpbacks"), the posterior part ("shorttails") or the entire vertebral column. Water temperature and time of vaccination are two of the factors that have been shown to induce development of platyspondyly. Berg *et al.* (2006) showed that early vaccination (and therefore higher water temperature) of relatively small salmon presmolts resulted in rapid development of intra-abdominal lesions and higher incidence of platyspondyly at slaughter. These fish were also the smallest compared with fish vaccinated later and at lower temperatures. Spinal deformities with a vaccine-related etiology were also shown by Aunsmo *et al.* (2008) and Haugarvoll *et al.* (2010). In a cohort study, Vågsholm and Djupvik (1998) showed that an increased period (from 2 to 5 months) from vaccination to seawater transfer was associated with an increased risk for development of skeletal lesions. These data clearly show that the negative impacts of vaccination can be reduced through good planning of the vaccination and knowledge of the biology of the fish.

13.8 AUTOIMMUNITY

In mice, systemic autoimmunity may be induced by the intra-abdominal injection of certain hydrocarbon oils, like the ones used as oil adjuvants. Systemic autoimmunity may also develop as a side-effect following the vaccination of Atlantic salmon with oil-adjuvanted vaccines (Koppang *et al.*, 2008). Also, several of the more diffuse side-effects observed in vaccinated fish may be related to the induction of systemic autoimmunity (Haugarvoll *et al.*, 2010). Systemic autoimmunity has several faces, including glomerulonephritis characterized by deposition of immune complexes in the basal membrane of the glomeruli, and the occurrence of different autoantibodies. The appearance of Mott cells is most likely also related to systemic autoimmunity.

13.9 LESIONS IN NON-SALMONID SPECIES

Several other farmed species are vaccinated against serious pathogens in their respective environments. Relevant species include sea bass and sea bream, tilapia, channel catfish, pangasius and Atlantic cod. Reports of side-effects following vaccination in these species are few, since adjuvanted vaccines are seldom used.

In sea bass, Afonso *et al.* (2005) demonstrated mobilization of neutrophils and macrophages 24–48 hours post-immunization with oil-adjuvanted vaccine. Following this initial response, a steady increase in the number of eosinophilic granular cells, lymphocytes, neutrophils and macrophages followed and were maintained for up to 60 days post-vaccination. Although macroscopically visible lesions were present 11 months after vaccination, lesions never reached the levels reported in salmon.

Although oil-adjuvanted vaccines may cause adverse side-effects in farmed cod, lesions are generally milder than in salmon and considered to be within levels that are acceptable, both from an animal welfare and consumer point of view. Due to the large size of the cod liver, the correct injection site is of great importance in order to minimize liver damage. In cod, lesions following vaccination are typically characterized by rapid encapsulation of the vaccine, and adhesions between visceral organs and the body wall are typically more moderate than in salmon. Furthermore, melanization of lesions and in muscle seldom occurs in cod (Maira *et al.*, 2007).

REFERENCES

Afonso, A., Gomes, S., da Silva, J., *et al.*, 2005. Side effects in sea bass (*Dicentrarchus labrax* L.) due to intraperitoneal vaccination against vibriosis and pasteurellosis. *Fish Shellfish Immunol* **19**: 1–16.

Aunsmo, A., Guttvik, A., Midtlyng, P.J., *et al.*, 2008. Association of spinal deformity and vaccine-induced abdominal lesions in harvest-sized Atlantic salmon, *Salmo salar* L. *J Fish Dis* **31**: 514–24.

Berg, A., Rødseth, O.M., Tangerås, A. and Hansen, T. 2006. Time of vaccination influences development of adhesions, growth and spinal deformities in Atlantic salmon *Salmo salar*. *Dis Aquat Org* **69**: 239–48.

Bjørge, M.H., Nordgreen, J., Janczak, A.M., *et al.*, 2011. Behavioural changes following intraperitoneal vaccination in Atlantic salmon (*Salmo salar*). *Appl Anim Behav Sci* **133**: 127–35.

Colquhoun, D.J., Skjerve, E. and Poppe, T.T. 1998. *Pseudomonas fluorescens*, infectious pancreatic necrosis virus and environmental stress as potential factors in the development of vaccine related adhesions in Atlantic salmon, *Salmo salar* L. *J Fish Dis* **21**: 355–64.

Fjelldal, P.G., Hansen, T., Breck, O., *et al.*, 2012. Vertebral deformities in farmed Atlantic salmon (*Salmo salar* L.): etiology and pathology. *J Appl Ichthyol* **28**: 433–40.

Haugarvoll, E., Bjerkås, I., Szabo, N.N., *et al.*, 2010. Manifestations of systemic autoimmunity in vaccinated salmon. *Vaccine* **28**: 4961–9.

Horne, M.T., Roberts, R.J., Tatner, M. and Ward, P. 1984. The effects of the use of potassium alum adjuvant in vaccines against vibriosis in rainbow trout, *Salmo gairdneri* Richardson. *J Fish Dis* **7**: 91–9.

Ingilæ, M., Arnesen, J.A., Lund, V. and Eggset, G. 2000. Vaccination of Atlantic halibut *Hippoglossus hippoglossus* L., and spotted wolffish *Anarhichas minor* L., against atypical *Aeromonas salmonicida*. *Aquaculture* **183**: 31–44.

Koppang, E.O., Haugarvoll, E., Hordvik, I., *et al.*, 2004. Granulomatous uveitis associated with vaccination in the Atlantic salmon. *Vet Pathol* **41**: 122–30.

Koppang, E.O., Haugarvoll, E., Hordvik, I., *et al.*, 2005. Vaccine-associated granulomatous inflammation and melanin accumulation in Atlantic salmon, *Salmo salar* L., white muscle. *J Fish Dis* **28**: 13–22.

Koppang, E.O., Bjerkås, I., Haugarvoll, E., *et al.*, 2008. Vaccination-induced systemic autoimmunity in farmed Atlantic salmon. *J Immunol* **181**: 4807–14.

Koskela, J., Rahkonen, R., Pasternack, M. and Knuutinen, H. 2004. Effect of immunization with two commercial vaccines on feed intake, growth and lysozyme activity in European whitefish (*Coregonus lavaretus* L.). *Aquaculture* **234**: 41–50.

Lillehaug, A. 1989. A survey on different procedures used for vaccinating salmonids against vibriosis in Norwegian fish farming. *Aquaculture* **83**: 217–26.

Lillehaug, A. 1991. Vaccination of Atlantic salmon (*Salmo salar* L.) against cold-water vibriosis – duration of protection and effect on growth rate. *Aquaculture* **92**: 99–107.

Lillehaug, A., Lunder, T. and Poppe, T.T. 1992. Field testing of adjuvanted furunculosis vaccines in Atlantic salmon, *Salmo salar* L. *J Fish Dis* **15**: 485–96.

Maira, C., Lystad, Y., Schrøder, M.B., *et al.*, 2007. Bieffektvurderinger hos torsk etter stikkvaksinering – bruk av en vurderingsskala tilpasset torsk. *Nor Fiskeoppdr* **32**: 52–5.

Midtlyng, P.J. and Lillehaug, A. 1998. Growth of Atlantic salmon *Salmo salar* after intraperitoneal administration of vaccines containing adjuvants. *Dis Aquat Org* **32**: 91–7.

Midtlyng, P.J., Reitan, L.J. and Speilberg, L. 1996. Experimental studies on the efficacy and side-effects of intraperitoneal vaccination of Atlantic salmon (*Salmo salar* L.) against furunculosis. *Fish Shellfish Immunol* **6**: 335–50.

Mulvey, B., Landolt, M.L. and Busch, R.A. 1995. Effects of potassium aluminium sulphate (alum) used in an *Aeromonas salmonicida* bacterin on Atlantic salmon, *Salmo salar* L. *J Fish Dis* **18**: 495–506.

Mutoloki, S., Brudeseth, B., Reite, O.B. and Evensen, Ø. 2006a. The contribution of *Aeromonas salmonicida* extracellular products to the induction of inflammation in Atlantic salmon (*Salmo salar* L.) following vaccination with oil-based vaccines. *Fish Shellfish Immunol* **20**: 1–11.

Mutoloki, S., Reite, O.B., Brudeseth, B., *et al.*, 2006b. A comparative immunopathological study of injection-site reactions in salmonids following intraperitoneal injection with oil-adjuvanted vaccines. *Vaccine* **24**: 578–88.

Olsen, A.B., Birkbeck, T.H., Nilsen, H.K., *et al.*, 2006. Vaccine-associated systemic *Rhodococcus erythropolis* infection in farmed Atlantic salmon *Salmo salar*. *Dis Aquat Org* **72**: 9–17.

Poppe, T.T. and Breck, O. 1997. Pathology of Atlantic salmon *Salmo salar* intraperitoneally immunized with oil-adjuvanted vaccine. A case report. *Dis Aquat Org* **29**: 219–26.

Pylkkö, P., Lyytikäinen, T., Ritola, O. and Pelkonen, S. 2000. Vaccination influences growth of Arctic charr. *Dis Aquat Org* **43**: 77–80.

Rønsholdt, B. and McLean, E. 1999. The effect of vaccination and vaccine components upon short-time growth and feed conversion efficiency in rainbow trout. *Aquaculture* **174**: 213–21.

Skrudland, A., Taksdal, T. and Kvellestad, A. 2002. Uhell og skade ved vaksinering av laks. *Nor Vet Tidsskr* **114**: 494–5.

Sørum, U. and Damsgård, B. 2004. Effects of anaesthetisation and vaccination on feed intake and growth in Atlantic salmon (*Salmo salar* L.). *Aquaculture* **232**: 333–41.

Vågsholm, I. and Djupvik, H.O. 1998. Risk factors for spinal deformities in Atlantic salmon, *Salmo salar* L. *J Fish Dis* **21**: 47–53.

14 Future Fish Vaccinology

Øystein Evensen

Norwegian School of Veterinary Science, Oslo, Norway

ABSTRACT

The majority of fish vaccines intended for injection are inactivated, whole virus/bacteria vaccines, often prepared with an adjuvant like mineral or vegetable oil. Immersion vaccines are usually non-adjuvanted and the majority of these vaccines are bacterin-based, while live vaccines, for injection or immersion, are used to a very limited extent. In the years to come we will see that the current vaccine formulations are refined to give reduced side-effects, local and systemic. It is also foreseen that the vaccine formulations and immunomodulating compounds can direct and improve the immune response, particularly against intracellular pathogens. DNA vaccines will also likely be part of the future vaccine portfolio. Immunization through the mucosal surfaces will be refined and improved in coming years, probably with a focus on improved local responses that can evoke an immune protection at the site of entry of the pathogen or the primary replication site. Vaccines against intracellular bacterial and viral pathogens will be one of the big challenges for the next 10 years of fish vaccine research. Use of DNA vaccine technology will likely play a role here, and so will new and improved formulations, oral boosting regimes, and possibly live vaccine preparations.

14.1 MOLECULAR TECHNOLOGIES

Advances in molecular biology have provided contributions to virological research, and with it also vaccines against virus infections. The techniques that make it possible to remove (knock-out), inactivate and insert genes in the virus, will allow the study of virulence mechanisms and components of importance for immunity. The novel techniques can be used to produce vaccines with certain advantages over conventional vaccines, particularly when the etiological agent is difficult to culture and it is sufficient that the genes of importance for immunity are known.

oystein.evensen@nmbu.no

Fish Vaccination, First Edition. Edited by Roar Gudding, Atle Lillehaug and Øystein Evensen.

14.2 RECOMBINANT VACCINES

There were great expectations of the new technologies of molecular biology and their potential application in recombinant vaccine technology. Expectations were, however, not fully met, and today we see few recombinant subunit vaccines used for vaccination of fish, but also for warm-blooded animals and even for humans. There are several reasons for this. Recombinant subunit vaccines have poor immunogenicity, as already mentioned. DNA vaccine technologies sparked new interest in the field of vaccinology, but also here we have seen several setbacks, not least related to the dose needed to elicit an immune response, and the variability between pathogens in terms of efficacy has discouraged many to embark on a long development plan for DNA vaccines. Safety aspects have also created some concern. It should be mentioned that therapeutic DNA vaccines possibly hold better promise in humans than prophylactic DNA vaccines. There are currently two licensed DNA vaccines, one of them against IHN in Atlantic salmon, and the other against melanoma in dogs (Bergman and Wolchok, 2008). There is also a DNA vaccine available against West Nile virus infections in condors (Chang *et al.*, 2007), and the first approved DNA vaccine was against West Nile virus infection of horses, but its sale has been discontinued.

14.2.1 Subunit vaccines

Escherichia coli strains are used as competent cells for propagation of plasmids encoding a protective antigen, with subsequent harvest of antigen at the end of the fermentation cycle. A classical example in fish vaccinology is the *E. coli*-based subunit vaccine against infectious pancreatic necrosis (IPN) in Atlantic salmon, licensed for the first time in 1995. *E. coli* is convenient for use, not least because this bacterium is widely used in molecular biological work and therefore many research laboratories have knowledge of the techniques and tools that are needed for proper expression of the transgene.

Recombinant vaccines have also been produced in *Saccharomyces cerevisiae*, including a subunit vaccine against infectious salmon anemia (ISA) in Chile. Other vectors may also be used for production of recombinant of vaccines, like silkworm, cabbage worm, plants and insect cells. There are currently no commercial vaccines available on the market based on these methods, but several experimental studies have been carried out, including IPN vaccines produced in cabbage worms (*Trichoplusia ni*) (Shivappa *et al.*, 2005), and plant-derived antigens expressing the capsid protein of nodavirus. The G-protein of viral hemorrhagic septicemia virus has been produced in *E. coli* (Lorenzen *et al.*, 1993), and the virus has also been propagated in insect cells (Lorenzen and Olesen, 1995). The latter has not been tested for their ability to induce immune responses, and recombinant proteins elicit a variable immune response and confer low protection (Lorenzen *et al.*, 1993).

Recombinant subunit vaccines have advantages over classical inactivated vaccines. A host organism is used for the production of the protective antigen(s). Multi-step, downstream purification processes are used to prepare recombinant vaccines after the antigen has been harvested from the vector organism. Recombinant subunit vaccines have particular advantages if it is difficult to cultivate the disease-causing microorganism. This applies to some viruses and other microorganisms. There is general agreement that recombinant subunit vaccines are safe for use, but of inferior immunogenicity compared with inactivated, whole cell/virus vaccines (Webster *et al.*, 1977). Potent adjuvants are therefore needed to improve immunogenicity.

There are few subunit vaccines available for use in farmed fish, and IPN and ISA vaccines are the best examples. For higher vertebrates some subunit recombinant vaccines have marketing authorization, but are still relatively limited in number. The vaccine against hepatitis B virus is one good example, and a vaccine against feline infectious leukemia containing a protein of FeLV virus, P45, produced in canary smallpox virus is also available on the market. It is not foreseen that the major advances in fish vaccinology will come within the field of recombinant subunit vaccines, but they will probably be the method of choice for some of the viruses that are difficult to grow like piscine reovirus (causing heart and skeletal muscle inflammation in Atlantic salmon) and piscine myocarditis virus (causing cardiomyopathy syndrome in Atlantic salmon).

14.2.2 Genetically modified vaccines

Live, attenuated vaccines based on numerous *in vitro* passages have been used for many decades for vaccination of higher vertebrates. Passage results in genome mutations that render the pathogen non-pathogenic, and the underlying mechanisms are not known. By use of molecular techniques, it is possible to attenuate microorganisms by removing/deleting specific genes or part of genes, thereby rendering the microorganism apathogenic.

Genetically modified vaccines are delivered to the animal as a live vaccine, and they will replicate as their pathogenic wild-type but at lower replication levels (Vaughan *et al.*, 1993; Marsden *et al.*, 1996, 1998). They will therefore stimulate an immune response that includes humoral and cellular immunity (Marsden *et al.*, 1998) and can also be used for induction of immune responses at mucosal surfaces. A broad immune response is one of the main benefits of genetically modified vaccines, and in general they confer moderate (Vivas *et al.*, 2004) to high degrees of protection against disease.

Live attenuated bacterial vaccines can be generated by rational design where genes encoding specific enzymes are mutated or deleted. This may be enzymes required to produce certain amino acids, and one example is the *aroA* gene (Vaughan *et al.*, 1993). Strains lacking this gene cannot produce aromatic amino acids. Attenuation can also occur by removing or altering genes encoding toxins that are important for the development of disease.

Genetic stability is the key point when evaluating safety of live attenuated vaccines. The risk of reversion to virulence or increase in virulence is considered to be higher for vaccines attenuated by traditional methods (passage) than for vaccines attenuated by molecular methods. The reasoning is that vaccines attenuated by traditional passage will usually have point mutations in the genome whereas vaccines generated by molecular techniques can "knock out" entire genes.

An example from fish-pathogenic bacteria is *Aeromonas salmonicida* that has been attenuated by removal of the *aroA* gene (Marsden *et al.*, 1996). This mutant has been shown to provide good short-term protection against furunculosis (Marsden *et al.*, 1998). The vaccine is currently not in used because adjuvanted, inactivated vaccines are considered a safer alternative and provide a high degree of protection, and there is also some doubt as to the longevity of protection (Figure 14.1).

Reverse genetics is the method of choice for attenuated virus vaccines, but of course not feasible for all virus species. There are examples where *Infectious hematopoietic necrosis virus* and *Viral hemorrhagic septicemia virus* (VHS) of the genus *Novirhabdovirus* have been rendered apathogenic by deleting the NV gene (Brémont, 2005). These NV-knock-out variants have then been used to immunize fish against IHN and VHS, respectively, and a high degree of

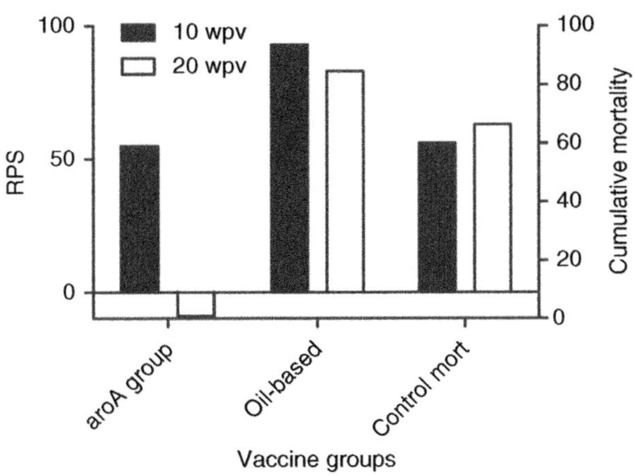

Fig. 14.1 Relative percent survival (RPS) in *aroA* and oil-based vaccine groups of Atlantic salmon (*Salmo salar* L.), challenged 10 and 20 weeks post-vaccination (wpv). RPS is good for both vaccines at 10 wpv, while at 20 wpv the *aroA*-vaccinated group shows a negative RPS value while the oil-based vaccine still obtains more than 80%. (Source: Evensen 2009, unpublished.)

protection has been obtained in rainbow trout and Japanese flounder. Improved protection can be achieved by use of prime-boost strategies. Further avirulent variants of *Salmon pancreas disease virus* (SPDV) made by reverse genetics have shown to give a high level of protection against sleeping disease in trout (Mérour *et al.*, 2013).

14.2.3 Vector vaccines

A third type of recombinant vaccine is produced when genes from one or more virulence factors or protective antigens of a pathogenic microorganism are transferred to a live avirulent microorganism. Vectors can be viruses or bacteria. Vaccinia virus was used to eradicate smallpox in humans and has later been used as a vaccine vector. It has a large genome so that foreign genes can be accepted, it is well characterized, and it is considered non-pathogenic.

A vector vaccine will stimulate a diverse immune response. Recombinant vector vaccines may stimulate humoral or cell-mediated immunity, which is usually not obtained for inactivated vaccines. An oral vaccine consisting of non-pathogenic intestinal bacteria colonizing the gut epithelial cells, and which simultaneously produces important antigens from a different microorganism, can stimulate production of a protective mucosal immunity. In diseases where unwanted antigens are important for disease development (e.g., feline infectious peritonitis or feline leukemia virus), vector vaccines can be used to exclude antigens that confer immunosuppression otherwise unwanted in the vaccine.

Vector vaccines have been tested to a very limited extent in finfish vaccinology. Immunization with vector vaccines will also result in the development of an immune response against the vector/vector antigens. Pre-existing antibodies against the vector virus can neutralize or inhibit viral vector such that the immune response against the foreign antigens is reduced. Vector vaccines are interesting candidates as carriers of foreign antigens also for finfish, and a replicon vaccine based upon the structural proteins of salmon pancreas disease virus has been shown to elicit protective immunity against ISA in Atlantic salmon (Wolf *et al.*, 2013).

Plants can also be used as vectors. This means that the vaccine can be administered in the feed, which will be an important asset for vaccines for animals. An oral vaccine reduces the need for both syringes and other equipment, and qualified personnel to carry out the vaccination. The protective effect of oral vaccines is still poor, which is an important limitation for the development of vector vaccines based on plants.

14.2.4 DNA vaccines

DNA vaccines have been described in a separate chapter. To what extent DNA vaccines will come into general use in aquaculture is not easy to predict. Their efficacy for many virus infections (Biering and Salonius, 2014) is well documented, and for these it is likely we will see additional vaccines being available in the market, like DNA vaccines against pancreas disease in salmonids. For this reason it is possible they will become part of the portfolio of vaccines available for use in aquaculture fish in the future.

The challenge for DNA vaccines is primarily related to genome integration, a safety issue. This primarily applies to the vaccinated animal, but has implications also for food safety. Questions have also been raised related to production of anti-DNA antibodies in the vaccinated animal, which give an autoimmunity condition, but studies so far lend very little support for this concern.

14.3 MARKER VACCINES

Under strict control regimes, traditional disease control measures include stamping out of infected animals. When identification of infected animals is based on serology, vaccination will often preclude differentiation between infected and vaccinated animals (Vannier *et al.*, 2007). The development of recombinant vaccines has made it possible to distinguish between the two categories. Such vaccines are referred to as marker vaccines or DIVA (differentiation between infected and vaccinated animals) vaccines. Such vaccines are usually genetically modified vaccines (gene-deleted vaccines) or they will lack an antigen against which the infected animal will mount an immune response. All four categories of recombinant vaccines may be used as marker vaccines. Marker vaccines have not been used in aquaculture so far.

14.4 MUCOSAL VACCINATION

The mucosal membranes are the gateway to systemic distribution for many pathogens. Stimulation of immunity in the mucosa with the purpose of halting an infection at an early stage has therefore been a sought-after strategy. Mucosal immunity in mammals is based upon IgA antibodies. In rainbow trout, IgT has been identified as the mucosal antibody (Zhang *et al.*, 2010). To what extent immunization in one compartment (like the gut) will result in protection in other compartments (like gills) remains to be proven. In general it has proved difficult to achieve good immunity against disease when primary immunization is performed via mucosal surfaces. Various types of vaccines that have been tested for their ability to stimulate mucosal immunity vaccines delivered by immersion have proven to elicit better immunity than oral vaccines. Inactivated vaccines generally elicit a poor immune response when given orally (Rombout and Viswanath, 2014).

It is foreseen that there will be more interest in the use of oral or mucosal vaccines in the future, particularly since there has been a lot of focus on side-effects from the use of adjuvanted injection vaccines and the need to boost primary vaccinations, delivered via injection routes or by mucosal surfaces.

14.5 VACCINES AGAINST PARASITIC DISEASES

Parasites cause major losses in all biological productions, and vaccines are only used to a limited extent to prevent infections with parasites (Vercruysse *et al.*, 2007). The reason is partly access to effective drugs for treatment, and partly due to the fact that it has proven difficult to obtain good levels of protection against parasites.

There are two main approaches that have been taken for developing vaccines against parasites: they can be based on live, attenuated parasites, or use subunit vaccines containing specific antigens produced by recombinant techniques cloned from endogenous proteins or enzymes often referred to as concealed antigens. Live, attenuated virus vaccines are not available for use in farmed fish. As regards a concealed antigen approach, this is best known from vaccine development against the tick, *Boophilus microplus*, in cattle, based on a protein, Bm86, as antigen (Willadsen *et al.*, 1992). This protein is part of the cell membranes in the intestine of the parasite. The host is not exposed to this protein as a consequence of infestation. By recombinant technology the antigen is delivered as a subunit vaccine to the host, and while the parasites suck blood, circulating antibodies will bind to the protein in the epithelial lineage of the gut and damage the intestinal functions of the parasite. The vaccine against *Boophilus* reduces losses and reduces the risk of other diseases that are transmitted by the parasite.

A similar approach has been used for the development of a vaccine against sea lice in salmonids, for *Lepeophtheirus salmonis* and *Caligus rogercrossey* infections. Preliminary studies are indicative of up to 40% reduction in the number of attached stages of the parasite (chalimus) compared with non-vaccinated animals. These studies have so far not been done in a full-scale production environment. In addition to this there are many challenges: the identification and production of appropriate antigens is one. Secondly, there is also some discussion as to what degree the attached stages of the sea lice consume blood. If not, circulating antibodies would have to be delivered to the skin mucus/surface. The more recent discovery that fish also have a mucosal immunoglobulin (IgT) bears some prospects that vaccines formulated to induce immune responses at mucosal sites would favor anti-parasite responses (Zhang *et al.*, 2010).

14.6 VACCINES FOR CONTROLLING REPRODUCTION

Farmed salmon escaping from captivity (so-called escapees) represent a potential threat to local strains of Atlantic salmon when they migrate up local rivers. For this reason, means to control sexual maturation through vaccination has been discussed as one opportunity. This can be achieved by immunizing with a synthetic analog of gonadotropin-releasing hormone (GnRH), which stimulates the production of antibodies against GnRH (Delves and Roitt, 2005). Since the antigen has low molecular weight, conjugation to a carrier protein and the use of adjuvant requires the level of antibodies against GnRH to be sufficiently high.

It will be possible to influence reproductive and other functions under endocrine control. An alternative is to use luteinizing hormone (LH) from the hypothalamus and pituitary as an antigen.

14.7 IMPROVED FORMULATIONS

Large strides have been made in fields related to new adjuvants and carrier molecules. One of the challenges is better stimulation of immunity on mucous membranes and skin. Protection of antigens in the front part of the gastrointestinal tract, and release of antigens near lymphoid tissue, is a goal. This can be made possible by entrapping the antigens in microcapsules composed of biodegradable polymers. One interesting observation is that the most significant contributions in this field have been the reduction of adjuvant used in injectable, oil-based fish vaccines over the last decade. Today, 50 μl is used regularly for injection, while when the first oil-based vaccines came into use, the injection volume was four times higher, so there has been a marked reduction over recent years. This reduction has made a significant contribution to the improved side-effect profile of the vaccines used in the Atlantic salmon market, particularly in Norway and Chile. For comparison we now inject 1.0–1.25 μl/g of live weight (40–50 g fish), while in humans the volume is 0.1 μl/g live weight (1 ml dose to a 10 kg child).

14.8 IMMUNOMODULATION

Cytokines are proteins produced by various cells such as lymphocytes, macrophages and other cells in the immune system. Some cytokines are involved in the regulation of immune response, both in terms of strength and character/profile. Cytokines also skew the immune response and arm immune effector cells. T helper (Th) cells play a central role in the immune system by producing several cytokines that direct the immune responses into different categories of responses. Overall these are defined as Th1, Th2 and Th17 (Mutoloki *et al.*, 2014). By molecular tools it is possible to produce cytokines to be used as immunomodulators or stimulants. There are, however, several challenges that must be solved before cytokines can be used as immunomodulating compounds in vaccines. Cytokines serve in a fine-tuned network, and overexpression can be deleterious to the host and thus promote disease rather than preventing it. Besides, cytokines are unstable compounds with a short half-life, making it difficult to achieve a prolonged effect of added cytokines.

Yet another area where there has been a lot of research over the last decade is pathogen receptor systems of various cells, typically toll-like receptors and various cytosolic receptors of dsRNA compounds and triphosphate RNA sensors. The ligands of these receptors are potential compounds to be used as immunomodulators in vaccines, like dsRNA (poly I:C), CpG, and other synthetic ligands that engage many of these receptor/sensor systems. These receptors/sensors are well conserved in lower vertebrates, and stimulation studies have been performed at cellular and organismic levels (Jørgensen, 2014). It is likely that we will see toll-like receptor ligands included as immunomodulators in the vaccine before cytokines come into use as immune adjuvants, but both carry the potential of being able to direct and modify responses to vaccine antigens, particularly when inactivated vaccine preparations are used.

14.9 CYTOKINES AND DAMPS (DANGER-ASSOCIATED MOLECULAR PATTERN) AS ADJUVANTS

In past years, a great number of cytokine genes have been identified in numerous fish species, but despite the fact that the use of cytokines as adjuvants has been widely explored in mammals, not many studies have focused on the possible use of cytokine genes as vaccine adjuvants in fish. This may be due to the fact that, for the majority of these molecules, many details concerning their immunological role are still lacking, and until we know what immune processes they are regulating, their use would be merely trial and error. In any case, some attempts to explore their potential have been made in some fish species.

Administration of IL-1ß-derived peptides to rainbow trout by IP injection induced reduced mortality of fish when exposed to VHSV after 2 days (Peddie *et al.*, 2003). The peptides also induced leukocyte migration into the peritoneal cavity 1–3 days post-injection, but its possible use as adjuvant was not further explored. The role of IL-1ß as an adjuvant was investigated in carp after IP injection of killed *A. hydrophila* in the absence and presence of recombinant C-terminal peptide of carp IL-1ß. It was found that the agglutinating antibody titer was significantly higher in the fish injected with killed bacteria plus recombinant IL-1ß peptide compared with killed bacteria alone, 3 weeks after vaccination (Yin and Kwang, 2000). The DAMP *Hsp70* (heat shock protein 70) gene was included in a DNA vaccine that also encoded for a *Streptococcus inia* antigen; this molecular vaccine showed promising results in a challenge experiment (Hu *et al.*, 2012).

Interleukin-8 (IL-8) is a CXC chemokine produced by many cell types in mammals, like macrophages, monocytes, epithelial cells, neutrophils and fibroblasts upon infection, or stimulated by cytokines like IL-1ß and tumor necrosis factor α (TNF-α). In mammals, chemokines have been widely used as experimental adjuvants in vaccines against viral infections, since not only do they attract more cells to the site of inflammation, but they also regulate the immune functions of the recruited cells. In fish, IL-8 has been characterized in rainbow trout among other species, and its chemo-attractant properties established (Harun *et al.*, 2008). In this species, a vaccine plasmid coding for the glycoprotein gene of VHSV was co-injected with a plasmid coding for rainbow trout IL-8 to explore its potential adjuvant effect (Jimenez *et al.*, 2006; Sanchez *et al.*, 2007). When the plasmid coding of IL-8 (pIL-8+) was administered together with the VHSV vaccine, an increase of IL-1ß in the spleen was found together with a greater cellular infiltration at the site of inoculation. Furthermore, fish injected with pIL-8+ alone showed a significantly higher expression of TNF-α, IL-11, TGF-ß and IL-18 in the spleen (Jimenez *et al.*, 2006). In a further study, the transcription of different inducible CC chemokines were studied in rainbow trout in response to both the VHSV DNA vaccine and/or pIL8+, demonstrating that when IL-8 is used as an adjuvant, the expression of other chemokines such as CK5A, CK6, CK7 and CK5B is also modulated (Sanchez *et al.*, 2007). All these results showed that IL-8 was able to modulate the early immune response and could be a potent vaccine adjuvant in fish against viral infections.

14.10 CONCLUDING REMARKS

In this summary we have not discussed the development of vaccines and assessment of host responses to vaccination in the context of host genome sequencing. The salmon genome is soon to become publicly available, and several model fish species have been fully sequenced. This is and will be a new era in fish vaccinology, particularly with the detailed fingerprinting of the protective immune response following immunization or natural infection. With new tools like high throughput sequencing and powerful analysis of transcriptome and proteome levels that likely will become available over the next decade, it is foreseen that the understanding of underlying fish responses to vaccination will also take a major step forward.

REFERENCES

Bergman, P.J. and Wolchok, J.D. 2008. Of Mice and Men (and Dogs): development of a xenogeneic DNA vaccine for canine oral malignant melanoma. *Cancer Ther* **6**: 817–26.

Biering, E. and Salonius, K. 2014. DNA vaccines, in *Fish Vaccination* (eds R. Gudding, A. Lillehaug and Ø. Evensen). Oxford, John Wiley & Sons, Ltd., 47–55.

Brémont, M. 2005. Reverse genetics on fish rhabdoviruses: tools to study the pathogenesis of fish rhabdoviruses. *Curr Top Microbiol Immunol* **292**: 119–41.

Chang, G.J., Davis, B.S., Stringfield, C. and Lutz, C. 2007. Prospective immunization of the endangered California condors (*Gymnogyps californianus*) protects this species from lethal West Nile virus infection. *Vaccine* **25**: 2325–30.

Delves, P.J. and Roitt, I.M. 2005. Vaccines for the control of reproduction – status in mammals, and aspects of comparative interest. *Dev Biol (Basel)* **121**: 265–73.

Harun, N.O., Zou, J., Zhang, Y.A., *et al*., 2008. The biological effects of rainbow trout (*Oncorhynchus mykiss*) recombinant interleukin-8. *Dev Comp Immunol* **32**: 673–81.

Hu, Y.H., Dang, W., Zhang, M. and Sun, L. 2012. Japanese flounder (*Paralichthys olivaceus*) Hsp70: adjuvant effect and its dependence on the intrinsic ATPase activity. *Fish Shellfish Immunol* **33**: 829–34.

Jimenez, N., Coll, J., Salguero, B.F.J. and Tafalla, C. 2006. Co-injection of interleukin 8 with the glycoprotein gene from viral haemorrhagic septicemia virus (VHSV) modulates the cytokine response in rainbow trout (*Oncorhynchus mykiss*). *Vaccine* **24**: 5615–26.

Jørgensen, J. 2014. The innate immune response in fish, in *Fish Vaccination* (eds R. Gudding, A. Lillehaug and Ø. Evensen). Oxford, John Wiley & Sons, Ltd., 85–103

Lorenzen, N. and Olesen, N.J. 1995. Multiplication of VHS virus in insect cells. *Vet Res* **26**: 428–32.

Lorenzen, N., Olesen, N.J., Vestergård-Jørgensen, P.E., *et al*., 1993. Molecular cloning and expression in *Escherichia coli* of the glycoprotein gene of VHS virus, and immunization of rainbow trout with the recombinant protein. *J Gen Virol* **74**: 623–30.

Marsden MJ, Vaughan LM, Fitzpatrick RM, *et al*., 1998. Potency testing of a live, genetically attenuated vaccine for salmonids. *Vaccine* **16**: 1087–94.

Marsden, M.J., Vaughan, L.M., Foster, T.J. and Secombes, C.J. 1996. A live (Δ*aroA*) *Aeromonas salmonicida* vaccine for furunculosis preferentially stimulates T-cell responses relative to B-cell responses in rainbow trout (*Oncorhynchus mykiss*). *Infect Immun* **64**: 3863–9.

Mérour, E., Lamoureux, A., Bernard, J., *et al*., 2013. A fully attenuated recombinant salmonid alphavirus becomes pathogenic through a single amino acid change in the E2 glycoprotein. *J Virol* **87**: 6027–30.

Mutoloki, S., Jørgensen, J. and Evensen, Ø. 2014. The adaptive immune response in fish, in *Fish Vaccination* (eds R. Gudding, A. Lillehaug and Ø. Evensen). Oxford, John Wiley & Sons, Ltd., 85–103.

Peddie, S., McLauchlan, P.E., Ellis, A.E. and Secombes, C.J. 2003. Effect of intraperitoneally administered IL-1beta-derived peptides on resistance to viral haemorrhagic septicaemia in rainbow trout *Oncorhynchus mykiss*. *Dis Aquat Org* **56**: 195–200.

Rombout, J.H.W.M. and Kiron, V. 2014. Mucosal vaccination of fish, in *Fish Vaccination* (eds R. Gudding, A. Lillehaug and Ø. Evensen). Oxford, John Wiley & Sons, Ltd., 56–67.

Sanchez, E., Coll, J. and Tafalla, C. 2007. Expression of inducible CC chemokines in rainbow trout (*Oncorhynchus mykiss*) in response to a viral haemorrhagic septicemia virus (VHSV) DNA vaccine and interleukin 8. *Dev Comp Immunol* **31**: 916–26.

Shivappa, R.B., McAllister, P.E., Edwards, G.H., *et al*., 2005. Development of a subunit vaccine for infectious pancreatic necrosis virus using a baculovirus insect/larvae system. *Dev Biol (Basel)* **121**: 165–74.

Vannier, P., Capua, I., Le Potier, M.F., *et al.*, 2007. Marker vaccines and the impact of their use on diagnosis and prophylactic measures. *Rev Sci Tech* **26**: 351–72.

Vaughan, L.M., Smith, P.R. and Foster, T.J. 1993. An aromatic-dependent mutant of the fish pathogen *Aeromonas salmonicida* is attenuated in fish and is effective as a live vaccine against the salmonid disease furunculosis. *Infect Immun* **61**: 2172–81.

Vercruysse, J., Schetters, T.P.M., Knox, D.P., *et al.*, 2007. Control of parasitic disease using vaccines: an answer to drug resistance? *Rev Sci Tech* **26**: 105–15.

Vivas, J., Riaño, J., Carracedo, B., *et al.*, 2004. The auxotrophic *aroA* mutant of *Aeromonas hydrophila* as a live attenuated vaccine against *A. salmonicida* infections in rainbow trout (*Oncorhynchus mykiss*). *Fish Shellfish Immunol* **16**: 193–206.

Webster, R.G., Glezen, P., Hannoun, C. and Laver, W.G. 1977. Potentiation of the immune response to influenza virus subunit vaccines. *J Immunol* **119**: 2073–7.

Willadsen, P., Kemp, D.H., Cobon, G.S. and Wright, I.G. 1992. Successful vaccination against *Boophilus microplus* and *Babesia bovis* using recombinant antigens. *Mem Inst Oswaldo Cruz* **87** (Suppl 3): 289–94.

Wolf, A., Hodneland, K., Frost, P., *et al.*, 2013. A hemagglutinin-esterase-expressing salmonid alphavirus replicon protects Atlantic salmon (*Salmo salar*) against infectious salmon anemia (ISA). *Vaccine* **31**: 661–9.

Yin, Z. and Kwang, J. 2000. Carp interleukin-1ß in the role of an immuno-adjuvant. *Fish Shellfish Immunol* **10**: 375–8.

Zhang, Y.A., Salinas, I., Li, J., *et al.*, 2010. IgT, a primitive immunoglobulin class specialized in mucosal immunity. *Nat Immunol* **11**: 827–35.

15 Vaccination against Vibriosis

Duncan J. Colquhoun and Atle Lillehaug

Norwegian Veterinary Institute, Oslo, Norway

ABSTRACT

Vaccination against classical vibriosis has been a success story that has inspired development of vaccines against other diseases in fish. Disease outbreaks of vibriosis may occur in a range of fish species exposed to seawater around the world. In addition to *Vibrio anguillarum*, the term "vibriosis" may also include infections with *V. ordalii*, *V. splendidus*, *V. vulnificus*, *V. salmonicida* and *Moritella viscosa*. In general, vibriosis vaccines are inactivated whole-cell bacterins, with LPS as the main antigenic component. These vaccines are administered by immersion/bath or intraperitoneal injection, with both methods providing significant levels of protection. Of the various recognized *V. anguillarum* serotypes, only serotypes O1, O2α and O2β are currently included in commercial vaccines. While commercial vaccines against *V. salmonicida* and *M. viscosa* are also available, vaccines against alternative *V. anguillarum* serotypes and other vibrios may be produced as autogenous vaccines.

15.1 VIBRIOSIS

Vaccination of fish against vibriosis represents one of the most comprehensively successful developments in disease prevention in modern aquaculture. This success relates both to the broad host-range and wide geographical distribution of the disease agent(s) involved, but most particularly it relates to the effectiveness of the vaccine products developed. Vibriosis vaccine research constituted some of the earliest experiments in the field of fish vaccinology.

The term "vibriosis" in relation to vaccinology has generally been used for infections caused by *Vibrio anguillarum* and *V. ordalii*; however, diseases in fish caused by other vibrios and closely related bacteria, which have been reclassified to other genera, are included in this outline. These include cold-water vibriosis caused by *V. salmonicida*, winter ulcers caused by *Moritella viscosa*, and infections with vibrios like *V. splendidus* and *V. vulnificus*.

duncan.colquhoun@vetinst.no

Fish Vaccination, First Edition. Edited by Roar Gudding, Atle Lillehaug and Øystein Evensen.

15.2 OCCURRENCE AND SIGNIFICANCE

Vibriosis (*V. anguillarum, V. ordalii*) is a disease affecting a wide range of fish species, both wild and farmed, around the world. The bacterial agents are strictly marine, and disease outbreaks only occur in seawater and brackish water, typically during the summer months in temperate areas, while water temperatures in the subarctic regions are too low. Manifestation of the disease is usually that of a hemorrhagic septicemia, and may include skin ulcers and abscesses. In wild fish, disease outbreaks have been reported in shoaling species like saithe (Egidius, 1987) and big scale sand smelt (Yiagnisis *et al.*, 2007). Vibriosis can cause devastating losses in marine aquaculture. Marine fish species and both Atlantic and Pacific salmonid species are at risk, with rainbow trout appearing to be particularly susceptible (Lillehaug *et al.*, 2003). Vibriosis outbreaks have been reported in several aquaculture species, including the Asian ayu (*Plecoglossus altivelis*) and yellowtail (*Seriola quinqueradiata*) (Sakata *et al.*, 1989), temperate water species like sea bass (*Dicentrarchus labrax*), sea bream (*Sparus aurata*) and turbot (*Scopththalmus maximus*) (Larsen *et al.*, 1994), and cold-water species like Atlantic cod (*Gadus morhua*) and halibut (Lillehaug *et al.*, 2003).

Cold-water vibriosis (*V. salmonicida*) is much less widespread than classical vibriosis, both regarding susceptible fish species and geographical distribution. The disease attacks almost exclusively Atlantic salmon, although occasional cases do occur from time to time in farmed rainbow trout and Atlantic cod. *V. salmonicida* has been an extremely serious fish pathogen in Norway, and cold-water vibriosis was the most common disease and reason for antibiotic prescription in the 1980s (Markestad and Grave, 1997). In the years prior to its peak in prevalence (1977–1984), *V. salmonicida*-related losses were estimated to have constituted more than 80% of disease-associated costs to the Norwegian aquaculture industry (Poppe *et al.*, 1985). Since introduction of the successful vaccine in 1987, the number of annual cases experienced in Norway has fallen drastically from more than 200 outbreaks in 1987 to close to none from the late 1990s onwards. Outside Norway, cold-water vibriosis has been described from Scotland (Bruno *et al.*, 1985), Iceland, the Faroe Isles (Dalsgaard *et al.*, 1988), the US and Canada (O'Halloran and Henry, 1993).

Winter-ulcer is a disease condition involving the bacterial species *Moritella viscosa*, which is related to the true vibrios. As with cold-water vibriosis, this disease appears to be restricted to the northern Atlantic, and is most frequently observed during the winter months. Its distribution as a serious pathogen of fish appears to be restricted to Norway and Iceland, where it affects sea-farmed Atlantic salmon (Lunder *et al.*, 1995), and to a lesser extent sea-farmed rainbow trout (Lillehaug *et al.*, 2003). Dermal circulatory disturbances, together with mechanical injuries, may play a role in disease development, predisposing for infection with the bacterium. This disease remains, despite widespread vaccination against *M. viscosa*, arguably the most economically significant bacterial disease in Norwegian aquaculture at the time of writing. Fish may display ulcers for long periods and may recover if the water temperature increases. As well as direct mortalities, losses are to a significant extent related to downgrading of the final fillet products due to ulceration/scarring.

Of the fish pathogenic vibrios, only *V. vulnificus* can cause serious disease in humans (Austin, 2010). The zoonotic aspect underlines, however, the importance of scientific competence in aquatic diagnostic bacteriology. *V. vulnificus* occurs as three recognized biotypes, of which biotypes 1 and 3 commonly cause disease in humans (Colodner *et al.*, 2004), while biotype 2 (serovars A and E) are almost, but not exclusively, associated with disease in fish

(Fouz *et al.*, 2010). *V. vulnificus* causes disease most commonly in farmed eels (Amaro *et al.*, 1992; Dalsgaard *et al.*, 1999), although other marine fish species can be affected (Li *et al.*, 2006). The bacterium seems to be ubiquitous in the marine environment in warm and temperate areas, and reports of disease problems in eel have been quite numerous in the Far East and Western Europe.

The list of remaining significant etiological agents of vibrios should include species such as *V. harveyi*, which is increasingly related to mortality in both marine fin-fish species and crustacean species (Robertson *et al.*, 1998), *V. alginolyticus* (Austin *et al.*, 1993), *V. splendidus* (Thomson *et al.*, 2005) and *V. tapetis* (Bergh and Samuelsen, 2007). It should be recognized, that as with *V. anguillarum*, these species are also ubiquitous members of the aquatic microbiota, and as such only a minority of strains are likely to be pathogenic.

15.3 ETIOLOGY

Vibrio spp. are gram-negative, curved or straight bacterial rods having a fermentative metabolism, and which are generally, but not exclusively, motile by sheathed polar flagellae (Farmer *et al.*, 2005). *Vibrio* spp. may be found in freshwater (Bockemuhl *et al.*, 1986; Ivanova *et al.*, 2001), but are usually associated with marine and brackish water environments. While disease caused by various *Vibrio* spp. has been identified in freshwater environments (Giorgetti and Ceschia, 1982; Fouz and Amaro, 2003; Kitao *et al.*, 2006), it is most commonly in marine and brackish water environments that some species of *Vibrio* occur as opportunistic pathogens of aquatic organisms, giving rise to systemic infections known collectively as vibriosis. Strictly speaking, all etiological agents of vibriosis should, therefore, reside within the genus *Vibrio*, in the Family *Vibrionaceae*, Order *Vibrionales*, of the Class *Gammaproteobacteria*. Bacterial nomenclature is, however, a dynamic field. As a result, bacterial species causing systemic disease in fish, previously classified as members of the genus *Vibrio*, have now been subsequently transferred to other genera within the family *Vibrionaceae*. Examples include *Vibrio viscosus*, now *Moritella viscosa* (Benediktsdottir *et al.*, 2000); and *Vibrio salmonicida*, now *Allivibrio salmonicida* (Urbanczyk *et al.*, 2007). The latter nomenclatural change has not been universally accepted by the scientific community, probably due to the possibility of confusion with another important fish pathogen, *Aeromonas salmonicida*, on abbreviation of both species to *A. salmonicida*. The term vibriosis will, therefore, for the purposes of the present chapter, be extended to include diseases caused by bacterial species currently residing within the Genus *Vibrio* and a single species now residing within the *Moritellaceae* (Table 15.1).

While the term vibriosis may correctly be used to describe disease caused by a wide variety of more or less related *Vibrio* species (Table 15.1), for many workers the term "classical vibriosis" is reserved for infections caused by *Vibrio anguillarum* and *V. ordalii*. The previously "grey" taxonomic position of *V. anguillarum* has recently been resolved with the proposed return of this bacterium to the genus *Vibrio* from the genus *Listonella* (Thompson *et al.*, 2011). *V. anguillarum* has a worldwide distribution, having been described as an agent of vibriosis in Europe, Asia, the Americas and Australasia (Munday *et al.*, 1992; Austin and Austin, 2007; Silva-Rubio *et al.*, 2008) in many different species of fish (Austin and Austin, 2007). Several serotyping schemes initially established for *V. anguillarum* were unified to a single system defining 23 serotypes (Pedersen *et al.*, 1999). In addition, strains not corresponding with known serotypes remain commonly identified, mainly from

Table 15.1 Main bacterial species associated with vibriosis in fish.

Bacterial species	**Main host species/group**	**Relevant references**
Vibrio anguillarum	Diverse species*	Austin *et al.* (1995)
		Grisez and Ollevier (1995)
		Kitao *et al.* (1984)
		Larsen *et al.* (1988)
		Larsen *et al.* (1994)
		Pedersen and Larsen (1995)
		Pedersen *et al.* (1999)
		Silva-Rubio *et al.* (2008)
		Song *et al.* (1988)
		Sørensen and Larsen (1986)
		Toranzo and Barja (1990)
Vibrio ordalii	Pacific salmon (*Oncorhynchus* spp.)	Colquhoun *et al.* (2004)
	Ayu (*Plectoglossus altivelis*)	Muroga *et al.* (1986)
	Atlantic salmon (*Salmo salar*)	Schiewe and Crosa (1981)
	Atlantic cod (*Gadus morhua*)	Schiewe *et al.* (1981)
Vibrio harveyi	Diverse marine fish and shrimp species	Austin and Zhang (2006)
Vibrio splendidus	Corkwing wrasse (*Symphodus melops*)	Jensen *et al.* (2003)
Vibrio tapetis	Corkwing wrasse (*Symphodus melops*)	Jensen *et al.* (2003)
Vibrio vulnificus	European eel (*Anguilla anguilla*)	Amaro and Biosca (1996)
Vibrio alginolyticus	Diverse species (warmer waters)	Balebona *et al.* (1998)
		Colorni *et al.* (1981)
		Kusada *et al.* (1986)
		Lee (1995)
Vibrio (Aliivibrio) salmonicida	Atlantic salmon (*Salmo salar*)	Lillehaug (1990)
	Rainbow trout (*Oncorhynchus mykiss*)	Lillehaug *et al.* (1990)
	Atlantic cod (*Gadus morhua*)	Schrøder *et al.* (1992)
Moritella viscosa (V. viscosus)	Atlantic salmon (*Salmo salar*)	Lunder *et al.* (1995)
	Rainbow trout (*Oncorhynchus mykiss*)	Grove *et al.* (2010)

*A degree of host specificity amongst serotypes has been identified.

environmental sources. By far the majority of fish pathogenic *V. anguillarum* isolates belong to serotypes O1 and O2 (including various subtypes), although serotype O3 has also been associated with disease in a range of fish species, including sea-bass, ayu, eels (Tiainen *et al.*, 1997) and salmonids in Chile (Silva-Rubio *et al.*, 2008). Evidence also exists for a degree of host-species specificity within certain serotypes of *V. anguillarum* (Colquhoun, unpublished results). As novel sero-/genotypes may be identified on introduction of new species of fish to aquaculture (Mikkelsen *et al.*, 2011), we may expect the diversity of known pathogenic *Vibrio* spp. to increase as aquaculture expands and diversifies.

V. ordalii, initially characterized as *V. anguillarum* biotype 2 (Schiewe and Crosa, 1981) prior to its description as an independent species (Schiewe *et al.*, 1981), is, in fact, very highly related to *V. anguillarum*, although possessing a considerably smaller genome (Naka *et al.*, 2011). The smaller genome suggests that *V. ordalii* may be undergoing genomic degradation consistent with evolutionary progression from an environmental to an obligate intracellular lifestyle (Naka *et al.*, 2011). While *V. ordalii* is also a well-established etiological agent of vibriosis, its reported distribution range is more restricted than *V. anguillarum*. *V. ordalii* has been reported as a pathogen of fish in North and South America, Japan, Australasia (Schiewe and Crosa, 1981; Wards *et al.*, 1991; Colquhoun *et al.*, 2004), and more recently Norway (http://www.vetinst.no/eng/Publications/Fish-Health-Report/The-Farmed-Fish-Health-Report-2005).

15.4 PATHOGENESIS

As with all infectious diseases, vibriosis is a result of the interplay between pathogen, host and environment. Water temperature is undoubtedly one of the major factors related to vibriosis outbreaks, with most cases involving wild and farmed fish associated with relatively high water temperatures during the summer months in temperate areas. The general association with high water temperatures is undoubtedly related both to increased bacterial virulence/activity, but also increased stress and reduced immunological capability in the affected fish populations. Handling of fish during grading or, paradoxically, vaccination, may also tip the balance in favor of the pathogen, resulting in outbreak of disease. Exceptions to the rule relating higher water temperatures to increased virulence are the diseases cold-water vibriosis and winter-ulcer caused by *V. salmonicida* and *M. viscosa*, respectively. These bacteria are associated with low temperatures and rarely cause disease above 10–11°C (Colquhoun *et al.*, 2002; Björnsdóttir *et al.*, 2011). In the case of *V. salmonicida*, it has been established that iron sequestration is greatly increased at low temperatures, with little or no siderophore production at temperatures above 10°C (Colquhoun and Sørum, 2001). The reasons for this relationship are no doubt also based on the host/pathogen balance, with reduced immunological activity of fish hosts at low temperatures.

Vibriosis can be generally described as disseminated systemic infections for which the macroscopically visible, and non-specific external signs, may include necrotic lesions and varying degrees of cutaneous hemorrhage on both body and fins, with or without exophthalmia. Internally, extensive inflammation, hemorrhage and often ascites may be observed. As vibriosis commonly manifests in a manner independent of the bacterial species involved, it is likely that many fish pathogenic vibrios share a number of basic virulence mechanisms, which may, together with more specific traits, result in a virulent phenotype. Species-specific pathogenesis is undoubtedly a complex interplay between many factors, few of which may be absolutely required for virulence. Extracellular toxins, such as proteases (Denkin and Nelson, 2004; Varina *et al.*, 2008) and hemolysins, undoubtedly play a role in vibriosis, as intramuscular injection of extracellular bacterial products has resulted in formation of lesions consistent with pathological changes observed during natural infections.

Despite characterization of many putative virulence factors in *Vibrio anguillarum*, much remains unknown (Naka *et al.*, 2011). Virulence in this bacterial species, recently reviewed (Frans *et al.*, 2011), has been related to factors including an operative flagellar system (Milton *et al.*, 1996; Ormonde *et al.*, 2000). Karlsen *et al.* (2008) demonstrated that flagellae in *V. salmonicida* were active in seawater, yet inactive under salinities equivalent to physiological levels within the host, suggesting a role in colonization. *V. anguillarum* and *V. alginolyticus* are highly chemotactic towards fish mucus, particularly in the intestine (O'Toole *et al.*, 1996; Bordas *et al.*, 1998), while Knudsen *et al.* (1999) identified serotype-specific binding of both *V. anguillarum* and *V. salmonicida* to salmon mucus. Denkin and Nelson (1999) showed that salmon mucus induces protease production in *V. anguillarum*. Both plasmid (Crosa *et al.*, 1977) and chromosomally bound iron sequestering systems (Lemos *et al.*, 1988) have been identified and associated with virulence in various vibrio species. Temperature-dependent siderophore-mediated iron sequestration was also identified in *V. salmonicida* (Colquhoun and Sørum, 2001). The ability to form biofilm is common to many types of bacteria, including vibrios, and may play a role in both colonization and persistence (Marco-Noales *et al.*, 2001). Biofilm-associated genes have been identified in *V. anguillarum* (Croxatto *et al.*, 2002; Wang *et al.*, 2002), *V. ordalii* (Naka *et al.*, 2011) and *V. alginolyticus* (Chen *et al.*, 2012). *Vibrio vulnificus* has been shown to establish a biofilm on the skin surface of affected eels, and *Vibrio harveyi* biofilms are described on various surfaces in association with shrimp disease (Karunasagar *et al.*, 1996). Tunsjø *et al.* (2009) suggest temperature-related adhesion as a possible virulence factor in *Moritella viscosa*, while the same authors also suggest a role for flagellae in colonization, and involvement of a putative tissue-necrotizing factor and a putative protease in tissue damage (Tunsjø *et al.*, 2011).

It would appear that the fish pathogenic vibrios are capable of rapid invasion of the tissues. The gill was identified as a portal of entry for *Moritella viscosa* (Løvoll *et al.*, 2009), while *V. salmonicida* was identified in the bloodstream of bath-challenged fish as little as two hours following challenge (Bjelland *et al.*, 2012). Colonization of the skin (Kanno *et al.*, 1990) and posterior intestine (Olsson *et al.*, 1996) with subsequent tissue invasion has been suggested for *V. anguillarum*.

15.5 VACCINES

Vibriosis vaccines are, for the most part, inactivated whole-cell bacterins designed for immersion or intraperitoneal injection. A number of vaccines can be administered by both routes. While oil-adjuvanted injectable vibriosis vaccines, considered to provide increased and extended levels of protection over non-adjuvanted formulations, have been recently and successfully introduced in marine fish, most injectable vibrio vaccines are delivered as a part of multicomponent vaccines, either non-adjuvanted or oil-adjuvanted. The highest valency currently available in the commercial market appears to be vaccines licensed for use in Atlantic salmon in Norway, which contain seven antigenic components, five of them bacterial including *V. anguillarum* serotypes O1 and O2a, *Vibrio salmonicida* and *Moritella viscosa*, in addition to *Aeromonas salmonicida*. The increased level of protection awarded by oil-adjuvanted vaccines is probably associated with a combination of the increased depot effect and slow antigen release from oil droplets, as well as general immune stimulation by the oil itself.

While commercial vaccine formulations are very well kept secrets, most, if not all, commercially available vibriosis vaccines are based on inactivated (either formalin inactivated or heat-killed) whole-cell broth-cultured bacterial cells. Manufacturers undoubtedly tailor culture conditions in terms of nutrient availability and culture temperature to optimize production of relevant antigens.

LPS (lipopolysaccharide) is definitely one of the most important antigenic components in vaccines against fish pathogenic vibrios, and one key feature of any vibrio vaccine is choice of the relevant LPS antigen (i.e., inclusion of the relevant bacterial species and serotype within the vaccine formulation). As little as 100 pg purified LPS from *V. ordalii* administered orally or 500 ng/ml administered as an immersion treatment (Velji *et al.*, 1990) protected juvenile coho salmon from infection. While there is undoubtedly a degree of cross-protection awarded by vibrios which may be quite broad, for example, *Vibrio salmonicida* vaccination appears to provide a degree of protection against *Aeromonas salmonicida* (Hoel *et al.*, 1998), maximum protection is widely recognized to be generated by inclusion of the species and serotype from which the field challenge is expected.

The majority of commercial vibriosis vaccines currently sold worldwide are directed at diseases caused by either *Vibrio anguillarum* or *Vibrio ordalii*. Despite the many *V. anguillarum* serotypes recognized, only serotypes O1, O2a (O2α) and O2b (O2β) appear to be considered serious enough pathogens to warrant production of vaccines on a commercial scale. In the case of Atlantic salmon farmed worldwide, vaccination strategies appear to be highly variable, with some countries vaccinating all sea-farmed Atlantic salmon (e.g., Norway) with vaccines containing serotypes O1 and O2a, while most other countries appear to vaccinate to a lesser degree (Håstein *et al.*, 2005). Routine vaccination of salmonids does not appear to be widely/currently performed in Scotland, the Faroe Islands or Ireland, Tasmania or New Zealand, while a proportion of stocks are vaccinated in Eastern and Western North America. *V. ordalii* is currently vaccinated against in a proportion of Atlantic salmon farmed in Chile and the northwest US. Two strains of *V. ordalii* are currently utilized in salmonid vaccines: Chilean and North American. These strains, although antigenically different, appear to share a degree of antigenic cross-reaction (Silva-Rubio *et al.*, 2010). Vaccination practices against vibriosis in sea-farmed rainbow trout vary from country to country, but when practiced, they are most commonly vaccinated against *V. anguillarum* serotype O1 (worldwide) and O2a.

Marine fish species appear to be susceptible to serotypes that also cause disease in salmonids (O1, O2a), although susceptibilities in such species vary considerably. Marine fish in the Mediterranean area and Japan are most often vaccinated against *V. anguillarum* serotype O1. Marine fish species also appear to be affected by serotypes that are apparently non-pathogenic or of low virulence in salmonids (e.g., serotype O2b).

Norway would appear to be almost alone in widespread vaccination of sea-farmed Atlantic salmon against cold-water vibriosis caused by *Vibrio salmonicida* and winter-ulcers caused by *Moritella viscosa*. Despite the presence of these bacterial species in other countries, only Iceland also vaccinates to any degree against these bacteria. While *Vibrio salmonicida* has never been subjected to analysis using modern molecular biological epidemiological assays, a degree of antigenic (Schrøder *et al.*, 1992) and plasmid variation has been described (Sørum *et al.*, 1990). A previously unrecognised diversity was recently identified in *M. viscosa* (Grove *et al.*, 2010), using a combination of phenotypic and genetic methods, with one strain having an affinity for Atlantic salmon. Whether the genetic diversity represents antigenic diversity in *M. viscosa*, and whether this diversity may be involved in the relatively poor protection awarded by current vaccines, is as yet unknown.

Vibriosis vaccines for use in market segments as yet unattractive to international commercial vaccine companies, such as initial culture of novel species, and small-scale culture of niche fish species, are commonly produced in university and other research laboratories, and also by companies specialising in autogenous vaccines. An immersion vaccine developed by the University of Valencia, Spain, for prevention of *V. vulnificus* serovars A and E (Esteve-Gassent *et al.*, 2004b) infections in eels, was demonstrated to be highly protective, but never entered commercial production due to the limited market represented by commercial eel farming.

While a number of experimental vaccines directed at protection against *Vibrio harveyi* and *Vibrio alginolyticus* have been produced experimentally, and a considerable number of scientific publications have focused on the feasibility of *V. harveyi* vaccines in particular, no commercial products appear to be available.

15.6 VACCINATION PROCEDURES

Vibriosis vaccines currently available (and utilized) today are either immersion- or intraperitoneal injection-based. Although intraperitoneal vaccination is generally acknowledged to provide better and more durable protection, the process is relatively expensive, and requires the vaccinated fish to be above a minimum size, dependent on fish species, but generally >20 g. The choice of route of administration is therefore based on the type and size/developmental stage of fish, as well as the value of the fish to be vaccinated.

As vibriosis is associated with the seawater stage of culture, high-value salmonid fish destined for marine ongrowth have the opportunity to be raised within a *Vibrio*-free freshwater environment to a size at which intraperitoneal vaccination is a practical alternative. This procedure also allows a sufficient period between vaccination and sea transfer for development of an optimal protective immune response. In this way, a single vaccination during the freshwater stage of culture is normally sufficient to award protection until harvest up to 18 months or more after sea transfer in salmonid species.

In the case of marine fish species, however, hatched into an environment containing many possibly pathogenic *Vibrio* spp. there is a need for vaccine protection as soon as the fish have immunologically matured. This means that an initial immersion vaccination is normally performed at an early stage (around 1 g), which is followed up with one or more booster immersion vaccinations or with intraperitoneal vaccination. Exposure to pathogenic microorganisms during early life-stages can be reduced significantly by use of water treatment systems like ozonisation or UV radiation (Liltved *et al.*, 1995) when the volume of water supply is modest. Risk of disease outbreaks will thus be lowered, making it possible to await development of immune competence before vaccination, and fingerlings transferred to sea-cage grow-out premises may be protected when they are confronted by a more "hostile" environment.

15.7 VACCINE EFFECT

Due to the diversity of vaccines available, and previously proven efficacy of vaccines against the various forms of vibriosis, little has been published in recent years relating to quantification of the protection awarded by modern vibrio vaccines. According to product information supplied with commercial vaccines, dip/immersion vaccines would appear to give relative percent survival (RPS) values of > 40%, while commercial injectable vibrio vaccines result in RPS values of > 75% for *Vibrio anguillarum*, > 90% reported for *V. salmonicida*, and notably lower levels (60–73%) of protection against the causative agent of winter-ulcer, *Moritella viscosa*.

It is generally acknowledged that the effect of vibriosis vaccines is good for most species of bacteria and fish involved, although variations in degree and duration of protection are reported. Immersion vaccination generally results in a satisfactory protection for a limited period, and the treatment must usually be repeated at least once, dependent on the vaccine, fish species and length of culture cycle involved prior to harvest. The greatest degree and duration of protection is undoubtedly awarded by intraperitoneal vaccination, particularly in association with oil-adjuvants. However, this method of vaccine delivery cannot always be used due to the requirement for protection in a fish size too small for IP vaccination, and inhibitory costs compared with product value.

Duration of protection is variable dependent on a number of factors, including method of administration, adjuvant type, water temperature, and so on. Manufacturers seem reluctant to provide "duration of protection" information on product information sheets. It is generally accepted, however, that initial immersion vaccination at a small fish size (around 1 g) should be repeated after approximately one month. This may depend on fish type, but a booster at around 5 g size may be indicated. Repeated immersion vaccinations, or a single IP injection at a suitable size, may be alternative relevant approaches to gain protection until market size. In eels, repeated revaccination may be required to provide protection against *V. vulnificus* until harvest (Esteve-Gassent *et al.*, 2004a). For vaccines delivered by IP injection, and in particular oil-adjuvanted vaccines, in anadromous fish species, a single IP vaccination should provide protection until harvest.

Vaccination against vibriosis caused by *V. anguillarum* and *V. ordalli* is generally successful, with few outbreaks of disease registered in vaccinated stocks. Losses to vibriosis are least in those species of fish that can be vaccinated in freshwater prior to seawater transfer, thus allowing development of a specific and protective response prior to challenge with the virulent bacteria. This relates to salmonid species, particularly Atlantic salmon and sea-farmed rainbow trout. In the case of marine fish, vaccination is generally highly effective, particularly in the case of oil-adjuvanted IP vaccines, provided the disease does not strike at or shortly after the application of the vaccine. For marine fish, held in an environment (i.e. un-treated seawater) in which the pathogenic strains may be already present, the vaccination procedure itself may prove so stressful that an outbreak of vibriosis is triggered prior to development of an immune response in the vaccinated fish.

Current vaccines against *Moritella viscosa* in sea-farmed Atlantic salmon do award significant protection in laboratory trials ($\geq 60\%$ RPS), and undoubtedly contribute to lower losses at sea. However, the disease continues to cause losses and the bacterium is regularly isolated from vaccinated stocks. Due to the large market in Norway, vaccine companies continue to research improved *M. viscosa* formulations.

15.8 SIDE-EFFECTS

Side-effects of vaccination are to a great extent related to the use of oil-adjuvanted vaccines (Midtlyng and Lillehaug, 1998). However, even dip vaccination may result in some degree of growth retardation (Lillehaug, 1991), probably due to handling stress during a time period when the fish are vulnerable, close to smoltification.

15.9 REGULATIONS

There are no particular regulatory concerns connected to vaccines against vibriosis and other vibrio infections in fish. The vibrio agents causing disease in aquaculture have a more or less worldwide distribution, and the vaccines are of basic technology, with inactivated bacterins constituting most products.

REFERENCES

Amaro, C. and Biosca, E. 1996. *Vibrio vulnificus* biotype 2, pathogenic for eels, is also an opportunist pathogen of humans. *Appl Environ Microbiol* **62**: 1454–7.

Amaro, C., Biosca, E.G., Esteve, C., *et al.*, 1992. Comparative study of phenotypic and virulence properties in *Vibrio vulnificus* biotype-1 and biotype-2 obtained from a European eel farm experiencing mortalities. *Dis Aquatic Org* **13**: 29–35.

Austin, B. 2010. Vibrios as causal agents of zoonoses. *Vet Microbiol* **140**: 310–17.

Austin, B. and Austin, D.A. 2007. *Bacterial Fish Pathogens. Disease of Farmed and Wild Fish.* 4th edn. Chichester, Springer Praxis.

Austin, B. and Zhang, Z.H. 2006. *Vibrio harveyi*: a significant pathogen of marine vertebrates and invertebrates. *Lett Appl Microbiol* **43**: 119–24.

Austin, B., Stobie, M., Robertson, P.A.W., *et al.*, 1993. *Vibrio alginolyticus* – the cause of gill disease leading to progressive low-level mortalities among juvenile turbot, *Scophthalmus maximus* L in a Scottish aquarium. *J Fish Dis* **16**: 277–80.

Austin, B., Alsina, M., Austin, D.A., *et al.*, 1995. Identification and typing of *Vibrio anguillarum*: a comparison of different methods. *Syst Appl Microbiol* **18**: 285–302.

Balebona, M.C., Zorilla, I., Morinigio, M.A. and Borrego, J.J. 1998. Survey of bacterial pathogens affecting farmed gilthead seabream (*Sparus aurata* L.) in southwestern Spain from 1990 to 1996. *Aquaculture* **166**: 19–35.

Benediktsdóttir, E., Verdonck, L., Sproer, C., *et al.*, 2000. Characterization of *Vibrio viscosus* and *Vibrio wodanis* isolated at different geographical locations: a proposal for reclassification of *Vibrio viscosus* as *Moritella viscosa* comb. nov. *Int J Syst Evol Microbiol* **50**: 479–88.

Bergh, O. and Samuelsen, O.B. 2007. Susceptibility of corkwing wrasse *Symphodus melops*, goldsinny wrasse *Ctenolabrus rupestis*, and Atlantic salmon *Salmo salar* smolt, to experimental challenge with *Vibrio tapetis* and *Vibrio splendidus* isolated from corkwing wrasse. *Aquacult Int* **15**: 11–18.

Bjelland, A.M., Johansen, R., Brudal, E., *et al.*, 2012. *Vibrio salmonicida* pathogenesis analyzed by experimental challenge of Atlantic salmon (*Salmo salar*). *Microb Pathog* **52**: 77–84.

Björnsdóttir, B., Guðmundsdóttir, T. and Guðmundsdóttir, B.K. 2011. Virulence properties of *Moritella viscosa* extracellular products. *J Fish Dis* **34**: 333–43.

Bockemuhl, J., Roch, K., Wohlers, B., *et al.*, 1986. Seasonal distribution of facultatively enteropathogenic vibrios (*Vibrio cholerae, Vibrio mimicus, Vibrio parahaemolyticus*) in the freshwater of the Elbe River at Hamburg. *J Appl Bacteriol* **60**: 435–42.

Bordas, M.A., Balebona, M.C., Rodriguez-Maroto, J.M., *et al.*, 1998. Chemotaxis of pathogenic *Vibrio* strains towards mucus surfaces of gilt-head sea bream (*Sparus aurata* L.). *Appl Environ Microbiol* **64**: 1573–5.

Bruno, D., Hastings, T.S., Ellis, A.E. and Wootten, R. 1985. Outbreak of a cold-water vibriosis in Atlantic salmon in Scotland. *Bull Eur Assoc Fish Patol* **5**: 62–3.

Chen, C., Wang, Q.B., Liu, Z.H., *et al.*, 2012. Characterization of role of the toxR gene in the physiology and pathogenicity of *Vibrio alginolyticus. Antonie Van Leeuwenhoek* **101**: 281–8.

Colodner, R., Raz, R., Meir, I., *et al.*, 2004. Identification of the emerging pathogen *Vibrio vulnificus* biotype 3 by commercially available phenotypic methods. *J Clin Microbiol* **42**: 4137–40.

Colorni, A., Paperna, I. and Gordin, H. 1981. Bacterial infections in gilthead seabream *Sparus aurata* cultured in Eilat. *Aquaculture* **23**: 257–67.

Colquhoun, D.J. and Sørum, H. 2001. Temperature dependent siderophore production in *Vibrio salmonicida. Microb Pathog* **31**: 213–19.

Colquhoun, D.J., Alvheim, K., Dommarsnes, K., *et al.*, 2002. Relevance of incubation temperature for *Vibrio salmonicida* vaccine production. *J Appl Microbiol* **92**: 1087–96.

Colquhoun, D.J., Aase, I.L., Wallace, C., *et al.*, 2004. First description of *Vibrio ordalii* from Chile. *Bull Eur Assoc Fish Patol* **24**: 185–8.

Crosa, J.H., Schiewe, M.H. and Falkow, S. 1977. Evidence for plasmid contribution to the virulence of fish pathogen *Vibrio anguillarum. Infect Immun* **18**: 509–13.

Croxatto, A., Chalker, V.J., Lauritz, J., *et al.*, 2002. VanT, a homologue of *Vibrio harveyi* LuxR, regulates serine, metalloprotease, pigment, and biofilm production in *Vibrio anguillarum*. *J Bacteriol* **184**: 1617–29.
Dalsgaard, I., Hoi, L., Siebeling, R.J. and Dalsgaard, A. 1999. Indole-positive *Vibrio vulnificus* isolated from disease outbreaks on a Danish eel farm. *Dis Aquat Org* **35**: 187–94.
Dalsgaard, I., Jürgens, O. and Mortensen, A. 1988. *Vibrio salmonicida* isolated from farmed Atlantic salmon in the Faroe Islands. *Bull Eur Assoc Fish Patol* **8**: 53–4.
Denkin, S.M. and Nelson, D.R. 1999. Induction of protease activity in *Vibrio anguillarum* by gastrointestinal mucus. *Appl Environ Microbiol* **65**: 3555–60.
Denkin, S.M. and Nelson, D.R. 2004. Regulation of *Vibrio anguillarum* empA metalloprotease expression and its role in virulence. *Appl Environ Microbiol* **70**: 4193–204.
Egidius, E. 1987. Vibriosis: Pathogenicity and pathology. A review. *Aquaculture* **67**: 15–28.
Esteve-Gassent, M.D., Fouz, B. and Amaro, C. 2004a. Efficacy of a bivalent vaccine against eel diseases caused by *Vibrio vulnificus* after its administration by four different routes. *Fish Shellfish Immunol* **16**: 93–105.
Esteve-Gassent, M.D., Fouz, B., Barrera, R. and Amaro, C. 2004b. Efficacy of oral reimmunisation after immersion vaccination against *Vibrio vulnificus* in farmed European eels. *Aquaculture* **231**: 9–22.
Farmer, J.J., Janda, J.M., Brenner, F.W., *et al.*, 2005. Genus I. *Vibrio* Pacini 1854, 411^{AL}, in *Bergey's Manual of Systematic Bacteriology*, Vol. 2 (ed. G.M. Garrity). The *Proteobacteria*, Part B, The *Gammaproteobacteria*. New York, Springer, 494–546.
Fouz, B. and Amaro, C. 2003. Isolation of a new serovar of *Vibrio vulnificus* pathogenic for eels cultured in freshwater farms. *Aquaculture* **217**: 677–82.
Fouz, B., Llorens, A., Valiente, E. and Amaro, C. 2010. A comparative epizootiologic study of the two fish-pathogenic serovars of *Vibrio vulnificus* biotype 2. *J Fish Dis* **33**: 383–90.
Frans, I., Michiels, C.W., Bossier, P., *et al.*, 2011. *Vibrio anguillarum* as a fish pathogen: virulence factors, diagnosis and prevention. *J Fish Dis* **34**: 643–61.
Giorgetti, G. and Ceschia, G. 1982. Vibriosis in rainbow trout, *Salmo gairdneri* Richardson, in freshwater in north-eastern Italy. *J Fish Dis* **5**: 125–30.
Grisez, L. and Ollevier, F. 1995. Comparative serology of the marine fish pathogen *Vibrio anguillarum*. *Appl Environ Microbiol* **61**: 4367–73.
Grove, S., Wiik-Nielsen, C.R., Lunder, T., *et al.*, 2010. Previously unrecognised division within *Moritella viscosa* isolated from fish farmed in the North Atlantic. *Dis Aquat Org* **93**: 51–61.
Håstein, T., Gudding, R. and Evensen, Ø. 2005. Bacterial vaccines for fish – an update of the current situation worldwide. *Dev Biol (Basel)* **121**: 55–74.
Hoel, K., Reitan, L.J. and Lillehaug, A. 1998. Immunological cross reactions between *Aeromonas salmonicida* and *Vibrio salmonicida* in Atlantic salmon (*Salmo salar* L.) and rabbit. *Fish Shellfish Immunol* **8**: 171–82.
Ivanova, E.P., Zhukova, N.V., Gorshkova, N.M. and Chaikina, E.L. 2001. Characterization of *Aeromonas* and *Vibrio* species isolated from a drinking water reservoir. *J Appl Microbiol* **90**: 919–27.
Jensen, S., Samuelsen, O.B., Andersen, K., *et al.*, 2003. Characterization of strains of *Vibrio splendidus* and *V. tapetis* from corkwing wrasse *Symphodus melops* suffering vibriosis. *Dis Aquat Org* **53**: 25–31.
Kanno, T., Nakai, T. and Muroga, K. 1990. Scanning electron-microscopy on the skin surface of ayu *Plecoglossus altivelis* infected with *Vibrio anguillarum*. *Dis Aquat Org* **8**: 73–5.
Karlsen, C., Paulsen, S.M., Tunsjø, H.S., *et al.*, 2008. Motility and flagellin gene expression in the fish pathogen *Vibrio salmonicida*: effects of salinity and temperature. *Microb Pathog* **45**: 258–64.
Karunasagar, I., Otta, S.K. and Karunasagar, I. 1996. Biofilm formation by *Vibrio harveyi* on surfaces. *Aquaculture* **140**: 241–5.
Kitao, T., Aoki, T. and Muroga, K. 1984. Three new serotypes of *Vibrio anguillarum*. *Bull Jap Soc Sci Fish* **50**: 1955.
Kitao, T., Aoki, T., Fukudome, M., *et al.*, 2006. Serotyping of *Vibrio anguillarum* isolated from diseased freshwater fish in Japan. *J Fish Dis* **6**: 175–81.
Knudsen, G., Sørum, H., Press, CMcL. and Olafsen, J.A. 1999. *In situ* adherence of *Vibrio* spp. to cryosections of Atlantic salmon, *Salmo salar* L., tissue. *J Fish Dis* **22**: 409–18.
Kusada, R., Yokoyama, J. and Kawai, K. 1986. Bacteriological study on cause of mass mortalities in cultured black seabream fry. *Bull Jap Soc Sci Fish* **52**: 1745–51.
Larsen, J.L., Rasmussen, H.B. and Dalsgaard, I. 1988. Study of *Vibrio anguillarum* strains from different sources with emphasis on ecological and pathobiological properties. *Appl Environ Microbiol* **54**: 2264–7.
Larsen, J.L., Pedersen, K. and Dalsgaard, I. 1994. *Vibrio anguillarum* serovars associated with vibriosis in fish. *J Fish Dis* **17**: 259–67.

Lee, K.K. 1995. Pathogenesis studies on *Vibrio alginolyticus* in the grouper, *Epinephalus malabaricus*, Bloch et Schneider. *Microb Pathog* **19**: 39–48.

Lemos, M.L., Salinas, P., Toranzo, A.E., *et al.*, 1988. Chromosome-mediated iron uptake system in pathogenic strains of *Vibrio anguillarum*. *J Bacteriol* **170**: 1920–5.

Li, G.F., Zhao, D.H., Huang, L., *et al.*, 2006. Identification and phylogenetic analysis of *Vibrio vulnificus* isolated from diseased *Trachinotus ovatus* in cage mariculture. *Aquaculture* **261**: 17–25.

Lillehaug, A. 1990. A field trial of vaccination against cold-water vibriosis in Atlantic salmon (*Salmo salar* L.). *Aquaculture* **84**: 1–12.

Lillehaug, A. 1991. Vaccination of Atlantic salmon (*Salmo salar* L) against cold-water vibriosis – duration of protection and effect on growth rate. *Aquaculture* **92**: 99–107.

Lillehaug, A., Sørum, R.H. and Ramstad, A. 1990. Cross-protection after immunization of Atlantic salmon, *Salmo salar* L., against different strains of *Vibrio salmonicida*. *J Fish Dis* **13**: 519–23.

Lillehaug, A., Lunestad, B.T. and Grave, K. 2003. Epidemiology of bacterial diseases in Norwegian aquaculture – a description based on antibiotic prescription data for the ten-year period 1991 to 2000. *Dis Aquat Org* **53**: 115–25.

Liltved, H., Hektoen, H. and Efraimsen, H. 1995. Inactivation of bacterial and viral fish pathogens by ozonation or Uv irradiation in water of different salinity. *Aquacult Eng* **14**: 107–22.

Løvoll, M., Wiik-Nielsen, C.R., Tunsjø, H.S., *et al.*, 2009. Atlantic salmon bath challenged with *Moritella viscosa* – pathogen invasion and host response. *Fish Shellfish Immunol* **26**: 877–84.

Lunder, T., Evensen, Ø., Holstad, G. and Håstein, T. 1995. Winter ulcer in the Atlantic salmon *Salmo salar*. Pathological and bacteriological investigations and transmission experiments. *Dis Aquat Org* **23**: 39–49.

Marco-Noales, E., Milan, M., Fouz, B., *et al.*, 2001. Transmission to eels, portals of entry, and putative reservoirs of *Vibrio vulnificus* serovar E (biotype 2). *Appl Environ Microbiol* **67**: 4717–25.

Markestad, A. and Grave, K. 1997. Reduction of antibacterial drug use in Norwegian fish farming due to vaccination. *Dev Biol Stand* **90**: 365–9.

Midtlyng, P.J. and Lillehaug, A. 1998. Growth of Atlantic salmon *Salmo salar* after intraperitoneal administration of vaccines containing adjuvants. *Dis Aquat Org* **32**: 91–7.

Mikkelsen, H., Lund, V., Larsen, R. and Seppola, M. 2011. Vibriosis vaccines based on various sero-subgroups of *Vibrio anguillarum* O2 induce specific protection in Atlantic cod (*Gadus morhua* L.) juveniles. *Fish Shellfish Immunol* **30**: 330–9.

Milton, D.L., O'Toole, R., Horstedt, P. and Wolf-Watz, H. 1996. Flagellin A is essential for the virulence of *Vibrio anguillarum*. *J Bacteriol* **178**: 1310–19.

Munday, B.L., Carson, J., Whittington, R. and Alexander, J. 1992. Serological responses and immunity produced in salmonids by vaccination with Australian strains of *Vibrio anguillarum*. *Immunol Cell Biol* **70**: 391–5.

Muroga, K., Jo, Y. and Masumura, K. 1986. *Vibrio ordalii* isolated from diseased ayu (*Plecoglossus altivelis*) and rockfish (*Sebastes schlegeli*). *Fish Pathol* **21**: 239–43.

Naka, H., Dias, G.M., Thompson, C.C., *et al.*, 2011. Complete genome sequence of the marine fish pathogen *Vibrio anguillarum* harboring the pJM1 virulence plasmid and genomic comparison with other virulent strains of *V. anguillarum* and *V. ordalii*. *Infect Immun* **79**: 2889–900.

O'Halloran, J. and Henry, R. 1993. *Vibrio salmonicida* (Hitra disease) in New Brunswick. *Bull Aquacult Assoc Can* **93**: 96–8.

Olsson, J.C., Jobörn, A., Westerdahl, A., *et al.*, 1996. Is the turbot, *Scophthalmus maximus* (L.) intestine a portal of entry for the fish pathogen *Vibrio anguillarum*? *J Fish Dis* **19**: 225–34.

Ormonde, P., Horstedt, P., O'Toole, R. and Milton, D.L. 2000. Role of motility in adherence to and invasion of a fish cell line by *Vibrio anguillarum*. *J Bacteriol* **182**: 2326–8.

O'Toole, R., Milton, D.L. and Wolf-Watz, H. 1996. Chemotactic motility is required for invasion of the host by the fish pathogen *Vibrio anguillarum*. *Mol Microbiol* **19**: 625–37.

Pedersen, K. and Larsen, J.L. 1995. Evidence for the existence of distinct populations of *Vibrio anguillarum* serogroup O1 based on plasmid contents and ribotypes. *Appl Environ Microbiol* **61**: 2292–6.

Pedersen, K., Grisez, L., van Houdt, R., *et al.*, 1999. Extended serotyping scheme for *Vibrio anguillarum* with the definition and characterization of seven provisional O-serogroups. *Curr Microbiol* **38**: 183–9.

Poppe, T.T., Håstein, T. and Salte, R. 1985. "Hitra disease" (Haemorrhagic syndrome) in Norwegian salmon farming: present status, in *Fish and Shellfish Pathology* (ed. A.E. Ellis). London, Academic Press, 223–9.

Robertson, P.A.W., Calderon, J., Carrera, L., *et al.*, 1998. Experimental *Vibrio harveyi* infections in *Penaeus vannamei* larvae. *Dis Aquat Org* **32**: 151–5.

Sakata, T., Matsuura, M. and Shimokawa, Y. 1989. Characteristics of *Vibrio damsela* isolated from diseased yellowtail *Seriola-quinqueradiata*. *Nippon Suisan Gakkaishi* **55**: 135–41.
Schiewe, M.H. and Crosa, J.H. 1981. Molecular characterisation of *Vibrio anguillarum* biotype 2. *Can J Microbiol* **27**: 1011–18.
Schiewe, M.H., Trust, T.J. and Crosa, J.H. 1981. *Vibrio ordalii* sp. nov.: A causative agent of vibriosis in fish. *Curr Microbiol* **6**: 343–8.
Schrøder, M.B., Espelid, S. and Jørgensen, T.Ø. 1992. Two serotypes of *Vibrio salmonicida* isolated from diseased cod (*Gadus morhua* L.); virulence, immunological studies and vaccination experiments. *Fish Shellfish Immunol* **2**: 211–21.
Silva-Rubio, A.A., Avendaño-Herrera, R., Jaureguiberry, B.B., *et al.*, 2008. First description of serotype O3 in *Vibrio anguillarum* strains isolated from salmonids in Chile. *J Fish Dis* **31**: 235–9.
Silva-Rubio, A., Acevedo, C., Magarinos, B., *et al.*, 2010. Antigenic and molecular characterization of *Vibrio ordalii* strains isolated from Atlantic salmon *Salmo salar* in Chile. *Dis Aquat Org* **79**: 27–35.
Song, Y.L., Chen, S.N. and Kou, G.H. 1988. Serotyping of *Vibrio anguillarum* strains isolated from fish in Taiwan. *Fish Pathol* **23**: 185–9.
Sørensen, U.B.S. and Larsen, J.L. 1986. Serotyping of *Vibrio anguillarum*. *Appl Environ Microbiol* 1986;**51**:593–597.
Sørum, H., Hvaal, A.B., Heum, M., *et al.*, 1990. Plasmid profiling of *Vibrio salmonicida* for epidemiologic studies of cold-water vibriosis in Atlantic salmon (*Salmo salar*) and cod (*Gadus morhua*). *Appl Environ Microbiol* **56**: 1033–7.
Thompson, F.L., Thompson, C.C., Dias, G.M., *et al.*, 2011. The genus *Listonella* MacDonell and Colwell 1986 is a later heterotypic synonym of the genus *Vibrio* Pacini 1854 (Approved Lists 1980) – a taxonomic opinion. *Int J Syst Evol Microbiol* **61**: 3023–7.
Thomson, R., Macpherson, H.L., Riaza, A. and Birkbeck, T.H. 2005. *Vibrio splendidus* biotype 1 as a cause of mortalities in hatchery-reared larval turbot, *Scophthalmus maximus* (L.). *J Appl Microbiol* **99**: 243–50.
Tiainen, T., Pedersen, K. and Larsen, J.L. 1997. *Vibrio anguillarum* serogroup O3 and *V. anguillarum*-like serogroup O3 cross-reactive species – comparison and characterization. *J Appl Microbiol* **82**: 211–18.
Toranzo, A.E. and Barja, J. 1990. A review of the taxonomy and seroepizootiology of *Vibrio anguillarum*, with special reference to aquaculture in the northwest of Spain. *Dis Aquat Org* **9**: 73–82.
Tunsjø, H.S., Paulsen, S.M., Berg, K., *et al.*, 2009. The winter ulcer bacterium *Moritella viscosa* demonstrates adhesion and cytotoxicity in a fish cell model. *Microb Pathog* **47**: 134–42.
Tunsjø, H.S., Wiik-Nielsen, C.R., Grove, S., *et al.*, 2011. Putative virulence genes in *Moritella viscosa*: activity during *in vitro* inoculation and *in vivo* infection. *Microb Pathog* **50**: 286–92.
Urbanczyk, H., Ast, J.C., Higgins, M.J., *et al.*, 2007. Reclassification of *Vibrio fischeri*, *Vibrio logei*, *Vibrio salmonicida* and *Vibrio wodanis* as *Aliivibrio fischeri* gen. nov., comb. nov., *Aliivibrio logei* comb. nov., *Aliivibrio salmonicida* comb. nov. and *Aliivibrio wodanis* comb. nov. *Int J Syst Evol Microbiol* **57**: 2823–9.
Varina, M., Denkin, S.M., Staroscik, A.M. and Nelson, D.R. 2008. Identification and characterization of epp, the secreted processing protease for the *Vibrio anguillarum* EmpA metalloprotease. *J Bacteriol* **190**: 6589–97.
Velji, M.I., Albright, L.J. and Evelyn, T.P.T. 1990. Protective immunity in juvenile coho salmon *Oncorhynchus kisutch* following immunization with *Vibrio ordalii* lipopolysaccharide or from exposure to live *V. ordalii* cells. *Dis Aquat Org* **9**: 25–9.
Wang, S.Y., Lauritz, J., Jass, J. and Milton, D.L. 2002. A ToxR homolog from *Vibrio anguillarum* serotype O1 regulates its own production, bile resistance, and biofilm formation. *J Bacteriol* **184**: 1630–9.
Wards, B.J., Patel, H.H., Anderson, C.D. and Delisle, G.W. 1991. Characterization by restriction endonuclease analysis and plasmid profiling of *Vibrio ordalii* strains from salmon (*Oncorhynchus tshawytscha* and *Oncorhynchus nerka*) with vibriosis in New-Zealand. *New Zeal J Mar Fresh* **25**: 345–50.
Yiagnisis, M., Vatsos, I.N., Kyriakou, C. and Alexis, M. 2007. First report of *Vibrio anguillarum* isolation from diseased big scale sand smelt, *Atherina boyeri* Risso 1810, in Limnos, Greece. *Bull Eur Assoc Fish Patol* **27**: 61–9.

16 Vaccination against Furunculosis

Paul J. Midtlyng

Norwegian School of Veterinary Science, Oslo, Norway

ABSTRACT

The term furunculosis is used to describe a lethal septicemia of salmonid species caused by the bacterium *Aeromonas salmonicida* subsp. *salmonicida*, but can also denote infections with atypical strains of the furunculosis bacterium occurring in a broad range of freshwater and marine species and most frequently manifesting with severe skin ulceration and wounds. The classical furunculosis bacterium (subsp. *salmonicida*) shows a remarkable genotypic and phenotypic uniformity worldwide, while the atypical *A. salmonicida* strains are much more diverse. Both classical and atypical furunculosis isolates possess a variety of cellular and extra-cellular pathogenicity and virulence factors that have been intensively studied over several decades. In general, none of these factors have proven alone responsible for the bacterium's ability to infect the host and cause mortality. Research to rank the protective antigens for both classical and atypical furunculosis bacteria has yielded inconsistent and apparently contradictory results, but evidence is accumulating to suggest that presence of the A-layer is perhaps the most important among the antigenic factors. Injectable, oil-adjuvanted vaccines against classical furunculosis are licensed in the largest salmonid farming markets, and frequently come in combination with other bacterial and viral antigens, while vaccines for immersion or oral administration, or live vaccine concepts have not been successful so far. Although classical furunculosis may provide some cross-protection, vaccines against atypical furunculosis need to be prepared with bacterial strains that are specific to the species and/or to the region in question, using oil-adjuvant technology.

16.1 INTRODUCTION

In a fish disease context, the term furunculosis may be used in the broad sense, denoting a variety of disease manifestations caused by bacteria belonging to the species *Aeromonas salmonicida*, occurring in a broad range of freshwater and marine fin-fish species. Many of

paul.midtlyng@aquamedic.no

Fish Vaccination, First Edition. Edited by Roar Gudding, Atle Lillehaug and Øystein Evensen.

these infections, however, fail to display the lead symptom that originally gave the disease its name (furuncles; hemorragic necrosis of skeletal muscle), and in the following, distinction will be made between classical furunculosis, a disease occurring predominantly in salmonid species being caused by *A. salmonicida* subspecies *salmonicida*, and disease conditions arising from infection with atypical *A. salmonicida* strains (*A. salmonicida* subspp. *achromogenes*, *masoui-cida*, *smithia* or *pectinolytica*), which are described from both salmonids and non-salmonids, and from numerous freshwater and marine species. This distinction is also made to allow a fruitful review of anti-furunculosis vaccination, where there are major differences in control practices between classical furunculosis and the atypical furunculosis infections. A recent and detailed description of furunculosis and the fish diseases caused by atypical furunculosis bacteria or motile Aeromonads can be found in Cipriano and Austin (2011). In the following, this chapter will therefore deal with the disease named classical furunculosis and its prevention and control by the use of vaccines. Some experiences from development of vaccines against disease caused by atypical *A. salmonicida* strains will be discussed towards the end of the chapter, but without going into great detail.

16.2 OCCURRENCE AND SIGNIFICANCE

Furunculosis of salmonids was first described as a potentially severe disease of freshwater reared brown trout (Emmerich and Weibel, 1894), and the authors were able to isolate a *Vibrio cholera*-like bacterium that was designated *Bacterium salmonicida*. Following this initial description, the disease and the isolation of an associated bacterium was soon reported from North America, England and Scotland, also causing epizootics in rivers. For decades, the published literature considered furunculosis a disease confined to fresh or brackish waters. However, the first furunculosis outbreak in marine reared salmon (Novotny, 1978) and reports of a new and more frequent disease manifestation in Scottish marine salmon farms (Munro and Waddell, 1984) signalled that, in parallel with the growth of marine production systems for salmon, a change in the manifestation patterns for this disease was emerging. This was confirmed by the dramatic epidemic spread of the disease from Norwegian marine salmon sites that had received latently infected smolts in 1985 (Egidius, 1987).

Classical furunculosis is probably the most intensively studied among diseases of fish, and one of relatively few animal diseases that has warranted its own book volume (Bernoth *et al.*, 1997), which is recommended for further in-depth reading about the disease and about furunculosis research. Today, the bacterium causing classical furunculosis has been reported from all regions where wild or farmed salmonids are cultured, with the exception of Australia and Chile. The occurrence and incidence of clinical disease are, however, highly dependent upon the prevailing practices of propagating or farming salmonid species, and in particular of vaccination practices (see below).

The clinical pattern of classical furunculosis is that of a septicemic infection with high mortality, chronic disease signs in survivors, little to no development of natural immunity, and recurrency of outbreaks most frequently from spring through late autumn and early winter. Prior to the introduction of effective vaccines, the cumulative losses due to furunculosis in European industrialized salmon farming were estimated in excess of 20% per year-class (Ellis, 1997b). It goes without saying that this situation had devastating consequences for the aquaculture industry, both in terms of direct financial losses, but also through prolonged withdrawal periods preventing timely harvest, and the development of antibiotic resistance that rendered furunculosis therapies increasingly ineffective.

16.3 ETIOLOGY

The causative agent of classical furunculosis, *A. salmonicida* subsp. *salmonicida*, is a gram-negative, non-motile, facultative anaerobic, short rod-shaped bacterium, growing readily on a range of non-selective agar media at 20–22°C, and tending to auto-agglutinate (Austin and Austin, 2007). Primary or subcultures dominated by subsp. *salmonicida* produce a characteristic brown diffusible pigment on trypticase soy or trypticase yeast agar (TSA/TYA), which is often used for confirmatory diagnosis. There are, however, reports of highly virulent non-pigmented isolates (Koppang *et al.*, 2000). As opposed to the atypical strains, subsp. *salmonicida* shows an astonishing phenotypical uniformity irrespective of clinical outbreak pattern, time of isolation, fish species or geographic origin, resembling a clonal distribution (Cipriano and Austin, 2011). This observation is in accordance with the presumption that movement or migration of clinically healthy, but latently infected fish have been the predominant route for geographic spread of the disease, an aspect noted very early on (Horne, 1928). While infection with the classical furunculosis bacterium is a necessary requirement, clinical outbreaks and illness are very often induced by various environmental, husbandry-related or other stressors that tend to lower the immune functions of the fish (Bernoth, 1997). The bacterium's reputation as an obligate parasite must be ascribed to the fact that under intensive farming conditions, latently infected salmonid populations hardly survive an entire farming cycle without experiencing clinical disease, if remaining unvaccinated. This is in contrast to free-living salmonid stocks, in which the occurrence of clinical outbreaks is far less frequent and highly dependent upon local conditions, such as water flow, temperature, and population density. Also the minimal dose (less than 50 cfu) required to induce mortality in experimentally inoculated naïve salmon supports this classification (Nordmo and Ramstad, 1997).

Furunculosis bacteria are not only shed by infected individuals, but are massively released from dead fish, and the disease is readily spread horizontally by fish-to-fish contact or waterborne transport. Moreover, suspended *A. salmonicida* associates easily with lipid droplets and tends to concentrate in the water surface, where salmonids are frequently moving (Enger, 1997). The risk for vertical transmission of furunculosis (from parents to offspring) is very low. When performed diligently, iodophor disinfection of eggs is effective to prevent vertical transmission of the infection to fry.

16.4 PATHOGENESIS AND VIRULENCE

The clinical appearance and pathology of acute classical furunculosis is that of a lethal bacterial septicemia, but with minimal inflammatory responses. External signs are rather non-specific; darkening, loss of appetite and lethargy, and sometimes small hemorrhages of the skin. Internal findings are hyperemia and diluted blood vessels, hemorrhages of serous surfaces, and swollen spleen and kidney. Individuals experiencing a sub-acute or chronic course of the disease tend to develop multiple necrotizing hemorrhages in the skeletal musculature, which may grow or combine to form larger intramuscular or subcutaneous furuncles. The histopathology of the disease is characterized by disseminated perivascular microcolonies surrounded by localized necrosis in heart, spleen and kidney, and acute toxic effects on hematopoietic tissue, kidney, liver and myocardial tissue (McCarthy and Roberts, 1980). All of these point to a pathogenesis dominated by the combined effects of several extracellular toxins produced by the furunculosis bacterium, causing severe coagulopathy (Salte *et al.*, 1993).

The body of research on *A. salmonicida* pathogenicity and virulence factors is large, and has been frequently reviewed (Ellis, 1991, 1997a). An overview of more recent papers, some of which also address these factors by use of experimental molecular genetic techniques, is provided in Table 16.1.

Surface elements are generally considered important for bacterial attachment and invasion. Molecular studies have shown that the expression of the relevant genes in *A. salmonicida* is disrupted, resulting in failure in the formation of polar or lateral flagella (Reith *et al.*, 2008). The presence of shorter fimbriae or pili at the *A. salmonicida* cell surface has, however, been confirmed, functionally supporting adhesion to gut mucus cells, but without showing essential functionality in host cell invasion (Boyd *et al.*, 2008; Danacay *et al.*, 2010).

Much attention has been given to the role of several outer membrane proteins for the virulence of *A. salmonicida*. Among the most studied is the crystalline surface protein array (S-layer; earlier named A-layer) that is formed by A-protein molecules and covers the outer cell membrane (Trust *et al.*, 1996; Noonan and Trust, 1997). Although there are some examples of bacterial strains devoid of this layer being pathogenic in experimental settings, it is present in nearly all virulent field strains of the bacterium, and has been shown to mediate resistance to macrophage killing. Also the iron-regulated outer membrane proteins of *A. salmonicida* have been well studied, although their essential role as protective antigens has not yet been confirmed (see below).

Table 16.1 Recent studies of the main pathogenic and virulence factors in *A. salmonicida* and evaluation of their role as protective antigens. (Source: Adapted from Ellis 1997a, 1997c; Tomás 2012; Beaz-Hidalgo and Figueras 2013.)

Pathogenic and virulence factors	References
Cell surface elements	
Fimbria/pili	Masada *et al.* (2002); Boyd *et al.* (2008); Danacay *et al.* (2010)
Outer membrane proteins (OMPs)	Hirst and Ellis (1994); Bricknell *et al.* (1999); O'Dowd *et al.* (1999); Ebanks *et al.* (2005)
S-layer (A-layer)	Ellis *et al.* (1988); Garduno *et al.* (2000); Lund *et al.* (2003a)
Porin protein	Lutwyche *et al.* (1995); Merino *et al.* (2005)
O-antigen (LPS)	Wang *et al.* (2006)
Polysaccharide capsule	Bricknell *et al.* (1997); Wang *et al.* (2004); Magnadóttir (2010)
Extracellular (secreted) toxins	
GCAT	Lee and Ellis (1990, 1991); Vipond *et al.* (1998)
Cytolysin (secreted LPS)	Ellis *et al.* (1988)
Serine protease	Ellis *et al.* (1988); Ellis (1991); Vipond *et al.* (1998)
Metalloprotease	Hussain *et al.* (2000); Prost (2001); Burr *et al.* (2005)
Intracellular machinery	
Toxin secretion systems	Burr *et al.* (2005); Danacay *et al.* (2006); Fast *et al.* (2009)
Iron acquisition systems	Ebanks *et al.* (2004, 2005); Najimi *et al.* (2009)
Quorum sensing systems	Bruhn *et al.* (2005); Schwenteit *et al.* (2011)

The summary of research on the extracellular products (ECPs) produced by the typical furunculosis bacterium, by Ellis (1997c), concluded that its extracellular toxins (GCAT complexing with secreted lipopolysaccharide (LPS), and the proteases) are mainly responsible for its ability to destroy tissues and kill the host. The effectiveness of the intracellular secretion systems, by which these toxins are released, has recently also been implicated as an important virulence factor (Danacay *et al.*, 2006). *A. salmonicida* grown *in vivo* or in certain culture media expresses an outer polysaccharide capsule (Garduno and Kay, 1995), presumably allowing the bacterium to avoid recognition by the host's immune system, and, together with the A-layer, to resist non-specific host defense mechanisms (Magnadóttir, 2010).

The port(s) of entry of the classical furunculosis bacteria remains to be definitively identified, but in a series of diligent experiments, Jutfelt *et al.* (2006, 2008) were able to show that the bacterium readily translocates across the salmon intestinal epithelium, and that the processes were influenced by the presence of the bacterium's extracellular products and secreted LPS.

16.5 ANTIGENS

The merits of nearly all of the *A. salmonicida* pathogenicity and virulence factors to act as antigens in anti-furunculosis vaccines were comprehensively discussed by Ellis (1997a), concluding that "the nature of the antigens and the immune parameters they elicit to achieve immunity to furunculosis are still not well-defined". Subsequent work has continued to produce divergent and in part apparently contradictory results, for example regarding the importance of the iron-regulated outer membrane proteins – IROMP – for virulence and vaccine protection (Hirst and Ellis, 1994; Vipond *et al.*, 1998; Bricknell *et al.*, 1999).

From the body of research dealing with furunculosis vaccination, there is good reason to question the conclusion drawn by Ellis (1997c) that the immune responses elicited to the *A. salmonicida* A-protein are not protective in nature. Opposite conclusions have since been presented by Lund *et al.* (2003a) and Romstad *et al.* (2013), as attenuated, S-layer deficient strains lost their ability to induce vaccine protection. After re-attachment, A-layer deficient strains have been shown to recover their virulence both *in vitro* (Garduno *et al.*, 2000) and *in vivo* (Arnesen *et al.*, 2010): results which serve to support a causative relationship. For the time being, it thus appears that the antigens for classical furunculosis vaccines should be produced from strains possessing all of the pathogenic and virulence factors listed above. The availability and annotation of the *A. salmonicida* genome sequences (Reith *et al.*, 2008; Charette *et al.*, 2012), and the future use of reverse genetics techniques, are likely to facilitate further discoveries of the bacterium's pathogenic and virulence mechanisms, and their relative contribution to infection and clinical illness. These methods will also facilitate a more precise clarification and ranking of the *A. salmonicida* antigens according to their contribution to vaccine protection.

16.6 VACCINES

The first results from a furunculosis vaccination trial were published by Duff (1942), who reported antibody development and improved survival to experimental challenge in groups of cutthroat trout (*Salmo clarkii*), being given feed supplemented with fresh, chloroform-killed cultures of the furunculosis bacterium. As reviewed by Midtlyng (1997) and Evelyn (1997), it took some 20 years, however, before successful anti-furunculosis vaccination was well documented, using an *A. salmonicida* bacterin prepared with mineral oil adjuvant (Krantz *et al.*, 1964). The first furunculosis vaccine to sustain the ups and downs of the fish vaccine markets was produced by a Canadian startup company (Paterson *et al.*, 1985). However, for a long time, furunculosis vaccines were generally considered premature and without major commercial use, until further scientific breakthroughs in virulence research and furunculosis immunology had been achieved (Horne and Ellis, 1988).

Following the introduction of classical furunculosis to the expanding Norwegian salmon industry, independent testing of available vaccines was initiated by the Norwegian Veterinary Institute in Oslo, yielding data showing significant protection after IP injection of alum-adjuvanted vaccines in salmon parr, both in experimental (Erdal and Reitan, 1992) and field trials (Lillehaug *et al.*, 1992). The level of protection was promising, but a significant drop in field protection was observed during the second summer after vaccination. During a large-scale testing of a wider range of candidate furunculosis vaccines and formulations starting in 1991, monovalent and trivalent (furunculosis, vibriosis, cold-water vibriosis) oil-adjuvanted formulations showed superior levels and duration of protection in experimental challenge trials after three and six months, and in a large-scale field study initiated the same year (Midtlyng, 1996; Midtlyng *et al.*, 1996b). After the encouraging 1991 experiences, mass vaccination was rapidly enforced by the Norwegian salmon aquaculture industry, resulting in strong additive herd immunity effect, which contributed to a remarkable drop in the use of antibacterial drugs (Markestad and Grave, 1997). Also in Scotland, furunculosis vaccination led to a major increase in the survival of salmon smolts from sea-transfer to harvest, from approximately 65% in the late 1980s, to above 90% in the year-classes transferred to sea in 1994 and following years (Munro and Gauld, 1997). In light of current industrial experiences, doubts initially voiced regarding the dominant contribution of oil-adjuvanted vaccines to furunculosis control (Smith and Hiney, 2000) have largely dissolved.

Although small-scale experiments have shown that oral and immersion vaccination against classical furunculosis may yield some degree of protection, waterborne challenge models and field experiences have demonstrated that these procedures yield insufficient duration of immunity to sustain the conditions of industrialized salmonid aquaculture (Midtlyng, 1996). Products for immersion or oral immunization against furunculosis are therefore not licensed commercially. Research to exploit live vaccine concepts against classical furunculosis has also been reported in the scientific literature, but the results have not been successfully pursued for licensing (Vaughan *et al.*, 1993; Thornton *et al.*, 1994; Marsden *et al.*, 1998; Grove *et al.*, 2003).

The injectable oil-adjuvanted bacterins have become completely dominant in furunculosis vaccine supply worldwide, coming in a variety of combinations with one or more *Vibrio* antigens, and for Atlantic salmon, often with further bacterial and/or viral components. As a consequence of the necessity to formulate furunculosis vaccines with oil adjuvants, the inclusion of new antigens into multivalent, oil-adjuvanted formulations is dominating the commercial vaccine development and supply for salmonids worldwide. However, other antigens would not necessarily need such a strong adjuvant to be effective. An alum-adjuvanted monovalent furunculosis vaccine is currently licensed only in Canada.

16.7 VACCINATION PROCEDURES

All commercially available furunculosis vaccines are recommended for administration intra-peritoneally, to heavily sedated or anesthetized fish, preferable at the pre-smolt or parr stage.

After use of injectable vaccines, studies have shown that 300–500 degree-days (no. of days times water temperature) or more are needed for anti-furunculosis immunity to develop (Midtlyng *et al.*, 1996b; Eggset *et al.*, 1997), and protection by oil-adjuvant formulations has been shown to last for more than 1500 degree-days (Midtlyng *et al.*, 1996b). The more or less complete absence of clinical outbreaks wherever mass vaccination against furunculosis is being performed demonstrates that the immunity induced by oil-adjuvanted vaccines against classical furunculosis endures throughout the entire production cycle.

In a study comparing different vaccination procedures, Midtlyng *et al.* (1996a) found that fish receiving the adjuvanted antigen by intraperitoneal injection were the only groups showing a notable antibody response, and head kidney leukocytes were activated. The effect lasted for at least 16 weeks post-immunization, while minimal effects were seen following non-parenteral vaccination procedures. These results led to a subsequent focus on development of injectable furunculosis vaccines, and subsequent discontinuation of immersion and oral vaccine development for licensing. There are, however, a number of subsequent papers reporting more favorable experiences from the use of non-oil furunculosis vaccine antigens and formulations, with or without oral boosting (Durbin *et al.*, 1999, Ackermann *et al.*, 2000; Bebak-Williams and Bullock, 2002; Irie *et al.*, 2005).

In modern Atlantic salmon farming, injection of furunculosis-containing multivalent vaccines normally takes place 6–8 weeks prior to transfer of autumn output smolts, and 4–5 months prior to sea-transfer of spring output smolts, differences being dictated by the water temperatures and sea-transfer timelines. In prospective breeders, the oil-emulsified vaccines can be administered into connective tissues without compromising vaccine protection, thus avoiding injection-site effects near the developing gonads (Treasurer and Cox, 2008). Anti-furunculosis immunization of salmonids after transfer to floating net pens is possible, but requires specialized equipment and technical skills for managing the netting, anesthesia and wake-up procedures without unintentional losses.

16.8 EFFECTS

Contrary to the belief in the late 1980s (Ellis *et al.*, 1988), the results presented by Midtlyng *et al.* (1996a,b) showed that antibody levels to *A. salmonicida* and good vaccine protection were associated, a finding that has subsequently been confirmed by others (Hoel *et al.*, 1998; Bricknell *et al.*, 1999; Villumsen *et al.*, 2012; Romstad *et al.*, 2012, 2013). The role of anti-furunculosis antibodies in protection was documented quite early by successful transfer of protection via hyperimmune serum (Spence *et al.*, 1965).

In the studies by Midtlyng *et al.* (1996b), the degree of protection conferred by a trivalent oil-adjuvanted furunculosis vaccine (*A. salmonicida* subsp. *salmonicida, V. anguillarum* O1α; *V. salmonicida*) reached 87% (% survival over saline controls). The protective level developed gradually, increasing strongly between 6 and 26 weeks post-immunization. Hoel *et al.* (1997) investigated which *Vibrio* species and mechanisms were responsible for the augmentation of furunculosis immunity in multivalent vaccine formulations. Using a factorial study design and analysis, it was found that the *V. salmonicida* bacterin was the strongest contributing factor, and the authors were able to show that antibodies raised against *V. salmonicida* reacted with *A. salmonicida* whole cells and to LPS, but not to the A-layer protein. Further investigations led the authors to conclude that cross-reaction between antibodies to cell-surface antigens, together with adjuvant effects on T-dependent antigens, were the likely underlying mechanisms (Hoel *et al.*, 1998).

Midtlyng *et al.* (1996a) were able to demonstrate that the use of oil-adjuvanted furunculosis vaccines in Atlantic salmon gave a lasting, non-specific activation of head kidney leucocytes. This effect should not be underestimated, considering that while the furunculosis bacterium is able to resist or even kill naïve (unstimulated) salmonid macrophages (Olivier *et al.*, 1992), macrophages that are activated by *A. salmonicida* antigen plus oil adjuvant are able to kill virulent *A. salmonicida* (Chung and Secombes, 1987).

In summary, it appears that strong activation of immune cells and high circulating antibody levels, as induced by the emulsified antigen, are both prerequisites for satisfactory protection against furunculosis. An important part of the immune mechanism is the so-called depot effect, denoting the fact that the antigen associated with oil droplets persists on the injection-site for a very long time. This antigen persistence coincides with the evolution of local inflammatory reactions, which, according to Mutoloki *et al.* (2004), tend to culminate from six to nine months post-immunization.

16.9 SIDE-EFFECTS

The immunity conferred by oil-adjuvanted furunculosis vaccines comes with adverse reactions, and in particular with the development of inflammatory and granulomatous lesions on the injection site. There is a large body of research describing these side-effects, and so only examples can be mentioned here: describing their pathology (Midtlyng, 1996; Poppe and Breck, 1997); attempting to quantify the outcomes (Midtlyng and Lillehaug, 1998; Rønsholt and McLean, 1999; Aunsmo *et al.*, 2008a); improving methodology (Aunsmo *et al.*, 2008b); and detailing the underlying tissue processes (Mutoloki *et al.*, 2006). In addition to inflammatory reactions that in some fish may leave visual scars or pigment on the processed product, furunculosis vaccines have been reported to cause reduced growth, but proving highly variable and depending on numerous geographic, temperature-related, and site-specific factors (Midtlyng and Lillehaug, 1998; Aunsmo *et al.*, 2008a). So far, nobody has been able to untangle the factors inducing these side-effects from the antigenic factors that are responsible for furunculosis vaccine protection.

16.10 VACCINATION AGAINST ATYPICAL FURUNCULOSIS

Infection with atypical *A. salmonicida* strains cause a variety of clinical manifestations of disease, and is described from all continents, including also Chile and Australia where classical furunculosis is considered absent. The species range of atypical furunculosis is extremely broad, and in many species the disease condition is named after the predominant clinical manifestation: contagious dermatitis (salmonids), goldfish ulcer disease, carp erythrodermatitis, and so on. Even though ulcers and cutaneous wounds are predominant in most species, acute courses of infection with septicemia, severe but non-specific organ pathology and high mortality do occur, much resembling epizootics of classical furunculosis. Comprehensive reviews of atypical furunculosis and the causative bacterial strains can be found in Wiklund and Dalsgaard (1998), Guðmundsdóttir (1998), and Guðmundsdóttir and Björnsdóttir (2007).

The fact that atypical furunculosis could not be easily controlled by copying classical furunculosis vaccine approaches has led research to continue on the virulence factors of atypical *A. salmonicida* strains, and their potential as vaccine antigens. Most of the publications are from

Table 16.2 Published studies on atypical furunculosis vaccination of freshwater and marine fish species.

Salmonids and coregonids	Guðmundsdóttir and Guðmundsdóttir (1997); Guðmundsdóttir *et al.* (1997); Guðmundsdóttir and Magnadóttir (1997); Lönnström *et al.* (2001); Pylkkö *et al.* (2002)
Cyprinids	Evenberg *et al.* (1988); Sinyakov *et al.* (2001); Maurice *et al.* (2004); Robertson *et al.* (2005)
Atlantic halibut	Ingilæ *et al.* (2000); Guðmundsdóttir *et al.* (2003); Lund *et al.* (2008b)
Spotted wolf-fish	Ingilæ *et al.* (2000); Lund *et al.* (2002, 2003b); Grøntvedt *et al.* (2003); Grøntvedt and Espelid (2004)
Atlantic cod	Mikkelsen *et al.* (2004); Lund *et al.* (2006, 2008a); Arnesen *et al.* (2010)
Turbot	Björnsdóttir *et al.* (2005); Santos *et al.* (2005)

Icelandic and Norwegian research groups. Like in classical furunculosis, much attention has been paid to the role of the S-layer (A-protein) and the secreted proteases for pathogenicity and virulence examples, being given by Lund and Mikkelsen (2004), and Gunnlaugsdóttir and Guðmundsdóttir (1997). The overall picture is that of remarkable diversity of the pathogenic and virulence factors, but in the majority of strains the factors leading to acute death and muscular tissue necrosis seem less prominent than in classical furunculosis. Despite the fact that inoculation with less than 100 cfu/fish of certain atypical strains may be lethal, for example for juvenile spotted wolf-fish, induction of mortality by bath exposure has proven notoriously difficult (Guðmundsdóttir and Magnadóttir, 1997; Lund *et al.*, 2008b). In turbot, doses between 10^7 and 10^9 cfu/fish were needed to induce high mortality (Santos *et al.*, 2005). In light of this, together with the observation that ulcerous clinical manifestation is typical, it appears that there are differences between typical and atypical furunculosis strains with regards to invasiveness and septicemic propagation.

There are some 20 recently published studies of atypical furunculosis vaccination in freshwater and marine species (Table 16.2), and for a comprehensive and detailed review, Guðmundsdóttir and Björnsdóttir (2007) is strongly recommended.

Summarizing this body of research, it appears that vaccine development for atypical furunculosis is even more challenging than for the classical variant of the disease. Although classical furunculosis vaccines have been reported to induce some degree of cross-protection to experimental challenge with atypical furunculosis in salmon (Guðmundsdóttir and Guðmundsdóttir, 1997), challenge studies performed in other species were discouraging (Lund *et al.*, 2002; Björnsdóttir *et al.*, 2005) or inconsistent (Lund *et al.*, 2008b). Furthermore, some degree of cross-protection has been seen when immunization and challenge were performed with a range of atypical furunculosis isolates from non-salmonid marine species. This led Norwegian researchers to suggest that vaccines against atypical furunculosis should be species-specific, possibly also containing several different antigenic strains, in order to reflect the antigenic diversity observed in practical aquaculture (Lund *et al.*, 2002, 2008b). This conclusion obviously represents a serious challenge to the economic viability of atypical vaccine development.

16.11 LEGAL ASPECTS AND REGULATIONS

Furunculosis in fish is not listed in the Aquatic Animal Health Code of the World Organization for Animal Health (OIE), nor is it subject to zoo-sanitary interventions under directive

91/67 EU, which specifies the requirements for trade and transfer of live aquatic animals in the European Union and the associated states, forming the European Economic Area. Some of these states, such as Norway and Sweden, have, however, maintained classical furunculosis on the list of diseases of national relevance, and retained certain legal instruments for use in the case of clinical outbreaks and epizootic events. In Norway, it is mandatory by regulation to vaccinate salmonids against furunculosis while in the hatchery. In Chile and Canada, both classical and atypical furunculosis are covered by fish disease legislation.

Potency testing of oil-adjuvanted furunculosis vaccines for the European markets should be performed according to the method described in the Pharmacopoeia Europa monograph, unless other methods have been documented and approved by the licensing authorities (Anonymous, 2008). However, these tests are based on IP challenge and have been repeatedly criticized for being unable to reveal subpotent formulations (Midtlyng, 2005). Work to develop an alternative potency test, based on antibody response measurements, is showing promising results (Romstad *et al.*, 2013), opening the possibility for replacement of the current method, involving the use of lethal study endpoints. Furunculosis vaccine for European markets, including formulations not involving oil adjuvants, must be documented following guidelines generally applying to veterinary vaccines (EMA/CVMP/IWP/206555/2010) and fish vaccines (EMA/CVMP/IWP/314550/2010).

Even though furunculosis vaccines are commonly licensed for the predominantly farmed salmonids only (Atlantic salmon and rainbow trout), legal use of these products is generally possible for other species, following the so-called "cascade" prescription. In Europe, this principle also allows the emergency use of furunculosis vaccines even in countries where no such vaccines have a regular marketing authorization. Also in Chile, emergency use of furunculosis vaccine licensed elsewhere can be authorized by Servicio Agricola y Ganadero (SAG). In the complete absence of available licensed vaccines, most countries allow immunization against atypical furunculosis to be pursued via manufacture and authority approval of autogenous vaccines, using pathogenic strains that are isolated in specific farms, regions or farming value chains that experience clinical disease problems.

REFERENCES

Ackermann, P.A., Iwama, G.K. and Thornton, J.C. 2000. Physiological and immunological effects of adjuvanted *Aeromonas salmonicida* vaccines on juvenile rainbow trout. *J Aquat Anim Health* **12**: 157–64.

Anonymous. 2008. Furunculosis vaccine (inactivated, oil-adjuvanted, injectable) for salmonids. *European Pharmacopoeia Monographs No. 1521.*

Arnesen, K.R., Mikkelsen, H., Schrøder, M.B. and Lund, V. 2010. Impact of reattaching various *Aeromonas salmonicida* A-layer proteins on vaccine efficacy in Atlantic cod (*Gadus morhua*). *Vaccine* **8**: 4703–8.

Aunsmo, A., Guttvik, A., Midtlyng, P.J., *et al.*, 2008a. Association of spinal deformity and vaccine induced abdominal lesions in harvest sized Atlantic salmon, *Salmo salar*. *J Fish Dis* **31**: 515–24.

Aunsmo, A., Larssen, R.B., Valle, P.S., *et al.*, 2008b. Improved field trial methodology for quantifying vaccination side-effects in farmed Atlantic salmon (*Salmo salar* L.). *Aquaculture* **284**: 19–24.

Austin, B. and Austin, D.A. 2007. *Bacterial Fish Pathogens. Disease of Farmed and Wild Fish*. 4th edn. Chichester, Springer Praxis.

Beaz-Hidalgo, R. and Figueras, M.J. 2013. *Aeromonas* spp. whole genomes and virulence factors implicated in fish disease. *J Fish Dis* **36**: 371–88.

Bebak-Williams, J. and Bullock, G.L. 2002. Vaccination against furunculosis in Arctic char: efficacy of a commercial vaccine. *J Aquat Anim Health* **14**: 294–7.

Bernoth, E.-M. 1997. Furunculosis, the history of the disease and of disease research, in *Furunculosis – Multidiciplinary Fish Disease Research* (eds E.-M. Bernoth, A.E. Ellis, P.J. Midtlyng, *et al.*,). London, Academic Press, 1–20.

Bernoth, E.-M., Ellis, A.E., Midtlyng, P.J., *et al.*, (eds) 1997. *Furunculosis – Multidiciplinary Fish Disease Research*. London, Academic Press.

Björnsdóttir, B., Guðmundsdóttir, S., Bambir, S.H. and Guðmundsdóttir, B.K. 2005. Experimental infection of turbot, *Scophthalmus maximus* (L.) by *Aeromonas salmonicida* subsp. *achromogenes* and evaluation of cross protection induced by a furunculosis vaccine. *J Fish Dis* **28**: 181–8.

Boyd, J.M., Danacay, A., Knickle, L.C., *et al.*, 2008. Contribution of type IV pili to the virulence of *Aeromonas salmonicida* subsp. *salmonicida* in Atlantic salmon (*Salmo salar* L.). *Infect Immun* **76**: 1445–55.

Bricknell, I.R., Bowden, T.J., Lomax, J. and Ellis, A.E. 1997. Antibody response and protection in Atlantic salmon (*Salmo salar*) immunized with an extracellular polysaccharide of *Aeromonas salmonicida*. *Fish Shellfish Immunol* **7**: 1–16.

Bricknell, I.R., King, J.A., Bowden, T.J. and Ellis, A.E. 1999. Duration of protective antibodies, and the correlation with protection in Atlantic salmon (*Salmo salar* L), following vaccination with an *Aeromonas salmonicida* vaccine containing iron-regulated outer membrane protein and secretory polysaccharide. *Fish Shellfish Immunol* **9**: 139–51.

Bruhn, J.B., Dalsgaard, I., Nielsen, K.F., *et al.*, 2005. Quorum sensing signal molecules (acylated homoserine lactones) in Gram-negative fish pathogenic bacteria. *Dis Aquat Org* **65**: 43–52.

Burr, S.E., Pugovkin, D., Wahli, T., *et al.*, 2005. Attenuated virulence of an *Aeromonas salmonicida* subsp. *salmonicida* type III secretion mutant in a rainbow trout model. *Microbiology* **151**: 2111–18.

Charette, S.J., Brochu, F., Boyle, B., *et al.*, 2012. Draft genome sequence of the virulent strain 01-B526 of the fish pathogen *Aeromonas salmonicida*. *J Bacteriol* **194**: 722–3.

Chung, S. and Secombes, C.J. 1987. Activation of rainbow trout macrophages. *J Fish Biol* **31A**: 51–6.

Cipriano, R.C. and Austin, B. 2011. Furunculosis and other aeromonad diseases, in *Fish Diseases and Disorders. Vol. 3: Viral, Bacterial and Fungal Infections*, 2nd edn (eds P.T.K. Woo and D.B. Bruno). Wallingford, CABI, 424–83.

Danacay, A., Knickle, L.C., Solanky, K.S., *et al.*, 2006. Contribution of the type III secretion system (TTSS) to virulence of *Aeromonas salmonicida* subsp. *salmonicida*. *Microbiology* **152**: 1847–56.

Danacay, A., Boyd, J.M., Fast, M.D., *et al.*, 2010. *Aeromonas salmonicida* type I pilus system contributes to host colonization but not invasion. *Dis Aquat Org* **88**: 199–206.

Duff, D.C.B. 1942. The oral immunization of trout against *Bacterium salmonicida*. *J Immunol* **44**: 87–94.

Durbin, M., McIntosch, D., Smith, P.D., *et al.*, 1999. Immunization against furunculosis in rainbow trout with iron-regulated outer membrane protein vaccines: relative efficacy of immersion, oral, and injection delivery. *J Aquat Anim Health* **11**: 68–75.

Ebanks, R.O., Dacanay, A., Goguen, M., *et al.*, 2004. Differential proteomic analysis of *Aeromonas salmonicida* outer membrane proteins in response to low iron and *in vivo* growth conditions. *Proteomics* **4**: 1074–85.

Ebanks, R.O., Goguen, M., McKinnon, S., *et al.*, 2005. Identification of the major outer membrane proteins of *Aeromonas salmonicida*. *Dis Aquat Org* **68**: 29–38.

Eggset, G., Mikkelsen, H. and Killie, J.E.A. 1997. Immunocompetence and duration of immunity against *Vibrio salmonicida* and *Aeromonas salmonicida* after vaccination of Atlantic salmon (*Salmo salar* L.) at low and high temperatures. *Fish Shellfish Immunol* **7**: 247–60.

Egidius, E. 1987. *Import of furunculosis to Norway with Atlantic salmon smolts from Scotland*. International Council for the Exploration of the Sea (ICES), Mariculture Committee Report no. C.M. 1987/F:8.

Ellis, A.E. 1991. An appraisal of the extracellular toxins of *Aeromonas salmonicida* subsp. *salmonicida*. *J Fish Dis* **14**: 265–77.

Ellis, A.E. 1997a. Furunculosis protective antigens and mechanisms, in *Furunculosis – Multidiciplinary Fish Disease Research* (eds E.-M. Bernoth, A.E. Ellis, P.J. Midtlyng, *et al.*,). London, Academic Press, 382–404.

Ellis, A.E. 1997b. Immunization with bacterial antigens: Furunculosis. *Dev Biol Stand* **90**: 107–16.

Ellis, A.E. 1997c. The extracellular toxins of *Aeromonas salmonicida* subsp. salmonicida, in *Furunculosis – Multidiciplinary Fish Disease Research* (eds E.-M. Bernoth, A.E. Ellis, P.J. Midtlyng, *et al.*,). London, Academic Press, 248–68.

Ellis, A.E., Burrows, A.S. and Stapleton, K.J. 1988. Lack of relationship between virulence of *Aeromonas salmonicida* and the putative virulence factors, A-layer, extracellular proteases, and extracellular hemolysins. *J Fish Dis* **11**: 309–23.

Emmerich, R. and Weibel, E. 1894. Über eine durch Bakterien erzeugte Seuche unter den Forellen. *Arch Hyg* **21**: 1–21.

Enger, Ø.E. 1997. Survival and inactivation of *Aeromonas salmonicida* outside the host – a most superficial way of life, in *Furunculosis – Multidiciplinary Fish Disease Research* (eds E.-M. Bernoth, A.E. Ellis, P.J. Midtlyng, *et al.*,). London, Academic Press, 159–77.

Erdal, J.I. and Reitan, L.J. 1992. Immune response and protective immunity after vaccination of Atlantic salmon (*Salmo salar* L.) against furunculosis. *Fish Shellfish Immunol* **2**: 99–108.

Evelyn, T.P.T. 1997. A historical review of fish vaccinology. *Dev Biol Stand* **90**: 3–12.

Evenberg, D., de Graaff, P., Lugtenberg, B. and van Muiswinkel, W.B. 1988. Vaccine-induced protective immunity against *Aeromonas salmonicida* tested in experimental carp erythrodermatitis. *J Fish Dis* **1**: 337–50.

Fast, M.D., Tse, B., Boyd, J.M. and Johnson, S.C. 2009. Mutation in the *Aeromonas salmonicida* subsp. *salmonicida* type III secretion system affect Atlantic salmon leucocyte activation and downstream immune responses. *Fish Shellfish Immunol* **27**: 721–8.

Garduno, R.A. and Kay, W.W. 1995. Capsulated cells of *Aeromonas salmonicida* grown *in vitro* have different functional properties than capsulated cells grown *in vivo*. *Can J Microbiol* **41**: 941–5.

Garduno, R.A., Moore, A.R., Olivier, G., *et al.*, 2000. Host cell invasion and intracellular residence by *Aeromonas salmonicida*: role of the S-layer. *Can J Microbiol* **46**: 660–68.

Grøntvedt, R.N. and Espelid, S. 2004. Vaccination and immune responses against atypical *Aeromonas salmonicida* in spotted wolffish (*Anarhichas minor* Olafsen) juveniles. *Fish Shellfish Immunol* **16**: 271–85.

Grøntvedt, R.N., Lund, V. and Espelid, S. 2003. Atypical furunculosis in spotted wolffish (*Anarhichas minor* O.) juveniles: bath vaccination and challenge. *Aquaculture* **232**: 69–80.

Grove, S., Høie, S. and Evensen, Ø. 2003. Distribution and retention of antigens of *Aeromonas salmonicida* in Atlantic salmon (*Salmo salar L.*) vaccinated with a Δ-*aroA* mutant or formalin-inactivated bacteria in oil-adjuvant. *Fish Shellfish Immunol* **15**: 349–58.

Guðmundsdóttir, B.K. 1998. Infections by atypical strains of the bacterium *Aeromonas salmonicida*: a review. *Búvisindi; Icel Agric Sci* **12**: 61–72.

Guðmundsdóttir, B.K. and Björnsdóttir, B. 2007. Vaccination against atypical furunculosis and winter ulcer disease of fish. *Vaccine* **25**: 5512–23.

Guðmundsdóttir, B.K. and Guðmundsdóttir, S. 1997. Evaluation of cross protection by vaccines against atypical and typical furunculosis in Atlantic salmon (*Salmo salar L.*). *J Fish Dis* **20**: 343–50.

Guðmundsdóttir, B.K. and Magnadóttir, B. 1997. Protection of Atlantic salmon (*Salmo salar* L.) against an experimental infection of *Aeromonas salmonicida* subsp. *achromogenes*. *Fish Shellfish Immunol* **7**: 55–69.

Guðmundsdóttir, B.K., Jonsdóttir, H., Steinthorsdóttir, V., *et al.*, 1997. Survival and humoral antibody response of in Atlantic salmon, *Salmo salar L.*, vaccinated against *Aeromonas salmonicida* subsp. *achromogenes*. *J Fish Dis* **20**: 351–60.

Guðmundsdóttir, S., Lange, S., Magnadóttir, B. and Guðmundsdóttir, B.K. 2003. Protection against atypical furunculosis in Atlantic halibut *Hippoglossus hippoglossus* (L.): comparison of a commercial furunculosis vaccine and an autogenous vaccine. *J Fish Dis* **26**: 331–8.

Gunnlaugsdóttir, B. and Guðmundsdóttir, B.K. 1997. Pathogenicity of atypical *Aeromonas salmonicida* in Atlantic salmon compared with protease production. *J Appl Bacteriol* **83**: 542–51.

Hirst, I.D. and Ellis, A.E. 1994. Iron-regulated outer membrane proteins of *Aeromonas salmonicida* are important protective antigens in Atlantic salmon against furunculosis. *Fish Shellfish Immunol* **4**: 29–45.

Hoel, K., Salonius, K. and Lillehaug, A. 1997. *Vibrio* antigens of polyvalent vaccines enhance the humoral immune response to *Aeromonas salmonicida* antigens in Atlantic salmon (*Salmo salar* L.). *Fish Shellfish Immunol* **7**: 71–80.

Hoel, K, Reitan, L.J. and Lillehaug, A. 1998. Immunological cross reactions between *Aeromonas salmonicida* and *Vibrio salmonicida* in Atlantic salmon (*Salmo salar L.)* and rabbit. *Fish Shellfish Immunol* **8**: 171–82.

Horne, J.H. 1928. Furunculosis in trout and the importance of carriers in the spread of the disease. *J Hyg* **28**: 67–78.

Horne, M.T. and Ellis, A.E. 1988. Commercial production and licensing of vaccines for fish, in *Fish Vaccination* (ed. A.E. Ellis). London, Academic Press, 47–54.

Hussain, I., Mackie, C., Cox, D., *et al.*, 2000. Suppression of the humoral immune response of Atlantic salmon, *Salmo salar* L. by the 64 kDa serine protease of *Aeromonas salmonicida*. *Fish Shellfish Immunol* **10**: 359–73.

Ingilæ, M., Arnesen, J.A., Lund, V. and Eggset, G. 2000. Vaccination of Atlantic halibut (*Hippoglossus hippoglossus* L.) and spotted wolffish (*Anarhichas minor* O.) against atypical *Aeromonas salmonicida*. *Aquaculture* **183**: 31–44.

Irie, T., Watarai, S., Iwasaki, T. and Kodama, H. 2005. Protection against experimental *Aeromonas salmonicida* infection in carp by oral immunisation with bacterial antigen entrapped liposomes. *Fish Shellfish Immunol* **18**: 235–42.

Jutfelt, F., Olsen, R.E., Glette, J., *et al.*, 2006. Translocation of viable *Aeromonas salmonicida* across the intestine of rainbow trout, *Oncorhynchus mykiss* (Walbaum). *J Fish Dis* **29**: 255–62.

Jutfelt, F., Sundh, H., Glette, J., *et al.*, 2008. The involvement of *Aeromonas salmonicida* virulence factors in bacterial translocation across the rainbow trout, *Oncorhynchus mykiss* (Walbaum) intestine. *J Fish Dis* **31**: 141–51.

Koppang, E.O., Fjølstad, M., Melgård, B., *et al.*, 2000. Non-pigment-producing isolates of *Aeromonas salmonicida* subspecies *salmonicida*: isolation, identification, transmission and pathogenicity in Atlantic salmon, *Salmo salar* L. *J Fish Dis* **23**: 39–48.

Krantz, G.E., Reddecliff, J.M. and Heist, C.E. 1964. Immune response of trout to *Aeromonas salmonicida*. Part I. Development of agglutinating antibodies and protective immunity. *Prog Fish Cult* **26**: 3–10.

Lee, K.K. and Ellis, A.E. 1990. Glycerophospholipid:cholesterol acyltransferase complexed with lipopolysaccharide (LPS) is a major lethal exotoxin and cytolysin of *Aeromonas salmonicida*: LPS stabilizes and enhances toxicity of the enzyme. *J Bacteriol* **172**: 5382–93.

Lee, K.K. and Ellis, A.E. 1991. Role of the lethal extracellular cytolysin of *Aeromonas salmonicida* in the pathology of furunculosis. *J Fish Dis* **14**: 453–60.

Lillehaug, A., Lunder, T. and Poppe, T.T. 1992. Field testing of adjuvanted furunculosis vaccines in Atlantic salmon, *Salmo salar L. J Fish Dis* **15**: 485–96.

Lönnström, L.-G., Rahkonen, R., Lundén, T., *et al.*, 2001. Protection, immune response and side-effects in European whitefish (*Coregonus lavaretus* L.) vaccinated against vibriosis and furunculosis. *Aquaculture* **200**: 271–84.

Lund, V. and Mikkelsen, H. 2004. Genetic diversity among A-proteins of atypical strains of *Aeromonas salmonicida*. *Dis Aquat Org* **61**: 257–62.

Lund, V., Arnesen, J.A. and Eggset, G. 2002. Vaccine development for atypical furunculosis in spotted wolffish *Anarhichas minor* O.: comparison of efficacy of vaccines containing different strains of atypical *Aeromonas salmonicida*. *Aquaculture* **204**: 33–44.

Lund, V., Arnesen, J.A., Coucheron, D., *et al.*, 2003a. The *Aeromonas salmonicida* A-layer protein is an important protective antigen in oil-adjuvanted vaccines. *Fish Shellfish Immunol* **15**: 367–72.

Lund, V., Espelid, S. and Mikkelsen, H. 2003b. Vaccine efficacy in spotted wolffish *Anarhichas minor*: relationship to molecular variation in A-layer protein of atypical *Aeromonas salmonicida*. *Dis Aquat Org* **56**: 31–42.

Lund, V., Børdal, S., Kjellsen, O., *et al.*, 2006. Comparison of antibody responses in Atlantic cod (*Gadus morhua* L.) to *Aeromonas salmonicida* and *Vibrio anguillarum*. *Dev Comp Immunol* **30**: 1145–55.

Lund, V., Arnesen, J.A., Mikkelsen, H., *et al.*, 2008a. Atypical furunculosis vaccines for Atlantic cod (*Gadus morhua*); vaccine efficacy and antibody responses. *Vaccine* **26**: 679–9.

Lund, V., Mikkelsen, H. and Schrøder, M.B. 2008b. Comparison of atypical furunculosis vaccines in spotted wolffish (*Anarhichas minor* O.) and Atlantic halibut (*Hippoglossus hippoglossus* L.) *Vaccine* **26**: 2833–40.

Lutwyche, P., Exner, M.M., Hancock, R.E.W. and Trust, T.J. 1995. A conserved *Aeromonas salmonicida* porin provides protective immunity to rainbow trout. *Infect Immun* **63**: 3137–42.

Magnadóttir, B. 2010. Immunological control of fish diseases. *Mar Biotechnol* **12**: 361–79.

Markestad, A. and Grave, K. 1997. Reduction of antibacterial drug use in Norwegian fish farming due to vaccination. *Dev Biol Stand* **90**: 365–9.

Marsden, M., Vaughan, L.M., Fitzpatrick, R.M., *et al.*, 1998. Potency testing of a live, genetically attenuated vaccine for salmonids. *Vaccine* **16**: 1087–94.

Masada, C.L., LaPatra, S.E., Morton, A.W. and Strom, M.S. 2002. An *Aeromonas salmonicida* type VI pilin is required for virulence in rainbow trout *Oncorhynchus mykiss*. *Dis Aquat Org* **51**: 13–25.

Maurice, S., Nussinovitch, A., Jaffe, N., *et al.*, 2004. Oral immunization of *Carassius auratus* with modified recombinant A-layer proteins entrapped in alginate beads. *Vaccine* **23**: 450–59.

McCarthy, D.H. and Roberts, R.J. 1980. Furunculosis of fish – the present state of our knowledge, in *Advances in Aquatic Microbiology* (eds M.R. Droop and H.W. Jannasch). London, Academic Press, 293–341.

Merino, S., Vilches, S., Canals, R., *et al.*, 2005. A C1q-binding 40kDa porin from *Aeromonas salmonicida*: cloning, sequencing, role in serum susceptibility and fish immunoprotection. *Microb Pathog* **38**: 227–37.

Midtlyng, P.J. 1996. A field study on intraperitoneal vaccination of Atlantic salmon (*Salmo salar L.*) against furunculosis. *Fish Shellfish Immunol* **6**: 553–65.

Midtlyng, P.J. 1997. Vaccination against furunculosis, in *Furunculosis – Multidiciplinary Fish Disease Research* (eds E.-M. Bernoth, A.E. Ellis, P.J. Midtlyng, G. Olivier and P.R. Smith). London, Academic Press, 382–404.

Midtlyng, P.J. 2005. Critical assessment of regulatory standards and tests for fish vaccines. *Dev Biol (Basel)* **121**: 219–26.

Midtlyng, P.J. and Lillehaug, A. 1998. Growth of Atlantic salmon *Salmo salar* after intraperitoneal administration of vaccines containing adjuvants. *Dis Aquat Org* **32**: 91–7.

Midtlyng, P.J., Reitan, L.J., Lillehaug, A. and Ramstad, A. 1996a. Protection, immune responses and side-effects in Atlantic salmon (*Salmo salar* L.) vaccinated against furunculosis by different procedures. *Fish Shellfish Immunol* **6**: 599–613.

Midtlyng, P.J., Reitan, L.J. and Speilberg, L. 1996b. Experimental studies on the efficacy and side-effects of intraperitoneal vaccination of Atlantic salmon (*Salmo salar L.*) against furunculosis. *Fish Shellfish Immunol* **6**: 335–50.

Mikkelsen, H., Schrøder, M.B. and Lund, V. 2004. Vibriosis and atypical furunculosis vaccines; efficacy and side-effects in Atlantic cod (*Gadus morhua* L). *Aquaculture* **242**: 81–91.

Munro, A.L.S. and Gauld, J.A. 1997. *Scottish fish farms annual production survey 1996*. SOAFD Marine Laboratory Aberdeen Report 1997.

Munro, A.L.S. and Waddell, I.F. 1984. *Furunculosis: experience of its control in the sea water cage culture of Atlantic salmon in Scotland*. International Council of the Exploration of the Sea, Mariculture Committee Report 1984; CM 1984 /F:32.

Mutoloki, S., Alexandersen, S. and Evensen, Ø. 2004. Sequential study of antigen persistence and concomitant inflammatory reactions relative to side-effects and growth of Atlantic salmon (*Salmo salar* L.) following intraperitoneal injection with oil-adjuvanted vaccines. *Fish Shellfish Immunol* **16**: 633–44.

Mutoloki, S., Brudeseth, B., Reite, O.B. and Evensen, Ø. 2006. The contribution of *Aeromonas salmonicida* extracellular products to the induction of inflammation in Atlantic salmon (*Salmo salar* L.) following vaccination with oil-based vaccines. *Fish Shellfish Immunol* **20**: 1–11.

Najimi, M., Lemos, M.L. and Osorio, C.R. 2009. Identification of iron regulated genes in the fish pathogen *Aeromonas salmonicida* subsp. *salmonicida*. Genetic diversity and evidence of conserved iron uptake systems. *Vet Microbiol* **133**: 377–82.

Noonan, B. and Trust, T.J. 1997. The synthesis, secretion and role in virulence of the paracrystalline surface protein layers of *Aeromonas salmonicida* and *A. hydrophila*. *FEMS Microbiol Lett* **154**: 1–7.

Nordmo, R. and Ramstad, A. 1997. Comparison of different challenge methods to evaluate the efficacy of furunculosis vaccines in Atlantic salmon, *Salmo salar* L. *J Fish Dis* **20**: 119–26.

Novotny, A. 1978. Vibriosis and furunculosis in marine cultured salmon in Puget Sound, Washington. *Mar Fish Rev* **40**: 52–5.

O'Dowd, A.M., Bricknell, I.R., Secombes, C.J. and Ellis, A.E. 1999. The primary and secondary antibody responses to IROMP antigens in Atlantic salmon (*Salmo salar* L) immunized with A^+ and A^- *Aeromonas salmonicida* bacterins. *Fish Shellfish Immunol* **9**: 125–38.

Olivier, G., Moore, A. and Fildes, J. 1992. Toxicity of *Aeromonas salmonicida* cells to Atlantic salmon, *Salmo salar*, peritoneal macrophages. *Dev Comp Immunol* **16**: 49–61.

Paterson, W.D., Lall, S.P., Airdrie, D., *et al.*, 1985. Prevention of disease in salmonids by vaccination and dietary modification. *Fish Pathol* **20**: 427–34.

Poppe, T.T. and Breck, O. 1997. Pathology of Atlantic salmon *Salmo salar* intraperitoneally immunized with oil-adjuvanted vaccine. A case report. *Dis Aquat Org* **29**: 219–26.

Prost, M. 2001. Extracellular proteases ECP of *Aeromonas salmonicida* and their significance in the pathogenesis and immunoprophylaxis of fish furunculosis. *Med Weter* **57**: 79–82.

Pylkkö, P., Lyytikainen, T., Ritola, O., *et al.*, 2002. Temperature effect on the immune defense functions of Arctic char *Salvelinus alpinus*. *Dis Aquat Org* **52**: 47–55.

Reith, M.E., Singh, R.K., Curtis, B., *et al.*, 2008. The genome of *Aeromonas salmonicida* subsp. *salmonicida* A449: insights into the evolution of a fish pathogen. *BMC Genomics* **9**: 427.

Robertson, P.A.W., Austin, D.A. and Austin, B. 2005. Prevention of ulcer disease in goldfish by means of vaccination. *J Aquat Anim Health* **17**: 203–9.

Romstad, A.B., Reitan, L.J., Midtlyng, P., *et al.*, 2012. Development of an antibody ELISA for potency testing of furunculosis (*Aeromonas salmonicida* subsp. *salmonicida*) vaccines in Atlantic salmon (*Salmo salar* L). *Biologicals* **40**: 67–71.

Romstad, A.B., Reitan, L.J., Midtlyng, P., *et al.*, 2013. Antibody responses correlate with antigen dose and *in vivo* protection for oil-adjuvanted, experimental furunculosis (*Aeromonas salmonicida* subsp. *salmonicida*) vaccines in Atlantic salmon (*Salmo salar* L.) and can be used for batch potency testing of vaccines. *Vaccine* **31**: 791–6.

Rønsholt, B. and McLean, E. 1999. The effect of vaccination and vaccine components upon short-term growth and feed conversion efficiency in rainbow trout. *Aquaculture* **174**: 213–21.

Salte, R., Norberg, K., Ødegård, O.R., *et al.*, 1993. Exotoxin-induced consumptive coagulopathy in Atlantic salmon *Salmo salar* L.; inhibitory effects of exogenous antithrombin and α-2 macroglobulin on *Aeromonas salmonicida* serine protease. *J Fish Dis* **16**: 561–8.

Santos, Y., Garcia-Marquez, S., Pereira, P.G., *et al.*, 2005. Efficacy of furunculosis vaccines in turbot, *Scophthalmus maximus* (L.): evaluation of immersion, oral and injection delivery. *J Fish Dis* **28**: 165–72.

Schwenteit, J., Gram, L., Nielsen, K.F., *et al.*, 2011. Quorum sensing in *Aeromonas salmonicida* subsp. *achromogenes* and the effect of the auto inducer synthease AsaI on bacterial virulence. *Vet Microbiol* **147**: 389–97.

Sinyakov, M., Dror, M., Margel, M. and Avtalion, R.R. 2001. Immunogenicity of the *Aeromonas salmonicida* A-protein in goldfish (*Carassius auratus* L.). *Isr J Aquacult – Bamidgeh* **53**: 110–14.

Smith, P. and Hiney, M. 2000. Oil-adjuvanted furunculosis vaccines in commercial fish farms: a preliminary epizootiological investigation. *Aquaculture* **190**: 1–9.

Spence, K.D., Pilcher, K.S. and Fryer, J.L. 1965. Active and passive immunization of certain salmonids fishes against *Aeromonas salmonicida*. *Can J Microbiol* **11**: 397–405.

Thornton, J.C., Garduno, R.A. and Kay, W.W. 1994. The development of live vaccines for furunculosis lacking the A-layer and O-antigen of *Aeromonas salmonicida*. *J Fish Dis* **17**: 195–204.

Tomás, J.M. 2012. The main *Aeromonas* pathogenic factors. *ISRN Microbiology*, article ID 256261.

Treasurer, J. and Cox, C. 2008. Intraperitoneal and dorsal median sinus vaccination effect on growth, immune response, and reproductive potential in farmed Atlantic salmon *Salmo salar*. *Aquaculture* **275**: 51–7.

Trust, T.J., Noonan, B., Chu, S.J., *et al.*, 1996. A molecular approach to understanding the pathogenesis of *Aeromonas salmonicida*; relevance to vaccine development. *Fish Shellfish Immunol* **6**: 269–76.

Vaughan, L.M., Smith, P.R. and Foster, T.J. 1993. An aromatic-dependent mutant of the fish pathogen *Aeromonas salmonicida* is attenuated in fish and is effective as a live vaccine against the salmonid disease furunculosis. *Infect Immun* **61**: 2172–81.

Villumsen, K.R., Dalsgaard, I., Holten-Andersen, L. and Raida, M.K. 2012. Potential role of specific antibodies as important vaccine induced protective mechanism against *Aeromonas salmonicida* in rainbow trout. *PLoS One* **7**: e46733.

Vipond, R., Bricknell, I.R., Durant, E., *et al.*, 1998. Defined deletion mutants demonstrate that the major secreted toxins are not essential for the virulence of *Aeromonas salmonicida*. *Infect Immun* **66**: 1990–98.

Wang, S., Laroque, S., Vinogradov, E., *et al.*, 2004. Structural studies of the capsular polysaccharide and lipopolysaccharide O-antigen of *Aeromonas salmonicida* strain 80204–1 produced under *in vitro* and *in vivo* growth conditions. *Eur J Biochem* **271**: 4507–16.

Wang, S., Li, J., Vinogradov, E. and Altman, E. 2006. Structural studies of the core region of *Aeromonas salmonicida* subsp. *salmonicida* lipopolysaccharide. *Carbohydr Res* **341**: 109–17.

Wiklund, T. and Dalsgaard, I. 1998. Occurrence and significance of atypical *Aeromonas salmonicida* in non-salmonid and salmonid species: a review. *Dis Aquat Org* **32**: 49–69.

17 Vaccination against Photobacteriosis

Jesús L. Romalde

Department of Microbiology and Parasitology, University of Santiago de Compostela, Spain

ABSTRACT

Photobacteriosis is a bacterial septicemia formerly called pasteurellosis or "pseudotuberculosis" due to the fact that, in the chronic form, the diseased fish showed white nodules in the internal organs, particularly spleen and kidney, which consist of bacterial accumulations. The halophilic bacterium *Photobacterium damselae* subsp. *piscicida* (previously *Pasteurella piscicida*) is the etiological agent of the disease. Photobacteriosis occurs on several continents, including Europe, Asia and America, affecting different economically relevant fish species such as white perch (*Morone americana*), striped bass (*M. saxatilis*), hybrid striped bass (*M. saxatilis x M. chrysops*), yellowtail (*Seriola quinqueradiata*), sea bream (*Sparus aurata*), sea bass (*Dicentrarchus labrax*) and sole (*Solea senegalensis*). Different vaccines have been formulated and used to prevent fish photobacteriosis. Thus, in European countries, sea bream and sea bass disease has been successfully controlled by vaccination with a commercially available ECP-enriched bacterin for more than ten years, and in Japan some vaccines are now available to protect yellowtail against this threatening pathogen.

17.1 OCCURRENCE AND SIGNIFICANCE

Photobacterium damselae subsp. *piscicida* was reported in white perch and striped bass in the upper region of Chesapeake Bay, USA, in 1963. Sniezsko *et al.* (1964) isolated from the blood and organs of moribund fish a unique bacterium which was placed into the genus *Pasteurella* on the basis of its morphological and biochemical characteristics. However, the taxonomic position of this microorganism was a matter of controversy that has only recently been clarified. Then, although this microorganism was assigned to different genera (Romalde, 2002), on the basis of rRNA studies and DNA-DNA hybridization, the approved name for the causal agent of fish pasteurellosis was established as *P. damselae* subsp. *piscicida* (Gauthier *et al.*, 1995).

jesus.romalde@usc.es

Fish Vaccination, First Edition. Edited by Roar Gudding, Atle Lillehaug and Øystein Evensen.

Although initially *P. damselae* subsp. *piscicida* was isolated from natural populations of white perch and striped bass, since 1969 this microorganism has caused significant losses in cultured juvenile yellowtail (*Seriola quinqueradiata*) in Japan. In 1970, *P. damselae* subsp. *piscicida* was thought to be responsible for heavy losses among wild menhaden (*Brevoortia tyranus*) and striped mullet (*Mugil cephalus*) in Galveston Bay, Texas (Lewis *et al.*, 1970). A few years later, pasteurellosis became a problem in yellowtail, ayu (*Plecoglosus altivelis*) and black sea bream (*Mylio macrocephalus*) cultures in Japan (Kusuda and Miura, 1972; Muroga *et al.*, 1977; Ohnishi *et al.*, 1982). Then, the disease spread to other fish species, and several epizootics were described in red sea bream (*Acanthopagrus schlegeli*) (Yasunaga *et al.*, 1983), red grouper (*Epinephelus akaara*) (Ueki *et al.*, 1990), and hybrid striped bass (*M. saxatilis x M. chrysops*) (Hawke *et al.*, 2003).

From 1990, *P. damselae* subsp. *piscicida* has caused economic losses in the marine culture of gilthead sea bream (*Sparus aurata*), sea bass (*Dicentrarchus labrax*) and sole (*Solea senegalensis*) in the Mediterranean countries of Europe (Ceschia *et al.*, 1990; Toranzo *et al.*, 1991; Balebona *et al.*, 1992; Zorrilla *et al.*, 1999; Baptista *et al.*, 1996). Recently, mortalities caused by this pathogen were registered in mullet (*Mugil cephalus*), mackerel (*Trachurus trachurus*) and red gurnard (*Aspitrigla cuculus*) in France (P. Daniel, personal comunication), as well as in cobia (*Rachycentron canadum*) in Taiwan (Liu *et al.*, 2003). In addition, the pathogen has been detected in apparently healthy mullets in Italy (Serracca *et al.*, 2011).

Pasteurellosis seems to be more prevalent during the summer months at higher water temperatures (greater than 23°C) and salinities (20–30‰) and when water quality is low (Fryer and Rohovec, 1984; Frerichs and Roberts, 1989; Magariños *et al.*, 2001). The different experiments performed by Janssen and Surgalla (1968) and Toranzo *et al.* (1982) showed that *P. damselae* subsp. *piscicida* remained viable in water for only 4–5 days. Both reports indicate that the water is not a primary reservoir. However, studies on survival in seawater and sediment showed that although this microorganism does not seem to persist for a long time in a culturable form away from fish, it possesses the capacity to enter into a viable but non-culturable state (Magariños *et al.*, 1994b). These results suggest that although *P. damselae* subsp. *piscicida* appears to be a very labile organism, the aquatic environment constitutes a reservoir and a vehicle of transmission for this pathogen. Moreover, it has been demonstrated that the dormant but viable cells of *P. damselae* subsp. *piscicida* maintain their pathogenic potential for fish, and that the non-culturable cells are capable of resuming rapid resuscitation and division when nutrient conditions are suitable.

Serological techniques have been used with effectiveness for the detection and diagnosis of this fish pathogen, as well as for the confirmation of its identity. These techniques, using specific antiserum, have confirmed the identity of the microorganisms presumptively assigned to *P. damselae* subsp. *piscicida*, and, in addition, they have demonstrated that the strains of this species, regardless of their geographic origin, are serologically homogenous (Magariños *et al.*, 1992a; Salati *et al.*, 1994), which makes it impossible to establish serotypes. This antigenic uniformity has facilitated the design of serological tools for diagnosis, many of them commercially available, which allow a rapid detection of this fish pathogen even from asymptomatic fish (Romalde *et al.*, 1995a,b, 1999), and also the development of effective vaccine formulations (Magariños *et al.*, 1994c, 1999; Bakopoulos *et al.*, 2003; Romalde *et al.*, 2005; Gravningen *et al.*, 2008).

17.2 ETIOLOGY

An exhaustive characterization of *Photobacterium damselae* subsp. *piscicida* shows that the microorganism is a non-motile, gram-negative, bipolar rod, oxidase and catalase positive, fermentative and sensitive to the vibriostatic agent O/129. It is a pleomorphic bacterium, changing from coccoidal to long rods depending on the culture conditions, with positive responses for arginine dihydrolase, lipase and phospholipase activities. This bacterium is negative for indole, nitrate reduction, urease, gelatinase, amylase and hydrogen sulfide production. Regarding the use of carbohydrates, this microorganism produces acid only from glucose, mannose, galactose and fructose. *P. damselae* subsp. *piscicida* can grow at temperatures from 15 to 32.5°C, although its optimum growth temperature is 22.5–30°C. These overall phenotypic results show that *P. damselae* subsp. *piscicida* constitutes a phenotypic homogenous group (Magariños *et al.*, 1992a). The classical description of *P. damselae* subsp. *piscicida* includes coccobacilli which are unencapsulated (Koike *et al.*, 1975). However, studies performed by Bonet *et al.* (1994) demonstrated that the majority of *P. damselae* subsp. *piscicida* strains constitutively produce capsular material composed of 99.6% carbohydrate and 0.4% protein that plays an important role in the pathogenesis of this microorganism.

Serologically, *P. damselae* subsp. *piscicida* constitutes a highly homogenous group (Kusuda and Fukuda, 1980; Nomura and Aoki, 1985; Magariños *et al.*, 1992a). This serological homogeneity was supported by lipopolysaccharide (LPS) profiles with all the strains showing the same electrophoretic patterns: O side-chains consisting of high molecular mass bands in a ladder-like pattern. In addition, similar patterns of total and outer membrane proteins were also observed for all the isolates. These LPS and membrane proteins were immunologically related among all the *P. damselae* subsp. *piscicida* isolates.

DNA fingerprinting methods such as ribotyping and different PCR techniques, AFLP (amplified fragment length polymorphism), RAPD (random amplified polymorphic DNA), ERIC (enterobacterial repetitive intergenic consensus sequences) and REP (repetitive extragenic palindromic sequences), showed the existence of two main clonal lineages within *P. damselae* subsp. *piscicida*, one including the European strains and the other the Japanese and US isolates (Magariños *et al.*, 1997, 2000; Thyssen *et al.*, 1999; Mancuso *et al.*, 2007). These results revealed the existence of genetic heterogeneity within this fish pathogen and proved to be applicable as epizootiological tools for this microorganism.

In recent years, the analysis of different regions of genoma using the SSH (suppression subtractive hybridization) methodology corroborated this high heterogeneity, in addition showing that an integrating conjugative element (ICE) can enable virulence gene transfer in this pathogen (Juíz-Río *et al.*, 2005; Osorio *et al.*, 2008).

Photobacterium damselae subsp. *piscicida* shows a different plasmid content depending on the strain analyzed. Thus, whereas in the majority of the European isolates a plasmid band of approximately 50 MDa has been detected, the Japanese isolates have a common 37-MDa plasmid band (Magariños *et al.*, 1992a).

17.3 PATHOGENESIS

The clinical signs of *P. damselae* subsp. *piscicida* infection have been previously described in detail (Kubota *et al.*, 1970; Fukuda and Kusuda, 1981) in yellowtail cultured in Japan, and are similar to those described for sea bream cultured in Galicia (northwestern Spain) and in the Mediterranean area (Toranzo *et al.*, 1991). Gross external signs of pasteurellosis are usually inconspicuous and there are generally no surface lesions. Only some affected fish may exhibit a darkening/decoloration of body color and/or slight hemorrhagic areas in the head and gills. Internally, the pathological changes may vary depending on whether the disease is acute or chronic. Whereas in the acute form, few gross pathological changes are observed, chronic lesions in internal organs are characterized by the presence of white tubercles or granulomas. The histopathological study of granulomatous deposits shows the presence of bacterial colonies and necrotic phagocytes. Moreover, the spleen, kidney and liver show accumulations of macrophages, many of which are necrotic, containing numerous intact bacteria (Nelson *et al.*, 1989; Noya *et al.*, 1995a). This fact may be indicative that *P. damselae* subsp. *piscicida* survives in host macrophages and is not degraded. Moreover, the gills also show degenerated macrophages containing *P. damselae* subsp. *piscicida* cells and necrosis of various cell types which would impair respiratory function (Noya *et al.*, 1995a).

Photobacterium damselae subsp. *piscicida* is highly pathogenic for different marine fish species without host specificity (Magariños *et al.*, 1995). Some authors have pointed out that the macrophages and neutrophils could be implicated in the differences in susceptibility of sea bass and sea bream to the disease on the basis of the fish age. Then, these host cell types only are functional in big fish phagocyting efficiently and killing the bacteria (Noya *et al.*, 1995b; Skarmeta *et al.*, 1995). In any case, the high pathogenicity reported for the different isolates indicates that this pathogen must possess important virulence mechanisms.

Regarding surface characteristics, it has been reported that *P. damselae* subsp. *piscicida* is moderately hydrophobic and weakly or non-hemagglutinating (Magariños *et al.*, 1996a). The analysis of its invasive properties revealed that this pathogen is moderately invasive. However, it is interesting to note that the bacterial cells are able to survive for at least 6 days within the host cells and to spread from cell to cell, originating destructive plaques in the fish cell monolayers. In addition, it has been demonstrated by cytochalasin D assays that the cytoskeleton of the host cell participates actively in the invasion process (Magariños *et al.*, 1996a).

The presence of a capsular material of polysaccharide nature in *P. damselae* subsp. *piscicida* isolates (Magariños *et al.*, 1996b) plays an important role in the virulence of the pathogen. In fact, the presence of this capsular material induces its resistance to the bactericidal action of the fish serum and results in lower LD_{50} values.

The ability of pathogenic bacteria to acquire iron is essential for their growth within the host, and essential, therefore, to cause infections. It has been reported (Magariños *et al.*, 1994a) that *P. damselae* subsp. *piscicida* also possesses an iron acquisition system. This system consists of a siderophore and at least three iron-regulated, high mass outer-membrane proteins. In addition, *P. damselae* subsp. *piscicida* cells were able to use hemin and hemoglobin as sole iron sources by direct binding of these compounds to iron-regulated membrane receptors (Magariños *et al.*, 1994a; do Vale *et al.*, 2002). It is currently known that the synthesis of the siderophore implicated in the virulence of *P. damselae* subsp. *piscicida* is codified by a pathogenicity island inserted in a mobile plasmid (Osorio *et al.*, 2008).

The extracellular products (ECPs) secreted by a variety of bacterial fish pathogens are important virulence factors since they can contribute to the development of the disease in terms of bacterial nutrition, or as aggressins enabling the bacteria to counteract the host's defense mechanisms. The ECPs of *P. damselae* subsp. *piscicida* strains have been shown to be lethal for different fish species, including gilthead sea bream, sea bass, turbot and rainbow trout.

In addition, these ECPs contained toxins with lethal effects for mice, and possessed strong phospholipase, cytotoxic, and hemolytic activities (Magariños *et al.*, 1992b).

The presence of an exotoxin of 56 kDa, plasmid-encoded AIP56, with apoptogenic activity against sea bass macrophages and neutrophils, has been also reported (do Vale *et al.*, 2005) and implicated in the virulence of *P. damselae* subsp. *piscicida*. By affecting both macrophages and neutrophils, the pathogen is able to evade the crucial host phagocytic defenses and, therefore, to multiplicate massively within the host. The apoptotic response involves activation of caspases and mitochondria, indicating the implication of both extrinsic and intrinsic apoptotic pathways (Costa-Ramos *et al.*, 2011). On the other hand, Liu *et al.* (2011) have purified a toxic metalloprotease with a molecular mass of 34.3 kDa and maximal activity at pH 6.0–8.0, which proved to be lethal to cobia with LD_{50} values of 6.8 mg protein/g body weight.

17.4 VACCINES

Chemotherapy was effective for the treatment of fish pasteurellosis until the 1980s. Since then, plasmid or chromosome-coded resistances to different antibiotics and other drugs have been observed (Magariños *et al.*, 1992b; Kim *et al.*, 1993). Moreover, it has been described that *P. damselae* subsp. *piscicida* has a period of intracellular parasitism within macrophages during infection (Kusuda and Salati, 1993), which can explain the ineffectiveness of chemotherapy in the treatment of some outbreaks of the disease.

In recent decades, different vaccine formulations have been designed to use as preventive measures against fish pasteurellosis (Romalde and Magariños, 1997). These vaccines usually contain whole cells of the pathogen grown in general culture media and inactivated by heat or using formalin. To improve the efficacy of such vaccines, ultrasound treatment was tested with immersion vaccination (Navot *et al.*, 2005), and mineral or non-mineral oil adjuvants were applied with injectable vaccines (Le Breton, 2009).

Further efforts to obtain better protection were focused on the use of novel culture media to obtain the bacterial cells (i.e., glucose and/or salt-enriched media, or iron-depleted media), the enrichment of the bacterins with extracellular products or LPS, or the use of bacterial components such as crude capsular polysaccharide (Magariños *et al.*, 1994c, 1999; Bakopoulos *et al.*, 2003; Gravningen *et al.*, 2008).

Some of these vaccines are commercially available in some countries from the Animal Health sections of manufacturers such as Pharmaq AS, Hipra SA, Merck, Novartis AG, or Pfizer Inc. Other veterinary companies, such as Acuitec SL, possess authorized laboratories to elaborate autovaccines.

Experimental vaccination studies using different stable siderophore-deficient and *aro*-A-deletion mutant strains have also been performed (Kusuda and Hamaguchi, 1988; Thune *et al.*, 2003), the latter formulation being patented in the US for hybrid striped bass.

The identification of proteins involved in the invasive process of *P. damselae* subsp. *piscicida* allowed the development of some formulations based on formalin-killed bacterin, cultured to overexpress such proteins (Barnes *et al.*, 2005), which were commercialized by Aqua Health, Canada, under the name Photogen. Such vaccines conferred promising dose-dependent protection in sea bass and yellowtail. Further research aims to localize the protective proteins in the ECPs of *P. damselae* subsp. *piscicida* and to prepare a subunit vaccine, although with limited results (Barnes *et al.*, 2005).

Recently, on the basis of immunoproteomic results, a Taiwanese research group has identified and cloned into *Escherichia coli* several proteins with the potential to be employed as bacterial subunit vaccines, since they confer better protection in cobia than the whole bacterial vaccine (Ho *et al.*, 2011).

17.5 VACCINATION PROCEDURES

Vaccination is becoming an increasingly important part of aquaculture, since it is considered a cost-effective method of controlling different threatening diseases. The term "vaccination strategy" has been defined to include the decision as to which diseases to vaccinate against, as well as the vaccine type, vaccination method, the timing of vaccination and the use of revaccination.

One important item for development and commercialization of vaccines includes application methods and procedures that can be integrated into the normal production protocols of the target fish species and are relevant to the typical ecology and epidemiology of the disease (i.e., seasonal occurrence, size of fish, host and geographic range of the disease).

Before attempting any vaccination strategy it is important to determine when the immune system is both morphologically and functionally mature. Strictly marine species like turbot, halibut, sea bream, sea bass or sole, in which after a short egg phase the immature and vulnerable larva is hatched into the marine environment, are much less immunologically developed at the time of hatching compared with salmonids, characterized by production of a few large yolky eggs, followed by a long egg incubation period. In addition, it is important to take into account that the time from hatching to the first feeding is extremely short in strictly marine fishes compared with salmonids.

Data on the earliest time to vaccinate marine species are scarce. Since in most marine species at the time of hatching the lymphoid system is still developing and will not become functionally mature until 70–100 days post-hatch, non-specific defense mechanisms constitute the most important part of the defense mechanisms of the larval fish. Therefore, in general, if the fish are vaccinated very early in age, the protection period will be limited and they will need a revaccination approximately a month later. In addition, if the disease occurs during the ongrowing period, a third vaccination must be given when fish reach 30–50 g. As mentioned before in this chapter, the best protection against photobacteriosis in sea bream and sea bass is obtained with an ECP-enriched bacterin, with a first dip immunization at larval stage (average 0.05 g) and a second vaccination of the fingerlings (1–2 g) in the hatchery, followed by an oral or an injection booster vaccination at the ongrowing site (Romalde *et al.*, 2005; Le Breton, 2009).

With regard to the use of immunostimulants for resistance against *P. damselae* subsp. *piscicida*, glucans can be used in the diet to prevent or reduce mortalities in gilthead sea bream due to pasteurellosis (Couso *et al.*, 2003). On the other hand, both positive and negative effects have been described for some dietary changes and/or supplements for the resistance of the fish to *P. damselae* subsp. *piscicida*. Thus, dietary arginine supplementation clearly increased the innate immune response of the Senegalese sole (Costas *et al.*, 2011), whereas the replacement of dietary fish oil by vegetable oils induced imbalances in fish immune response, leading to a lower potential response against infections (Montero *et al.*, 2010).

Photobacteriosis has been associated with high temperatures. Magariños *et al.* (2001) showed that gilthead sea bream larvae obtained from asymptomatic carrier broodstock are also carriers, and can develop pasteurellosis when the water temperature is higher than 18°C. Maintaining the temperature below such values, although slightly retarding the fish growth, helped to control the disease (Magariños *et al.*, 2001).

In summary, a combination of vaccination, control of water temperature, and use of glucans in the diet, contribute to a better prevention of the photobacteriosis caused by *P. damselae* subsp. *piscicida*.

17.6 EFFECT

In the last 20 years, different studies employing heat- or formalin-killed cells have assessed the effectiveness of immunization in preventing photobacteriosis (Romalde and Magariños, 1997). However, the formulations evaluated showed problems of reproducibility and difficulties in production on a large scale. Fukuda and Kusuda (1981) evaluated the passive immunization, but the results showed a short period of protection.

The best protection against photobacteriosis in sea bream and sea bass was obtained with an ECP-enriched bacterin, achieving relative percent survival (RPS) values higher than 75% in fish vaccinated between 0.5 and 2 g (Magariños *et al.*, 1994c). This vaccine is also effective at larval stages (50-day-old fish) with RPS values of 84–90% (Magariños *et al.*, 1999). This licenced vaccine (DI) is commercially available and successfully employed in several European countries.

Further studies in sole (Romalde *et al.*, 2005) showed that fish immunization with this bacterin is highly effective in the prevention of the disease. Similar results were obtained when this formulation was employed in divalent vaccines against photobacteriosis and vibriosis for this fish species as well as for sea bream (Moriñigo *et al.*, 2002; Arijo *et al.*, 2005), and in formulations against photobacteriosis and lactococcosis for yellowtail and amberjack (*Seriola dumerili*) (Wada *et al.*, 2008). However, an antagonistic effect among the different antigens of *P. damselae* subsp. *piscicida* and *Tenacibaculum maritimum* was detected when these microorganisms were employed in the composition of divalent formulations to prevent photobacteriosis and tenacibaculosis (Romalde *et al.*, 2005).

17.7 SIDE-EFFECTS

As mentioned in other chapters in this book, side-effects of vaccination are to a great extent related to the use of oil-adjuvanted vaccines or to handling stress. To our knowledge there is only one study on the specific side-effects in sea bass due to intraperitoneal vaccination against pasteurellosis (Afonso *et al.*, 2005). These authors found a steady increase in lymphocytes/small cells and a high concentration of neutrophils and macrophages in groups IP-injected with oil-adjuvanted formulations. However, with the exception of some macroscopic granulomas, all the lesions observed were moderate, which led the authors to hypothesize that in sea bass the pathological effects due to IP vaccination are less severe than in other fish species.

17.8 REGULATIONS

There are no particular regulatory concerns related to vaccines against photobacteriosis in fish, since the commonly used vaccines are of basic technology, namely inactivated bacterins.

REFERENCES

Afonso, A., Gomes, S., da Silva, J., *et al.*, 2005. Side effects in sea bass (*Dicentrarchus labrax* L.) due to intraperitoneal vaccination against vibriosis and pasteurellosis. *Fish Shellfish Immunol* **19**: 1–16.

Arijo, S., Rico, R., Chabrillon, M., *et al.*, 2005. Effectiveness of a divalent vaccine for sole, *Solea senegalensis* (Kaup), against *Vibrio harveyi* and *Photobacterium damselae* subsp. *piscicida*. *J Fish Dis* **28**: 33–8.

Bakopoulos, V., Volpatti, D., Gusmani, L., *et al.*, 2003. Vaccination trials of sea bass, *Dicentrarchus labrax* (L.), against *Photobacterium damsela* subsp. *piscicida*, using novel vaccine mixtures. *J Fish Dis* **26**: 77–90.

Balebona, M.C., Moriñigo, M.A., Sedano, J., *et al.*, 1992. Isolation of *Pasteurella piscicida* from sea bass in southwestern Spain. *Bull Eur Assoc Fish Pathol* **12**: 1–3.

Baptista, T., Romalde, J.L. and Toranzo, A.E. 1996. First epizootic of pasteurellosis in Portugal affecting cultured gilthead sea bream (*Sparus aurata*). *Bull Eur Assoc Fish Pathol* **16**: 92–5.

Barnes, A.C., dos Santos, N.M.S. and Ellis, A.E. 2005. Update on bacterial vaccines: *Photobacterium damselae* subsp. *piscicida*. *Dev Biol (Basel)* **121**: 75–84.

Bonet, R., Magariños, B., Romalde, J.L., *et al.*, 1994. Capsular polysacaccharide expressed by *Pasteurella piscicida* grown *in vitro*. *FEMS Microbiol Lett* **124**: 285–90.

Ceschia, G., Giorgetti, G. and Bovo, G. 1990. Grave epizoozia da *Pasteurella piscicida* in specie eurihaline del Nord Adriatico. *Boll Soc Ital Patol Ittica* **4**: 11–17.

Costa-Ramos, C., do Vale, A., Ludovico, P., *et al.*, 2011. The bacterial exotoxin AIP56 induces fish macrophage and neutrophil apoptosis using mechanisms of the extrinsic and intrinsic pathways. *Fish Shellfish Immunol* **30**: 173–81.

Costas, B., Conceição, L.E.C., Dias, J., *et al.*, 2011. Dietary arginine and repeated handling increase disease resistance and modulate innate immune mechanisms of Senegalese sole (*Solea senegalensis* Kaup, 1858). *Fish Shellfish Immunol* **31**: 838–47.

Couso, N., Castro, R., Magariños, B., *et al.*, 2003. Effect of oral administration of glucans on the resistance of gilthead sea bream to pasteurellosis. *Aquaculture* **219**: 99–109.

do Vale, A., Magariños, B., Romalde, J.L., *et al.*, 2002. Binding of haemin by the fish pathogen *Photobacterium damselae* subsp. *piscicida*. *Dis Aquat Org* **48**: 109–15.

do Vale, A., Silva, M.T., dos Santos, N.M., *et al.*, 2005. AIP56, a novel plasmid-encoded virulence factor of *Photobacterium damselae* subsp. *piscicida* with apoptogenic activity against sea bass macrophages and neutrophils. *Mol Microbiol* **58**: 1025–38.

Frerichs, G.N. and Roberts, R.J. 1989. The bacteriology of teleosts, in *Fish Pathology* (ed. R.J. Roberts). London, Bailliere Tindall, 289–319.

Fryer, J.L. and Rohovec, J.S. 1984. Principal bacterial diseases of cultured marine fish. *Helgoländer Meeresunters* **37**: 533–45.

Fukuda, Y. and Kusuda, R. 1981. Efficacy of vaccination for pseudotuberculosis in cultured yellowtail by various routes of administration. *Bull Jap Soc Sci Fish* **47**: 147–50.

Gauthier G, Lafay B, Ruimi R, *et al.*, 1995. Small subunit rRNA sequences and whole DNA relatedness concur for the reassignment of *Pasteurella piscicida* (Sniezsko *et al*.,.) Janssen and Surgalla to the genus *Photobacterium* as *Photobacterium damselae* subsp. *piscicida* comb. nov. *Int J Syst Bacteriol* **45**: 139–44.

Gravningen, K., Sakai, M., Mishiba, T. and Fujimoto, T. 2008. The efficacy and safety of an oil-based vaccine against *Photobacterium damsela* subsp. *piscicida* in yellowtail (*Seriola quinqueradiata*): a field study. *Fish Shellfish Immunol* **24**: 523–9.

Hawke, J.P., Thune, R.L., Cooper, R.K., *et al.*, 2003. Molecular and phenotypic characterization of strains of *Photobacterium damselae* subsp. *piscicida* from hybrid striped bass cultured in Louisiana, USA. *J Aquat Anim Health* **15**: 189–201.

Ho, L.-P., Lin, J.H.-Y., Liu, H.-C., *et al.*, 2011. Identification of antigens for the development of a subunit vaccine against *Photobacterium damselae* ssp. *piscicida*. *Fish Shellfish Immunol* **30**: 412–19.

Janssen, W.A. and Surgalla, M.J. 1968. Morphology, physiology, and serology of *Pasteurella* species pathogenic for white perch. *J Bacteriol* **96**: 1606–10.

Juíz-Río, S., Osorio, C.R., de Lorenzo, V. and Lemos, M.L. 2005. Subtractive hybridization reveals a high genetic diversity in the fish pathogen *Photobacterium damselae* subsp. *piscicida*: evidence of a SXT-like element. *Microbiology* **151**: 2659–69.

Kim, E.-H., Yoshida, T. and Aoki, T. 1993. Detection of R plasmids encoded with resistance to florfenicol in *Pasteurella piscicida*. *Fish Pathol* **28**: 165–70.

Koike, Y., Kuwahara, A. and Fujiwara, H. 1975. Characterization of *Pasteurella piscicida* isolated from white perch and cultivated yellowtail. *Jap J Microbiol* **19**: 241–7.

Kubota, S.S., Kimura, M. and Egusa, S. 1970. Studies of a bacterial tuberculoidosis of the yellowtail. I. Symptomatology and histopathology. *Fish Pathol* **4**: 11–18.

Kusuda, R. and Fukuda, Y. 1980. Agglutinating antibody titers and serum protein changes of yellowtail after immunization with *Pasteurella piscicida* cells. *Bull Jap Soc Sci Fish* **46**: 103–8.

Kusuda, R. and Hamaguchi, M. 1988. The efficacy of attenuated live bacterin of *Pasteurella piscicida* against pseudotuberculosis in yellowtail. *Bull Eur Assoc Fish Pathol* **8**: 51–3.

Kusuda, R. and Salati, F. 1993. Major bacterial diseases affecting mariculture in Japan. *Annu Rev Fish Dis* **3**: 69–85.

Kusuda, R. and Miura, W. 1972. Characteristics of a *Pasteurella* sp. pathogenic for pond cultured ayu. *Fish Pathol* **7**: 51–7.

Le Breton, A.D. 2009. Vaccines in Mediterranean aquaculture: practice and needs. *Op Mediterr* **86**: 147–54.

Lewis, D.H., Grumbles, L.C., McConnell, S. and Flowers, A.I. 1970. *Pasteurella*-like bacteria from an epizootic in menhaden and mullet in Galveston Bay. *J Wild Dis* **6**: 160–62.

Liu, P.C., Liu, J.Y. and Lee, K.K. 2003. Virulence of *Photobacterium damselae* subsp. *piscicida* in cultured cobia *Rachycentron canadum*. *J Basic Microbiol* **43**: 499–507.

Liu, P.C., Chuang, W.H. and Lee, K.K. 2011. Purification of a toxic metalloprotease produced by the pathogenic *Photobacterium damselae* subsp. *piscicida* isolated from cobia (*Rachycentron canadum*). *Z Naturforsch* **66**: 287–95.

Magariños, B., Romalde, J.L., Bandín, I., *et al.*, 1992a. Phenotypic, antigenic and molecular characterization of *Pasteurella piscicida* strains isolated from fish. *Appl Environ Microbiol* **58**: 3316–22.

Magariños, B., Santos, Y., Romalde, J.L., *et al.*, 1992b. Pathogenic activities of live cells and extracellular products of the fish pathogen *Pasteurella piscicida*. *J Gen Microbiol* **138**: 2491–8.

Magariños, B., Romalde, J.L., Lemos, M.L., *et al.*, 1994a. Iron uptake by *Pasteurella piscicida* and its role in pathogenicity for fish. *Appl Environ Microbiol* **60**: 2990–98.

Magariños, B., Romalde, J.L., Barja, J.L. and Toranzo, A.E. 1994b. Evidence of a dormant but infective state of the fish pathogen *Pasteurella piscicida* in seawater and sediment. *Appl Environ Microbiol* **60**: 180–86.

Magariños, B., Romalde, J.L., Santos, Y., *et al.*, 1994c. Vaccination trials on gilhead sea bream (*Sparus aurata*) against *Pasteurella piscicida*. *Aquaculture* **120**: 201–8.

Magariños, B., Toranzo, A.E. and Romalde, J.L. 1995. Different susceptibility of gilthead sea bream and turbot to *Pasteurella piscicida* infection by the water route. *Bull Eur Assoc Fish Pathol* **15**: 88–90.

Magariños, B., Romalde, J.L., Noya, M., *et al.*, 1996a. Adherence and invasive capacities of the fish pathogen *Pasteurella piscicida*. *FEMS Microbiol Lett* **138**: 29–34.

Magariños, B., Bonet, R., Romalde, J.L., *et al.*, 1996b. Influence of the capsular layer on the virulence of *Pasteurella piscicida* for fish. *Microb Pathogen* **21**: 289–97.

Magariños, B., Osorio, C.R., Toranzo, A.E. and Romalde, J.L. 1997. Applicability of ribotyping for intraspecific classification and epidemiological studies of *Photobacterium damselae* subsp. *piscicida*. *Syst Appl Microbiol* **20**: 634–9.

Magariños, B., Romalde, J.L., Barja, J.L., *et al.*, 1999. Protection of gilthead sea bream against pasteurellosis at the larval stages. *Bull Eur Assoc Fish Pathol* **19**: 159–61.

Magariños, B., Toranzo, A.E., Barja, J.L. and Romalde, J.L. 2000. Existence of two geographically-linked clonal lineages in the bacterial fish pathogen *Photobacterium damselae* subsp. *piscicida* evidenced by random amplified polymorphic DNA analysis. *Epidemiol Infect* **125**: 213–19.

Magariños, B., Couso, N., Noya, M., *et al.*, 2001. Effect of temperature on the development of pasteurellosis in carrier gilthead sea bream (*Sparus aurata*). *Aquaculture* **195**: 17–21.

Mancuso, M., Avendaño-Herrera, R., Zaccone, R., *et al.*, 2007. Evaluation of different DNA-based fingerprinting methods for typing *Photobacterium damselae* subsp. *piscicida*. *Biol Res* **40**: 85–92.

Montero, D., Mathlouthi, F., Tort, L., *et al.*, 2010. Replacement of dietary fish oil by vegetable oils affects immunity and expression of pro-inflammatory cytokines genes in gilthead sea bream *Sparus aurata*. *Fish Shellfish Immunol* **29**: 1073–81.

Moriñigo, M.A., Romalde, J.L., Chabrillon, M., *et al.*, 2002. Effectiveness of a divalent vaccine for gilthead sea bream (*Sparus aurata*) against *Vibrio alginolyticus* and *Photobacterium damselae* subsp. *piscicida*. *Bull Eur Assoc Fish Pathol* **22**: 298–303.

Muroga, K., Sugiyama, T. and Ueki, N. 1977. Pasteurellosis in cultured black sea bream, *Mylio macrocephalus*. *J Fac Fish Anim Husb Hiroshima Univ* **16**: 17–21.

Navot, N., Kimmel, E. and Avtalian, R.R. 2005. Immunisation of fish by bath immersion using ultrasound. *Dev Biol (Basel)* **121**: 135–42.

Nelson, J.S., Kawahara, E., Kawai, K. and Kusuda, R. 1989. Macrophage infiltration in pseudotuberculosis of yellowtail, *Seriola quinqueradiata*. *Bull Mar Sci Fish Kochi Univ* **11**: 17–22.

Nomura, J. and Aoki, T. 1985. Morphological analysis of lipopolysaccharide from Gram negative fish pathogenic bacteria. *Fish Pathol* **20**: 193–7.

Noya, M., Magariños, B., Toranzo, A.E. and Lamas, J. 1995a. Sequential pathology of experimental pasteurellosis in gilthead sea bream, *Sparus aurata*. A light- and electron-microscopic study. *Dis Aquat Org* **21**: 177–86.

Noya, M., Magariños, B. and Lamas, J. 1995b. Interactions between peritoneal exudate cells (PECs) of gilthead sea bream (*Sparus aurata*) and *Pasteurella piscicida*. *A morphological study*. *Aquaculture* **131**: 11–21.

Ohnishi, K., Watanabe, K. and Jo, Y. 1982. *Pasteurella* infection in young black sea bream. *Fish Pathol* **16**: 207–10.

Osorio, C.R., Marrero, J., Wozniak, R.A.F., *et al.*, 2008. Genomic and functional analysis of ICE*Pda*Spa1, a fish-pathogen-derived SXT-related integrating conjugative element that can mobilize a virulence plasmid. *J Bacteriol* **190**: 3353–61.

Romalde, J.L. 2002. *Photobacterium damselae* subsp. *pisicida*: an integrated view of a bacterial fish pathogen. *Int Microbiol* **5**: 3–9.

Romalde, J.L. and Magariños, B. 1997. Immunization with bacterial antigens: pasteurellosis. *Dev Biol (Basel)* **90**: 167–77.

Romalde, J.L., Magariños, B., Fouz, B., *et al.*, 1995a. Evaluation of BIONOR mono-kits for rapid detection of bacterial fish pathogens. *Dis Aquat Org* **21**: 25–34.

Romalde, J.L., le Breton, A., Magariños, B. and Toranzo, A.E. 1995b. Use of BIONOR Aquarapid-Pp kit for the diagnosis of *Pasteurella piscicida* infections. *Bull Eur Ass Fish Pathol* **15**: 64–6.

Romalde, J.L., Magariños, B., Lores, F., *et al.*, 1999. Assessment of a magnetic bead-EIA based kit for the rapid diagnosis of fish pasteurellosis. *J Microbiol Methods* **38**: 147–54.

Romalde, J.L., Ravelo, C., López-Romalde, S., *et al.*, 2005. Vaccination strategies to prevent emerging diseases for Spanish aquaculture. *Dev Biol (Basel)* **121**: 85–95.

Salati, F., Giorgetti, G. and Kusuda, R. 1994. Comparison among strains of *Pasteurella piscicida* from Japan, Italy and USA. *Riv Itali Acquac* **29**: 133–9.

Serracca, L., Ercolini, C., Rossini, I., *et al.*, 2011. Occurrence of both subspecies of *Photobacterium damselae* in mullets collected in the river Magra (Italy). *Can J Microbiol* **57**: 437–40.

Skarmeta, A.M., Bandín, I., Santos, Y. and Toranzo, A.E. 1995. *In vitro* killing of *Pasteurella piscicida* by fish macrophages. *Dis Aquat Org* **23**: 51–7.

Sniezsko, S.F., Bullock, G.L., Hollis, E. and Boone, J.G. 1964. *Pasteurella* sp. from an epizootic of white perch (*Roccus americanus*) in Chesapeake Bay tidewaters areas. *J Bacteriol* **88**: 1814–15.

Thune, R.L., Fernández, D.H., Hawke, J.P. and Miller, R. 2003. Construction of a safe, stable, efficacious vaccine against *Photobacterium damselae* ssp. *piscicida*. *Dis Aquat Org* **57**: 51–8.

Thyssen, A., Goris, J., Pedersen, K., *et al.*, 1999. Phenotypic and genotypic characterization of *Photobacterium damselae* subsp. *piscicida*, in *Proceedings of the 9th International Conference of the EAFP: Diseases of Fish and Shellfish*, Rhodes, Greece.

Toranzo, A.E., Barja, J.L. and Hetrick, F.M. 1982. Survival of *Vibrio anguillarum* and *Pasteurella piscicida* in estuarine and fresh waters. *Bull Eur Ass Fish Pathol* **3**: 43–5.

Toranzo, A.E., Barreiro, S., Casal, J.F., *et al.*, 1991. Pasteurellosis in cultured gilthead sea bream (*Sparus aurata*): first report in Spain. *Aquaculture* **99**: 1–15.
Ueki, N., Kayano, Y. and Muroga, K. 1990. *Pasteurella piscicida* in juvenile red grouper. *Fish Pathol* **25**: 43–4.
Wada, Y., Oyamatsu, T., Ng, J., *et al.*, 2008. Bivalent vaccine protects yellowtails, amberjack against pasteurellosis. *Glob Aquac Advocate* **11** (May–June): 51–2.
Yasunaga, N., Katai, K. and Tsukahara, J. 1983. *Pasteurella piscicida* from an epizootic of cultured red sea bream. *Fish Pathol* **18**: 107–10.
Zorrilla, I., Balebona, M.C., Moriñigo, M.A., *et al.*, 1999. Isolation and characterization of the causative agent of pasteurellosis, *Photobacterium damselae* ssp. *piscicida*, from sole, *Solea senegalensis* (Kaup). *J Fish Dis* **22**: 167–72.

18 Vaccination against Enteric Septicemia of Catfish

Phillip H. Klesius and Julia W. Pridgeon

USDA-ARS, Aquatic Animal Health Research Laboratory, Alabama, USA

ABSTRACT

Edwardsiella ictaluri is an important aquaculture pathogen that causes enteric septicemia of catfish (ESC) as well as non-ictalurid fish species. An attenuated live vaccine against ESC has been commercially licensed for mass immunization through bath immersion. The commercially available attenuated live vaccine against ESC was produced through a rifampicin-resistance strategy. In addition, another attenuated live vaccine against ESC was developed through a novobiocin-resistance strategy. Inactivated ESC vaccine is not commercially available in the US. The occurrence, significance, etiology, pathogenesis, vaccine, vaccination procedures, vaccine effects and efficacies are reviewed in this chapter.

18.1 SIGNIFICANCE

Edwardsiella ictaluri, the causative agent of enteric septicemia of catfish (ESC), is one of the most economically important diseases of cultured channel catfish (Hawke, 1979; Hawke *et al.*, 1981). In 2002, Wagner and coworkers reported that ESC and columnaris were the two most predominant catfish diseases in the US. Cultured yellow catfish (*Pelteobagrus fulvidraco*) were reported to be infected with *E. ictaluri* in China (Ye *et al.*, 2009; Liu *et al.*, 2010). Up to 50% annual cumulative mortalities were observed in cultured yellow catfish. Natural outbreaks of *E. ictaluri* infection were observed in cultured Tra catfish (*Pangasius hypophthalmus*) in Vietnam (Ferguson *et al.*, 2001; Crumlish *et al.*, 2002; Dung *et al.*, 2008). *Edwardsiella ictaluri* was also identified as the etiological agent of cultured Tra catfish in Indonesia (Yuasa *et al.*, 2003). ESC outbreaks are becoming increasingly important in the cultured catfish industry in Southeast Asia. In the US, ESC causes economic losses estimated at US$50–80 million annually (Russo *et al.*, 2009). ESC outbreaks cause severe economic losses through decreased production, treatment costs and mortality.

phillip.klesius@ars.usda.gov

Fish Vaccination, First Edition. Edited by Roar Gudding, Atle Lillehaug and Øystein Evensen.

18.2 OCCURRENCE

Edwardsiella ictaluri has a limited host range compared with *E. tarda*. Originally *E. ictaluri* was believed to be specific to ictalurids (Plumb, 2000). However, non-ictalurids have also been found to be susceptible to ESC. The host range of *E. ictaluri* is greater than originally documented (Waltman *et al.*, 1985). Besides channel catfish, Tra catfish and yellow catfish mentioned above, ESC has also been reported in brown bullhead (*Ameriurus nebulosus*), white catfish (*I. catus*), and rosy barb (*Puntius conchonius*) (Hawke *et al.*, 1979, 1981; Humphrey *et al.*, 1986). Green knife fish *Eigemannia virens* and *Danio devario* were found to be diseased by *E. ictaluri* (Kent and Lyons, 1982; Waltman *et al.*, 1985). Walking catfish *Clarias batrachua*, tadpole madtom *Noturus gyrinus*, rainbow trout *Oncorhynchus mykiss* and harlequin tetra *Rosbara hetermorpha* were found to have ESC or ESC-like signs (Kasornchandra *et al.*, 1987; Reid and Boyle, 1989; Klesius *et al.*, 2003; Keskin *et al.*, 2004). A mortality rate of 60% was observed in channel catfish infected by the *E. ictaluri* isolated from tadpole madtom through intraperitoneal (IP) injection (Klesius *et al.*, 2003). Zebrafish (*Danio rerio*) has been used as a model for ESC (Petrie-Hanson *et al.*, 2007). It was found that zebrafish exposed to *E. ictaluri* had lower mortality (13.3%) than that observed in channel catfish (100%). In addition, the following fish species have been experimentally infected with *E. ictaluri*: Chinook salmon (*Oncorhynclus tshawytsha*), tilapia (*Oreochromis aureus*), and European catfish (*Silurus gianis*) (Plumb and Sanchez, 1983; Plumb and Huge, 1987; Baxa *et al.*, 1990). However, no natural infections have been reported in these fish species. Previously, *E. ictaluri* was considered to be serologically and biochemically homogenous (Plumb and Klesius, 1988; Plumb and Vinitnantharat, 1993; Waltman *et al.*, 1986; Bertolini *et al.*, 1990).

18.3 ETIOLOGY

Enteric septicemia of catfish typically occurs in the acute form, with signs of abnormal swimming behavior, pale gills, exophthalmia, enlarged abdomens, and rapid mortality. In its chronic form, ESC typically has a slower progression and causes a "hole-in-the-head" lesion that may remain localized or progress to septicemia and death. Fish surviving acute ESC may develop chronic ESC. During the course of infection, *E. ictaluri* can be recovered from brain, head kidney and cranial lesions. ESC may occur in all life stages including fingerling, juvenile and food-size catfish stages. In the US, ESC usually occurs in cultured catfish during spring and fall seasons, when the mortality rates peak (Plumb and Sanchez, 1983). Klesius (1992a) speculated that the rapid change in water temperature from temperatures of 11–17°C (Bly and Clem, 1991) to 20–30°C could be associated with increased horizontal transmission of *E. ictaluri* and thus more ESC outbreaks. The optimal temperature for *E. ictaluri* growth is about 25–30°C.

The etiology of ESC remains poorly understood. Klesius (1992b) showed that healthy channel catfish exposed to *E. ictaluri* and subsequently treated with Romet-30 could be carriers of *E. ictaluri* and may be a reservoir of infection for fish that are susceptible to ESC. Thus, asymptomatic carriers of *E. ictaluri* are likely to transmit to other cultured catfish, especially when the fish of different life stages are present in continuous batch production. In another study, Klesius (1994) observed that cannibalizing of *E. ictaluri*-infected fish, or the shedding of *E. ictaluri* from dead fish, or both, were mechanisms whereby horizontal transmission of ESC among channel catfish occurs. Other means of *E. ictaluri* transmission are believed to occur via water and from mud of ponds containing channel catfish infected with the pathogen (Plumb and Quinlan, 1986). Transmission may also occur via nets and equipment contaminated with *E. ictaluri* and infected fish carcasses that remain in ponds. Newton *et al.* (1989) demonstrated that experimental immersion challenge of catfish with *E. ictaluri* may be a source of infection to other fish.

Environmental, host and microbial factors are believed to influence frequencies of ESC outbreaks in catfish production. The poor pond management practices that include poor water quality, unconsumed feed, excretions, dead fish carcasses, a high density of fish and poor nutrition or feeding practices are likely responsible for ESC outbreaks. Other practices such as crowding of fish-farming sites, lack of sanitation barriers and the overuse of antimicrobial drugs are likely risks to introduction of pathogens. The increased risk of transfer of drug-resistant microbes to terrestrial animals and man is a major health issue. Intensive production practices have led to higher risk of ESC outbreaks in the catfish industry worldwide. In China, intensive practices may be responsible for increased mortality rates and losses of income in the yellow catfish production (Deng *et al.*, 2008). ESC occurs at about the same time as *Flavobacterium columnare* disease. *E. ictaluri* and parasite *Ichthyophthirus multifillis* are also major pathogens of catfish. In a recent study, Xu *et al.* (2012) demonstrated that Ich parasitized catfish showed significantly higher mortality when exposed to *E. ictaluri* than non-parasitized catfish. Ich infection enhanced the susceptibility of channel catfish to bacterial invasion and increased fish mortality. This is an example of co-infection by two pathogens that may augment the virulence of catfish pathogens.

18.4 PATHOGENESIS

E. ictulari may invade and cause ESC by several routes. Two possible routes of *E. ictaluri* infections were determined to be the gut and nares of catfish (Shotts *et al.*, 1986). *E. ictaluri* may invade the nares and migrate into the olfactory nerve, then into the brain meninges and to the skull and skin (Morrison and Plumb, 1994). Infection may progress up the olfactory nerves and cause neurological signs. The mechanism may be the attachment of bacterial lectins to specific sugar moieties, such as d-mannose, N-acetylneuraminic acid of the nasal mucosa (Wolfe *et al.*, 1994). Another possible route was demonstrated by immersion exposure of channel catfish to ^{35}S-labeled *E. ictaluri* for 1 h (Nusbaum and Morrison, 1996). They found that *E. ictaluri* accumulate on and enter via the gills. They hypothesized that *E. ictaluri* could enter the blood circulation through gill macrophages. From there, it would promptly be transported to the anterior kidney via the circulation, where it would be internalized within the resident macrophage population. Another study demonstrated that primary entry of *E. ictaluri* was via abraded skin and was followed by systematic infection of channel catfish (Menanteau-Ledouble *et al.*, 2011). They also found that higher numbers of *E. ictaluri* were detected following bath immersion. *E. ictaluri* seems to be able to invade the skin of catfish through the muscle layers. They concluded that skin abrasion cause catfish to be more susceptible to ESC. Santander *et al.* (2011) found that *E. ictaluri* cyclic adenosine 3′5′-monophosphate receptor protein (Crp) mutants were able to colonize gills, spleen and kidney following immersion challenge of channel catfish.

Using Illumina RNA-sequence technology, Li and coworkers (2012) determined the transcriptomic responses in the intestine of catfish following challenge with *E. ictaluri*. They were able to identify a number of catfish genes and quantify the transcript levels of 1633 differentially expressed genes at 3 hours, 24 hours and 3 days following exposure. The study revealed the importance of actin-cytoskeletal polymerization and junctional regulation in *E. ictaluri* entry and subsequent inflammatory responses in catfish.

18.5 VIRULENCE FACTORS

A variety of virulence factors have been identified in *Edwardsiella ictaluri*. Lipopolysaccharide (LPS) plays a role in virulence (Weete *et al.*, 1988; Newton and Triche, 1993a; Klesius and Shoemaker, 1999; Lawrence *et al.*, 2001, 2003; Arias *et al.*, 2003; Thune *et al.*, 2007). Saeed and Plumb (1986) demonstrated that LPS from *E. ictaluri* was able to stimulate strong antibody titers in catfish but with no protection following *E. ictaluri* challenge. Flagella were identified as a virulence factor of *E. ictaluri* (Newton and Triche, 1993b; Panangala *et al.*, 2009a). The *E. ictaluri* genome was shown to encode at least four distinct flagellin proteins, which are very similar to *Serratia marcescens* flagellin proteins. Another type of virulence factor was identified as outer membrane proteins (Newton *et al.*, 1990; Klesius and Horst, 1991; Vinitnantharat *et al.*, 1993; Bader *et al.*, 2004). Two outer membrane components were identified as 35 and 58.5 kDa proteins in the extracellular products or exoantigens of *E. ictaluri* (Klesius and Horst, 1991; Klesius, 1993). The extracellular proteins were identified as major immunodominant antigens capable of producing a strong serum antibody response. Klesius and Sealey (1996) were able to show that the extracellular products of *E. ictaluri* are able to stimulate chemotactic and chemokinetic responses of channel catfish macrophages.

Hemolysins and chondroitinase were described as possible virulence factors of *E. ictaluri*. However, the wild-type *E. ictaluri* was found not to be different to hemolysin-deficient *E. ictaluri* mutant in their hemolytic activity (Williams and Lawrence, 2005). In a preliminary study, Copper *et al.* (1996) suggested a role for chondroitin sulfatase in the virulence of *E. ictaluri*. They produced an *E. ictaluri* chondroitinase-deficient mutant that did not cause ESC in catfish. Previously, Waltman *et al.* (1986) showed that *E. ictaluri* was capable of degrading chondroitin sulfate, which may be responsible for the formation of the hole-in-the-head lesion characteristic of ESC.

18.6 VACCINES AND IMMUNITY

The majority of vaccines available for fish are killed bacterial prophylactics or bacterins. In the US there are only 10 licensed fish vaccines including 5 killed bacterins, 1 killed viral, 1 live attenuated viral, and 3 live attenuated bacterial prophylactics. Table 18.1 lists the current US-licensed fish vaccines. The majority of vaccines are for use in salmonids. Two vaccines are available for use in catfish. No fish vaccines are currently licensed for tilapia, barramundi, yellow perch, marine species and other US raised fish. Fish producers have fewer vaccines available for immunization than producers in poultry and the livestock industries. There is a recognized need to develop fish vaccines as well as to improve the efficacy of available vaccines against bacterial and viral diseases.

Table 18.1 USDA-licensed fish vaccines, as of February 2013.

Name of the product	Product code	Date license issued
Novartis Animal Health, Inc.		
Aeromonas Salmonicida Bacterin	Code 2035.02	01JUN05
Arthrobacter Vaccine, Live Culture	Code 1K11.00	01JUN05
Aeromonas Salmonicida-Vibrio Anguillarum-Ordalii- Salmonicida Bacterin	Code 2138.02	01JUN05
Flavobacterium Columnare Bacterin	Code 2974.00	01JUN05
Infectious Salmon Anemia Virus Vaccine, Killed Virus	Code 4A45.20	01JUN05
Yersinia Ruckeri Bacterin	Code 2638.00	01JUN05
Vibrio Anguillarum-Ordalii Bacterin	Code 2858.03	01JUN05
Cyprinid Herpesvirus Type 3 Vaccine, Modified Live Virus	Code 1443.20	01JUN05
Merck Animal Health, Inc.		
Edwardsiella Ictaluri Vaccine, Avirulent Live Culture	Code 1531.00	26OCT09
Flavobacterium Columnare Vaccine, Avirulent Live Culture	Code 17F1.00	26OCT09

Table 18.2 Positive and negative characteristics of *Edwardsiella ictaluri* bacterins.

Positive characteristics	Negative characteristics
Safe	Injection administration
Full antigenic complement	Short duration of protective immunity
Altered proteins by formalin inactivation	
Cross-protection against field strains	Boosters may be required
Low production costs	Antibody-mediated immunity
Fermentation	
Long shelf life	No or little protection against intracellular pathogens
Lyophilized	

The positive and negative characteristics of *Edwardsiella ictaluri* bacterins are given in Table 18.2. A number of *E. ictaluri* bacterins have been developed and evaluated in catfish (Plumb, 1988; Vinitnantharat and Plumb, 1992, 1993; Plumb *et al.*, 1994; Nusbaum and Morrison,1996; Thune *et al.*, 1992, 1997a,b). *E. ictaluri* bacterins were shown to be safe. However, currently there is no licensed killed *E. ictaluri* vaccine for use in the US catfish industry. This may be due to the fact that killed *E. ictaluri* vaccines were found not to be efficacious against ESC, with often equivocal results in the field. The *E. ictaluri* bacterins were found to stimulate specific antibody titers without protection against ESC (Klesius and Sealy, 1995; Thune *et al.*, 1997a).

The positive and negative characteristics of live attenuated *E. ictaluri* vaccines are summarized in Table 18.3. The development and use of live attenuated bacterial vaccines are becoming more attractive due to their many advantages, despite concerns raised regarding their safety.

Table 18.3 Positive and negative characteristics of live attenuated *Edwardsiella ictaluri* vaccine.

Positive characteristics	Negative characteristics
Loss of virulence	Safety and regulations may be an issue in EU countries
Altered LPS	
Full antigenic complement	
Cellular immunity	
In vivo capacity for the mutant to replicate in the fish	
Replication in host for 7–10 days	
Bacteriological detectable marker	
Long duration of protective immunity	
Fry immunization in hatchery at 7–10 days post-hatch	
Cross-immunity against field strains	
Easy and mass delivery	
Low production costs	
Fermentation	

The principal reason behind the concern that live attenuated vaccines are considered more risky than killed vaccine is their possible reversion from the weakened state to a virulent state. However, this risk appears to be unfounded as no reversion has been documented for the AQUAVAC-ESC® attenuated vaccine which has been used in the US catfish industry for more than 10 years. A risk/benefit analysis on the use of live attenuated *E. ictaluri* vaccine may reveal the potential preventive benefits that outweigh the decision to preclude these vaccines from the market. Favre and Viret (2006) have provided a framework on European regulations for biosafety assessment of human oral attenuated vaccines that provides valuable insight into the assessment of attenuated vaccines in veterinary practice. Incorporation of specific genetic markers such as synthetic antibiotic resistance into the attenuated vaccine strain will allow the wild-type parent strain to be distinguished from the attenuated vaccine strain by appropriate bacteriological methods. This is important for monitoring the biosafety of the attenuated vaccine in the field.

Earlier results provided guidance for the design of a live attenuated *E. ictaluri* vaccine (Klesius *et al.*, 2001). Radiation and foreign host mutagenesis were first attempted to produce an *E. ictaluri* mutant. Attempts to produce *E. ictaluri* mutants using gamma radiation and inoculation of chicken eggs with *E. ictaluri* were not successful (Klesius, personal communication). Norqvist *et al.* (1989) produced a live attenuated *Vibrio anguillarum* mutant (Van1000) using antibiotic mutagenesis with rifampin (200 μg/ml) and streptomycin (100 μg/ml). The rifampin (rifampicin)-streptomycin mutant was able to stimulate protective immunity against the homologous as well as a heterologous strain of *V. anquillarum*. The live attenuated vaccine induced protection by a single bath vaccination for at least 17 weeks. The live attenuated *V. anquillarum* vaccine was also used to induce protection against *Aeromonas salmonicida* challenge at 12 weeks. They concluded that the Van1000 strain was a safe, live attenuated vaccine.

Schurig *et al.* (1991) produced a live attenuated *Brucella abortus* vaccine that was found to be efficacious against bovine brucellosis. They produced this live attenuated vaccine using multiple passages of increasing concentration of rifampicin. Rifampicin was found to inhibit bacterial DNA-dependent RNA polymerase (Wehrli *et al.*, 1968).

Klesius and Shoemaker (1999) demonstrated that slight differences exist between *E. ictaluri* strains in their ability to induce protection immunity to ESC. Catfish immunized with live exposure to the strain EILO were significantly protected against ESC following challenge with the majority of *E. ictaluri* strains from channel catfish. The findings were important to the development of an efficacious ESC vaccine. The 18 *E. ictaluri* were shown to possess a high degree of homogeneity (70% similar or higher) in their protein profiles and 95% similarity in their FAME profiles (Panangala *et al.*, 2006, 2009b). In addition, *E. ictaluri* was able to protect catfish against secondary *E. ictaluri* challenge (Shoemaker and Klesius, 1997), which suggested that protective immunity against ESC was cell mediated.

Klesius and Shoemaker (1999) produced a live attenuated *E. ictaluri* mutant using rifampicin with a non-channel catfish *E. ictaluri* EILO strain from an *E. ictaluri* diseased walking catfish. This live attenuated vaccine was shown to be able to immunize large numbers of fish by bath immersion with minimum stress (Shoemaker *et al.*, 1999, 2009; Klesius *et al.*, 2001; Klesius and Shoemaker, 2000). The live attenuated vaccine was found to be efficacious in catfish and was licensed by USDA to Intervet/Schering-Plough Animal Health as AQUAVAC-ESC® (Klesius and Shoemaker, 2000). The AQUAVAC-ESC® is labeled for use on 7–10 day post-hatched or older catfish by bath immersion (Klesius and Shoemaker, 1999; Wise *et al.*, 2000, Wise, 2006). The relative percent survival (RPS) was 57–94% between 10 to 48 days post-hatch. The loss of virulence was associated with an alternation in the LPS component (Klesius and Shoemaker, 1999; Arias *et al.*, 2003).

This vaccine was efficacious in eyed egg of channel catfish by bath immersion (Klesius *et al.*, 2000, 2004; Shoemaker *et al.*, 2002, 2007). The RPS was 57% when the immunized fingerlings were challenged 60 days post-immunization. However, when the immunized fry were booster-immunized by immersion at 7 days post-hatch, the RPS declined to 27.3%. These results indicated that an additional antigen load from the booster immunization compromised the immune protection conferred by the attenuated vaccine. Attenuated vaccines have been reported to lead to immunosuppression (Salmbandamurthy and Jacobs, 2005). It was believed that the persistence of the attenuated vaccine strain in the egg and fry resulted in the successful immunization of eyed eggs and their fry. The results also showed that eyed catfish eggs were safely immunized with no adverse mortality.

Eyed catfish eggs were immunized by immersion with either monovalent *F. columnare* attenuated vaccine or bivalent attenuated *F. columnare* and *E. ictaluri* vaccines (Shoemaker *et al.*, 2007). The RPS of monovalent attenuated vaccine was 76.8% at 137 days post-immunization following *F. columnare* challenge. The RPS of bivalent attenuated vaccine challenged with *F. columnare* was 56.7% at 109 days post-immunization, and when challenged with *E. ictaluri*, the RPS was 66.7% at 116 days post-immunization. Attenuated vaccines may be very effective at protection of fish following immunization at the nursery or fingerling stages.

Live attenuated *E. ictaluri* vaccines activate immune responses that closely mimic a natural infection because the majority of the antigens are expressed *in vivo*. The vaccine activates both innate and acquired immune systems. While stimulating antibody and cellular responses, live attenuated vaccines induce both local and systemic immune responses (Carrias *et al.*, 2008). Live attenuated vaccines are generally more potent than killed vaccines in activating cellular immunity. Shoemaker *et al.* (1997), using a low dose of *E. ictaluri*, showed that macrophages from vaccinated fish were more efficient in killing *E. ictaluri*. These investigators showed that opsonization of *E. ictaluri* by serum from immunized fish increased killing by macrophages from vaccinated fish compared with macrophages from non-immunized fish. *E. ictaluri* was able to survive and replicate within catfish macrophages and can result in macrophage lysis (Russo *et al.* 2009). They also reported that macrophages from vaccinated catfish were more efficient in phagocytosis and killing of *E. ictaluri* in contrast to non-vaccinated catfish.

To understand why the live attenuated *E. ictaluri* vaccine was able to protect channel catfish, a study was conducted by Pridgeon *et al.* (2010). Using the polymerase chain reaction (PCR) subtractive cDNA hybridization technique, 41 expressed sequence tags (ESTs) were isolated from the live attenuated strain versus the virulent parent strain *E. ictaluri*. The results showed that 33 ESTs were upregulated at least three-fold in the attenuated strain versus the parent strain; 22% of the upregulated genes were found to be involved in protective immunity against ESC. In another study, Pridgeon *et al.* (2012a) revealed that 167 functionally known genes of catfish upregulated, whereas 40 were down-regulated when compared *E. ictaluri* attenuated vaccinated and control fish. Microarray analysis showed that lysozyme C was upregulated the most in vaccinated fish at 48 h post vaccination. Down-regulated genes were myotubularin related protein 1a and cytochrome P450 2J27. Pridgeon and coworkers (2012a) concluded that these differentially regulated genes may play an important roles in catfish immunity following live attenuated vaccination. Global gene expression profiles in catfish after immersion vaccination with AQUA-ESC vaccine revealed that 52 unique genes were found to be upregulated (Pridgeon *et al.*, 2012b). Microarray analysis found that apolipoprotein A-1 was upregulated at 48 h post-vaccination.

Live attenuated vaccines activate strong and long-memory T-cells (Salerno-Goncalves and Sztein, 2006), stimulate the production of cytokines, and produce cytotoxic T-lymphocytes (Secombes, 2008). The pathway is initiated by first interactions between naïve CD_4 T-cells and antigen presenting cells that lead to cytokine production. This is followed by pathways that activate and differentiate T-helper cell subsets, which release different types of cytokines that finally stimulate specific immunity against a pathogen.

Generally, attenuated bacterial vaccines are protective against many wild-type strains encountered in the field (Klesius and Shoemaker, 1999). This is an advantage over a killed bacterial vaccine that is usually limited in its capacity to provide cross-protection against different strains. Killed vaccines are able to stimulate specific antibody response (Seder and Hill, 2000). Formalin-killed *E. ictaluri* vaccine has not been efficacious (Nusbaum and Morrison, 1996). This may be due to the mode of action of formalin, which may result in alteration of surface antigens of *E. ictaluri* (Bader *et al.*, 1997) or the loss of the ability of *E. ictaluri* to enter the host fish (Nusbaum and Morrison, 1996). Furthermore, killed vaccines stimulate short-lived immunity, whereas attenuated vaccines produce long-term immunity. It is believed that this longer duration of immunity is the result of replication of the attenuated bacteria within the tissues of the fish (Norqvist *et al.*, 1989). It is believed that the longer the attenuated strain persists in the host, the more protection is achieved (Salmbandarmurthy and Jacobs, 2005). This might be due to the strength of the immune response induced by the attenuated live vaccine, and/or the functions of the antigens expressed by the live vaccines. Duration of immunity following bath immersion exposure to live attenuated bacteria has been reported to last more than 4 months (Klesius and Shoemaker, 1999; Shoemaker *et al.*, 2009). Since live attenuated bacterial vaccines are more effective in eliciting stronger cellular

Table 18.4 Live attenuated *Edwardsiella ictaluri* vaccines.

Vaccine	Fish	Attenuation method	Delivery	Fish age or size	RPS (weeks post-vaccination)
E. ictaluri (1)	Catfish	Rifampicin-resistant	Immersion	7–10 d	60–100 (4)
E. ictaluri (2)	Catfish	Novobiocin-resistant	Injection	10 g	93–100 (4–6)
			Immersion		90 (4–6)
E. ictaluri (3)	Catfish	aroA-deletion	Immersion	8 m	54.1–63.8 (4)
E. ictaluri (4)	Catfish	purA-deletion	Immersion	5 g	67 (3)
E. ictaluri (5)	Catfish	LPS deletion	Injection	6 m	94 (4)
			Immersion		0 (4)

(Source: (1) Klesius and Shoemaker 1999; (2) Pridgeon *et al.* 2011; (3) Thune *et al.* 1999; (4) Lawrence *et al.* 1997; (5) Lawrence *et al.* 2001.)

immune responses, they are more potent against intracellular gram-negative pathogens such as *E. ictaluri*.

Attenuated mutants have been produced using auxotrophy, transposon insertion and by chemical/drug mutagenesis (Table 18.4). Auxotropic mutants were produced by inactivation of the aroA gene by the insertion of a DNA fragment containing an antibiotic resistant gene (Thune *et al.*, 1999). After allelic exchange using a suicide vector, aroA mutants were selected for their loss of survival in fish due to their need for aromatic metabolites (Thune *et al.*, 1999). The aroA attenuated vaccine was shown to have 5 $\log_{10}$ loss of virulence over the wild type. However, no viable mutant cells were detected in catfish following immersion immunization at 48–72 h. Furthermore, the aroA-attenuated vaccine was found to be less efficacious (RPS: 54.1–63.8) against ESC (Thune *et al.*, 1999). A purA mutant of *E. ictaluri* was produced and evaluated for its attenuation, persistence and efficacy in catfish (Lawrence *et al.*, 1997). Attenuation resulted in 5 $\log_{10}$ loss of virulence compared with the wild type. The purA mutant was detected following immersion immunization for 48 h. The RPS for vaccinated catfish challenged with wild-type *E. ictaluri* was 63.3%.

Transposon mutagenesis was also used to produce *E. ictaluri* mutants that were deficient in lipopolysaccharide O side-chains (O LPS). The O LPS attenuated mutant was shown to be highly attenuated (Lawrence *et al.*, 2001). The attenuated mutant was detectable for 14 days in catfish following immunization by immersion exposure (Lawrence and Barnes, 2005). Intraperitoneal injection produced protection (RPS 90%), whereas bath immersion exposure resulted in a RPS of 0%. The live attenuated RE-33 (Klesius and Shoemaker, 1999) vaccine by immersion exposure had a RPS of 100%, whereas the RPS of the O LPS mutant vaccine was 0% (Lawrence and Barnes, 2005).

The efficacy of live attenuated *E. ictulari* vaccine was determined in channel catfish by bath immersion and intraperitoneal injection (Pridgeon and Klesius, 2011). This novel vaccine was produced from a virulent strain of *E. ictaluri* through selection for novobiocin resistance. Novobiocin was shown to bind to DNA gyrase, and block adenosine triphosphatase (ATPase) activity (Sugino *et al.*, 1978). Pridgeon and Klesius (2011) determined that the RPS of the attenuated vaccine was greater than 90% at 15, 30 and 60 days post-immunization given by bath immersion. The RPS of this vaccine in channel catfish immunized by IP injection was 100, 93 and 100% respectively, at 15, 30 and 60 days post-immunization. They concluded that this vaccine is a safe and efficacious vaccine against ESC in channel catfish.

Santander *et al.* (2011) showed that deletion of the crp gene in *E. ictaluri* was an effective strategy to develop immersion live attenuated antibiotic-sensitive vaccines against ESC. They found the *E. ictaluri* crp-10 mutant was attenuated, colonized lymphoid tissues and conferred protection against *E. ictaluri* infection in zebrafish and catfish. Catfish were found to be 92% and 100% protected against ESC following bath immersion and oral administration, respectively. Catfish were protected for at least 6 weeks post-immunization by bath immersion.

18.7 REGULATIONS (US)

Development and biosafety evaluation of vaccines in the US is regulated by the USDA, Animal and Plant Inspection Service, Center for Veterinary Biologics. Acceptance of vaccine requires comprehensive assessments of all criteria of vaccine development. This assessment includes biological safety to both aquatic animals and environment, and the assessment of purity and efficacy of the vaccine. The US protocols for studies of host animal immunogenicity/efficacy, safety, backpassage, shed/spread, immunological interference, and other areas can be found at http://www.aphis.usda.gov/animal_health/vet_biologics. This requirement applies to conventionally derived modified live vaccine products and those derived by recombinant DNA technology.

18.8 VACCINATION PRACTICES

Vaccines should not only reduce fish mortality and morbidity, but also provide additional economic benefits such as promoting faster growth rates and improved feed conversion. From an economic standpoint, profits of US$3000 to $4000 per ha were experienced for AQUAVAC-ESC® vaccinated over non-vaccinated catfish in field trials (Wise and Terhune, 2001). The use of this attenuated vaccine has also been found to improve survival and to increase profits for catfish held longer in nursery ponds before being released into fingerling ponds (Carrias *et al.*, 2008). The added economic benefits to the producer using this or similar attenuated vaccine is obvious.

The decision whether to vaccinate against a certain pathogen or not depends upon the producers' willingness to risk a disease outbreak (Thorarinsson and Powell, 2006). Vaccination is a form of insurance policy against a disease outbreak occurring and its economic impact to the producer. The risk of a major economic loss occurring becomes greater in relation to the production time. A disease outbreak with high mortality and morbidity at the food size stage will have considerably greater impact than at the fingerling stage. The loss of 50% of fish or more, at or about the food size stage, may lead to a substantial losses, even leading to the closure of the farm. Vaccination with attenuated vaccines would reduce the disease risk and provide additional profits that may offset the cost of vaccination. If a particular disease occurs with some frequency on a farm, a decision against vaccination is the highest form of risk-taking. A good vaccination strategy that is applied on a regular basis will result in a reduction in disease outbreaks over time and consequently result in greater profits. Treating disease outbreaks with drugs generally does not achieve this beneficial outcome.

In a study of the live attenuated vaccine usage, Bebak and Wagner (2012) found that 9.7% of the total fingerling operation used the live attenuated *E. ictaluri* vaccine in 2009. Producers that used vaccinated fish were larger, with a mean of 510.6 acres. Of the producers stocking fish vaccinated against ESC, 41.9% thought that survival was better in vaccinated fish. From the survey on producers' expectations regarding the percentage of vaccinated fish that would be protected against ESC, 52.4% responded that they expected 100% of their fish to be protected.

REFERENCES

Arias, C.R., Shoemaker, C.A., Evans, J.J. and Klesius, P.H. 2003. A comparative study of *Edwardsiella ictaluri* parent (EILO) and *E. ictulari* rifampicin-mutant (RE-33) isolates using lipopolysaccharide, outer membrane proteins, fatty acids, Biolog, API 20E and genomic analysis. *J Fish Dis* **26**: 415–21.

Bader, J.A., Vinitnantharat, S. and Klesius, P.H. 1997. Comparison of whole cell antigens of pressure- and formalin-killed *Flexibacter columnare* from channel catfish (*Ictalurus punctutus*). *Am J Vet Res* **58**: 985–8.

Bader, J.A., Shoemaker, C.A. and Klesius, P.H. 2004. Immune response induced by N-lauroylsarcosine extracted outer membrane proteins of an isolate *Edwardsiella ictaluri* in channel catfish. *Fish Shellfish Immunol* **16**: 281–428.

Baxa, D.W., Groff, J.M., Wishkovsky, A. and Hedrick, R.P. 1990. Susceptibility of nonictalurid fishes to experimental infection with *Edwardsiella ictaluri*. *Dis Aquat Org* **8**: 113–17.

Bebak J, Wagner B. Use of vaccination against enteric septicemia of catfish and columnaris disease by the US catfish industry. *J Aquat Anim Health* 2012; 24: 30–36.

Bertolini, J.M., Capriano, R.C., Pyle, S.W. and McLaughlin, J.J.A. 1990. Serological investigation of the fish pathogen *Edwardsiella ictaluri*, cause of septicemia of catfish. *J Wildl Dis* **26**: 246–52.

Bly, J.E. and Clem, L.W. 1991. Temperature-mediated processes in teleost immunity: *in vitro* immunosuppression induced by *in vivo* low temperature in channel catfish. *Vet Immunol Immunopathol* **28**: 365–77.

Carrias, A.A., Terhune, J.S., Sayles, C.A. and Chappel, C.A. 2008. Effects of an extended hatchery phase and vaccination against enteric septicemia of catfish on the production of channel catfish, *Ictalurus punctatus* fingerlings. *J World Aquat Soc* **39**: 259–66.

Copper, R.K., Shotts, E.B. and Nolan, L.K. 1996. Use of a minitransposon to study chondroitinase activity association with *Edwardsiella ictaluri*. *J Aquat Anim Health* **8**: 319–24.

Crumlish, M., Dung, T.T., Turnbull, J.F., *et al.*, 2002. Identification of *Edwardsiella ictaluri* from diseased freshwater catfish, *Pangasius hypophthalmus* (Sauvage), cultured in the Mekong Delta, Vietnam. *J. Fish Dis* **25**: 733–6.

Deng, X.Y., Luo, W., Tan, S.H., *et al.*, 2008. Isolation and identification of bacteriosis pathogen-*Edwardsiella tarda* from yellow catfish (*Pelteobagrus fulvidraco*) with red head disease. *Oceanol Limnol Sinica* **39**: 511–15.

Dung, T.T., Haesebrouck, F., Tuan, N.A., *et al.*, 2008. Antimicrobial susceptibility pattern of *Edwardsiella ictaluri* isolates from natural outbreaks of bacillary necrosis of *Pangasianodon hypophthalmus* in Vietnam. *Microbiol Drug Resist* **14**: 311–16.

Favre, D. and Viret, J.-F. 2006. Biosafety evaluation of recombinant live oral bacterial vaccines in the context of European regulation. *Vaccine* **24**: 3856–64.

Ferguson, H.W., Turnbull, J.F., Shinn, A.K., *et al.*, 2001. Bacillary necrosis in farmed *Pangasius hypophthalmus* (Sauvage) from the Mekong Delta, Vietnam. *J Fish Dis* **24**: 509–13.

Hawke, J. 1979. A bacterium associated with disease of pond cultured channel catfish, *Ictalurus punctatus*. *J Fish Res Board Canada* **36**: 1508–12.

Hawke, J., McWhorter, A., Steignwalt, A. and Brenners, D. 1981. *Edwardsiella ictulari* sp nov., the cause agent of enteric septicemia of catfish. *Int J Sys Bacteriol* **31**: 396–400.

Humphrey, J.D., Lancaster, C., Gudkovs, N. and McDonald, W. 1986. Exotic bacterial pathogens *Edwardsiella* tarda and *Edwardsiellia ictaluri* from imported ornamental fish *Betta splendens* and *Puntius conchonius*, respectively: isolation and quarantine significance. *Aust Vet J* **63**: 368–71.

Kasornchandra, J., Roger, W.A. and Plumb, J.A. 1987. *Edwardsiella ictaluri* from walking catfish, *Clarias batrahus L.* in Thailand. *J Fish Dis* **10**: 137–8.

Kent, M. and Lyons, J. 1982. *Edwardsiella ictaluri* in the green knife fish, *Eigemannia virescens*. *Fish Health News* **2**: 2.
Keskin, O., Secer, S., Izgur, M., *et al.*, 2004. *Edwardsiella ictaluri* infection in rainbow trout (*Oncorhynchus mykiss*). *Turkish J Vet Anim Sci* **28**: 649–53.
Klesius, P.H. 1992a. Carrier state of channel catfish infected with *Edwardsiella ictaluri*. *J Aquat Anim Health* **4**: 227–30.
Klesius, P. 1992b. Immune system of channel catfish: an overture of immunity to *Edwardsiella ictaluri*. *Annu Rev Fish Dis* 325–38.
Klesius, P.H. 1993. Rapid enzyme-linked immunosorbent test for detecting antibodies to *Edwardsiella ictaluri* in channel catfish, *Ictalurus punctatus*, using exoantigen. *J Aquat Anim Health* **36**: 359–69.
Klesius, P.H. 1994. Transmission of *Edwardsiella ictaluri* from infected, dead to noninfected channel catfish. *J Aquat Anim Health* **6**: 180–82.
Klesius, P.H. and Horst, M.H. 1991. Characterization of a major outer-membrane antigen of *Edwardsiella ictaluri*. *J Aquat Anim Health* **3**: 181–7.
Klesius, P.H. and Sealey, W.M. 1995. Characteristics of serum antibody in enteric septicemia of catfish. *J Aquat Anim Health* **7**: 205–10.
Klesius, P.H. and Sealey, W.M. 1996. Chemotactic and chemokinetic responses of channel catfish macrophages to exoantigen from *Edwardsiella ictaluri*. *J Aquat Anim Health* **8**: 314–18.
Klesius, P.H. and Shoemaker, C.A. 1999. Development and use of modified live *Edwardsiella ictaluri* vaccine against enteric septicemia of catfish. *Adv Vet Med* **41**: 523–37.
Klesius, P.H. and Shoemaker, C.A. 2000. Modified live *Edwardsiella ictaluri* against enteric septicemia in channel catfish. US Patent No. 6,019,981.
Klesius, P.H., Shoemaker, C.A. and Evans, J.J. 2000. *In ovo* methods for utilizing live *Edwardsiella ictaluri* against enteric septicemia in channel catfish. US Patent No. 6,153,202.
Klesius, P.H., Shoemaker, C.A., Evans, J.J. and Lim, C. 2001. Vaccines: prevention of diseases in aquatic animals, in *Nutrition and Fish Health* (eds C. Lim and C. Webster). Binghamton, New York, Haworth Press, 317–35.
Klesius, P., Lovy, J., Evans, J., *et al.*, 2003. Isolation of *Edwardsiella ictaluri* from tadpole madtom in a southwestern New Jersey River. *J Aquat Anim Health* **15**: 295–301.
Klesius, P.H., Evans, J.J. and Shoemaker, C.A. 2004. Warmwater fish vaccinology in catfish production. *Anim Health Res Rev* **5**: 305–11.
Lawrence, M.L. and Barnes, M.M. 2005. Tissue persistence and vaccine efficacy of an O side chain mutant strain of *Edwardsiella ictaluri*. *J Aquat Anim Health* **17**: 228–32.
Lawrence, M.L., Copper, R.K. and Thune, R.L. 1997. Attenuation, persistence and vaccine potential of an *Edwardsiella ictaluri* purA mutant. *Infect Immun* **65**: 4642–751.
Lawrence, M.L., Barnes, M.M. and Williams, M.L. 2001. Phenotype and virulence of a transponson-derived lipopolysaccharide O side-chain mutant strain of *Edwardsiella ictulari*. *J Aquat Anim Health* **13**: 291–9.
Lawrence, M.L., Barnes, M.M., Azadi, P. and Reeks, B.Y. 2003. The *Edwardsiella ictaluri* O polysaccharide biosynthesis gene cluster and the role of O polysaccharide in resistance to normal catfish serum and catfish neutrophils. *Microbiology* **149**: 1402–21.
Li, C., Zhang, Y., Wang, R., *et al.*, 2012. RNA-seq analysis of mucosal immune response reveals signatures of intestinal barrier disruption and pathogen entry following *Edwardsiella ictaluri* infection in channel catfish, *Ictalurus punctatus*. *Fish Shellfish Immunol* **32**: 816–27.
Liu, J.Y., Li, A.H., Zhou, D.R., *et al.*, 2010. Isolation and characterization of *Edwardsiella ictaluri* strains as pathogens from diseased yellow catfish *Pelteobagrus fulvidraceo* (Richardson) cultured in China. *Aquac Res* **41**: 1835–44.
Menanteau-Ledouble, S., Karsi, A. and Lawrence, M.L. 2011. Importance of skin adhesion as a primary site adhesion for *Edwardsiella ictaluri* and impact on invasion and systematic infection in channel catfish *Ictalurus punctatus*. *Vet Microbiol* **148**: 425–30.
Morrison, E.E. and Plumb, J.A. 1994. Olfactory organ of channel catfish as a site of experimental *Edwardsiella ictaluri* infection. *J Aquat Anim Health* **6**: 101–9.
Newton, J.C. and Triche, P.L. 1993a. Electrophoretic and immunochemical characterization of lipopolysaccharide of *Edwardsiella ictaluri* from channel catfish. *J Aquat Anim Health* **5**: 246–53.
Newton, J.C. and Triche, P.L. 1993b. Isolation and characterization of flagella from *Edwardsiella ictaluri*. *J Aquat Anim Health* **5**: 16–22.

Newton, J.C., Wolfe, L.G., Grizzle, J.M. and Plumb, J.A. 1989. Pathology of experimental enteric septicemia in channel catfish, *Ictalurus punctatus* (Rafinesque), following immersion exposure to *Edwardsiella ictaluri*. *J Fish Dis* **12**: 335–47.

Newton, J.C., Blevins, W.T., Wilt, G.R. and Wolfe, L.G. 1990. Outer membrane protein profiles of *Edwardsiella ictulari* from fish. *Am J Vet Res* **51**: 264–73.

Norqvist, A., Hagstrom, A. and Wolf, H. 1989. Protection of rainbow trout against vibriosis and furunculosis by the use of attenuated strains of *Vibrio anguillarum*. *Appl Environ Microbiol* **55**: 1400–405.

Nusbaum, K.E. and Morrison, E.E. 1996. Entry of 35S-labeled *Edwardsiella ictaluri* into channel catfish. *J Aquat Anim Health* **8**: 146–9.

Panangala, V.S., Shoemaker, C.A., McNulty, S.T., *et al*., 2006. Intra- and interspecific phenotypic characteristics of fish-pathogenic *Edwardsiella ictaluri* and *E. tarda*. *Aquac Res* **37**: 49–60.

Panangala, V.S., Russo, R., Van Santen, V.L., *et al*., 2009a. Organization and sequence of four flagellin-encoding genes of *Edwardsiella ictaluri*. *Aquac Res* **40**: 1135–47.

Panangala, V.S., Shoemaker, C.A., Klesius, P.H., *et al*., 2009b. Cross-protection elicited in channel catfish (*Ictalurus punctatus* Rafinesque) immunized with low dose of virulent *Edwardsiella ictaluri* strains. *Aquac Res* **40**: 915–26.

Petrie-Hanson, L., Romano, C.L., Mackey, R.B., *et al*., 2007. Evaluation of zebrafish *Danio rerio* as a model for enteric septicemia of catfish (ESC). *J Aquat Anim Health* **19**: 151–8.

Plumb, J.A. 1988. Vaccination against *Edwardsiella ictaluri*, in *Fish Vaccination* (ed. A.E. Ellis). London, Academic Press, 152–61.

Plumb, J.A. 2000. Catfish bacterial diseases, in *Health Maintenance and Principal Microbial Diseases of Cultured Fishes* (ed. J.A. Plumb). Ames, Iowa State University Press, 187–94.

Plumb, J.A. and Sanchez, D. 1983. Susceptibility of five species of fish to *Edwardsiella ictaluri*. *J Fish Dis* **6**: 261–6.

Plumb, J.A. and Quinlan, E.E. 1986. Survival of *Edwardsiella ictaluri* in pond water and bottom mud. *Prog Fish Cult* **48**: 212–14.

Plumb, J.A. and Huge, V. 1987. Susceptibility of European catfish (*Silurus gianis*) to *Edwardsiella ictaluri*. *J Appl Ichthyol* **3**: 45–8.

Plumb, J.A. and Klesius, P.H. 1988. An assessment of the antigenic homogeneity of *Edwardsiella ictaluri* using monoclonal antibody. *J Fish Dis* **11**: 499–510.

Plumb, J.A. and Vinitnantharat, S. 1993. Vaccination of channel catfish, *Ictalurus punctatus* (Rafinesque) by immersion and oral booster against *Edwardsiella ictaluri*. *J Fish Dis* **16**: 65–71.

Plumb, J.A., Vinitnantharat, S. and Paterson,W.D. 1994. Optimum concentration of *Edwardsiella ictaluri* vaccine in feed for oral vaccination of channel catfish. *J Aquat Anim Health* **6**: 118–21.

Pridgeon, Y. and Klesius, P. 2011. Development of a novobiocin-resistant *Edwardsiella ictaluri* as a novel vaccine in channel catfish (*Ictalurus punctatus*). *Vaccine* **29**: 5631–7.

Pridgeon, Y., Russo, R., Shoemaker, C. and Klesius, P. 2010. Identification of *in vitro* upregulated genes in a modified live vaccine strain of *Edwardsiella ictaluri* compared to a virulent parent strain. *Comp Immunol Microbiol Infect Dis* **33**(6): e31–40.

Pridgeon, Y., Yeh, H.H., Shoemaker, C., *et al*., 2012a. Global gene expression in channel catfish after vaccination with an attenuated *Edwardsiella ictaluri*. *Fish Shellfish Immunol* **32**: 524–33.

Pridgeon, Y., Yeh, H.H., Shoemaker, C. and Klesius, P. 2012b. Global transcription analysis of vaccinated channel catfish following challenge with virulent *Edwardsiella ictaluri*. *Vet Immunol Immunopathol* **146**: 53–61.

Reid, W.S. and Boyle, J.A. 1989. Plasmid homologies in *Edwardsiella ictaluri*. *Appl Environ Microbiol* **55**: 3253–5.

Russo, R., Shoemaker, C.A., Panangala, V.S. and Klesius, P.H. 2009. *In vitro* and *in vivo* interaction of macrophages from vaccination and non-vaccination channel catfish (*Ictalurus punctatus*) to *Edwardsiella ictaluri*. *Fish Shellfish Immunol* **26**: 543–52.

Saeed, M.O. and Plumb, J.A. 1986. Immune response of channel catfish to lipopolysaccharides and whole cell *Edwardsiella ictaluri* vaccine. *Dis Aquat Org* **2**: 21–6.

Salerno-Goncalves, R. and Sztein, M.B. 2006. Cell-mediated immunity and challenges for vaccine development. *Trends Microbiol* **14**: 536–42.

Salmbandamurthy, V.K. and Jacobs, W.R. 2005. Live attenuated mutants of *Mycobacterium tuberculosis* as candidate vaccines against tuberculosis. *Microbiol Infect* **5**: 955–61.

Santander, J., Mitra, A. and Curtiss, R. 2011. Phenotype, virulence and immunogenicity of *Edwardsiella ictaluri* cyclic adenosine 3′5′ monophosphate receptor protein (Crp) mutants in catfish host. *Fish Shellfish Immunol* **31**: 1142–53.

Schurig, G.G., Roop II, R.M., Bagchi, T., *et al.*, 1991. Biological properties of RB51; a stable rough strain of *Brucella abortus*. *Vet Microbiol* **28**: 171–88.

Secombes, C. 2008. Will advances in fish immunology change vaccination strategies? *Fish Shellfish Immunol* **25**: 409–16.

Seder, R.A. and Hill, A.V.S. 2000. Vaccines against intracellular infections requiring cellular immunity. *Nature* **406**: 793–7.

Shoemaker, C.A. and Klesius, P.H. 1997. Protective immunity against enteric septicemia in channel catfish, *Ictalurus punctatus* (Rafineque), following controlled exposure to *Edwardsiella ictaluri*. *J Fish Dis* **20**: 101–8.

Shoemaker, C.A., Klesius, P.H. and Plumb, J.A. 1997. Killing of *Edwardsiella ictaluri* by macrophages from channel catfish immune and susceptible to enteric septicemia of catfish. *Vet Immunol Immunopathol* **58**: 181–90.

Shoemaker, C.A., Klesius, P.H. and Bricker, J.M. 1999. Efficacy of a modified live *Edwardsiella ictaluri* vaccine in channel catfish as young as seven days post hatch. *Aquaculture* **176**: 189–93.

Shoemaker, C.A., Klesius, P.H. and Evans, J.J. 2002. *In ovo* method for utilizing live *Edwardsiella ictaluri* vaccine against enteric septicemia in channel catfish. *Aquaculture* **203**: 221–2.

Shoemaker, C.A., Klesius, P.H. and Evans, J.J. 2007. Immunization of eyed channel catfish, *Ictalurus punctatus*, eggs with monovalent *Flavobacterium columnare* vaccine and bivalent *F. columnare* and *Edwardsiella ictaluri* vaccine. *Vaccine* **25**: 1126–31.

Shoemaker, C.A., Klesius, P.H., Evans, J.J. and Arias, C.R. 2009. Use of modified live vaccines in aquaculture. *J World Aquac* **40**: 573–85.

Shotts, E.B., Blazer, V.S. and Waltman, W.D. 1986. Pathogenesis of experimental *Edwardsiella ictaluri* infections in channel catfish (*Ictalurus punctatus*). *Can J Fish Aquat Sci* **43**: 36–42.

Sugino, A., Higgins, N.P., Brown, P.O., *et al.*, 1978. Energy coupling in DNA gyrase and the mechanism of action of novobiocin. *Proc Natl Acad Sci USA* **75**: 4838–42.

Thorarinsson, R. and Powell, D.B. 2006. Effects of disease risk, vaccine efficacy, and market price on the economics of fish vaccination. *Aquaculture* **256**: 42–9.

Thune, R.L., Hawke, J.P. and Johnson, M.C. 1992. Studies on vaccination of channel catfish *Ictalurus punctatus*, against *Edwardsiella ictaluri*. *J Appl Aquac* **3**: 11–24.

Thune, R.L., Hawke, J.P., Fernandez, D.H., *et al.*, 1997a. Immunization with bacterial antigens: edwardsiellosis. *Dev Biol Stand* **90**: 125–34.

Thune, R.L., Collins, L.A. and Pena, M.A. 1997b. A comparison of immersion, immersion/oral combination and injection vaccination of channel catfish *Ictalurus punctatus* against *E. ictaluri*. *J World Aquac Soc* **28**: 193–201.

Thune, R.L., Fernandez, D.H. and Battista, R. 1999. An aroA mutant of *Edwardsiella ictaluri* is safe and efficacious as a live attenuated vaccine. *J Aquat Anim Health* **11**: 358–72.

Thune, R.L., Fernandez, D.L., Benoit, J.L., *et al.*, 2007. Signature-tagged mutagenesis of *Edwardsiella ictaluri* identifies virulence-related genes, including a *Salmonella* pathogenicity island 2 class of type III secretion systems. *Appl Environ Microbiol* **73**: 7934–46.

Vinitnantharat, S. and Plumb, J.A. 1992. Kinetics of the immune response of channel catfish to *Edwardsiella ictaluri*. *J Aquat Anim Health* **4**: 207–14.

Vinitnantharat, S. and Plumb, J.A. 1993. Protection of channel catfish *Ictalurus punctatus* following natural exposure to *Edwardsiella ictaluri* and effects of feeding antigen on antibody titer. *Dis Aquat Org* **15**: 31–4.

Vinitnantharat, S., Plumb, J.A. and Brown, A.E. 1993. Isolation and purification of an outer membrane of *Edwardsiella ictaluri* and its antigenicity to channel catfish (*Ictalurus punctatus*). *Fish Shellfish Immunol* **3**: 401–9.

Wagner, B.A., Wise, D.J., Khoo, L.H. and Terhune, J.S. 2002. The epidemiology of bacterial diseases in food-size channel catfish. *J Aquat Anim Health* **14**: 263–72.

Waltman, W.D., Shotts, E.B. and Blazer, V.S. 1985. Recovery of *Edwardsiella ictaluri* from danio (*Danio devario*). *Aquaculture* **46**: 63–6.

Waltman, W.D., Shotts, E.B. and Hsu, T.C. 1986. Biochemical characteristics of *Edwardsiella ictaluri*. *Appl Environ Microbiol* **51**: 101–4.

Weete, J.D., Blevins, W.T., Chitrakorn, S., *et al.*, 1988. Chemical characterization of lipopolysaccharide from *Edwardsiella ictaluri* from channel catfish. *Can J Microbiol* **34**: 1224–9.

Wehrli, W., Knusel, P., Schmid, K. and Staehelin, M. 1968. Interaction of rifamycin with bacterial RNA polymerase. *Proc Natl Acad Sci USA* **61**: 667–73.

Williams, M.L. and Lawrence, M.L. 2005. Identification and characterization of a two-component hemolysin from *Edwardsiella ictaluri*. *Vet Microbiol* **108**: 281–9.

Wise, D.J. 2006. Vaccination shown to improve production efficiencies. *Catfish J*: 6–7.

Wise, D.J. and Terhune, J. 2001. The relationship between vaccine dose and efficacy in channel catfish *Ictalurus punctutus* vaccinated with live attenuated strain of *Edwardsiella ictaluri* (RE-33). *J World Aquac Soc* **32**: 177–83.

Wise, D.J., Klesius, P.H., Shoemaker, C.A. and Wolters, W.R. 2000. Vaccination of mixed and full-sib families of channel catfish *Ictalurus punctatus* against enteric septicemia of catfish with a live attenuated *Edwardsiella ictaluri* isolate (RE-33). *J World Aquac Soc* **31**: 206–12.

Wolfe, K., Plumb, J.A. and Morrison, E.E. 1994. Lectin binding characteristics of the olfactory mucosa of channel catfish: potential factors in attachment of *Edwardsiella ictulari*. *J Aquat Anim Health* **10**: 348–60.

Xu, D.H., Shoemaker, C.A., Martins, M.L., *et al.*, 2012. Enhanced susceptibility of channel catfish to the bacterium *Edwardsiella ictaluri* after parasitism by *Ichthyophthirius multifiliis*. *Vet Microbiol* **158**: 216–19.

Ye, S., Qiao, H.L.G. and Zhangshi, L. 2009. First case of *Edwardsiella ictaluri* infection in China farmed yellow catfish *Pelteobagrus fulvidraco*. *Aquaculture* **292**: 6–10.

Yuasa, K., Kholidin, E.B. and Panigoro Nand Hatai, K. 2003. First isolation of *Edwardsiella ictaluri* from cultured striped catfish *Pangasius hypophthalmus* in Indonesia. *Fish Pathol* **38**: 181–3.

19 Vaccination against Yersiniosis

Andrew Bridle and Barbara Nowak
NCMCRS University of Tasmania, Tasmania, Australia

ABSTRACT

Yersiniosis is a disease caused by *Yersinia ruckeri*, which mostly affects salmonids during their hatchery stage. Vaccines against yersiniosis have been commercially available for more than 40 years. These vaccines are inactivated bacterins, and are mostly applied by immersion. Boosters are often required to ensure longevity of protection. Since the late 1980s, biotype 2 variants of *Y. ruckeri* started to cause infections and are now the major variants causing yersiniosis throughout the US and Europe. This emergence of new variants resulted in the changes in the biotypes used for vaccine production.

19.1 YERSINIOSIS

Yersiniosis in fish is caused by infection with *Yersinia ruckeri*, a member of the family *Enterobacteriaceae*. The term "yersiniosis" is synonymous with enteric redmouth disease (ERM), a disease of fish caused by overt infection with *Yersinia ruckeri*. ERM was first described in the late 1950s when it was affecting rainbow trout in the Hagerman Valley of Idaho (Rucker, 1966). Yersiniosis is now endemic across all the major salmonid farming areas of the world. *Yersinia ruckeri* was most likely introduced from the US to Europe in the late 1970s or the early 1980s (Horne and Barnes, 1999). In response to the increasing geographic distribution of *Y. ruckeri* and its ability to cause disease in species other than rainbow trout, the use of ERM to describe the disease has largely been replaced by the term "yersiniosis". A vaccine against ERM was one of the first commercial fish vaccines licensed in the US in the 1970s.

B.Nowak@utas.edu.au

Fish Vaccination, First Edition. Edited by Roar Gudding, Atle Lillehaug and Øystein Evensen.

19.2 OCCURRENCE AND SIGNIFICANCE

Yersinia ruckeri is widespread in freshwater and fish. It has been isolated from samples from Europe, North and South Americas, South Africa, Asia, Australia and New Zealand. Yersiniosis has been reported from a variety of fish, including salmonids, eels, goldfish, sole, sturgeon, Nile tilapia and turbot. Yersiniosis is a serious issue in salmonid-farming countries, causing up to 30–79% mortality if left untreated (Horne and Barnes, 1999). Most outbreaks affect small-size rainbow trout (northern hemisphere) or Atlantic salmon (Australia) in hatcheries after transfer to flow-through tanks or ponds where the presence of pathogens and water quality, in particular temperature, cannot be controlled. However, the disease can affect production in larger fish, for example, smolt during transfer to marine grow-out sites.

There are considerable differences between yersiniosis in most countries where it is mostly a disease of rainbow trout, and Australia where it affects farmed Atlantic salmon. Until recently the Hagerman strain (causing enteric redmouth or ERM, which is considered to be exotic to Australia) has been the main *Yersinia ruckeri* strain of concern in the northern hemisphere. More recently an emerging vaccine-insensitive group has been reported and attributed to the emergence of non-motile, Tween 80-negative, biotype 2 isolates (Austin *et al.*, 2003). It has been suggested that the biotype 2 phenotype has arisen independently in different clonal groups in mainland Europe and the UK (Wheeler *et al.*, 2009).

19.3 ETIOLOGY

Yersinia ruckeri is a member of the family *Enterobacteriaceae*; it is a gram-negative non-spore-forming, non-encapsulated rod, and facultative anaerobe with variable motility. Although within the same genus as *Yersinia pestis*, the infamous etiological agent of the bubonic plague, *Y. ruckeri* causes disease only in fish. Based on 16S rRNA phylogenetic analysis, its divergence from the rest of the *Yersinia* genus has provided doubt as to its taxonomic assignment within the genus. Before phylogenetic analyses were performed, controversy surrounded the taxonomic assignment of *Y. ruckeri*, as early descriptions of this fish pathogen found phenotypic similarities more common to other genera of *Enterobacteriaceae* than *Yersinia*. However, subsequent analyses of many isolates of *Y. ruckeri* have left no doubt as to the validity of its position within the genus *Yersinia*.

Recent use of high throughput whole-genome sequencing technologies has allowed the comparative genomic analysis of the entire *Yersinia* genus, and confirmed that *Y. ruckeri* is the most evolutionary distant member of the genus (Chen *et al.*, 2010). This study showed the total genome size of *Y. ruckeri* as 3.58–3.89 Mbp, substantially less than the 4.6–4.8 Mbp obtained for the other species within the genus. Phylogenetic analyses using the core protein set of each species split the genera into three clades: *Y. ruckeri*, the most evolutionary distant, the sole member of clade 1; the second clade containing *Y. pestis* and *Y. pseudotuberculosis*; and the third clade containing the remainder of the enterocolitica-like species.

Biochemical characteristics within the species are highly uniform and typical of other members of the *Enterobacteriaceae* family. *Y. ruckeri* is glucose-fermentative, oxidase-negative and nitrate-reductive, but nonetheless routine biochemical tests including kits, such as the rapid API 20E system, can be used to distinguish *Y. ruckeri* from other species (Frerichs, 1993). Initial research using isolates from disease outbreaks suggested that *Y. ruckeri* was a homogenous bacterial species (Ross *et al.*, 1966; Busch, 1973). Similarly, early molecular characterization of isolates using multilocus isoenzyme electrophoresis of 15 enzyme loci found 42 of 47 isolates with the same type, suggesting very low genetic diversity and the clonal nature of the species (Schill *et al.*, 1984). More recently a wealth of high-resolution phenotypic and molecular techniques including serotyping, antibiotic resistance typing, biotyping, pulsed-field gel electrophoresis (PFGE) and outer membrane protein (OMP) profiling have provided evidence of high genetic diversity (Wheeler *et al.*, 2009; Bastardo *et al.*, 2011; Tinsley *et al.*, 2011a). Although likely in need of revision, serological typing is still the most commonly adopted method of intraspecies classification. The intraspecies isolates are classified according to five different serotypes (O1, O2, O5, O6 and O7) using antiserum specific to heat-stable O-antigens (Davies, 1990). Serotype O1 can be divided into two subgroups, O1a and O1b, while serotype O2 can be divided into three subgroups, O2a, O2b and O2c (Romalde *et al.*, 1993).

Of great importance is the emergence of a non-motile variant of the O1 serotype that lacks secreted phospholipase activity and first appeared in the 1980s (Davies and Frerichs, 1989). Initially termed EX5, this variant defined a new biotype, biotype 2, and caused disease in trout vaccinated against the then-predominant motile O1 serotype (biotype 1) (Austin *et al.*, 2003). Biotype 2 variants of *Y. ruckeri* now represent the major disease-causing variants of yersiniosis throughout the US and Europe, where very successful bacterin-based vaccines based on the Hagerman strain O1a, biotype 1, have been used for over 30 years.

19.4 PATHOGENESIS

Worldwide, yersiniosis causes significant losses in salmonid aquaculture (Tobback *et al.*, 2007). Despite this, there is a general lack of information about yersiniosis and its pathogenicity is not well understood (Tobback *et al.*, 2007). Virulent strains cause systemic septicemia and death (Tobback *et al.*, 2009a). High numbers of bacteria are present in the gills immediately after infection, resulting in a rapid spread of *Y. ruckeri* in the internal organs, indicating that gills may be an important site of entry and suggesting that virulence of *Y. ruckeri* is related to immune evasion (Tobback *et al.*, 2009a). This is further supported by the fact that *Y. ruckeri* is a facultative intracellular pathogen and can survive in macrophages (Ryckaert *et al.*, 2010). Immersion challenge resulted in high numbers of the pathogen being detected in the intestinal tract of rainbow trout at 24 to 72 hours post-infection, followed by systemic infection by 5 days post-infection (Mendez and Guijarro, 2013).

Y. ruckeri can produce extracellular products (ECPs), including hemolysins, which have been shown to play a role in pathogenesis (Romalde and Toranzo, 1993). A hemolysin/cytolysin *YhlA* has been proposed to play an important role in the pathogenicity of *Y. ruckeri* as it lyses erythrocytes and cultured fish cells, and contributes to the acquisition of iron from the host (Fernandez *et al.*, 2007a). *Y. ruckeri* virulence factors were investigated *in vitro* (Tobback *et al.*, 2009b). A high level of adherence capability to gill and intestinal mucus and resistance to serum were characteristic of virulent strains of *Y. ruckeri*.

A number of *Y. ruckeri* genes were suggested to play a role in the pathogenesis of yersiniosis. Iron acquisition by the siderophore ruckerbactin, proteolytic and hemolytic activities, and resistance to immune mechanisms, were proved to be involved in the virulence of *Y. ruckeri* (Fernandez *et al.*, 2007b). The BarA-UvrY two-component system (TCS) contributes to the pathogenesis of *Y. ruckeri* in rainbow trout, possibly by regulating the invasion of epithelial cells and sensitivity to oxidative stress induced by immune cells (Dahiya and Stevenson, 2010). Application of *in vivo* expression technology (IVET) to *Y. ruckeri* allowed the identification of two adjacent genes that represent a novel bacterial system involved in the uptake and degradation of L-cysteine, a system which is involved in the virulence of *Y. ruckeri* (Mendez *et al.*, 2011).

Y. ruckeri infection of rainbow trout results in upregulation of a number of pro- and anti-inflammatory cytokine genes in the spleen, including IL1 family members, IL-2 (Diaz-Rosales *et al.*, 2009), IL-17 family members (Wang *et al.*, 2009), and IL-6, IL-8, IL-10, and IL-11 (Raida and Buchmann, 2008). However, the upregulation of at least some of the interleukins including IL1beta, IL-8 and IL-10 in blood of immersion-challenged rainbow trout did not result in protection and was positively correlated to the bacterial load in the blood (Raida *et al.*, 2011b).

Recently, cathelicidins have been shown to have an important role in the pathogenesis of yersiniosis in Atlantic salmon (Bridle *et al.*, 2011, 2012). Cathelicidins are antimicrobial peptides, and two genes have been described in Atlantic salmon: asCATH1 and asCATH2 (Chang *et al.*, 2006). Atlantic salmon cathelicidins were significantly upregulated during yersiniosis (Bridle *et al.*, 2011). For example, in the spleen of infected fish, asCATH1 expression was maintained at approximately 30-fold higher than the expression in the control fish at 72 and 96 h. Expression of asCATH2 more than doubled in fold increase from 48-fold at 72 h post-infection to 98-fold at 96 h. Both asCATH1 and 2 were upregulated to a greater extent and earlier in the spleen compared with the gills. However, different strains of *Y. ruckeri* have different virulence and can produce different disease outcomes (Tobback *et al.*, 2009b). The extent of cathelicidin response seen during yersiniosis may therefore be specific to the Tasmanian O1b serotype of *Y. ruckeri* (Bridle *et al.*, 2011).

19.5 VACCINES

Licensed in 1976, a bacterin produced from formalin-killed *Y. ruckeri* was the first vaccine against ERM and the first commercialized fish vaccine. Prepared as an inactivated whole cell bacterin, this vaccine has been predominantly used for immersion vaccination of hatchery-size fish. While usually recommended to be delivered via immersion, several commercial yersiniosis vaccines may be delivered by injection without oil-adjuvant or as an oral preparation during a booster immunization.

The emergence of biotype 2 isolates causing yersiniosis outbreaks in salmonids vaccinated against the original biotype 1 isolates has driven the recent development of commercial yersiniosis vaccines incorporating a bivalent antigen design. The bivalent yersiniosis vaccines contain the original 'Hagerman' O1 biotype 1 strain, with a biotype 2 or EX5-like strain. Antigenic and cross-protection studies of biotype 1 and biotype 2 isolates of *Y. ruckeri* in rainbow trout have confirmed the O-antigen as the dominant immunogenic molecule, and explained the limited protection conferred against biotype 2 isolates by the monovalent (biotype 1) vaccine (Tinsley *et al.*, 2011b). Furthermore, protection against biotype 1 isolates is equally as effective, if not more effective, in trout immunized with the bivalent vaccine compared with the monovalent vaccine (Deshmukh *et al.*, 2012).

Since the pioneering work of Klontz (1963), who demonstrated that a bacterin prepared from *Y. ruckeri* when administered orally could provide an RPS of 87%, many experimental vaccines have been tested. The O-antigen of the lipopolysaccharide is a known immunogen, and along with other subcellular components is able to confer high levels of protection against yersiniosis when isolated from both *Y. ruckeri* and probiotic species such as *Aeromonas sobria* and *Bacillus subtilus* and IP-injected into trout (Abbass *et al.*, 2010). Furthermore, Fernandez *et al.* (2003) tested the protective ability of immunization with a toxoid of the Yrp1 protease against yersiniosis. Intramuscular injection of this toxoid conferred high protection against yersiniosis.

A more controversial approach has been the use of a live attenuated vaccine created by inducing a mutation in the aroA gene, rendering the gene dysfunctional. The aroA gene encodes the enzyme 5-enolpyruvylshikimate-3-phosphate synthase, which is involved in the biosynthesis of aromatic amino acids. Although Temprano *et al.* (2005) found that this approach provided superior protection to the currently used bacterin-based vaccines, concerns regarding the environmental safety of genetically modified organisms have and are likely to continue to limit the commercial use of live attenuated vaccines.

Although bacterin-based vaccines against yersiniosis have been commercially used and studied for more than 30 years, the exact mechanisms that confer protection are still poorly understood. Specific antibodies are generally accepted to be important in vaccination; however, specific antibody-mediated protection against yersiniosis has never been clearly established. Proof of antibody-mediated protection is scarce, as only one study, performed by Olesen (1991), was able to successfully passively immunize trout against yersiniosis using trout serum. The importance of antibody-mediated protection was also highlighted in a later study by Lee *et al.* (2000), in which anti *Y. ruckeri* IgY antibodies produced in chicken eggs were able to protect trout against infection when administered by IP injection 4 hours before challenge with *Y. ruckeri*. More recently a study in trout found that plasma-specific IgM antibody titers and bactericidal activity increased significantly following immersion vaccination against yersiniosis, and that fewer *Y. ruckeri* were found in the blood of vaccinated trout 3–14 days post-challenge (Raida *et al.*, 2011a). An increase in IgM titre was also reported after IP injection of rainbow trout with a commercial vaccine against yersiniosis (Raida and Buchmann, 2007). The potential contribution of other humoral or cellular factors during the vaccine-induced host response may explain repeated failures to demonstrate protection against yersiniosis via passive immunization. Moreover, it is plausible that the recently identified ability of *Y. ruckeri* to reside within macrophages (Ryckaert *et al.*, 2010) may aid *Y. ruckeri* to elude antibody-mediated host protective responses.

19.6 VACCINATION PROCEDURES

The first report of successful vaccination of trout against yersiniosis was by Klontz (1963) using a bacterin prepared from *Y. ruckeri* and administered orally. Further work by Ross and Klontz (1965) and later by Anderson and Ross (1972) led to the adoption of immersion as the administration method of choice. Although Anderson and Nelson (1974) showed that IP injection of the bacterin conferred superior protection, very little has changed in terms of the administration of bacterin-based yersiniosis vaccines. As yersiniosis is still predominantly a disease that occurs in salmonid hatcheries, the benefits of immersion vaccination in terms of ease of administration to fry and juvenile fish mean that it has remained as the delivery method of choice. Immersion vaccination is usually implemented in the form of a 30–60 s dip of fish weighing 5 g or less. However, in the hatchery there are times when booster vaccination is required to ensure adequate duration of protection, and this is only feasible by means of oral delivery of vaccine that is either incorporated into or coated onto feed. While IP injection has long been known to provide the most effective protection in terms of RPS values and duration of protection (Anderson and Nelson, 1974), it is impractical for small fish (< 20 g).

The use of a bath with a more dilute concentration (1:100), usually over a period of at least 1 hour, has been used as an alternate form of immersion vaccination. The use of this technique is often based on a belief by some aquaculturists that a longer bath immersion technique is less stressful to the fish and prevents aspects of the stress response negating the efficacy of the vaccine. Until recently the Tasmanian salmonid industry routinely performed immersion vaccinations via a bath, and only converted to using the more common dip form of immersion after a study by Costa *et al.* (2011) found serious shortcomings in the duration of protection afforded by bath vaccinations.

Yersiniosis is a common problem within salmonid hatcheries and is likely to affect fish from very early stages of development, well before they have reached the recommended weight of 5 g for immersion vaccination suggested by several commercial yersiniosis vaccine producers. In an attempt to address this issue, booster immunizations are administered according to fish size and the period of year. Small fish are more easily booster immunized by immersion or oral delivery, while larger fish may be injected if the water temperature is not too high. Hatchery salmonids are usually vaccinated when they weigh 1–3 g and again at 5 g. Additional booster treatments are recommended to ensure high levels of protection during the rest of the production cycle. Recent outbreaks in Atlantic salmon transferred to marine sites in both Europe and Australia have given aquaculturists a reason to re-evaluate the cost-benefit analysis of intraperitoneal injection against yersiniosis, or incorporating them into existing injection formulations and regimes. Along with excellent levels of protection, injection of yersiniosis vaccines has the added benefit of not requiring an adjuvant, therefore avoiding the issues surrounding tissue damage from oil-based adjuvants.

19.7 VACCINE EFFECT

Relative percent survival (RPS) figures of 70–100% are commonly afforded by bacterin-based yersiniosis vaccines administered by immersion, and obviously depend on the species of fish, size of fish, infection challenge dose and duration post-vaccination or booster. Even the earliest experimental work by Klontz (1963) found that simple formalin-killed whole cells of *Y. ruckeri*, when administered orally, could provide a RPS of 87%. Soon after, immersion vaccines of similarly prepared bacterins were also shown to provide excellent levels of protection in trout against yersiniosis (Ross and Klontz, 1965; Anderson and Ross, 1972). Not only do these monovalent bacterins provide high levels of protection against biotype 1 strains, but the duration of protection after a single 20–60 s dip immersion of 3–10 g fish is often 120–300 days, after which it starts to decline (Johnson *et al.*, 1982).

More recently, yersiniosis outbreaks in fish vaccinated using the original monovalent vaccine and attributed to the emergence of biotype 2 strains have led to the development and need to characterize the efficacy of newly developed vaccines against these strains. Fortunately, bacterins produced from biotype 2 strains and a combination of these in conjunction with biotype 1 strains have been experimentally proven to provide effective protection against yersiniosis. In a study assessing the cross-protective abilities of these vaccines against biotype 1 and 2 strains, RPS values of 87–100% were demonstrated in trout challenged by IP injection with several biotype 2 strains, 28 days after vaccination with a commercial bivalent vaccine (Tinsley *et al.*, 2011b). When vaccinated with a monovalent vaccine and challenged with the same biotype 2 strains, RPS values were significantly lower and ranged from 72–100%. The monovalent and bivalent vaccines provided good protection against a biotype 1 strain, with RPS values of 81% and 92%, respectively. Both monovalent and bivalent vaccines were administered by a 30 s dip immersion using a 1:10 dilution of the vaccine. A study by Deshmukh *et al.* (2012) also assessed the cross-protective abilities of the same commercial monovalent and bivalent vaccines in trout against both biotypes, but focused on assessment of longer-term protection. Injection challenge with a biotype 2 strain at 4 and 6 months post-vaccination with the monovalent vaccine resulted in relatively low RPS values of 13.5% and 29.5%, respectively. When vaccinated with the bivalent vaccine and challenged at 4 and 6 months post-vaccination, RPS values of 42.5% and 52% were obtained. These studies demonstrate the protective benefits of the bivalent vaccine and highlight the need for booster regimes to ensure effective duration of protection.

Immersion vaccination against yersiniosis resulted in a differential expression of 17 genes in the gills of Atlantic salmon; this biosignature was considered as a predictor of vaccine-induced protection (Bridle *et al.*, 2012). These genes included some involved in detoxification and repair (alcohol dehydrogenase class-3 and thioredoxin interacting protein) and others involved in immune response (two Ig heavy chain transcripts, hepcidin, thymopoetin, E3 ubiquitin-protein ligase, SAM and SH3 domain containing protein 1, myelin, lymphocyte protein, LIM, actin binding protein and TRIM). Immunoglobulin heavy chain gene and selenoprotein were significantly upregulated in gills of Atlantic salmon following vaccination and 72 h post-challenge, indicating protective host response (Bridle *et al.*, 2012).

19.8 SIDE-EFFECTS

There are no reports of side-effects of vaccines against yersiniosis. This is possibly due to the application of the vaccine without an adjuvant (Håstein *et al.*, 2005). Side-effects of vaccination are usually related to the use of oil-adjuvanted vaccines (Midtlyng and Lillehaug, 1998; Koppang *et al.*, 2005). While not usually considered a side-effect, the prevalence of asymptomatic carriers appears to be high in vaccinated fish, at least in Atlantic salmon (Bridle, unpublished). This suggests that while the vaccination protects from disease and mortality, the infection can still persist in a high proportion of the population.

19.9 REGULATIONS

Licensing of fish vaccines is regulated by laws and regulations outlined in the European Pharmacopoeia monographs and guidance documents (Galligani *et al.*, 2005). Regulatory frameworks are country-specific, and while there are some efforts to harmonise requirements, licensing and permit requirements differ between countries and regions. In the EU, wherever relevant European Pharmacopoeia monographs exist, vaccine tests and procedures must comply with the published standards (Midtlyng, 2005). There are a number of vaccines against yersiniosis licensed or permitted in different countries. In Australia, vaccine against yersiniosis is not registered, but used under a permit, which means that the vaccine must be used under veterinary supervision. Imports of vaccines manufactured in different countries can be restricted. For example, there is a ban on importation to Australia of veterinary vaccines manufactured in facilities that store and/or handle pathogens exotic to Australia or other diseases of biosecurity significance to Australia.

REFERENCES

Abbass, A., Sharifuzzaman, S. and Austin, B. 2010. Cellular components of probiotics control *Yersinia ruckeri* infection in rainbow trout, *Oncorhynchus mykiss* (Walbaum). *J Fish Dis* **33**: 31–7.

Anderson, D.P. and Ross, A.J. 1972. Comparative study of Hagerman redmouth disease oral bacterins. *Prog Fish Cult* **34**: 226–8.

Anderson, D.P. and Nelson, J.R. 1974. Comparison of protection in rainbow trout (*Salmo gairdneri*) inoculated with and fed Hagerman redmouth bacterins. *J Fish Res Board Can* **31**: 214–16.

Austin, D.A., Robertson, P.A.W. and Austin, B. 2003. Recovery of a new biogroup of *Yersinia ruckeri* from diseased rainbow trout (*Oncorhynchus mykiss*, Walbaum). *System Appl Microbiol* **26**: 127–31.

Bastardo, A., Bohle, H., Ravelo, C., *et al.*, 2011. Serological and molecular heterogeneity among *Yersinia ruckeri* strains isolated from farmed Atlantic salmon *Salmo salar* in Chile. *Dis Aquat Org* **93**: 207–14.

Bridle, A., Nosworthy, E., Polinski, M. and Nowak, B.F. 2011. Evidence of an antimicrobial-immunomodulatory role of Atlantic salmon cathelicidins during infection with *Yersinia ruckeri*. *PLoS One* **6**: e23417.

Bridle, A.R., Koop, B.F. and Nowak, B.F. 2012. Identification of surrogates of protection against yersiniosis in immersion vaccinated Atlantic salmon. *PLoS One* **7**: e40841.

Busch, R.A. 1973. *The serological surveillance of salmonid populations for presumptive evidence of specific disease association*. PhD thesis, University of Idaho.

Chang, C.I., Zhang, Y.A., Zou, J., *et al.*, 2006. Two cathelicidin genes are present in both rainbow trout (*Oncorhynchus mykiss*) and Atlantic salmon (*Salmo salar*). *Antimicrob Agents Chemother* **50**: 185–95.

Chen, P.E., Cook, C., Stewart, A.C., *et al.*, 2010. Genomic characterization of the *Yersinia* genus. *Genome Biol* **11**: R1.

Costa, A.A., Leef, M.J., Bridle, A.R., *et al.*, 2011. Effect of vaccination against yersiniosis on the relative percent survival, bactericidal and lysozyme response of Atlantic salmon, *Salmo salar*. *Aquaculture* **315**: 201–6.

Dahiya, I. and Stevenson, R.M.W. 2010. The UvrY response regulator of the BarA-UvrY two-component system contributes to *Yersinia ruckeri* infection of rainbow trout (*Oncorhynchus mykiss*). *Arch Microbiol* **192**: 541–7.

Davies, R. 1990. O-serotyping of *Yersinia ruckeri* with special emphasis on European isolates. *Vet Microbiol* **22**: 299–307.

Davies, R. and Frerichs, G.N. 1989. Morphological and biochemical differences among isolates of *Yersinia ruckeri* obtained from wide geographical areas. *J Fish Dis* **12**: 357–65.

Deshmukh, S., Raida, M.K., Dalsgaard, I., *et al.*, 2012. Comparative protection of two different commercial vaccines against *Yersinia ruckeri* serotype O1 and biotype 2 in rainbow trout (*Oncorhynchus mykiss*). *Vet Immunol Immunopathol* **145**: 379–85.

Diaz-Rosales, P., Bird, S., Wang, T.H., *et al.*, 2009. Rainbow trout interleukin-2: cloning, expression and bioactivity analysis. *Fish Shellfish Immunol* **27**: 414–22.

Fernandez, L., Lopez, J., Secades, P., *et al.*, 2003. *In vitro* and *in vivo* studies of the Yrp1 protease from *Yersinia ruckeri* and its role in protective immunity against enteric red mouth disease of salmonids. *Appl Environ Microbiol* **69**: 7328–35.

Fernandez, L., Prieto, M. and Guijarro, J.A. 2007a. The iron- and temperature-regulated haemolysin *yhia* is a virulence factor of *Yersinia ruckeri*. *Microbiology* **153**: 483–9.

Fernandez, L., Mendez, J. and Guijarro, J.A. 2007b. Molecular virulence mechanisms of the fish pathogen *Yersinia ruckeri*. *Vet Microbiol* **125**: 1–10.

Frerichs, G.N. 1993. Isolation and identification of fish bacterial pathogens, in *Bacterial Diseases of Fish* (eds V. Inglis, R.J. Roberts and N.R. Bromage). Oxford, Blackwell Scientific Publications, 270–72.

Galligani, G., David-Andersen, I. and Fossum, B. 2005. Regulatory constraints as seen from the pharmaceutical industry. *Dev Biol (Basel)* **121**: 235–41.

Håstein, T., Gudding, R. and Evensen, Ø. 2005. Bacterial vaccines for fish – an update of the current situation worldwide. *Dev Biol (Basel)* **121**: 55–74.

Horne, M.T. and Barnes, A.C. 1999. Enteric redmouth disease (*Yersinia ruckeri*), in *Fish Diseases and Disorders, Viral, Bacterial and Fungal Infections*, 2nd edn (eds P.T.K. Woo and D.W. Bruno). Wallingford, CABI, 455–77.

Johnson, K., Flynn, J. and Amend, D. 1982. Duration of immunity in salmonids vaccinated by direct immersion with *Yersinia ruckeri* and *Vibrio anguillarum* bacterins. *J Fish Dis* **5**: 207–13.

Klontz, G.W. 1963. Oral immunization of rainbow trout against redmouth, in *Proceedings of the Northwest Fish Cultural Conference*, Olympia, Washington 5–6 December, p.121.

Koppang, E.O., Haugarvoll, E., Hordvik, I., *et al.*, 2005. Vaccine-associated granulomatous inflammation and melanin accumulation in Atlantic salmon, *Salmo salar* L., white muscle. *J Fish Dis* **28**: 13–22.

Lee, S.B., Mine, Y. and Stevenson, R.M.W. 2000. Effects of hen egg yolk immunoglobulin in passive protection of rainbow trout against *Yersinia ruckeri*. *J Agric Food Chem* **48**: 110–15.

Mendez, J. and Guijarro, J.A. 2013. *In vivo* monitoring of *Yersinia ruckeri* in fish tissues: progression and virulence gene expression. *Environ Microbiol Reports* **5**: 179–85.

Mendez, J., Reimundo, P., Perez-Pascual, D., *et al.*, 2011. A novel *cdsAB* operon is involved in the uptake of L-Cysteine and participates in the pathogenesis of *Yersinia ruckeri*. *J Bacteriol* **193**: 944–51.

Midtlyng, P.J. 2005. Critical assessment of regulatory standards and tests for fish vaccines. *Dev Biol (Basel)* **121**: 219–26.

Midtlyng, P.J. and Lillehaug, A. 1998. Growth of Atlantic salmon *Salmo salar* after intraperitoneal administration of vaccines containing adjuvants. *Dis Aquat Org* **32**: 91–7.

Olesen, N.J. 1991. Detection of the antibody-response in rainbow-trout following immersion vaccination with *Yersinia ruckeri* bacterins by Elisa and passive-immunization. *J Appl Ichthyol* **7**: 36–43.

Raida, M.K. and Buchmann, K. 2007. Temperature-dependent expression of immune-relevant genesin rainbow trout following *Yersinia ruckeri* vaccination. *Dis Aquat Org* **77**: 41–52.

Raida, M.K. and Buchmann, K. 2008. Development of adaptive immunity in rainbow trout, *Oncorhynchus mykiss* (Walbaum) surviving an infection with *Yersinia ruckeri*. *Fish Shellfish Immunol* **25**: 533–41.

Raida, M.K., Nylen, J., Holten-Andersen, L. and Buchmann, K. 2011a. Association between plasma antibody response and protection in rainbow trout *Oncorhynchus mykiss* immersion vaccinated against *Yersinia ruckeri*. *PLoS One* **6**: e18832.

Raida, M.K., Holten-Andersen, L. and Buchmann, K. 2011b. Association between *Yersinia ruckeri* infection, cytokine expression and survival in rainbow trout (*Oncorhynchus mykiss*). *Fish Shellfish Immunol* **30**: 1257–64.

Romalde, J.L. and Toranzo, A.E. 1993. Pathological activities of *Yersinia-ruckeri*, the enteric redmouth (ERM) bacterium. *FEMS Microbiol Lett* **112**: 291–300.

Romalde, J.L., Magariños, B., Barja, J.L. and Toranzo, A.E. 1993. Antigenic and molecular characterization of *Yersinia ruckeri*. Proposal for a new intraspecies classification. *System Appl Microbiol* **16**: 411–19.

Ross, A.J. and Klontz, G.W. 1965. Oral immunization of rainbow trout (*Salmo gairdneri*) against an etiologic agent of redmouth disease. *J Fish Res Board Can* **22**: 763–70.

Ross, A.J., Rucker, R.R. and Ewing, W.H. 1966. Description of a bacterium associated with redmouth disease of rainbow trout (*Salmo gairdneri*). *Can J Microbiol* **12**: 763–70.

Rucker, R. 1966. Redmouth disease of rainbow trout (*Salmo gairdneri*). *Bull Off Int Epiz* **65**: 825–30.

Ryckaert, J., Bossier, P., D'Herde, K., *et al.*, 2010. Persistence of *Yersinia ruckeri* in trout macrophages. *Fish Shellfish Immunol* **29**: 648–55.

Schill, W.B., Phelps, S.R. and Pyle, S.W. 1984. Multilocus electrophoretic assessment of the genetic structure and diversity of *Yersinia ruckeri*. *Appl Environ Microbiol* **48**: 975–9.

Temprano, A., Riano, J., Yugueros, J., *et al.*, 2005. Potential use of a *Yersinia ruckeri* O1 auxotrophic aroA mutant as a live attenuated vaccine. *J Fish Dis* **28**: 419–27.

Tinsley, J.W., Austin, D.A., Lyndon, A. and Austin, B. 2011a. Novel non-motile phenotypes of *Yersinia ruckeri* suggest expansion of the current clonal complex theory. *J Fish Dis* **34**: 311–17.

Tinsley, J.W., Lyndon, A.R. and Austin, B. 2011b. Antigenic and cross-protection studies of biotype 1 and biotype 2 isolates of *Yersinia ruckeri* in rainbow trout, *Oncorhynchus mykiss* (Walbaum). *J Appl Microbiol* **11**: 8–16.

Tobback, E.A., Decostere, A., Hermans, K., *et al.*, 2007. *Yersinia ruckeri* infections in salmonid fish. *J Fish Dis* **30**: 257–68.

Tobback, E., Decostere, A., Hermans, K., *et al.*, 2009a. Route of entry and tissue distribution of *Yersinia ruckeri* in experimentally infected rainbow trout *Oncorhynchus mykiss*. *Dis Aquat Org* **84**: 219–28.

Tobback, E., Decostere, A., Hermans, K., *et al.*, 2009b. *In vitro* markers for virulence in *Yersinia ruckeri*. *J Fish Dis* **33**: 197–209.

Wang, T., Martin, S.A. and Secombes, C.J. 2009. Two interleukin-17C-like genes exist in rainbow trout *Oncorhynchus mykiss* that are differentially expressed and modulated. *Dev Comp Immunol* **34**: 491–500.

Wheeler, R.W., Davies, R.L., Dalsgaard, I., *et al.*, 2009. *Yersinia ruckeri* biotype 2 isolates from mainland Europe and the UK likely represent different clonal groups. *Dis Aquat Org* **84**: 25–33.

20 Vaccination against Streptococcosis and Lactococcosis

Julia W. Pridgeon and Phillip H. Klesius

USDA-ARS, Aquatic Animal Health Research Laboratory, Alabama, USA

ABSTRACT

Streptococcosis and lactococcosis are hyperacute systemic diseases that can occur in both cultured and wild fish species in various aquatic environments of all countries that sustain an active aquaculture. The causative agents of streptococcosis and lactococcosis are gram-positive bacteria belonging to the genus *Streptococcus* and *Lactococcus*, respectively, including *S. agalactiae*, *S. iniae*, and *L. garvieae*. Their occurrence, significance, etiology, pathogenesis, vaccines, vaccination procedures, vaccine effects and side-effects are included in this review, with a focus on their vaccine development.

20.1 OCCURRENCE

Streptococcosis and lactococcosis are hyperacute systemic diseases that can occur in both cultured and wild fish species in various aquatic environments (freshwater, estuarine, and marine). Many fish species are affected by streptococcosis/lactococcosis, including tilapia, catfish, carp, grouper, mullet, pomfret, trout, salmon, flounder, sea bream, red porgy, barramundi, rabbitfish, hybrid striped bass, yellowtail, sturgeon, amberjack, and rockfish. Therefore, streptococcosis and lactococcosis are important bacterial diseases in all countries that sustain an active aquaculture industry.

20.2 SIGNIFICANCE

Streptococcus and *Lactococcus* are major bacterial pathogens causing infectious diseases not only in fish, but also in humans and other vertebrates such as pigs and cattle. For example, *S. agalactiae* (group B streptococcus) is an important cause of disease in infants, pregnant women, the elderly and immune-suppressed adults (Heath, 2011). In addition, *S. agalactiae*

julia.pridgeon@ars.usda.gov

Fish Vaccination, First Edition. Edited by Roar Gudding, Atle Lillehaug and Øystein Evensen.

is responsible for many cases of mastitis in dairy animals (Watts *et al.*, 1984). In aquaculture, *S. agalactiae* affects both cultured and wild fish species in various aquatic environments (freshwater, estuarine, and marine). Outbreaks of streptococcosis can cause massive mortality in fish farms. For example, in August and September of 2001, *S. agalactiae* was responsible for a massive fish kill at Kuwait Bay, causing a loss of over 2500 metric tons of wild mullet (*Liza klunzingeri*) (Glibert *et al.*, 2002). In 2009, streptococcosis outbreaks were responsible for 50–70% mortality of tilapia in some farms in China (Lu, 2010). In addition, *S. agalactiae* was reported to be the causative agent of disease outbreaks from 2007 to 2011 in Queensland, Australia, in giant Queensland grouper (*Epinephelus lanceolatus*), which can grow to 4 m and weigh up to 400 kg (Bowater *et al.*, 2012). In Taiwan, lactococcosis outbreaks in 1997 and 1998 caused significant mortality to rainbow trout and grey mullet (Chen *et al.*, 2002). In Turkey, between May and June of 2001, lactococcosis outbreak caused by *Lactococcus garvieae* was responsible for 80% mortality in rainbow trout (weight of 100–150 g) (Diler *et al.*, 2002). In August 2003, a disease outbreak caused by *L. garvieae* caused 25% to 40% mortality among 3 to 4 month old cultured flounder in a farm in Hebei province of China (Fang *et al.*, 2006). In Iran, of the 108 gram-positive isolates cultured from diseased rainbow trout in seven provinces from 2008 to 2009, 49 samples (45%) were identified as *S. iniae*, 37 samples (35%) matched with *Lactococcus garvieae*, and 22 samples (19%) were identified as members of genus *Streptooccus* (Haghighi Karsidani *et al.*, 2010), suggesting that the rainbow trout farms in Iran are severely affected by both streptococcosis and lactococcosis. Annual economic losses to the aquaculture industry due to *S. iniae* infection alone has been estimated to be US$10 million in the US and $100 million globally (Shoemaker *et al.*, 2001).

20.3 ETIOLOGY

Streptococcosis and lactococcosis are caused by gram-positive bacteria belonging to the genus *Streptococcus* and *Lactococcus*, respectively. Both *Streptococcus* and *Lactococcus* belong to the *Streptococcaceae* family (Bacteria; Firmicutes; Lactobacillales). Various *Streptococcus* and *Lactococcus* species have been reported as fish pathogens, including *S. agalactiae* (Glibert *et al.*, 2002), *S. iniae* (Al Harbi, 2011), *S. dysgalactiae* (Pourgholam *et al.*, 2011), *S. phocae* (Gonzalez-Contreras *et al.*, 2011), *S. parauberis* (Park *et al.*, 2009), *S. ictaluri* (Shewmaker *et al.*, 2007), *S. milleri* (Austin and Robertson, 1993), *L. garvieae* (Fang *et al.*, 2006), and *L. lactis* (Gürpinar and Savasan, 2010).

Streptococcus was first reported in the bacterial flora of normal fish in Norway in 1943 (Thjøtta and Sømme, 1943). *Streptococcus* of alpha-hemolytic (Foo *et al.*, 1985), beta-hemolytic (Kusuda *et al.*, 1976; Minami *et al.*, 1979), and gamma-hemolytic or non-hemolytic (Rasheed and Plumb, 1984) have all been reported to cause diseases in fish. Serotypes of *S. agalactiae* isolated from diseased fish are either type Ia, type Ib, or type II (Bowater *et al.*, 2012; Guo *et al.*, 2012). Both biotype I and biotype II of *Streptococcus iniae* (Sheehan *et al.*, 2009) have been reported to cause streptococcosis in fish.

The etiological agent of lactococcosis is *Lactococcus garviae*. In 1991, *Enterococcus seriolicida* (synonym of *Lactococcus garvieae*: Eldar *et al.*, 1996) was isolated from diseased yellowtails and eels in Japan (Kusuda *et al.*, 1991). In 2002, *L. garvieae* was reported to be the causative agent of disease outbreaks in grey mullet (*Mugil cephalus*) in Taiwan (Chen *et al.*, 2002). In 2003, *Lactococcus garvieae* infection was reported in wild wrasse *Coris aygula* in the Red Sea (Colorni *et al.*, 2003). In 2004, *L. garvieae* was reported to be an emerging pathogen in cultured rainbow trout in Portugal (Pereira *et al.*, 2004) and rockfish (*Sebastes schlegeli*) in Japan (Kobayashi *et al.*, 2004). In 2006, *L. garvieae* was reported to be responsible for a 2003 disease outbreak in flounder *Paralichthys olivaceus* cultured in China (Fang *et al.*, 2006). In 2007, a series of *Lactococcus garvieae* outbreaks were reported in rainbow trout cultured in Greece (Savvidis *et al.*, 2007). In 2010, *L. garvieae* was reported to be one of the main fish pathogens responsible for a disease outbreak in rainbow trout cultured in Iran (Haghighi Karsidani *et al.*, 2010). In 2011, *L. garvieae* was reported in diseased rainbow trout cultured in Spain (Aguado-Urda *et al.*, 2011). Both *Streptococcus* and *Lactococcus* bacteria are known to be able to cause disease outbreaks in human and other animals (Wang *et al.*, 2007; MacFarquhar *et al.*, 2010). However, the origins of these bacteria are currently unknown.

20.4 PATHOGENESIS

Several studies have been performed to understand the pathogenesis of streptococcosis and lactococcosis. Studies on the effect of exotoxin on streptococcal infections in cultured yellowtails (*Seriola spp.*) demonstrated that bacteria-free exotoxin extracts were able to induce mortality in fish (Kimura and Kusuda, 1979, 1982). However, inoculation with either low virulence or virulent bacteria alone failed to produce the disease in the fish (Kimura and Kusuda, 1979, 1982). Cytolysin produced by *S. iniae* is reported to confer hemolytic phenotype on blood agar media (Fuller *et al.*, 2002). Studies of transposon mutants have demonstrated that *S. iniae* streptolysin S expression is required for local tissue necrosis (Fuller *et al.*, 2002). Large-scale screening of 1128 signature-tagged transposon mutants through a zebrafish model allowed identification of several putative capsule synthesis genes for successful *S. iniae* infection (Miller and Neely, 2005). In addition, capsule gene cpsD (required for capsule polymerization and export in group B *Streptococcus*) was demonstrated to be a virulence factor of *S. iniae* through a gene deletion strategy in hybrid striped bass (Locke *et al.*, 2007a). Capsule polysaccharide was also demonstrated to be a virulence factor for *S. iniae* in Japanese flounder (Shutou *et al.*, 2007). Random transposon mutagenesis and high-throughput screening in a hybrid striped bass model revealed that phosphoglucomutase was a virulence factor for *S. iniae* (Buchanan *et al.*, 2005). It was demonstrated that the deletion mutant of phosphoglucomutase was severely attenuated and cleared more rapidly in the blood of hybrid striped bass (Buchanan *et al.*, 2005). Streptolysin S, a secreted pore-forming cytotoxin, was also demonstrated to be a virulence factor of *S. iniae* in hybrid striped bass (Locke *et al.*, 2007b). M-like protein was also reported to play a significant role in the virulence of *S. iniae* (Locke *et al.*, 2008). Using both whole-genome pyrosequencing and transposon mutagenesis, a polysaccharide deacetylase was demonstrated to play a role in the pathogenesis of *S. iniae*, including adherence and invasion to the fish host, lysozyme resistance, and survival in fish blood (Milani *et al.*, 2010). Although different virulence factors have been reported, the exact pathogenetic mechanisms of streptococcosis and lactococcosis remain to be elucidated.

20.5 VACCINES

Currently, at least one vaccine is commercially available for aquaculture to fight *S. agalactiae* infections. In 2011, Merck Animal Health Inc. obtained regulatory approval in Brazil to begin marketing AQUAVAC® Strep Sa, an inactivated oil-adjuvant vaccine that provides protection against *Streptococcus agalactiae* infections in tilapia and other susceptible fish species. However, AQUAVAC® Strep Sa is only available for administration by injection to fish weighing more than 15 grams, which is rather labor-intensive. In addition, the fish that farmers obtain from the hatchery are 1 to 2 weeks old, weighing 3–5 g or less. Therefore, a *S. agalactiae* vaccine that is safe and efficacious to smaller fish is urgently needed. Experimentally, formalin-killed cells along with concentrated extracellular products (greater than 3 kDa) of a single isolate of *S. agalactiae* have been reported to offer significant protection to 30 g tilapia, but not to 5 g tilapia, with a relative percent survival (RPS) of 80% in vaccinated fish compared with non-vaccinated fish at 30 days post-vaccination (Evans *et al.*, 2004). However, the RPS dropped to 60%, 55%, and 46% at 47, 90, and 180 days post-vaccination, respectively (Pasnik *et al.*, 2005). It was also reported that a formalin-killed *S. agalactiae* vaccine was able to increase the antibody titer in vaccinated fish compared with control fish. However, vaccination by either intraperitoneal injection or by a combination of intraperitoneal injection and oral booster vaccination (one and two doses per month) failed to protect Nile tilapia from *S. agalactiae* infections (Manjaiang *et al.*, 2007). In addition, when 85 *S. agalactiae* strains with 10 distinct pulsed-field gel electrophoresis (PFGE) genotypes (A–J) were used to develop an inactivated whole-cell bacterial vaccine, it was found that the protective immunity of *S. agalactiae* was not only associated with their serotypes, but also related to their PFGE genotypes (Chen *et al.*, 2012). To provide broader protection to fish against infections caused by *S. agalactiae*, a polyvalent attenuated vaccine consisting of 30 isolates of *S. agalactiae* was developed through a sparfloxacin-resistance strategy (Pridgeon and Klesius, 2013). The polyvalent vaccine provided significant ($P < 0.001$) protection to both 3–5 g and 15–20 g Nile tilapia against challenges with 30 parent isolates of *S. agalactiae* (Pridgeon and Klesius, 2013).

Besides *S. agalactiae*, *S. iniae* is also an important fish pathogen in aquaculture. A bacterin vaccine is currently available in Asia to protect tilapia from *S. iniae* infection (Sommerset *et al.*, 2005). However, no *S. iniae* vaccine is currently available for use in other parts of the world. The most extensively studied *S. iniae* vaccines are bacterins (Eldar *et al.*, 1997; Bercovier *et al.*, 1997; Romalde *et al.*, 1999). These formalin-killed *S. iniae* bacterins have been previously used successfully as vaccines to protect rainbow trout in Israel. However, recently it has been reported that these bacterins are unable to protect fish from infection by variant isolates (serotypes) of *S. iniae* (Bachrach *et al.*, 2001; Eyngor *et al.*, 2008). Other vaccines consisting of both formalin-killed *S. iniae* and concentrated extracellular products of *S. iniae* have been reported to partially protect Nile tilapia (*Oreochromis niloticus* L.) from *S. iniae* infection (Klesius *et al.*, 1999, 2000, 2006; Shoemaker *et al.*, 2006). *Streptococcus iniae* putative secretory antigen DNA vaccine was also reported to offer protection to turbot under laboratory conditions, with a RPS of 73.9% and 92.3%, respectively, when challenged with high and low doses (producing a cumulative mortality of 92% and 52%, respectively, in the control groups) of *S. iniae* (Sun *et al.*, 2010). In addition to bacterin and DNA vaccines, live attenuated *S. iniae* strains defective in phosphoglucomutase and M-like protein have been reported to offer protection against homologous *S. iniae* challenge (Buchanan *et al.*, 2005; Locke *et al.*, 2008). However, it is not clear whether they offer protection against heterologous *S. iniae*. Recently, a highly efficacious attenuated novobiocin-resistant *Streptococcus iniae* vaccine (named ISNO) has been reported to protect tilapia for at least 6 months against a virulent *S. iniae* strain (Pridgeon and Klesius, 2011). In addition, ISNO is able to offer protection against heterologous virulent strains of *S. iniae* (F3CB, 102F1K, 405F1K, IF6, and ARS60) at 2 month post-vaccination, with RPS of 78%, 90%, 100%, 100%, and 100%, respectively (Pridgeon and Klesius, 2011). Furthermore, ISNO vaccine has a wide range of efficacious immunization dosages, with RPS values of 81%, 94%, 100%, 100%, 100%, and 100% at vaccination dosages of 10^2, 10^3, 10^4, 10^5, 10^6, and 10^7 CFU/fish, respectively (Pridgeon and Klesius, 2011). In addition to *S. agalactiae* and *S. iniae*, other *Streptococcus* bacteria such as *S. dysgalactiae* and *S. phocae* are also emerging as important pathogens in aquaculture. Currently, no vaccine is commercially available to protect fish from infections by *S. dysgalactiae* or *S. phocae*.

For *Lactococcus garvieae* infections, vaccines are commercially available for rainbow trout in Italy, France, and UK (Sommerset *et al.*, 2005). A commercial vaccine for *L. garvieae* is also available for amberjack/yellowtail in Japan (Sommerset *et al.*, 2005). It was reported that formalin-inactivated *L. garvieae* was able to protect trout for five months under laboratory conditions and three months under field conditions, with protection rates of 70–80% (Bercovier *et al.*, 1997). Similarly, formalin-killed *L. garvieae* cells of KG- phenotype (capsulated phenotype) or of KG+ phenotype cells (unencapsulated phenotype) were reported to confer long-term protection to yellowtails when these vaccines were administered by intraperitoneal injection (Ooyama *et al.*, 1999). In addition, studies have been performed to compare different adjuvants of *L. garvieae* vaccine to the aqueous bacterin vaccine alone (Ravelo *et al.*, 2006). It was found that both the aqueous and the non-mineral oil adjuvanted vaccine (Aquamun) yielded good protection at 4 weeks after immunization, with RPS above 80% (Ravelo *et al.*, 2006). However, at three months after vaccination, the non-adjuvanted vaccine offered only 40% protection, whereas the Aquamun-adjuvanted vaccine offered 92% protection (Ravelo *et al.*, 2006). It was also found that the Aquamun-adjuvanted *L. garvieae* vaccine offered high protection at 6 and 8 months post-vaccination (with RPS of 90% and 83%, respectively) (Ravelo *et al.*, 2006). Similarly, when formalin-inactivated *L. garvieae* bacterin vaccines were combined with Freund's incomplete adjuvant, the vaccines were found to provide longer protection against virulent *L. garvieae* infections in rainbow trout compared with that without the adjuvant (Kubilay *et al.*, 2008). In addition to formalin-killed *L. garvieae* bacterin vaccine, live attenuated *L. garvieae* as an experimental vaccine has also been reported. An attenuated *L. garvieae* strain lacking a virulence-associated capsule on its cell surface as a live vaccine has been reported to confer long-lasting protection to yellowtail, *Seriola quinqueradiata* (Ooyama *et al.*, 2006).

20.6 VACCINATION PROCEDURES AND VACCINE EFFECT

Three major procedures (i.e., injection, immersion, and oral feeding) commonly used for other vaccines are also used for streptococcosis/lactococcosis vaccines. Streptococcosis bacterin vaccine administered by intraperitoneal (IP) injection was reported to offer higher protection to yellowtail than that administered by oral feeding (Iida *et al.*, 1982). Formalin-killed bacterin vaccines of beta-hemolytic *Streptococcus sp.* offered significant protection to rainbow trout against virulent *Streptococcus sp.* through both IP injection and bath immersion routes, with RPS of 70% or greater (Sakai *et al.*, 1987). In addition to the typical intraperitoneal injection route, intramuscular injection routes can also be used to vaccinate fish. However, the intramuscular injection route was found to be less efficient than the intraperitioneal injection route in some cases. For example, when formalin-killed *S. iniae* ARS-10 vaccine was administered to tilapia by intraperitoneal injection, the RPS was 45.6% after fish were challenged with the homologous isolate *S. iniae* ARS-10. However, the RPS was only 17.7% when the same vaccine was administered by intramuscular injection (Klesius *et al.*, 2000). Similarly, the formalin-killed *S. iniae* ARS-10 vaccine offered 93.7% protection to tilapia against challenge by a heterologous isolate *S. iniae* ARS-60 through intraperitoneal injection, whereas the same vaccine only offered 59.5% protection against the heterologous isolate ARS-60 when administered by intramuscular injection (Klesius *et al.*, 2000).

Comparison of IP injection and bath immersion procedures for the same vaccine revealed that IP injection typically offers better protection than bath immersion. For example, formalin-killed bacterin vaccine of *S. agalactiae* (ARS-KU-MU-11B) offered 30 g tilapia 80% protection by IP injection. However, bath immunization of 30 g tilapia resulted in RPS values that were half those achieved with IP vaccination (Evans *et al.*, 2004). In addition to the typical injection and immersion vaccination procedures, oral feeding of vaccine is also used. When formalin-killed bacterin vaccine of *Streptococcus* sp was evaluated in cultured yellowtail in three vaccination procedures (IP injection, oral feeding, and hyperosmotic infiltration), IP injection was found to be the best, followed by hyperosmotic infiltration and oral feeding (Iida *et al.*, 1982). When formalin-killed bacterin vaccine of *S. iniae* was administered to rainbow trout, IP injection offered 74–100% protection, whereas immersion and oral feeding routes offered 30–45% and 9–29% protection, respectively (Soltani *et al.*, 2007).

Oral vaccinations with encapsulated and non-encapsulated antigens were also evaluated as alternative immunization procedures against trout lactococcosis (Kawai and Hatamoto, 1999). It was found the alginate-encapsulated vaccine (RPS of 50%) offered the best protective rates of oral immunization procedures (Kawai and Hatamoto, 1999). However, oral feeding of alginate-encapsulated vaccine should not be used as the primary immunization method since it was not as effective as injection (Kawai and Hatamoto, 1999). When trout were primarily immunized by an aqueous-based *L. garvieae* bacterin vaccine by IP injection followed by a booster oral feeding of encapsulated vaccine, the RPS was increased to 87% (Kawai and Hatamoto, 1999).

For live bacterial vaccine, bath immersion could be as effective as injection. For example, live attenuated *S. iniae* vaccine ISNO offered 88% protection to tilapia against virulent *S. iniae* challenge when administered by bath immersion (Pridgeon and Klesius, 2011). When ISNO was administered to tilapia by IP injection, it offered 100% protection to tilapia against *S. iniae* infection (Pridgeon and Klesius, 2011).

In addition to the three typical vaccination methods, a new administration method, percutaneous administration by immersion with application of a multiple puncture instrument, was also developed (Nakanishi *et al.*, 2002). For the vaccination of juvenile rainbow trout against β-hemolytic *Streptococcus*, this simple and convenient method was found to be as effective as intraperitoneal injection. Small skin lesions were produced using a multiple puncture instrument while fish were immersed in a vaccine suspension containing formalin-killed *Streptococcus iniae*. Upon challenge, 2 weeks after vaccination, mortality of fish vaccinated by this method was 40%, which was equal to that obtained by IP injection, whereas non-vaccinated control fish and fish vaccinated by immersion (without multiple puncture) each had 80% mortality (Nakanishi *et al.*, 2002).

Streptococcosis bacterin vaccine was reported to be highly effective in turbot (*Scophthalmus maximus*), with RPS of 100% by IP injection (Romalde *et al.*, 1999). Formalin-killed *S. iniae* with concentrated extracellular product (ECP) as vaccine was reported to offer 91% protection in tilapia, *Oreochromis niloticus*, by IP injection (Klesius *et al.*, 1999). IP-injected, formalin-killed *S. agalactiae* plus ECP vaccine was able to offer 80% and 25% protection to 30 g and 5 g tilapia, respectively (Evans *et al.*, 2004). When adjuvanted with Aquamun, formalin-killed *Lactococcus garvieae* vaccine was reported to offer 92% protection in rainbow trout at 3 months post-vaccination (Ravelo *et al.*, 2006). A formalin-killed vaccine of *Streptococcus sp.*, when administered by IP injection along with Freund's complete adjuvant, offered sea bass 100%, 92%, and 74% protection rates at 10, 20, and 30 days post-vaccination, respectively (Wanman *et al.*, 2007). A putative secretory antigen Sia10 DNA vaccine was reported to offer protection to turbot, with RPS of 73.9% and 92.3%, respectively, when challenged with high and low doses (producing a cumulative mortality of 92% and 52%, respectively, in the control groups) of *S. iniae* (Sun *et al.*, 2010). Live attenuated *S. iniae* strains defective in phosphoglucomutase and M-like protein were reported to offer significant protection against homologous *S. iniae* challenge (Buchanan *et al.*, 2005; Locke *et al.*, 2008). An attenuated *S. iniae* vaccine (ISNO) was reported to protect tilapia for at least 6 months against a virulent *S. iniae* strain (Pridgeon and Klesius, 2011). In addition, ISNO was reported to protect tilapia against heterologous virulent strains of *S. iniae* (F3CB, 102F1K, 405F1K, IF6, and ARS60) at 2 months post-vaccination, with RPS of 78%, 90%, 100%, 100%, and 100%, respectively (Pridgeon and Klesius, 2011).

20.7 SIDE-EFFECTS

Non-adjuvanted killed streptococcosis/lactococcosis vaccines usually offer protection for a limited period of time. To increase their duration of protection, oil adjuvants are usually added to the aqueous vaccines. However, adjuvanted vaccines have been reported to retard fish growth (Midtlyng and Lillehaug, 1998). In addition, vaccination could cause intra-abdominal adhesions and injection site lesions (Ronsholdt and McLean, 1999). Therefore, the focus of future vaccine formulation should consider not only the effects of formulation parameters on antigen retention, but also the stresses that could be inflicted upon the fish.

20.8 REGULATIONS

Fish vaccines are considered as "biologics" in the US. Therefore, they are regulated and licensed by the Center for Veterinary Biologics, USDA Animal and Plant Inspection Service (APHIS). APHIS regulates veterinary biologics (vaccines, bacterins, antisera, diagnostic kits, and other products of biological origin) to ensure that the veterinary biologics available for the diagnosis, prevention, and treatment of animal diseases are pure, safe, potent, and effective. APHIS regulation on biologics can be found at www.aphis.usda.gov/animal_health/vet_biologics/vb_regs_and_guidance.shtml. The Code of Federal Regulations regarding fish vaccines can be found at www.aphis.usda.gov/animal_health/vet_biologics/vb_cfr.shtmlon.

REFERENCES

Aguado-Urda, M., Lopez-Campos, G.H., Gibello, A., *et al.*, 2011. Genome sequence of *Lactococcus garvieae* 8831, isolated from rainbow trout lactococcosis outbreaks in Spain. *J Bacteriol* **193**: 4263–4.

Al Harbi, A.H. 2011. Molecular characterization of *Streptococcus iniae* isolated from hybrid tilapia [*Oreochromis niloticus* x *Oreochromis aureus*]. *Aquaculture* **312**: 15–18.

Austin, B. and Robertson, P.A. 1993. Recovery of *Streptococcus milleri* from ulcerated koi carp (*Cyprinus carpio* L.) in the UK. *Bull Eur Assoc Fish Pathol* **13**: 207–9.

Bachrach, G., Zlotkin, A., Hurvitz, A., *et al.*, 2001. Recovery of *Streptococcus iniae* from diseased fish previously vaccinated with a streptococcus vaccine. *Appl Environ Microbiol* **67**: 3756–8.

Bercovier, H., Ghittino, C. and Eldar, A. 1997. Immunization with bacterial antigens: infections with streptococci and related organisms. *Dev Biol Stand* **90**: 153–60.

Bowater, R.O., Forbes-Faulkner, J., Anderson, I.G., *et al.*, 2012. Natural outbreak of *Streptococcus agalactiae* (GBS) infection in wild giant Queensland grouper, *Epinephelus lanceolatus* (Bloch), and other wild fish in northern Queensland, Australia. *J Fish Dis* **35**: 173–86.

Buchanan, J.T., Stannard, J.A., Lauth, X., *et al.*, 2005. *Streptococcus iniae* phosphoglucomutase is a virulence factor and a target for vaccine development. *Infect Immun* **73**: 6935–44.

Chen, M., Wang, R., Li, L.P., *et al.*, 2012. Screening vaccine candidate strains against *Streptococcus agalactiae* of tilapia based on PFGE genotype. *Vaccine* **30**: 6088–92.

Chen, S., Liaw, L., Su, H., *et al.*, 2002. *Lactococcus garvieae*, a cause of disease in grey mullet, *Mugil cephalus* L., in Taiwan. *J Fish Dis* **25**: 727–32.

Colorni, A., Ravelo, C., Romalde, J.L., *et al.*, 2003. *Lactococcus garvieae* in wild red sea wrasse *Coris aygula* (Labridae). *Dis Aquat Org* **56**: 275–8.

Diler, O., Altun, S., Adiloglu, A.K., *et al.*, 2002. First occurrence of streptococcosis affecting farmed rainbow trout (*Oncorhynchus mykiss*) in Turkey. *Bull Eur Assoc Fish Pathol* **22**: 21–6.

Eldar, A., Ghittino, C., Asanta, L., *et al.*, 1996. *Enterococcus seriolicida* is a junior synonym of *Lactococcus garvieae*, a causative agent of septicemia and meningoencephalitis in fish. *Curr Microbiol* **32**: 85–8.

Eldar, A., Horovitcz, A. and Bercovier, H. 1997. Development and efficacy of a vaccine against *Streptococcus iniae* infection in farmed rainbow trout. *Vet Immunol Immunopathol* **56**: 175–83.

Evans, J.J., Klesius, P.H. and Shoemaker, C.A. 2004. Efficacy of *Streptococcus agalactiae* (group B) vaccine in tilapia (*Oreochromis niloticus*) by intraperitoneal and bath immersion administration. *Vaccine* **22**: 3769–73.

Eyngor, M., Tekoah, Y., Shapira, R., *et al.*, 2008. Emergence of novel *Streptococcus iniae* exopolysaccharide-producing strains following vaccination with nonproducing strains. *Appl Environ Microbiol* **74**: 6892–7.

Fang, H., Chen, C. and Zhang, X. 2006. *Lactococcus garvieae* as a pathogen in flounder (*Paralichthys olivaceus* Temminck et Schlegel). *J Fish Sci China* **13**: 403–9.

Foo, J.T., Ho, B. and Lam, T.J. 1985. Mass mortality in *Siganus canaliculatus* due to streptococcal infection. *Aquaculture* **49**: 185–96.

Fuller, J.D., Camus, A.C., Duncan, C.L., *et al.*, 2002. Identification of a streptolysin S-associated gene cluster and its role in the pathogenesis of *Streptococcus iniae* disease. *Infect Immun* **70**: 5730–39.

Glibert, P.M., Landsberg. J.H., Evans, J.J., *et al.*, 2002. A fish kill of massive proportion in Kuwait Bay, Arabian Gulf, 2001: the roles of bacterial disease, harmful algae, and eutrophication. *Harmful Algae* **1**: 215–31.

Gonzalez-Contreras, A., Magariños, B., Godoy, M., *et al.*, 2011. Surface properties of *Streptococcus phocae* strains isolated from diseased Atlantic salmon, *Salmo salar* L. *J Fish Dis* **34** :203–15.

Guo, Y., Zhang, D., Fan, H., *et al.*, 2012. Molecular epidemiology of *Streptococcus agalactiae* isolated from tilapia in Southern China. *J Fish China* **36**: 399–406.

Gürpinar, S. and Savasan, S. 2010. Investigation of Gram-positive bacterial infections in culture fisheries in the Aegean Region. *Etlik Vet Mikrobiyol Derg* **21**: 31–6.

Haghighi Karsidani, S., Soltani, M., Nikbakhat-Brojeni, G., *et al.*, 2010. Molecular epidemiology of zoonotic streptococcosis/lactococcosis in rainbow trout (*Oncorhynchus mykiss*) aquaculture in Iran. *Iran J Microbiol* **2**: 198–209.

Heath, P.T. 2011. An update on vaccination against group B streptococcus. *Exp Rev Vaccines* **10**: 685–94.

Iida, T., Wakabayashi, H. and Egusa, S. 1982. Vaccination for control of streptococcal disease in cultured yellowtail. *Fish Pathol* **16**: 201–6.

Kawai, K. and Hatamoto, K. 1999. Encapsulation of oral delivery vaccine against *Lactococcus garvieae* infection in yellowtail *Seriola quinqueradiata*. *Bull Mar Sci Fish Kochi Univ* **19**: 71–8.

Kimura, H. and Kusuda, R. 1979. Studies on the pathogenesis of streptococcal infection in cultured yellowtails *Seriola spp.*: effect of the cell free culture on experimental streptococcal infection. *J Fish Dis* **2**: 501–10.

Kimura, H. and Kusuda, R. 1982. Studies on the pathogenesis of streptococcal infection in cultured yellowtails, *Seriola spp.*: effect of crude exotoxin fractions from cell-free culture on experimental streptococcal infection. *J Fish Dis* **5**: 471–8.

Klesius, P.H., Shoemaker, C.A. and Evans, J.J. 1999. Efficacy of a killed *Streptococcus iniae* vaccine in tilapia (*Oreochromis niloticus*). *Bull Eur Assoc Fish Pathol* **19**: 39–41.

Klesius, P.H., Shoemaker, C.A. and Evans, J.J. 2000. Efficacy of single and combined *Streptococcus iniae* isolate vaccine administered by intraperitoneal and intramuscular routes in tilapia (*Oreochromis niloticus*). *Aquaculture* **188**: 237–46.

Klesius, P.H., Evans, J.J., Shoemaker, C.A. and Pasnik, D.J. 2006. A vaccination and challenge model using calcein marked fish. *Fish Shellfish Immunol* **20**: 20–28.

Kobayashi, T., Ishitaka, Y., Imai, M. and Kawaguchi, Y. 2004. Pathological studies on *Lactococcus garvieae* infection of cultured rockfish *Sebastes schlegeli*. *Suisan Zoshoku* **52**: 359–64.

Kubilay, A., Altun, S., Ulukoy, G., *et al.*, 2008. Immunization of rainbow trout (*Oncorhynchus mykiss*) against *Lactococcus garvieae* using vaccine mixtures. *Isr J Aquac* **60**: 268–73.

Kusuda, R., Kawai, K., Toyoshima, T. and Komatsu, I. 1976. A new pathogenic bacterium belonging to the genus *Streptococcus* isolated from an epizootic disease of cultured yellowtails. *Nippon Suisan Gakkaishi* **42**: 1345–52.

Kusuda, R., Kawai, K., Salati, F., *et al.*, 1991. *Enterococcus seriolicida sp. nov.*, a fish pathogen. *Int J Syst Bacteriol* **41**: 406–9.

Locke, J.B., Colvin, K.M., Datta, A.K., *et al.*, 2007a. *Streptococcus iniae* capsule impairs phagocytic clearance and contributes to virulence in fish. *J Bacteriol* **189**: 1279–87.

Locke, J.B., Colvin, K.M., Varki, N., *et al.*, 2007b. *Streptococcus iniae* beta-hemolysin streptolysin S is a virulence factor in fish infection. *Dis Aquat Org* **76**: 17–26.

Locke, J.B., Aziz, R.K., Vicknair, M.R., *et al.*, 2008. *Streptococcus iniae* M-like protein contributes to virulence in fish and is a target for live attenuated vaccine development. *PloS One*: e2824.

Lu, M. 2010. Review of research on streptococcosis in tilapia. *S China Fish Sci* **6**: 75–9.

MacFarquhar, J.K., Jones, T.F., Woron, A.M., *et al.*, 2010. Outbreak of late-onset group B *Streptococcus* in a neonatal intensive care unit. *Am J Infect Control* **38**: 283–8.

Manjaiang, P., Areechon, N., Srisapoome, P. and Mahasawas, S. 2007. Application of vaccine to prevent disease caused by *Streptococcus agalactiae* in Nile tilapia (*Oreochromis niloticus*). *Proceedings of the 45th Kasetsart University Annual Conference*, Bangkok, 174–82.

Midtlyng, P.J. and Lillehaug, A. 1998. Growth of Atlantic salmon *Salmo salar* after intraperitoneal administration of vaccines containing adjuvants. *Dis Aquat Org* **32**: 91–7.

Milani, C.J., Aziz, R.K., Locke, J.B., *et al.*, 2010. The novel polysaccharide deacetylase homologue Pdi contributes to virulence of the aquatic pathogen *Streptococcus iniae*. *Microbiology* **156**: 543–54.

Miller, J.D. and Neely, M.N. 2005. Large-scale screen highlights the importance of capsule for virulence in the zoonotic pathogen *Streptococcus iniae*. *Infect Immun* **73**: 921–34.

Minami, T., Nakamura, M., Ikeda, Y. and Ozaki, H. 1979. A beta-hemolytic *Streptococcus* isolated from cultured yellowtail. *Fish Pathol* **1**: 33–8.

Nakanishi, T., Kiryu, I. and Ototake, M. 2002. Vaccine development of a new vaccine delivery method for fish: percutaneous administration by immersion with application of a multiple puncture instrument. *Vaccine* **20**: 3764–9.

Ooyama, T., Kera, A., Okada, T., *et al.*, 1999. The protective immune response of yellowtail *Seriola quinqueradiata* to the bacterial fish pathogen *Lactococcus garvieae*. *Dis Aquat Org* **37**: 121–6.

Ooyama T, Shimahara Y, Nomoto R, *et al.*, 2006. Application of attenuated *Lactococcus garvieae* strain lacking a virulence-associated capsule on its cell surface as a live vaccine in yellowtail *Seriola quinqueradiata* Temminck and Schlegel. *J Appl Ichthyol* **22**: 149–52.

Park, Y., Nho, S., Shin, G., *et al.*, 2009. Antibiotic susceptibility and resistance of *Streptococcus iniae* and *Streptococcus parauberis* isolated from olive flounder (*Paralichthys olivaceus*). *Vet Microbiol* **136**: 76–81.

Pasnik, D.J., Evans, J.J. and Klesius, P.H. 2005. Duration of protective antibodies and correlation with survival in Nile tilapia *Oreochromis niloticus* following *Streptococcus agalactiae* vaccination. *Dis Aquat Org* **66**: 129–34.

Pereira, F., Ravelo, C., Toranzo, A.E. and Romalde, J.L. 2004. *Lactococcus garvieae*, an emerging pathogen for the Portuguese trout culture. *Bull Eur Assoc Fish Pathol* **24**: 274–9.

Pourgholam, R., Laluei, F., Saeedi, A.A., *et al.*, 2011. Distribution and molecular identification of some causative agents of streptococcosis isolated from farmed rainbow trout (*Oncorhynchus mykiss*, Walbaum) in Iran. *Iran J Fish Sci* **10**: 109–22.

Pridgeon, J.W. and Klesius, P.H. 2011. Development and efficacy of a novobiocin-resistant *Streptococcus iniae* as a novel vaccine in Nile tilapia (*Oreochromis niloticus*). *Vaccine* **29**: 5986–93.

Pridgeon, J.W. and Klesius, P.H. 2013. Development of live attenuated *Streptococcus agalactiae* as potential vaccines by selecting for resistance to sparfloxacin. *Vaccine* **31**: 2705–12.

Rasheed, V. and Plumb, J.A. 1984. Pathogenicity of a non-haemolytic group B *Streptococcus* sp. in gulf killifish (*Fundulus grandis* Baird and Girard). *Aquaculture* **37**: 97–105.

Ravelo, C., Magarinos, B., Herrero, M.C., *et al.*, 2006. Use of adjuvanted vaccines to lengthen the protection against lactococcosis in rainbow trout (*Oncorhynchus mykiss*). *Aquaculture* **251**: 153–8.

Romalde, J.L., Magariños, B. and Toranzo, A.E. 1999. Prevention of streptococcosis in turbot by intraperitoneal vaccination: a review. *J Appl Ichthyol* **15**: 153–8.

Ronsholdt, B. and McLean, E. 1999. The effect of vaccination and vaccine components upon short-term growth and feed conversion efficiency in rainbow trout. *Aquaculture* **174**: 213–21.

Sakai, M., Kubota, R., Atsuta, S. and Kobayashi, M. 1987. Vaccination of rainbow trout *Salmo gairdneri* against beta-hemolytic streptococcal disease. *Nippon Suisan Gakkaishi* **53**: 1373–6.

Savvidis, G.K., Anatoliotis, C., Kanaki, Z. and Vafeas, G. 2007. Epizootic outbreaks of lactococcosis disease in rainbow trout, *Oncorhynchus mykiss* (Walbaum), culture in Greece. *Bull Eur Assoc Fish Pathol* **27**: 223–8.

Sheehan, B., Labrie, L., Lee, Y., *et al.*, 2009. Streptococcal diseases in farmed tilapia. *Aqua Asia Paci* **5**(6): 26–9.

Shewmaker, P.L., Camus, A.C., Bailiff, T., *et al.*, 2007. *Streptococcus ictaluri* sp. nov., isolated from channel catfish *Ictalurus punctatus* broodstock. *Int J Syst Evol Microbiol* **57**: 1603–6.

Shoemaker, C.A., Klesius, P.H. and Evans, J.J. 2001. Prevalence of *Streptococcus iniae* in tilapia, hybrid striped bass, and channel catfish on commercial fish farms in the United States. *Am J Vet Res* **62**: 174–7.

Shoemaker, C.A., Vandenberg, G.W., Désormeaux, A., *et al.*, 2006. Efficacy of a *Streptococcus iniae* modified bacterin delivered using Oralject™ technology in Nile tilapia (*Oreochromis niloticus*). *Aquaculture* **255**: 151–6.

Shutou, K., Kanai, K. and Yoshikoshi, K. 2007. Virulence attenuation of capsular polysaccharide-deleted mutants of *Streptococcus iniae* in Japanese flounder *Paralichthys olivaceus*. *Fish Pathol* **42**: 41–8.

Soltani, M., Alishahi, M., Mirzargar, S. and Nikbakht, G. 2007. Vaccination of rainbow trout against *Streptococcus iniae* infection: comparison of different routes of administration and different vaccines. *Iran J Fish Sci* **7**: 129–40.

Sommerset, I., Krossøy, B., Biering, E. and Frost, P. 2005. Vaccines for fish in aquaculture. *Exp Rev Vaccines* **4**: 89–101.

Sun, Y., Hu, Y., Liu, C. and Sun, L. 2010. Construction and analysis of an experimental *Streptococcus iniae* DNA vaccine. *Vaccine* **28**: 3905–12.

Thjøtta, T. and Sømme, O.M. 1943. *The Bacterial Flora of Normal Fish*. Oslo. (Det norske videnskapsakademi i Oslo. I. Matematisk-naturvidenskapelig klasse. Skrifter 1942, no. 4).

Wang, C.Y., Shie, H.S., Chen, S.C., *et al.*, 2007. *Lactococcus garvieae* infections in humans: possible association with aquaculture outbreaks. *Int J Clin Pract* **61**: 68–73.

Wanman, C.H., Tanmark, N. and Supamattaya, K. 2007. Production of killed vaccine from *Streptococcus sp.* and its application in sea bass (*Lates calcarifer*). *Songklanakarin J Sci Tech* **29**: 1251–61.

Watts, J.L., Nickerson, S.C. and Pankey, J.W. 1984. A case study of *Streptococcus* group G infection in a dairy herd. *Vet Microbiol* **9**: 571–80.

21 Vaccination against Piscirickettsiosis

Sergio H. Marshall[1] and Jaime A. Tobar[2]

[1]Institute of Biology, Faculty of Sciences, Pontifical Catholic University of Valparaíso, Valparaíso, Chile
[2]Centrovet-Virbac Ltda., Santiago, Chile

ABSTRACT

Piscirickettsiosis, or salmonid rickettsial septicemia (SRS), caused by *Piscirickettsia salmonis*, has severely challenged the sustainability of the Chilean salmon industry since its appearance in 1989. *P. salmonis* is a facultative gram-negative bacterium for which several aspects of its lifecycle relevant for vaccine development (e.g., virulence and pathogenesis) remain poorly understood. Vaccination plays a pivotal role in this strategy, although its efficiency as a procedure will rely on an adequate interpretation of the biological and immunological features of the target pathogen. At present, although this is not the case for *P. salmonis* and because it has become a serious problem in confined salmon-rearing in Chile, a number of vaccines have been designed and commercialized, so far with moderate effect.

21.1 OCCURRENCE AND SIGNIFICANCE

Piscirickettsia salmonis is the etiological agent of salmonid rickettsial septicemia (SRS), which infects salmonids and other fish species. Coho salmon was the only species affected before the turn of the century. The disease has since spread to all cultivated salmonids, and to other commercial fish species (Chen *et al.*, 1994; Athanassopoulou *et al.*, 2004; Arkush *et al.*, 2005; McCarthy *et al.*, 2005; Rojas *et al.*, 2009).

Although strict management strategies have helped, the problem still remains. Chile has been the most affected geographic area, and although a number of classical vaccines and other prophylactic approaches have been evaluated, the appearance of continuous epizootics is a clear signal that new and efficient strategies are necessary in order to prevent geographic and host-range spread.

At present, recurrent episodes occur, resulting in high mortality and, more importantly, significant damage of muscle tissue, which constitutes the exportable resource (Marshall,

smarshal@ucv.cl

Fish Vaccination, First Edition. Edited by Roar Gudding, Atle Lillehaug and Øystein Evensen.

unpublished). This is a clear indication that, on the one hand, we are dealing with a highly versatile, genetically variable and highly adaptable microorganism, and on the other, that the biology and lifecycle of this bacterium in the environment is not fully understood. The available information originates entirely from *in vitro* experiments, carried out under optimal laboratory conditions, quite different from those faced by the bacteria in the field. There are no reports explaining how it survives or persists in harsh marine environments where it is highly infective. Indeed, it was recently reported that *P. salmonis* is able to survive at low densities in seawater for at least 40 days, an indicator of resistance which unfortunately is not clearly understood (Olivares and Marshall, 2010).

After the initial description in Chile, *P. salmonis* was identified in diseased salmonids in western Canada, Norway and Ireland (Brocklebank *et al.*, 1992; Evelyn, 1992; Olsen *et al.*, 1993; Rodger and Drinan, 1993; Palmer *et al.*, 1997; Almendras and Fuentealba, 1997; Fryer and Hedrick, 2003).

As with all forms of intensive confined cultures where a single species is reared at high population densities, infectious disease agents are able to transmit easily between host individuals, and large economic losses can result from disease outbreaks. This is the case in salmon production in Chile, and *P. salmonis* constituting its largest threat. Husbandry methods are designed and put in practice to minimize these losses by employing a variety of strategies implemented by the authorities, but central to all of these is provision of an optimal culture environment that does not jeopardize the animals health and well-being.

21.2 ETIOLOGY

The bacterium was initially described as a strictly intracellular, non-motile, non-encapsulated, pleomorphic, but generally coccoid bacterium, with a diameter of 0.2 to 1.5 mm (Bravo and Campos, 1989; Mauel *et al.*, 1999). Unfortunately, this information severely hampered its study at the molecular level since the bacteria were only grown in different cell lines (Peña *et al.*, 2010). The situation changed when the bacterium was recently reclassified as a facultative intracellular organism, able to grow in cell-free media (Mauel *et al.*, 2008; Mikalsen *et al.*, 2008; Gómez *et al.*, 2009; Yáñez *et al.*, 2012).

The genus *Piscirickettsia* is a member of the family *Piscirickettsaceae*, within the order *Thiotrichales* belonging to the Gammaproteobacteria group. This family contains six phylogenetically related but phenotypically diverse genera (*Cycloclasticus*, *Hydrogenovibrio*, *Sulfurivirga*, *Thioalkalimicrobium*, *Thiomicrospira* and *Piscirickettsia*). The genus *Piscirickettsia* comprises a single species called *Piscirickettsia salmonis* (Fryer and Lannan, 2005). The wild-type strain, LF89 (ATCC VR-1361), was the first gram-negative intracellular bacterium isolated from fish. This organism was initially described in 1989 in coho salmon (*Oncorhynchus kisutch*) affected by high mortality (70–90%) in southern Chile (Bravo and Campos, 1989). Phenotypically, the bacterium was initially classified as a member of the Alphaproteobacteria in the order *Rickettsiales* within the family *Rickettsiaceae*, and related to the genera *Rickettsia*, *Wolbachia*, *Anaplasma*, and *Ehrlichia* (Fryer *et al.*, 1990). Analysis of the 16S rRNA has allowed reclassification of *P. salmonis* to the Gammaproteobacteria group within the order *Thiotrichales*, constituting *Piscirickettsia salmonis* gen. nov., sp. nov. (Fryer *et al.*, 1992).

To date, the molecular characterization of *P. salmonis* has been poorly reported, and the genome sequence of this pathogen has not been annotated. Most of the molecular studies of *P. salmonis* have focused on the search for antigenic molecules for development of new vaccines. Several molecular chaperones have been characterized by different authors as being relevant for vaccine development: HSP60 (ChaP.s/GroEL), HSP70 (DnaK), HSP10 (GroES), and HSP16 (Wilhelm *et al.*, 2005, 2006; Marshall *et al.*, 2007). Additionally, the OspA antigen has been characterized and used as a recombinant vaccine to moderate effect (Kuzyk *et al.*, 2001a).

Presumptive diagnosis is based on clinical and pathological observations, and confirmed following histopathological examination, isolation in tissue culture combined with either immunofluorescence or immunoperoxidase staining, as well as dot blot DNA hybridization (Noga, 2010). In addition, polymerase chain reaction techniques are available for the rapid identification of *P. salmonis* in clinically affected animals (Marshall *et al.*, 1998).

21.3 PATHOGENESIS

The reclassification of the bacterium as well as its culture potential in cell-free media has favored a better analysis and understanding of pathogenesis of the disease. Some of the following factors might be important in antigen selection of vaccines against piscirickettsiosis: the bacteria's ability to attach firmly to target surfaces, including eggs, by means of complex membrane extensions, named the "piscirickettsial attachment complex" (PAC) (Larenas *et al.*, 2003); its primary infection of host macrophages, which appears to be the site of expansion (McCarthy *et al.*, 2005; Rojas *et al.*, 2009); the detection of a highly immunogenic protein named ChaPs with protective potential (Marshall *et al.*, 2007); the description of highly infective small isoforms of *P. salmonis* (sP.s) both *in vivo* and *in vitro* which have been proposed to comprise the master infective units of the bacterium (Rojas *et al.*, 2008; Marshall *et al.*, 2012); the capacity to induce apoptosis in macrophages *in vitro* as a possible *in vivo* strategy to evade the host immune system (Rojas *et al.*, 2010); the partial analysis of the bacterial genome, which reveals the presence of insertion sequences indicative of high genomic plasticity (GenBank: AF184152; Marshall *et al.*, 2011), as well as two operons coding for toxin-antitoxin proteins, known to be strict regulators of host cell activity (Gómez *et al.*, 2011, GenBank: JQ023629); confirmation that the bacteria skips phagosome-lysosome fusion in fish macrophages as an efficient survival strategy (Gómez *et al.*, 2013); and finally, and most importantly for its implications for vaccine development, the fact that the bacterium under different stress conditions generates biofilm (Marshall *et al.*, 2012) and expresses most genes of a type IV secretion system, both traits have been directly associated with bacterial pathogenic potential (Gómez *et al.*, 2013).

Information relating to the biological behavior of *P. salmonis* will be even more important when genomic sequences from different isolates are completed (Marshall *et al.*, 2011). Several draft genome sequences exist, but none are as yet completed or annotated.

21.4 VACCINES AND VACCINATION

Vaccine development against piscirickettsiosis has been the subject of extensive studies in salmonid fish, with a focus on vaccine composition, challenge design and evaluation parameters (Bravo and Midtlyng, 2007). However, little or no field results are available relating to their efficacy under farm conditions. Despite the economic risk in including unvaccinated control groups, the variation between salmon farms at several levels, including biosafety, weather and water conditions, salmonid species, and fish densities, make vaccine evaluation in the field difficult.

21.5 CURRENT VACCINE STATUS

The first *P. salmonis* vaccines were formulated as formalin-inactivated bacterins, using cell-culture derived organisms grown in CHSE-214 cells, derived from Chinook salmon embryonic cell culture (Fryer, 1992; Gaggero, 1995). Normally, bacterin vaccines have been designed as emulsion preparations applied by intraperitoneal injection in pre-smolt salmon, in order to let vaccinated fish to establish protective immunity before seawater transfer. Bacterins have induced variable protection depending on formulation, bacterial processing, antigen dosage, challenge dose and challenge time post-vaccination, making specific assesment and value for vaccine protection difficult. However, it is clear that antigenic dosage and the time after challenge are the main factors that influence the outcome of bacterin vaccines (Kuzyk *et al.*, 2001a; Birkbeck *et al.*, 2004b; Tobar *et al.*, 2011; Wilda *et al.*, 2012).

The first bacterin-vaccination studies showed the potential of formalin-inactivated *P. salmonis* bacterins as immunogenic agents against SRS. Protection was improved when bacteria were heat-inactivated prior to formulation. Initial bacterin antigens were prepared in classical fish cell lines, which are known to give a very limited bacterial yield. Moreover, considering the addition of adjuvants at a minimum of 20% v/v, bacterin concentrations could reach doses ranging between 10^3-10^4 $TCID_{50}$/fish. Using this scheme, 18 g coho salmon vaccinated with such formulations and challenged 210 degree-days after vaccination gave poor RPS, ranging from −30% to 15% (Kuzyk *et al.*, 2001a). Subsequent improvements to *P. salmonis* culture methodology enabled manufacturers to produce higher bacterial titers (Birkbeck *et al.*, 2004a), which were used for additional bacterin trials in vaccines containing doses 4–5 orders of magnitude greater than previously. Challenge at approximately 2000 degree-days of 100 g Atlantic salmon showed improved RPS values, varying between 70.7% and 49.6% depending on whether the bacterin was formalin- or heat-inactivated (Birkbeck *et al.*, 2004b). This study, besides suggesting the existence of heat-labile, immunosuppressive *P. salmonis* proteins, also supports the notion that high antigen concentrations are essential for protection.

Commercial vaccines have shown promising results under controlled conditions. Survival of 30 g Atlantic salmon vaccinated intraperitoneally with a commercial vaccine (Centrovet Ltda., Santiago, Chile), was reported to be dependent upon time post-vaccination, giving survival rates that ranged from 45% to 90% when challenge was performed at 300 or 600 degree-days after vaccination, respectively (Tobar *et al.*, 2011). Another commercial bacterin vaccine (Recalcine SA, Santiago, Chile), evaluated in 30 g Atlantic salmon and challenged at ~370 degree-days after vaccination, gave a RPS_{60} value, which represents the RPS calculation when control groups reached 60% of mortality, equivalent to 86.4% (Wilda *et al.*, 2012).

Recombinant antigens have also been identified and evaluated. The first description of an efficacious recombinant antigen was the outer membrane protein OspA, discovered using an outer-membrane-directed expression library in *E. coli*. Serum from convalescent fish was used as a probe for antigen identification (Kuzyk *et al.*, 2001a,2001b) and identified a small protein, toxic for *E. coli* expression, which was antigenically optimized using known T-cell epitopes and a fusion partner to avoid toxicity. Antigenic preparations gave high protection in IP challenge (RPS ranging from 50–80%) and were the basis for new recombinant antigen discovery and optimization. Besides the importance of serum from convalescent fish as a screening method for antigen discovery, also subsequently demonstrated for a *Flavobacterium psychrophilum* recombinant vaccine (Crump *et al.*, 2007), the fact that serum-reactive *P. salmonis* proteins behave as good candidates for recombinant vaccines indicates at least the partial need for humoral immunity in obtaining efficient *P. salmonis* protection (Kuzyk *et al.*, 2001a; Wilda *et al.*, 2012).

Other recombinant vaccines evaluated have used multiple antigen formulations, including in its formulation heat-shock proteins, which have been reported as potent adjuvants for vaccines in several animal models (Wilhelm *et al.*, 2005). RPS values after IP challenge varied between 10% and 85% depending on antigenic composition, and serum from convalescent fish recognized recombinant proteins (Wilhelm *et al.*, 2006). Among the antigens identified and studied, the authors described *fliC*, gene important for bacterial flagellum assembly, which although not recognized by fish serum, could help explain the dissemination of *P. salmonis* in water. However, more studies are necessary in order to determine whether *P. salmonis* could exhibit motility under certain environmental conditions.

The bacterins and recombinant vaccines described so far corresponds to injectable vaccines. These vaccines generally provide cost-effective results, reduce uncertainty regarding individual vaccination, and induce the longest-lasting immunity in farmed fish to date (Sommerset, 2005). However, some important issues still need to be addressed, such as side-effect induction (Midtlyng *et al.*, 1996), and particularly in salmon, the duration of immunity.

So far live vaccines have not been evaluated using attenuated *P. salmonis* cells. However, *Arthrobacter davidanieli*, a non-pathogenic bacterium, has been described as being able to induce immunity not only against piscirickettisosis, but also against bacterial kidney disease caused by *Renibacterium salmoninarum*. A vaccine is licensed in Chile and Canada (Novartis Animal Health), and has been reported to induce good protection levels for BKD (80% RPS) and significant reduction of mortality due to piscirickettsiosis under farm conditions (Salonius *et al.*, 2005). Although its mechanism of action has not been described, it has been proposed that this live bacterium could behave as an immunostimulant rather than a specific-immunity inducer (Wietz *et al.*, 2012).

Oral vaccination in fish has been studied from the early 1980s (Vandenberg, 2004; Rombout *et al.*, 2011). Extensive studies have been performed in order to elucidate the basis of fish mucosal protection. However, few oral vaccines for fish are available (Plant and LaPatra, 2011). An oral vaccine against SRS was recently developed and licensed in Chile, showing earlier inducement of protection, but a shorter protection window compared with conventional, oil-based bacterins. Oral vaccination has been demonstrated to induce specific anti-*P. salmonis* IgM antibodies correlating with a reported 85–90% survival of vaccinated fish when vaccine was applied either by feed alone, or as a booster following IP vaccination (Tobar *et al.*, 2011). Additionally, the vaccine has been shown to extend the protection given by an initial IP vaccination, enabling salmon farmers to boost or re-vaccinate fish during the seawater stage with no handling required. The oral delivery route seems another option for non-stressful vaccination, and the coming challenge will be to improve the duration of immunity.

21.6 FUTURE PERSPECTIVES

The efficacy of vaccines against piscirickettsiosis represents one of the most discussed subjects in fish aquaculture. A possible difficulty in the unification of efficacy criteria seems to be the diversity of challenge methods published in the literature, including variations in the time after vaccination when challenge is performed, fish size, water conditions, and the unit by which the efficacy is measured (Smith *et al.*, 1997; Kuzyk *et al.*, 2001a; Birkbeck *et al.*, 2004b; Salonius *et al.*, 2005; Wilhelm *et al.*, 2006; Tobar *et al.*, 2011; Wilda *et al.*, 2012). In order to efficiently develop vaccines it is necessary to design assays with common criteria, which should be strongly based upon the fish susceptibility period and, in the case of anadromous species such as salmon, include the smoltification process and freshwater stages as an important consideration for immunity onset.

Bacterial challenge in vaccine/control trials is complex, with different outcomes depending upon strain type, dose and route of administration (Smith *et al.*, 1997). Additionally, animal welfare issues for vaccine evaluation and the three Rs principle have highlighted the need for additional, objective protection indicators (Midtlyng *et al.*, 2011). Although this is difficult to establish for intracellular pathogens such as *P. salmonis*, some effort has been made. Recently, a vaccine research group has developed a partially validated method for evaluation of specific anti-*P. salmonis* antibodies as a predictor for degree of vaccine protection. The antibody titer was found to strongly correlate with RPS values using an emulsion bacterin vaccine, in a dose–response fashion (Wilda *et al.*, 2012). Considering *P. salmonis* as an intracellular pathogen, it seems at first surprising that humoral immunity could correlate with protection. However, these results are consistent with other vaccination trials with *P. salmonis* vaccines (Kuzyk *et al.*, 2001a; Wilhelm *et al.*, 2006; Tobar *et al.*, 2011). It also applies to other vaccines for salmon against intracellular pathogens, such as the vaccine against infectious salmon anemia (Lauscher *et al.*, 2011). However, the role of the cellular immune response as a predictor for protection against piscirickettsiosis must not be excluded.

New commercial vaccines must bring long-lasting and/or a higher degree of protection under field conditions, as well as being environmentally safe, and not induce side-effects in vaccinated fish. Additionally, vaccines must be applied in a non-stressful fashion. In this respect the oral vaccination route has been demonstrated to be promising.

Alternatives to overcoming such issues are represented by different methods for immunization, such as oral, live or DNA vaccines, which could either enhance immunity duration by allowing re-vaccination in field conditions when injectable vaccine is not practical, or induce a longer-lasting immunity, through mechanisms that are poorly understood to date (Lepa *et al.*, 2010).

DNA vaccines have not been evaluated in depth, although initial reports show promising results at both the immunological and practical level. Conventional eukaryotic promoters driving expression of a random genomic *P. salmonis* library have shown a quantifiable reduction in mortality as well as the induction of specific IgM levels in a dose- and prime/boost-dependent fashion (Miquel *et al.*, 2003), suggesting that with appropriate antigenic research, development of a successful vaccine formulation is possible. More recently, Hsp60 and Hsp70, two different heat-shock proteins from *P. salmonis* cloned in a conventional mammalian expression vector, yielded RPS_{60} values of 40.9–54.5% with proportional antibody titers, suggesting that classical mammalian promoters could be expressed in Atlantic salmon, and that DNA vaccines work and could be optimized by appropriate research.

Considering the actual results for fish DNA vaccinology, the advances in genomic sequencing, and development of improved bioinformatic tools and antigenic prediction, this option represents a reasonable strategy to improve actual vaccines against SRS. To make this strategy a commercial reality, more research must be done regarding safety aspects, in order to efficiently control, follow and validate the safety of DNA vaccine vectors for farmed fish.

REFERENCES

Almendras, F.E. and Fuentealba, I.C. 1997. Salmonid rickettsial septisemia caused by *Piscirickettsia salmonis*: a review. *Dis Aquat Org* **29**: 137–44.

Arkush, K.D., McBride, A.M., Mendonca, H.L., *et al.*, 2005. Genetic characterization and experimental pathogenesis of *Piscirickettsia salmonis* isolated from white seabass *Atractoscion nobilis*. *Dis Aquat Org* **63**: 139–49.

Athanassopoulou, F., Groman, D., Prapas, T.H. and Sabatakou, O. 2004. Pathological and epidemiological observations on rickettsiosis in cultured sea bass (*Dicentrarchus labrax* L.) from Greece. *J Appl Ichth* **20**: 525–9.

Birkbeck, T.H., Griffen, A.A., Reid, H.I., *et al.*, 2004a. Growth of *Piscirickettsia salmonis* to high titers in insect tissue culture cells. *Infect Immun* **72**: 3693–4.

Birkbeck, T.H., Rennie, S., Hunter, D., *et al.*, 2004b. Infectivity of a Scottish isolate of *Piscirickettsia salmonis* for Atlantic salmon *Salmo salar* and immune response of salmon to this agent. *Dis Aquat Org* **60**: 97–103.

Bravo, S. and Campos, M. 1989. Síndrome del salmon Coho. *Chile Pesquero* **54**: 47–8.

Bravo, S. and Midtlyng, P.J. 2007. The use of fish vaccines in the Chilean salmon industry 1999–2003. *Aquaculture* **270**: 36–42.

Brocklebank, J.R., Speare, D.J., Armstrong, R.D. and Evelyn, T. 1992. British Columbia-septicemia suspected to be caused by a rickettsia-like agent in farmed Atlantic salmon. *Can Vet J* **33**: 407–8.

Chen, S.C., Tung, M.C., Chen, S.P., *et al.*, 1994. Systemic granulomas caused by a rickettsia-like organism in Nile tilapia, *Oreochronuis niloticus* (L.), from southern Taiwan. *J Fish Dis* **17**: 591–9.

Crump, E.M., Burian, J., Allen, P.D., *et al.*, 2007. Identification of a ribosomal L10-like protein from *Flavobacterium psychrophilum* as a recombinant vaccine candidate for rainbow trout fry syndrome. *J Mol Microbiol Biotechnol* **13**: 55–64.

Evelyn, T.P.T. 1992. Salmonid rickettsial septicemia, in *Diseases of Seawater Netpen-Reared Salmonid Fishes in the Pacific Northwest* (ed. M.L. Kent). *Can Spec Pub Fish Aquat Sci* **116**: 18–19.

Fryer, J.L. and Hedrick, R.P. 2003. *Piscirickettsia salmonis*: a Gram-negative intracellular bacterial pathogen of fish. *J Fish Dis* **26**: 251–62.

Fryer, J.L. and Lannan, C.N. 2005. Family II. *Piscirickettsiaceae* fam. nov, in *Bergey's Manual of Systematic Bacteriology*, 2nd edn, vol. 2 (The *Proteobacteria*) part B (The *Gammaproteobacteria*) (eds D.J. Brenner, N.R. Krieg, J.T. Staley and G.M. Garrity). New York, Springer, 180.

Fryer, J.L., Lannan, C.N., Garcés, H.L., *et al.*, 1990. Isolation of Rickettsiales-like organism from diseased coho salmon (*Oncorhynchus kisutch*) in Chile. *Fish Pathol* **25**: 107–14.

Fryer, J.L., Lannan, C.N., Giovannoni, S.J. and Wood, N.D. 1992. *Piscirickettsia salmonis* gen. nov. sp. nov. the causative agent of an epizootic disease in salmonid fishes. *Int J Sys Evol Micro* **42**: 120–26.

Gaggero, A., Castro, H. and Sandino, A.M. 1995. First isolation of *Piscirickettsia salmonis* from coho salmon, *Oncorhynchus kisutch* (Walbaum), and rainbow trout, *Oncorhynchus mykiss* (Walbaum), during the freshwater stage of their life cycle. *J Fish Dis* **18**: 277–80.

Gómez, F., Henríquez, V. and Marshall, S.H. 2009. Additional evidence of the facultative intracellular nature of the fish bacterial pathogen *Piscirickettsia salmonis*. *Arch Med Vet* **41**: 261–7.

Gómez, F.A., Cárdenas, C., Henríquez, V. and Marshall, S.H. 2011. Characterization of a functional toxin/anti-toxin module in the genome of the fish pathogen *Piscirickettsia salmonis*. *FEMS Microbiol Lett* **317**: 83–92.

Gómez, F.A., Tobar, J.A., Henríquez, V., *et al.*, 2013. Evidence of the presence of a functional Dot/Icm Type IV-B secretion system in the fish bacterial pathogen *Piscirickettsia salmonis*. *PloS One* **8**: 1–11.

Kuzyk, M.A., Burian, J., Machander, D., *et al.*, 2001a. An efficacious recombinant subunit vaccine against the salmonid rickettsial pathogen *Piscirickettsia salmonis*. *Vaccine* **19**: 2337–44.

Kuzyk, M.A., Burian, J., Thornton, J.C. and Kay, W.W. 2001b. OspA, a lipoprotein antigen of the obligate intracellular bacterial pathogen *Piscirickettsia salmonis*. *J Mol Microbiol Biotechnol* **3**: 83–93.

Larenas, J.J., Bartholomew, J., Troncoso, O., *et al.*, 2003. Experimental vertical transmission of *Piscirickettsia salmonis* and *in vitro* study of attachment and mode of entrance into the fish ovum. *Dis Aquat Org* **56**: 25–30.

Lauscher, A., Krossøy, B., Frost, P., *et al.*, 2011. Immune responses in Atlantic salmon (*Salmo salar*) following protective vaccination against infectious salmon anemia (ISA) and subsequent ISA virus infection. *Vaccine* **29**: 6392–401.

Lepa, A., Siwicki, A.K. and Terech-Majewska, E. 2010. Application of DNA vaccines in fish. *Pol J Vet Sci* **13**: 213–15.

Marshall, S.H., Heath, S., Henríquez, V. and Orrego, C. 1998. Minimally invasive detection of *Piscirickettsia salmonis* in cultivated salmonids via the PCR. *Appl Environ Microbiol* **64**: 3066–9.

Marshall, S.H., Conejeros, P., Zahr, M., *et al.*, 2007. Immunological characterization of a bacterial protein isolated from salmonid fish naturally infected with *Piscirickettsia salmonis*. *Vaccine* **25**: 2095–2102.

Marshall, S.H., Henríquez, V., Gómez, F.A. and Cárdenas, C. 2011. ISPsa2, the first mobile genetic element to be described and characterized in the bacterial facultative intracellular pathogen *Piscirickettsia salmonis*. *FEMS Microbiol Lett* **314**: 18–24.

Marshall, S.H., Gómez, F.A., Ramírez, R., *et al.*, 2012. Biofilm generation by *Piscirickettsia salmonis* under growth stress conditions: a putative *in vivo* survival/persistence strategy in marine environments. *Res Microbiol* **163**: 557–66.

Mauel, M.J., Giovannoni, S.J. and Fryer, J.L. 1999. Phylogenetic analysis of *Piscirikettsia salmonis* by 16S, internal transcribed spacer (ITS) and 23S ribosomal DNA sequencing. *Dis Aquat Org* **35**: 115–23.

Mauel, M.J., Ware, C. and Smith, P.A. 2008. Culture of *Piscirickettsia salmonis* on enriched blood agar. *J Vet Diagn Invest* **20**: 213–14.

McCarthy, U.M., Bron, J.E., Brown, L., *et al.*, 2005. Survival and replication of *Piscirickettsia salmonis* in rainbow trout head kidney macrophages. *Fish Shellfish Immunol* **25**: 477–84.

Midtlyng, P.J., Reitan, L.J. and Speilberg, L. 1996. Experimental studies on the efficacy and side-effects of intraperitoneal vaccination of Atlantic salmon (*Salmo salar* L.) against furunculosis. *Fish Shellfish Immunol* **6**: 335–50.

Midtlyng, P.J., Hendriksen, C., Balks, E., *et al.*, 2011. Three Rs approaches in the production and quality control of fish vaccines. *Biologicals* **39**: 117–28.

Mikalsen, J., Skjærvik, O., Wiik-Nielsen, J., *et al.*, 2008. Agar culture of *Piscirickettsia salmonis*, a serious pathogen of farmed salmonid and marine fish. *FEMS Microbiol Lett* **278**: 43–7.

Miquel, A., Müller, I., Ferrer, P., *et al.*, 2003. Immunoresponse of coho salmon immunized with a gene expression library from *Piscirickettsia salmonis*. *Biol Res* **36**: 313–23.

Noga, E.J. 2010. *Fish Disease Diagnosis and Treatment* (2nd edn). Iowa, Wiley-Blackwell.

Olivares, J. and Marshall, S.H. 2010. Determination of minimal concentration of *Piscirickettsia salmonis* in water columns to establish a fallowing period in salmon farms. *J Fish Dis* **33**: 261–6.

Olsen, A.B., Evensen, Ø., Speilberg, L., *et al.*, 1993. Ny laksesykdom forårsaket av rickettsie. *Norsk Fiskeoppdrett* **12**: 40–41.

Palmer, R., Ruttledge, M., Callanan, K. and Drinan, E. 1997. A piscirickettsiosis-like disease in farmed Atlantic salmon in Ireland – isolation of the agent. *Bull Eur Assoc Fish Pathol* **17**: 68–72.

Peña, A.A., Bols, N.C. and Marshall, S.H. 2010. An evaluation of potential reference genes for stability of expression in two salmonid cell lines after infection with either *Piscirickettsia salmonis* or IPNV. *BMC Res Notes* **3**: 101–10.

Plant, K.P. and LaPatra, S.E. 2011. Advances in fish vaccine delivery. *Dev Comp Immunol* **35**: 1256–62.

Rodger, H.D. and Drinan, E.M. 1993. Observation of a rickettsia-like organism in Atlantic salmon, *Salmo salar* L., in Ireland. *J Fish Dis* **16**: 361–9.

Rojas, V., Olivares, J., Del Río, R. and Marshall, S.H. 2008. Characterization of a novel and genetically different small infective variant of *Piscirickettsia salmonis*. *Microb Pathog* **44**: 370–78.

Rojas, V., Galanti, N., Bols, N.C. and Marshall, S.H. 2009. Productive infection of *Piscirickettsia salmonis* in macrophages and monocyte-like cells from rainbow trout, a possible survival strategy. *J Cell Biochem* **108**: 631–7.

Rojas, V., Galanti, N., Bols, N.C., *et al.*, 2010. *Piscirickettsia salmonis* induces apoptosis in macrophages and monocyte-like cells from rainbow trout. *J Cell Biochem* **110**: 468–76.

Rombout, J.H., Abelli, L., Picchietti, S., *et al.*, 2011. Teleost intestinal immunology. *Fish Shellfish Immunol* **31**: 616–26.

Salonius, K., Siderakis, C., MacKinnon, A.M. and Griffiths, S.G. 2005. Use of *Arthrobacter davidanieli* as a live vaccine against *Renibacterium salmoninarum* and *Piscirickettsia salmonis* in salmonids. *Dev Biol (Basel)* **121**: 189–97.

Smith, P.A., Contreras, J.R., Larenas, J.J., *et al.*, 1997. Immunization with bacterial antigens: piscirickettsiosis. *Dev Biol (Basel)* **90**: 161–6.

Sommerset, I., Krossøy, B., Biering, E. and Frost, P. 2005. Vaccines for fish in aquaculture. *Exp Rev Vaccines* **4**: 89–101.

Tobar, J.A., Jerez, S., Caruffo, M., *et al.*, 2011. Oral vaccination of Atlantic salmon (*Salmo salar*) against salmonid rickettsial septicaemia. *Vaccine* **29**: 2336–2340.

Vandenberg, G.W. 2004. Oral vaccines for finfish: academic theory or commercial reality? *Anim Health Res Rev* **5**: 301–4.

Wietz, M., Månsson, M., Bowman, J.S., *et al.*, 2012. Wide distribution of closely related, antibiotic-producing *Arthrobacter* strains throughout the Arctic Ocean. *Appl Environ Microbiol* **78**: 2039–42

Wilda, M., Lavoria, M.Á., Giráldez, A., *et al.*, 2012. Development and preliminary validation of an antibody filtration-assisted single-dilution chemiluminometric immunoassay for potency testing of *Piscirickettsia salmonis* vaccines. *Biologicals* **40**: 415–20.

Wilhelm, V., Soza, C., Martínez, R., *et al.*, 2005. Production and immune response of recombinant Hsp60 and Hsp70 from the salmon pathogen *Piscirickettsia salmonis*. *Biol Res* **38**: 69–82.

Wilhelm, V., Miquel, A., Burzio, L.O., *et al.*, 2006. A vaccine against the salmonid pathogen *Piscirickettsia salmonis* based on recombinant proteins. *Vaccine* **24**: 5083–91.

Yáñez, A.J., Valenzuela, K., Silva, H., *et al.*, 2012. Broth medium for the successful culture of the fish pathogen *Piscirickettsia salmonis*. *Dis Aquat Org* **97**: 197–205.

22 Vaccination against Bacterial Kidney Disease

Diane G. Elliott[1], Gregory D. Wiens[2], K. Larry Hammell[3] and Linda D. Rhodes[4]

[1]US Geological Survey, Western Fisheries Research Center, Seattle, Washington, USA
[2]USDA-ARS, National Center for Cool and Cold Water Aquaculture, Kearneysville, West Virginia, USA
[3]University of Prince Edward Island, Charlottetown, Canada
[4]NOAA, Northwest Fisheries Science Center, Seattle, Washington, USA

ABSTRACT

Bacterial kidney disease (BKD) of salmonid fishes, caused by *Renibacterium salmoninarum*, has presented challenges for development of effective vaccines, despite several decades of research. The only vaccine against BKD that is commercially licensed is an injectable preparation containing live cells of *Arthrobacter davidanieli* (proposed nomenclature), a non-pathogenic environmental bacterium with a relatively close phylogenetic relationship to *R. salmoninarum*. The stimulatory effect of the live vaccine is believed to be associated with an *Arthrobacter* surface carbohydrate that is similar to the exopolysaccharide of *R. salmoninarum*. Significant protection of Atlantic salmon (*Salmo salar*) against BKD, but limited or no protection of Chinook salmon (*Oncorhynchus tshawytscha*) against the disease, has been observed following intraperitoneal injection of the vaccine. Further research is needed for development of more efficacious BKD vaccines for a wider range of salmonid species.

22.1 INTRODUCTION

Bacterial kidney disease (BKD) caused by *Renibacterium salmoninarum* has been recognized as a serious disease in salmonid fishes since the 1930s (Belding and Merrill, 1935; Smith, 1964; Evelyn, 1988) and the potential for salmonids to mount an immune response against the bacterium was first reported in the early 1970s (Evelyn, 1971). Despite years of research, however, only a single vaccine has been licensed for prevention of BKD, and has demonstrated variable efficacy (Rhodes *et al.*, 2004b; Alcorn *et al.*, 2005; Salonius *et al.*, 2005; Burnley *et al.*, 2010). Therefore, in addition to a presentation of the current status of BKD vaccination,

dgelliott@usgs.gov

Fish Vaccination, First Edition. Edited by Roar Gudding, Atle Lillehaug and Øystein Evensen.

a discussion of potential future directions for BKD vaccine development is included in this chapter. This discussion is focused on the unique characteristics of *R. salmoninarum* and its biology, as well as aspects of the salmonid immune system that might be explored specifically to develop more effective vaccines for BKD prevention.

22.2 OCCURRENCE

R. salmoninarum and BKD have been reported from many areas of the world where wild or cultured salmonids are present, including North America, Chile, Europe and Japan. Several extensive reviews have been written about the disease and the pathogen (Fryer and Sanders, 1981; Austin and Austin, 1987; Elliott *et al.*, 1989; Evelyn, 1993; Evenden *et al.*, 1993; Fryer and Lannan, 1993; Pascho *et al.*, 2002).

All salmonids are considered to be vulnerable to BKD, but susceptibility varies among species. Pacific salmon such as sockeye (*Oncorhynchus nerka*), chum (*O. keta*), and Chinook salmon (*O. tshawytscha*) exhibit greater susceptibility than Atlantic salmon (*Salmo salar*), whereas freshwater and anadromous trout species such as rainbow and steelhead (*Oncorhynchus mykiss*) and brown trout (*Salmo trutta*), and char species such as bull trout (*Salvelinus confluentus*) and lake trout (*S. namaycush*), are more refractory (Kawamura *et al.*, 1977; Sanders *et al.*, 1978; Sakai *et al.*, 1991; Starliper *et al.*, 1997; Meyers *et al.*, 2003; Jones *et al.*, 2007).

Clinical BKD has only been observed in salmonid fishes (Fryer and Lannan, 1993; Pascho *et al.*, 2002). However, *R. salmoninarum* has been detected by culture, immunological assays and/or molecular tests in non-salmonid fish species as well as bivalve molluscs (Sakai and Kobayashi, 1992; Kent *et al.*, 1998; Starliper and Morrison, 2000; Eissa *et al.*, 2006; Polinski *et al.*, 2010; Rhodes *et al.*, 2011). The demonstration for non-salmonids to serve as potential reservoirs or vectors emphasizes the opportunity for horizontal transmission, which may be particularly important as a local reservoir of infection or for transfer between river catchments with species, such as eels, that can migrate short distances, including over land (Chambers *et al.*, 2008).

Fish with subclinical infections of *R. salmoninarum* are found in both cultured and free-ranging populations (Lovely *et al.*, 1994; Elliott *et al.*, 1997; Suzuki and Sakai, 2007), and the occurrence of these cases among cultured fish significantly influences management options (Murray *et al.*, 2011). Increasingly sensitive detection methods have identified a greater prevalence of infected salmonids (Elliott *et al.*, 1997; Bruno *et al.*, 2007; Sandell and Jacobson, 2011). While species differences in BKD susceptibility may need to be incorporated into vaccine strategies, sites with intensive salmonid culture should conduct epidemiological evaluations to ensure those strategies are logically consistent with management practices (Murray *et al.*, 2012).

22.3 SIGNIFICANCE

Outbreaks of BKD are most often reported in fish culture facilities, and spread of the disease has been aided by the expansion of salmonid culture (Evenden *et al.*, 1993). Clinical BKD has also been recorded in free-ranging fish (Smith, 1964; Pippy, 1969; MacLean and Yoder, 1970;

Mitchum *et al.*, 1979; Banner *et al.*, 1986; Holey *et al.*, 1998; Faisal *et al.*, 2010), including naturally spawning populations without a history of supplementation with hatchery-reared fish (Evelyn *et al.*, 1973; Souter *et al.*, 1987).

Although BKD losses as high as 80% and 40% have been reported for stocks of Pacific and Atlantic salmon, respectively (Evenden *et al.*, 1993), the chronic nature of the disease has hindered accurate estimates of BKD mortality, especially in feral fish populations. Clinical BKD in wild salmon usually goes undetected because they are more vulnerable to predation (Mesa *et al.*, 1998). Smoltification has been shown to dramatically increase the proliferation of infection and disease outbreaks for populations in which BKD is endemic (Mesa *et al.*, 1999), likely contributing to mortality observed in marine farms and to strong associations observed with movements of smolts from particular freshwater facilities (Murray *et al.*, 2012). In addition, immunosuppression by *R. salmoninarum* in infected fish may contribute to mortality that is ultimately attributed to secondary pathogens. Although difficult to quantify, impacts of BKD in aquaculture may include decreased growth and production loss, and significant costs associated with control and treatment of the disease (Burnley *et al.*, 2010; Munson *et al.*, 2010).

BKD is considered among the most difficult of bacterial fish diseases to control (Elliott *et al.*, 1989). Efforts aimed at BKD prevention and control have included investigations of chemotherapeutics, management practices, and vaccines. Anti-BKD chemotherapeutants have been identified and applied with partial success (e.g., Austin, 1985; Brown *et al.*, 1990; Moffitt, 1991, 1992; Lee and Evelyn, 1994; Moffitt and Kiryu, 1999; Fairgrieve *et al.*, 2005), but do not fully eliminate the pathogen (Wolf and Dunbar, 1959; Austin, 1985; Moffitt, 1992; Moffitt and Kiryu, 1999), and potential for emergence of antibiotic resistance exists (Bell *et al.*, 1988; Rhodes *et al.*, 2008). Improvements in hygiene, husbandry, and biosecurity in fish culture facilities may decrease BKD impacts (Maule *et al.*, 1996; Pascho *et al.*, 2002; Munson *et al.*, 2010; Murray *et al.*, 2012), and practices such as segregation or culling of infected broodstock have demonstrated effectiveness for reducing prevalence and severity of BKD in subsequent generations (Pascho *et al.*, 1991; Guðmundsdóttir *et al.*, 2000; Meyers *et al.*, 2003; Munson *et al.*, 2010). Vaccination against BKD is not widely practiced (Sommerset *et al.*, 2005; Bravo and Midtlyng, 2007), but is viewed as a potentially valuable measure for BKD prevention (Pascho *et al.*, 2002; Rhodes *et al.*, 2004b).

22.4 ETIOLOGY

Renibacterium salmoninarum is a non-motile, non-spore-forming, strongly gram-positive rod that usually occurs in pairs (Sanders and Fryer, 1980). Growth is aerobic and optimal at 15–18°C. The genome of the American Type Culture Collection strain ATCC 33209 is composed of a single, circular chromosome of 3,155,250 DNA base-pairs and is predicted to contain 3507 open-reading frames (ORFs; Wiens *et al.*, 2008). The sequenced strain lacks integrated phage or associated plasmids but contains 80 insertion sequence elements interspersed throughout the genome. Approximately 21% of the predicted ORFs are inactivated via frameshifts, point mutations, insertion sequences, and putative deletions. The *R. salmoninarum* genome has extended regions of synteny to the *Arthrobacter* sp. strain FB24 and *Arthrobacter aurescens* TC1 genomes, but the genome is much smaller, suggesting that significant genome reduction has occurred since divergence from the last common ancestor.

The presence of only two ribosomal loci and the numerous pseudogenes within the metabolic pathways may account for the slow generation (doubling) time of approximately 24 hours.

The biochemical properties and cell wall composition of *R. salmoninarum* isolates are conserved (Bruno and Munro, 1986a; Fiedler and Draxl, 1986). These include an inability to produce acid from sugars (Sanders and Fryer, 1980) and a cysteine requirement for growth (Ordal and Earp, 1956; Daly and Stevenson, 1985). The genome of *R. salmoninarum* ATCC 33209 lacks apparent functional genes critical to the *de novo* synthesis of amino acids serine, glycine, cysteine, asparagine and methionine (Wiens *et al.*, 2008). Genome analyses also suggest core central metabolic pathways are functional, including glycolysis, pentose phosphate, tricarboxylic acid (Krebs) cycle, and pyruvate cycle. *R. salmoninarum* may be able to utilize several sugars and polyols, as the organism contains genes to import and utilize glucose, fructose, arabinose, gluconate, glycerol and citrate. It also appears to be able to utilize a variety of carbon substrates for energy, including pyruvate, lactate, succinate, malate, glycerol-3-phosphate, proline, butanoyl-CoA and fatty acids. *R. salmoninarum* apparently is incapable of synthesizing both unsaturated and saturated fatty acids because it lacks *fabA* and *fabZ* homologs, suggesting it has to scavenge these compounds from the salmonid host.

R. salmoninarum produces catalase activity (Ordal and Earp, 1956) and the genome encodes enzymes that confer resistance to oxygen radicals, including superoxide dismutase, peroxidases and thioredoxin peroxidase (Wiens *et al.*, 2008). Proteolytic activity (Ordal and Earp, 1956; Smith, 1964; Rockey *et al.*, 1991), deoxyribonuclease (DNAse), and β-hemolytic activities against salmonid erythrocytes have been described (Bruno and Munro, 1986a; Evenden *et al.*, 1993). Two specific hemolysins have been biochemically identified, and one has been cloned and designated *hly* (Evenden *et al.*, 1993; Grayson *et al.*, 1995, 2001). Genome analysis identified three additional candidate hemolysins encoded by ORFs RSal33209_0811, RSal33209_3195, and RSal33209_3047 (Wiens *et al.*, 2008). Their role in virulence evolution and fish adaption is unknown.

The *R. salmoninarum* genome contains an ORF encoding a SrtD homolog, which is a member of a group of cysteine transpeptidases that are produced by gram-positive bacteria and promote covalent anchoring of proteins to the peptidoglycan surface of the cell envelope. Bioinformatics analyses of the genome identified eight ORFs that contain putative sortase cleavage motifs. Treatment of *R. salmoninarum* with sortase inhibitors decreased bacterial adherence to fibronectin and fish cells *in vitro*, suggesting that some of these proteins have a role in attachment (Sudheesh *et al.*, 2007).

R. salmoninarum is generally considered to be antigenically homogenous, as measured using polyclonal antisera (Bullock *et al.*, 1974; Getchell *et al.*, 1985; Fiedler and Draxl, 1986). However, limited antigenic variation has been described in the p57 (MSA) protein, and the cause of this variation mapped to a single nucleotide mutation occurring in both the *msa*1 and *msa*2 genes of 5 of 8 isolates from Norway (Wiens *et al.*, 2002). The antigenic-variant strains also shared other sequence variation characteristics including one tandem repeat in the ETRA locus, a sequovar-four 16-23S rRNA intervening DNA sequence, a larger *Xho*I fragment in the *msa*1 5' region, and an absent *msa*3 gene. These results indicate that limited antigenic and genomic variation exists among strains, and this variation appears geographically restricted in distribution, which can be advantageous for development of vaccines with broad applicability.

22.5 PATHOGENESIS

Although focal *R. salmoninarum* infections with lesions confined to the skin, ocular or postorbital tissues, or brain have been reported (Hendricks and Leek, 1975; Hoffmann *et al.*, 1984; Speare, 1997; Ferguson, 2006), classical BKD is a slowly progressing systemic infection that rarely manifests as clinical disease until fish are 6 to 12 months of age (Evelyn, 1993). The disease appears histologically as a chronic granulomatous inflammation (Wolke, 1975; Bruno, 1986), and while kidney hematopoietic tissue may be particularly affected, granulomas typically are found in all infected tissues. The granulomas in Pacific salmon are characteristically diffuse with poorly defined borders, whereas those in Atlantic salmon are more encapsulated and contain numerous epithelioid macrophages (Evelyn, 1993). Evidence indicates that the bacterium can survive and perhaps multiply within macrophages (Young and Chapman, 1978; Bruno, 1986; Bandín *et al.*, 1993; Flaño *et al.*, 1996; Dale *et al.*, 1997).

The dual modes of *R. salmoninarum* transmission, horizontal and vertical, likely aid in persistence of the pathogen (Evelyn, 1993) and complicate management strategies. The exact mechanisms of horizontal transmission are not known, but entry sites are believed to include the gastrointestinal tract after ingestion of infected fish carcasses (Wood and Wallis, 1955), or fecal material containing the bacterium (Balfry *et al.*, 1996), or the eyes and skin through sites of injury (Hendricks and Leek, 1975; Hoffmann *et al.*, 1984; Hayakawa *et al.*, 1989; Elliott and Pascho, 2001). Horizontal transmission of *R. salmoninarum* can occur in both freshwater (Mitchum and Sherman, 1981; Bell *et al.*, 1984) and seawater (Murray *et al.*, 1992; Evelyn, 1993). At the population level, horizontal transmission is observed as spatial and temporal clustering in which cases occur based on movements within the aquaculture industry or within a single company, exposure to wild fish reservoirs, or exposure to infection from trout farms (Murray *et al.*, 2012). Vertical transmission of *R. salmoninarum* from parent to progeny occurs in association with the egg, with at least some of the bacteria carried intra-ovum (Evelyn *et al.*, 1984, 1986). Subsequent horizontal transmission among progeny, and within hatcheries generally, likely contributes to both farmed and enhancement populations having increased prevalence of infection leading to further bacterial propagation in later life stages (Fenichel *et al.*, 2009).

The immunosuppressive capacity of *R. salmoninarum* has been well demonstrated *in vitro* and *in vivo*. *In ovo* exposure can increase susceptibility to disease and mortality, suggesting induced tolerance (Brown *et al.*, 1996). The highly abundant, 57 kDa extracellular major soluble antigen (MSA or p57 protein) of *R. salmoninarum* has been strongly implicated as a principal mediator of immunosuppressive activities such as reducing antibody production and cytokine interference (Turaga *et al.*, 1987; Fredriksen *et al.*, 1997). MSA interacts directly with immune cells (Campos-Perez *et al.*, 1997; Wiens *et al.*, 2002), and its removal enhances antibody production and decreases susceptibility to infection (Wood and Kaattari, 1996; Piganelli *et al.*, 1999b). Virulence correlates with MSA protein abundance (Senson and Stevenson, 1999; O'Farrell *et al.*, 2000) or functional MSA gene copy number (Rhodes *et al.*, 2004a; Coady *et al.*, 2006). MSA exhibits characteristics of a dominant virulence factor, and removal or neutralization should be considered in vaccine design.

There has been no clear correlation between the humoral (antibody) response to *R. salmoninarum* bacterins and protection from BKD (Paterson *et al.*, 1981; Sakai *et al.*, 1989; Piganelli *et al.*, 1999b; Alcorn *et al.*, 2005), and formation of antigen–antibody complexes may result in some of the deleterious pathological effects of BKD (Sami *et al.*, 1992). Research suggests that for this pathogen, cell-mediated, rather than humoral, immunity is more valuable in protecting against infection and disease (Hardie *et al.*, 1996; Kaattari and Piganelli, 1997; Ellis, 1999). For example, production of macrophage-activating cytokines by primed head kidney leukocytes (presumably T-helper-like lymphocytes) has been shown to result in macrophage activation and inhibition of *R. salmoninarum* growth *in vitro*, concomitant with increased generation of macrophage respiratory burst products (Hardie *et al.*, 1996).

Responses to infection depend upon exposure history, host genetics, and bacterial phenotype. While vertical transmission may induce immunotolerance, *R. salmoninarum* can elicit an anamnestic response (Jansson *et al.*, 2003), a promising feature for vaccination. Variation in heritable resistance to infection in Chinook salmon suggests a potential for selection for increased BKD resistance (Beacham and Evelyn, 1992; Johnson *et al.*, 2003; Hard *et al.*, 2006), a prediction that may have been fulfilled in Great Lakes stocks that have undergone repeated epizootics over the past 40 years (Purcell *et al.*, 2008). Mechanisms for resistance may include greater control of serum iron by transferrin (Suzumoto *et al.*, 1977) or stronger innate immune response (Ellis, 1999). However, pathology due to host response can be as debilitating as direct bacterial damage. Glomerulonephritis mediated by antigen–antibody complexes in type III hypersensitivity (Lumsden *et al.*, 2008) is a hallmark of BKD morbidity (Sami *et al.*, 1992; O'Farrell *et al.*, 2000; Metzger *et al.*, 2010). Expression patterns for immune genes exhibit few differences between salmon stocks with phenotypic differences in survival (Metzger *et al.*, 2010). In contrast, early upregulation of interferon-inducible-like genes are observed in response to a bacterial strain with reduced MSA (Rhodes *et al.*, 2009), suggesting possible immune indicators that could be exploited in vaccine development.

22.6 VACCINES

Most vaccine development efforts to date have focused on whole cell or lysed bacterin reagents, and heat or formalin treatment has been used for inactivation. Early efforts to develop bacterins as BKD vaccines demonstrated variable protection against acute challenge or a variable immune response (Paterson *et al.*, 1981; McCarthy *et al.*, 1984). While surface proteins are important for eliciting immunity, retention of MSA on killed cells confers little or no protection to Pacific salmon through either an oral or intraperitoneal route (Sakai *et al.*, 1993; Wood and Kaattari, 1996; Piganelli *et al.*, 1999b; Alcorn *et al.*, 2005). Approaches to reducing MSA in bacterin preparations include selecting strains that express low levels of MSA (Rhodes *et al.*, 2004b) and heat treatment (Piganelli *et al.*, 1999a,1999b; US Patent No. 5,871,751). A promising aspect of bacterins with reduced MSA is a low, yet detectable, therapeutic effect for fish already infected with *R. salmoninarum* (Rhodes *et al.*, 2004b).

In addition to use in bacterins, attenuated *R. salmoninarum* strains with reduced or normal cell-associated MSA have also been tested as live vaccines (Griffiths *et al.*, 1998; Daly *et al.*, 2001; Rhodes *et al.*, 2004b). Intraperitoneal vaccination with attenuated *R. salmoninarum* strains with normal cell-associated MSA showed greater protection of Atlantic salmon than a strain with reduced MSA following *R. salmoninarum* challenge by intraperitoneal injection (Daly *et al.*, 2001), although protection was incomplete.

Attempts to isolate avirulent strains of *R. salmoninarum* for use as vaccine candidates resulted in the discovery of *Arthrobacter davidanieli* (proposed nomenclature) as a vaccine that provides significant protection in Atlantic salmon (Griffiths *et al.*, 1998; Salonius *et al.*, 2005; Burnley *et al.*, 2010). Laboratory test results suggested that this vaccine provides greater protection for Atlantic salmon against BKD than live attenuated *R. salmoninarum* vaccines (Griffiths *et al.*, 1998). In contrast to results in Atlantic salmon, however, the live *Arthrobacter* vaccine has demonstrated limited (Rhodes *et al.*, 2004b) or no (Alcorn *et al.*, 2005) efficacy in Pacific salmon. This *Arthrobacter* species is marketed as the live vaccine Renogen®[1] in several countries, and is the only commercially licensed BKD vaccine. The relatively close phylogenetic relationship between *Arthrobacter* and *R. salmoninarum* probably underpins Renogen's immunogenicity against BKD (Wiens *et al.*, 2008). The stimulatory effect of the live vaccine is believed to be associated with an *Arthrobacter* surface carbohydrate that is similar to the exopolysaccaride of *R. salmoninarum* (Griffiths *et al.*, 1998).

Adjuvants used in conjunction with BKD vaccines have ranged from Freund's complete or incomplete adjuvant, to DNA adjuvants, to no adjuvant at all (e.g., Pascho *et al.*, 1997; Griffiths *et al.*, 1998; Piganelli *et al.*, 1999b; Daly *et al.*, 2001; Rhodes *et al.*, 2004b; Alcorn *et al.*, 2005). Although there has been little evidence that adjuvants potentiate the efficacy of BKD vaccines, a directed study of adjuvants for BKD vaccines has not yet been conducted.

22.7 VACCINATION PROCEDURES

Whereas most vaccines tested for protection against BKD have been delivered by intraperitoneal injection (or less commonly, intramuscular injection), use of oral formulations has also been investigated. Research by Piganelli *et al.* (1999b) suggested that oral administration of formalin-killed *R. salmoninarum* cells, depleted of MSA by heat treatment and encapsulated in enteric-coated microspheres, provided better protection of coho salmon (*Oncorhynchus kisutch*) against a waterborne *R. salmoninarum* challenge than similarly delivered untreated cells, or intraperitoneal injection of MSA-depleted cells.

The licensed vaccine Renogen® consists of a lyophilized culture of *Arthrobacter* cells that is resuspended in sterile saline (0.9% NaCl) diluent before administration. When vaccination with Renogen® occurs in commercial settings, the vaccine is administered by intraperitoneal injection separately from other antigenic components, usually using a double-barrel delivery system that provides vaccine through a single injection site, mixing vaccines only at the time of injection (Figure 22.1) (Burnley *et al.*, 2010). This separation of the BKD component may restrict its adaptability when considering vaccine combinations that include antigenic components provided by other vaccine companies. All vaccination is performed on pre-smolt stages, ensuring that the individual fish size is sufficient to handle the intraperitoneal injection procedure, which provides antigenic stimulation by the time smolts are transferred to seawater. The manufacturer of the commercial *Arthrobacter* BKD vaccine recommends a minimum period of 400 degree-days between vaccination and exposure to pathogens.

Field tests of vaccines at commercial fish farms involve logistical and participation challenges that include: randomization, inclusion of controls, blind assessments, and allocation of

[1] Any use of trade names is for descriptive purposes only and does not imply endorsement by the US Government or the publishers.

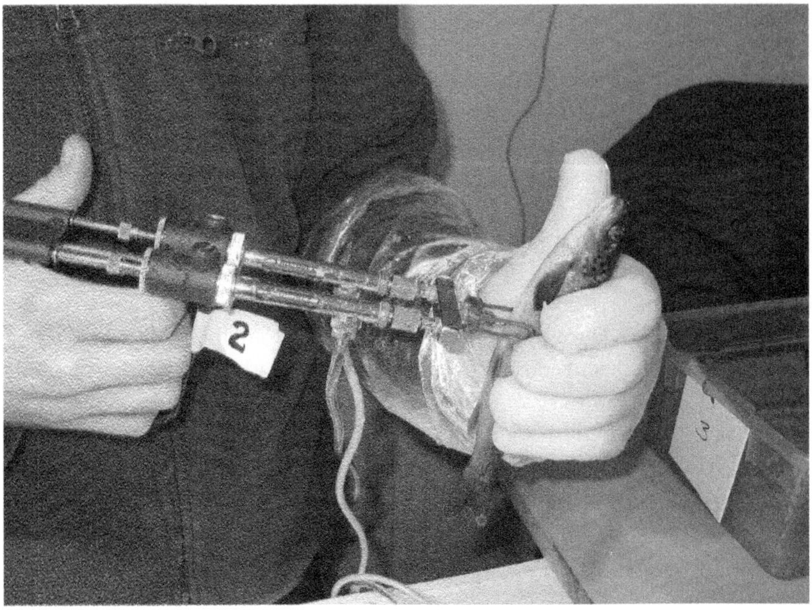

Fig. 22.1 Double-barrel vaccination apparatus used for large-scale administration of commercial BKD vaccine (which contains live cells of *Arthrobacter* sp.) in conjunction with delivery of formalin-inactivated vaccines against other pathogens. (Source: K.L. Hammell.)

vaccine to large groups (i.e., cage or site units of concern; Burnley *et al.*, 2010). Interpretation of vaccine effect is frequently complicated by unrelated disease events, such as sea lice burdens, or antibacterial treatments in commercial facilities.

Because infection can occur early in oocyte development (Bruno and Munro, 1986b; Rhodes, unpublished), a focus on mass vaccination of progeny as early as possible after hatching may provide better protection against both vertical and horizontal transmission. Although some DNA vaccines have shown multi-year protection (Kurath *et al.*, 2006), the typical short-lived immunity to bacterins observed in salmonids (Johnson *et al.*, 1982) would indicate the use of boosters, particularly for fish first vaccinated at a small size. While horizontal transmission may be mediated primarily through gastrointestinal mucosa (Balfry *et al.*, 1996) rather than gill epithelia (McIntosh *et al.*, 2000), indicating applicability of oral immunization, an immersion vaccine could stimulate multi-organ mucosal immunity.

22.8 VACCINE EFFECTS AND SIDE-EFFECTS

Few studies have been published on the efficacy of the licensed Renogen® BKD vaccine, but have shown mixed results depending on the fish species vaccinated. In juvenile Atlantic salmon, relative percent survival (RPS) of vaccinated groups compared with unvaccinated groups ranged between 72% and 91% following a laboratory challenge by intraperitoneal injection of *R. salmoninarum* (Salonius *et al.*, 2005). Field studies with natural BKD exposure of Atlantic salmon during marine cage culture also showed significantly higher survival in groups that received Renogen® in addition to vaccines against other pathogens, in comparison with reference groups that only received the non-BKD vaccines (Salonius *et al.*, 2005; Burnley *et al.*, 2010). Salonius *et al.* (2005) reported a RPS of 80% in Renogen®-vaccinated groups compared with reference groups during a two-month BKD outbreak, and Burnley *et al.* (2010) determined that the Renogen®-vaccinated group had a significantly reduced risk of dying in comparison with the reference group (hazard ratio = 0.68, $P = 0.018$) during a 240-day BKD outbreak. In contrast, Rhodes *et al.* (2004b) demonstrated limited protection of juvenile Chinook salmon against an acute intraperitoneal *R. salmoninarum* challenge following Renogen® vaccination, with low RPS values (0.4–15.0%) and modest but significant increases in median survival (4–13 days, $P = 0$–0.04) compared with controls. Alcorn *et al.* (2005) showed no significant difference ($P > 0.05$) in survival between Renogen®-injected and control Chinook salmon following a 285-day challenge by cohabitation with *R. salmoninarum*-infected Chinook salmon.

Duration of protection of BKD vaccines has received little attention. Significantly higher survival was reported for Renogen®-vaccinated Atlantic salmon compared with controls about 23 months (Salonius *et al.*, 2005) and 27 months (Burnley *et al.*, 2010) after vaccination in field studies with natural BKD outbeaks, but it is likely that the fish were exposed to *R. salmoninarum* long before the first BKD mortalities were recorded at about 21 and 19 months post-vaccination, respectively. Burnley *et al.* (2010) noted that initial *R. salmoninarum* exposure of fish in their study may have occurred shortly after seawater transfer 4 months post-vaccination because of the practice (since discontinued) of holding harvest-sized fish at the same sea-cage site as smolts. Holding more than one year class of fish at the same site may have provided continuous immune stimulation via *R. salmoninarum* shed by the older fish as clinical disease developed.

Although commercial vaccines may augment BKD control strategies for Atlantic salmon producers in areas potentially affected, they are generally not relied upon to any great extent. Prevention strategies focus efforts on blocking vertical transmission by separating broodstock from marine production fish and by repeated testing or containment of brood fish in high biosecurity systems to prevent potential exposure. Frequent monitoring for the emergence of clinical BKD in farm populations facilitates decisions on treatment with oral antibiotics during early stages of the disease when a greater proportion of the population is still feeding. Even though vaccination against BKD provides a benefit in mortality reduction during clinical outbreaks (Burnley *et al.*, 2010), farm management apparently considers this an unwarranted cost over other prevention and control practices in endemic areas.

The potential for BKD vaccines to confer protection on individuals already exposed in endemic situations, or those asymptomatically infected through vertical transmission, is unknown. Vaccination of juvenile Atlantic salmon with Renogen® was reported to be unsuccessful for amelioration of BKD when natural *R. salmoninarum* infection rates in the population (as determined by bacteriological culture) were 30–40% at the time of vaccination (Salonius *et al.*, 2005). In an experiment conducted with juvenile Chinook salmon naturally infected with *R. salmoninarum*, however, survival was significantly higher in comparison with mock-vaccinated controls, in groups vaccinated with either Renogen® alone or Renogen® combined with killed cells of an *R. salmoninarum* strain with reduced MSA, with the combination vaccine showing the greatest therapeutic effect (Rhodes *et al.*, 2004b).

Increases in growth and growth efficiency expected when a vaccine provides some level of protection against a chronic infection such as BKD remain unproven. Although Salonius *et al.*

(2005) reported a 16% greater harvest weight in Renogen®-vaccinated Atlantic salmon than in salmon vaccinated against other pathogens 23 months after vaccination, Burnley *et al.* (2010) observed no significant differences in weight gain at harvest, 27 months after vaccination, between Renogen®-vaccinated Atlantic salmon and those that had been administered vaccines against other pathogens. In both of the above field studies, natural BKD mortality occurred among all groups.

In addition to reported efficacy of Renogen® for protection of Atlantic salmon against BKD, protection has also been reported against salmonid rickettsial septicemia (SRS) caused by *Piscirickettsia salmonis*, an obligate intracellular gram-negative bacterium. Significantly lower SRS mortality has been demonstrated for Renogen®-vaccinated coho salmon in comparison with controls in laboratory and field studies (Salonius *et al.*, 2005).

Fish vaccine side-effects such as intra-abdominal adhesions and reduced growth are most often associated with the use of oil-adjuvanted vaccines (Midtlyng, 1996; Midtlyng and Lillehaug, 1998). Some experimental BKD vaccines have included oil adjuvants, but the commercial live vaccine Renogen® is injected without an adjuvant.

22.9 REGULATIONS

The commercial vaccine Renogen® has been licensed in Canada, the US, and Chile for vaccination of salmonids against BKD, but the vaccine has not been licensed in Europe or Japan (Sommerset *et al.*, 2005). Economic consideration of the cost of vaccine licensing relative to the size of the market for a BKD vaccine has probably deterred commercial licensing efforts in some countries. Some locations, such as Scotland, have BKD eradication programs that render vaccines unusable (Murray *et al.*, 2012). Because the Renogen® vaccine contains live cells of a non-pathogenic environmental bacterium, lack of potential for reversion to virulence has been easy to demonstrate, and the vaccine has been more readily accepted for licensing than a vaccine containing attenuated *R. salmoninarum* cells (Salonius *et al.*, 2005).

22.10 FUTURE DIRECTIONS

Vaccines of greater efficacy for BKD prevention could be valuable tools for management of this disease in more salmonid species. Characteristics of the bacterium and the host response pertinent to vaccine performance have been discussed in previous sections, and some of the research directions that could be explored for improvement of BKD vaccines are outlined below.

22.10.1 DNA vaccines and protein subunit vaccines

The availability of the *R. salmoninarum* genome sequence makes it possible to select genes that may be candidates for DNA vaccination. Limited research showed significant protection of rainbow trout (*Oncorhynchus mykiss*) against an *R. salmoninarum* injection challenge following intramuscular vaccination with expression vectors containing either DNA coding for MSA or a random mix of DNA fragments from the *R. salmoninarum* genome (Gomez-Chiarri *et al.*, 1996). Many extracellular or outer membrane proteins may be obscured by MSA, but could be expressed individually or in combination in DNA vaccine constructs. More than 440

ORFs appear to possess a leader peptide sequence characteristic of a Sec-dependent secretion pathway, and both a putative sortase gene and potential sortase substrate genes have been identified (Wiens *et al.*, 2008). Sortases and their surface protein substrates are important virulence determinants of gram-positive bacteria, with functions in adhesion to host cells, colonization, and immune evasion (Sudheesh *et al.*, 2007; Maresso and Schneewind, 2008). Immunization of mice with recombinant sortase (Gianfaldoni *et al.*, 2009) or sortase substrate proteins (Stranger-Jones *et al.*, 2006) has been shown to provide protection against challenge with virulent strains of *Streptococcus pneumoniae* and *Staphylococcus aureus*, respectively.

22.10.2 Adjuvants

Freund's adjuvants and oil-based adjuvants cause injection site pathologies such as inflammation and adhesions (Mutoloki *et al.*, 2006), but avoiding lesions is desirable for both fish health and marketability. Unmethylated CpG dinucleotide sequences in bacterial (and viral) DNA can be highly immunostimulatory in vertebrates, and this is the underlying mechanism of DNA adjuvants (Higgins *et al.*, 2007). When a bacterium breaches physical host barriers such as skin or gastrointestinal mucosa, conserved bacterial CpG motifs are recognized by host cell toll-like receptors (TLRs), which play a key role in initiation of innate immune responses, and influence later antigen-specific adaptive immunity. The stimulatory effect is sequence-dependent, and there have been few studies with fish (Rhodes *et al.*, 2004b; Pedersen *et al.*, 2006). Exploration for DNA sequences that are immunostimulatory for fish may uncover adjuvants that can potentiate the effectiveness of DNA vaccines or bacterins for BKD prevention. The availability of cloned TLRs from trout and salmon (Rebl *et al.*, 2010) can facilitate the systematic screening for ligands, such as bacterial unmethylated CpG islands, that bind either the fish-specific TLRs or conserved vertebrate TLRs.

22.10.3 *In vitro* testing of vaccine candidates

The identification of potential vaccine candidates in the *R. salmoninarum* genome underscores the need to develop high-throughput methods for vaccine evaluation and/or surrogate measures of immunity that predict progression to clinical disease. Although primary head kidney cells of salmonids exhibit proinflammatory and immune gene expression responses to infection (Grayson *et al.*, 2002), an immortalized or transformed salmonid macrophage line would improve capacity and speed of screening ORFs for potential vaccine candidates. A macrophage cell line has been established and characterized from goldfish (*Carassius auratus*; Wang *et al.*, 1995), and salmonid cell lines exhibiting some characteristics of macrophages have also been established (Ganassin and Bols, 1998; Collet and Collins, 2009).

22.10.4 Endpoints for vaccine screening in fish

Testing of BKD vaccines could be streamlined to enable screening of larger numbers of vaccine candidates by measuring biomarkers that are predictive of disease outcome, rather than using mortality as the endpoint. For a chronic disease such as BKD, protracted challenge trials (typically > 3 months in duration) are needed to assess mortality. Prognostic biomarkers that could be evaluated much earlier in the disease process could shorten the time required for vaccine evaluation. For example, upregulation of expression of certain immune genes including TNF-alpha (Grayson *et al.*, 2002), iNOS (Metzger *et al.*, 2010), interferon-inducible genes (Rhodes *et al.*, 2009), and interferon-gamma (Figure 22.2) have been associated with early

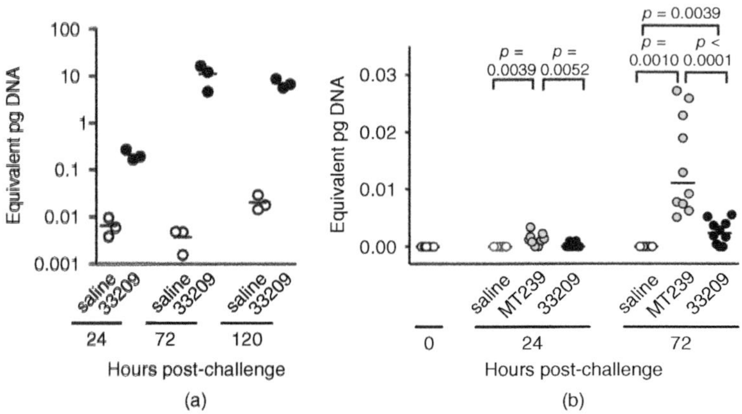

Fig. 22.2 Rapid gene expression of interferon gamma (IFNγ), a cytokine associated with cellular immunity, in response to experimental challenge with *R. salmoninarum*. (a) IFNγ expression in juvenile rainbow trout kidney (mean wt = 24 ± 6 g) elevated after challenge with the virulent ATCC type strain 33209 relative to mock challenged fish. Each horizontal bar is the median for three fish. Primer and probe sequences have been previously described (Wiens and Vallejo, 2010). (b) IFNγ expression in juvenile Chinook salmon kidney by 3 days after challenge is significantly higher in response to the attenuated MT239 strain compared with the virulent 33209 strain or saline control. Each horizontal bar is the median for 10 fish; *p* values from the Kruskal-Wallis test. (Primer and probe sequences for B: forward primer, 5-CACCTGCAGAACCTGTGGG-3′; reverse primer, 5′-AACTCGGACAGAGCCTTCCC-3′; probe, 5′6-FAM-CATCGAGACCAGTGACACCACAGTCCA-BHQ1-3′.) (Source: (a) G.D. Wiens, unpublished; (b) L.D. Rhodes, unpublished.)

host responses to *R. salmoninarum*, and their expression may be useful to monitor an effective response in a post-vaccination challenge. Because early response biomarkers may lack specificity due to the complexity of the host-pathogen dynamic during infection, however, such biomarkers may have better predictive capabilities if they are combined with or normalized against bacterial load estimates, which could also be determined by rapid molecular assays (Suzuki and Sakai, 2007; Metzger *et al.*, 2010).

REFERENCES

Alcorn, S., Murray, A.L., Pascho, R.J. and Varney, J. 2005. A cohabitation challenge to compare the efficacies of vaccines for bacterial kidney disease (BKD) in Chinook salmon *Oncorhynchus tshawytscha*. *Dis Aquat Org* **63**: 151–60.

Austin, B. 1985. Evaluation of antimicrobial compounds for the control of bacterial kidney disease in rainbow trout, *Salmo gairdneri* Richardson. *J Fish Dis* **8**: 209–20.

Austin, B. and Austin, D.A. 1987. *Bacterial Fish Pathogens: Disease in Farmed and Wild Fish*. Chichester, Ellis Horwood.

Balfry, S.K., Albright, L.J. and Evelyn, T.P.T. 1996. Horizontal transfer of *Renibacterium salmoninarum* among farmed salmonids via the fecal-oral route. *Dis Aquat Org* **25**: 63–9.

Bandín, I., Ellis, A.E., Barja, J.L. and Secombes, C.J. 1993. Interaction between rainbow trout macrophages and *Renibacterium salmoninarum in vitro*. *Fish Shellfish Immunol* **3**: 25–33.

Banner, C.R., Long, J.J., Fryer, J.L. and Rohovec, J.S. 1986. Occurrence of salmonid fish infected with *Renibacterium salmoninarum* in the Pacific Ocean. *J Fish Dis* **9**: 273–5.

Beacham, T.D. and Evelyn, T.P.T. 1992. Population and genetic variation in resistance of Chinook salmon to vibriosis, furunculosis, and bacterial kidney disease. *J Aquat Anim Health* **4**: 153–67.

Belding, D.L. and Merrill, B. 1935. A preliminary report upon a hatchery disease of the Salmonidae. *Trans Am Fish Soc* **65**: 76–84.

Bell, G.R., Higgs, D.A. and Traxler, G.S. 1984. The effect of dietary ascorbate, zinc, and manganese on the development of experimentally induced bacterial kidney disease in sockeye salmon (*Oncorhynchus nerka*). *Aquaculture* **36**: 293–311.

Bell, G.R., Traxler, G.S. and Dworschak, C. 1988. Development *in vitro* and pathogenicity of an erythromycin-resistant strain of *Renibacterium salmoninarum*, the causative agent of bacterial kidney disease in salmonids. *Dis Aquat Org* **4**: 19–25.

Bravo, S. and Midtlyng, P.J. 2007. The use of fish vaccines in the Chilean salmon industry 1999–2003. *Aquaculture* **270**: 36–42.

Brown, L.L., Albright, L.J. and Evelyn, T.P.T. 1990. Control of vertical transmission of *Renibacterium salmoninarum* by injection of antibiotics into maturing female coho salmon *Oncorhynchus kisutch*. *Dis Aquat Org* **9**: 127–31.

Brown, L.L., Iwama, G.K. and Evelyn, T.P.T. 1996. The effect of early exposure of coho salmon (*Oncorhynchus kisutch*) eggs to the p57 protein of *Renibacterium salmoninarum* on the development of immunity to the pathogen. *Fish Shellfish Immunol* **6**: 149–65.

Bruno, D.W. 1986. Histopathology of bacterial kidney disease in laboratory infected rainbow trout, *Salmo gairdneri* Richardson, and Atlantic salmon, *Salmo salar* L., with reference to naturally infected fish. *J Fish Dis* **9**: 523–37.

Bruno, D.W. and Munro, A.L.S. 1986a. Uniformity in the biochemical properties of *Renibacterium salmoninarum* isolates obtained from several sources. *FEMS Microbiol Lett* **33**: 247–50.

Bruno, D.W. and Munro, A.L.S. 1986b. Observations on *Renibacterium salmoninarum* and the salmonid egg. *Dis Aquat Org* **1**: 83–7.

Bruno, D., Collet, B., Turnbull, A., *et al*., 2007. Evaluation and development of diagnostic methods for *Renibacterium salmoninarum* causing bacterial kidney disease (BKD) in the UK. *Aquaculture* **269**: 114–22.

Bullock, G.L., Stuckey, H.M. and Chen, P.K. 1974. Corynebacterial kidney disease of salmonids: growth and serological studies on the causative bacterium. *Appl Microbiol* **28**: 811–14.

Burnley, T.A., Stryhn, H., Burnley, H.J. and Hammell, K.L. 2010. Randomized clinical field trial of a bacterial kidney disease vaccine in Atlantic salmon, *Salmo salar* L. *J Fish Dis* **33**: 545–57.

Campos-Perez, J.J., Ellis, A.E. and Secombes, C.J. 1997. Investigation of factors influencing the ability of *Renibacterium salmoninarum* to stimulate rainbow trout macrophage respiratory burst activity. *Fish Shellfish Immunol* **7**: 555–66.

Chambers, E., Gardiner, R. and Peeler, E.J. 2008. An investigation into the prevalence of *Renibacterium salmoninarum* in farmed rainbow trout, *Oncorhynchus mykiss* (Walbaum), and wild fish populations in selected river catchments in England and Wales between 1998 and 2000. *J Fish Dis* **31**: 89–96.

Coady, A.M., Murray, A.L., Elliott, D.G. and Rhodes, L.D. 2006. Both msa genes in *Renibacterium salmoninarum* are needed for full virulence in bacterial kidney disease. *Appl Environ Microbiol* **72**: 2672–8.

Collet, B. and Collins, M.D. 2009. Comparative gene expression profile in two Atlantic salmon cell lines TO and SHK-1. *Vet Immunol Immunopathol* **130**: 92–5.

Dale, O.B., Gutenberger, S.K. and Rohovec, J.S. 1997. Estimation of variation of virulence of *Renibacterium salmoninarum* by survival analysis of experimental infection of salmonid fish. *J Fish Dis* **20**: 177–83.

Daly, J.G. and Stevenson, R.M. 1985. Charcoal agar, a new growth medium for the fish disease bacterium *Renibacterium salmoninarum*. *Appl Environ Microbiol* **50**: 868–71.

Daly, J.G., Griffiths, S.G., Kew, A.K., *et al*., 2001. Characterization of attenuated *Renibacterium salmoninarum* strains and their use as live vaccines. *Dis Aquat Org* **44**: 121–6.

Eissa, A.E., Elsayed, E.E., McDonald, R. and Faisal, M. 2006. First record of *Renibacterium salmoninarum* in the sea lamprey (*Petromyzon marinus*). *J Wildl Dis* **42**: 556–60.

Elliott, D.G. and Pascho, R.J. 2001. Evidence that coded-wire-tagging procedures can enhance transmission of *Renibacterium salmoninarum* in Chinook salmon. *J Aquat Anim Health* **13**: 181–93.

Elliott, D.G., Pascho, R.J. and Bullock, G.L. 1989. Developments in the control of bacterial kidney disease of salmonid fishes. *Dis Aquat Org* **6**: 201–15.

Elliott, D.G., Pascho, R.J., Jackson, L.M., *et al*., 1997. *Renibacterium salmoninarum* in spring-summer Chinook salmon smolts at dams on the Columbia and Snake Rivers. *J Aquat Anim Health* **9**: 114–26.

Ellis, A.E. 1999. Immunity to bacteria in fish. *Fish Shellfish Immunol* **9**: 291–308.

Evelyn, T.P.T. 1971. The agglutinin response in sockeye salmon vaccinated intraperitoneally with a heat-killed preparation of the bacterium responsible for salmonid kidney disease. *J Wildl Dis* **7**: 328–35.

Evelyn, T.P.T. 1988. Bacterial kidney disease in British Columbia, Canada: comments on its epizootiology and methods for its control on fish farms. *AQUA NOR 87 Trondheim International Conference*. Trondheim, Norske Fiskeoppdretternes Salgslag A/L, 51–7.

Evelyn, T.P.T. 1993. Bacterial kidney disease – BKD, in *Bacterial Diseases of Fish* (eds V. Inglis, R.J. Roberts and N.R. Bromage). New York, Halsted Press, 177–95.

Evelyn, T.P.T., Hoskins, G.E. and Bell, G.R. 1973. First record of bacterial kidney disease in an apparently wild salmonid in British Columbia. *J Fish Res Board Can* **30**: 1578–80.

Evelyn, T.P.T., Ketcheson, J.E. and Prosperi-Porta, L. 1984. Further evidence for the presence of *Renibacterium salmoninarum* in salmonid eggs and for the failure of povidone-iodine to reduce the intra-ovum infection rate in water-hardened eggs. *J Fish Dis* **7**: 173–82.

Evelyn, T.P.T., Prosperi-Porta, L. and Ketcheson, J.E. 1986. Experimental intra-ovum infection of salmonid eggs with *Renibacterium salmoninarum* and vertical transmission of the pathogen with such eggs despite their treatment with erythromycin. *Dis Aquat Org* **1**: 197–202.

Evenden, A.J., Grayson, T.H., Gilpin, M.L. and Munn, C.B. 1993. *Renibacterium salmoninarum* and bacterial kidney disease - the unfinished jigsaw. *Annu Rev Fish Dis* **3**: 87–104.

Fairgrieve, W.T., Masada, C.L., McAuley, W.C., *et al.*, 2005. Accumulation and clearance of orally administered erythromycin and its derivative, azithromycin, in juvenile fall Chinook salmon *Oncorhynchus tshawytscha*. *Dis Aquat Org* **64**: 99–106.

Faisal, M., Loch, T.P., Brenden, T.O., *et al.*, 2010. Assessment of *Renibacterium salmoninarum* infections in four lake whitefish (*Coregonus clupeaformis*) stocks from northern Lakes Huron and Michigan. *J Great Lakes Res* **36**: 29–37.

Fenichel, E.P., Tsao, J.I. and Jones, M.L. 2009. Modeling fish health to inform research and management: *Renibacterium salmoninarum* dynamics in Lake Michigan. *Ecol Appl* **19**: 747–60.

Ferguson, H.W. 2006. *Systemic Pathology of Fish: a Text and Atlas of Normal Tissues in Teleosts and their Responses in Disease*. 2nd edn. London, Scotian Press.

Fiedler, F. and Draxl, R. 1986. Biochemical and immunochemical properties of the cell surface of *Renibacterium salmoninarum*. *J Bacteriol* **168**: 799–804.

Flaño, E., Kaattari, S.L., Razquin, B. and Villena, A.J. 1996. Histopathology of the thymus of coho salmon *Oncorhynchus kisutch* experimentally infected with *Renibacterium salmoninarum*. *Dis Aquat Org* **26**: 11–18.

Fredriksen, A., Endresen, C. and Wergeland, H.I. 1997. Immunosuppressive effect of a low molecular weight surface protein from *Renibacterium salmoninarum* on lymphocytes from Atlantic salmon (*Salmo salar* L). *Fish Shellfish Immunol* **7**: 273–82.

Fryer, J.L. and Sanders, J.E. 1981. Bacterial kidney disease of salmonid fish. *Annu Rev Microbiol* **35**: 273–98.

Fryer, J.L. and Lannan, C.N. 1993. The history and current status of *Renibacterium salmoninarum*, the causative agent of bacterial kidney disease in Pacific salmon. *Fish Res* **17**: 15–33.

Ganassin, R.C. and Bols, N.C. 1998. Development of a monocyte-macrophage-like cell line, RTS11, from rainbow trout spleen. *Fish Shellfish Immunol* **8**: 457–76.

Getchell, R.G., Rohovec, J.S. and Fryer, J.L. 1985. Comparison of *Renibacterium salmoninarum* isolates by antigenic analysis. *Fish Pathol* **20**: 149–59.

Gianfaldoni, C., Maccari, S., Pancotto, L., *et al.*, 2009. Sortase A confers protection against *Streptococcus pneumoniae* in mice. *Infect Immun* **77**: 2957–61.

Gomez-Chiarri, M., Brown, L.L. and Levine, R.P. 1996. Protection against *Renibacterium salmoninarum* infection by DNA-based immunization, in *Aquaculture Biotechnology* (eds E. Donaldson and D. McKinlay). Proceedings, 2nd International Congress on the Biology of Fish, San Francisco, 155–7. Available at http://www.fishbiologycongress.org/1996.html

Grayson, T.H., Evenden, A.J., Gilpin, M.L., *et al.*, 1995. A gene from *Renibacterium salmoninarum* encoding a product which shows homology to bacterial zinc-metalloproteases. *Microbiology* **141**: 1331–41.

Grayson, T.H., Gilpin, M.L., Evenden, A.J. and Munn, C.B. 2001. Evidence for the immune recognition of two haemolysins of *Renibacterium salmoninarum* by fish displaying clinical symptoms of bacterial kidney disease (BKD). *Fish Shellfish Immunol* **11**: 367–70.

Grayson, T.H., Cooper, L.F., Wrathmell, A.B., *et al.*, 2002. Host responses to *Renibacterium salmoninarum* and specific components of the pathogen reveal the mechanisms of immune suppression and activation. *Immunology* **106**: 273–83.

Griffiths, S.G., Melville, K.J. and Salonius, K. 1998. Reduction of *Renibacterium salmoninarum* culture activity in Atlantic salmon following vaccination with avirulent strains. *Fish Shellfish Immunol* **8**: 607–19.

Guðmundsdóttir, S., Helgason, S., Sigurjónsdóttir, H., *et al.*, 2000. Measures applied to control *Renibacterium salmoninarum* infection in Atlantic salmon: a retrospective study of two sea ranches in Iceland. *Aquaculture* **186**: 193–203.

Hard, J.J., Elliott, D.G., Pascho, R.J., *et al.*, 2006. Genetic effects of ELISA-based segregation for control of bacterial kidney disease in Chinook salmon (*Oncorhynchus tshawytscha*). *Can J Fish Aquat Sci* **63**: 2793–808.

Hardie, L.J., Ellis, A.E. and Secombes, C.J. 1996. *In vitro* activation of rainbow trout macrophages stimulates inhibition of *Renibacterium salmoninarum* growth concomitant with augmented generation of respiratory burst products. *Dis Aquat Org* **25**: 175–83.

Hayakawa, Y., Harada, T., Hatai, K., *et al.*, 1989. Histopathology of BKD (bacterial kidney disease) occurred in sea-cultured coho salmon (*Oncorhynchus kisutch*). *Fish Pathol* **24**: 17–21.

Hendricks, J.D. and Leek, S.L. 1975. Kidney disease postorbital lesions in Chinook salmon (*Oncorhynchus tshawytscha*). *Trans Am Fish Soc* **104**: 805–7.

Higgins, D., Marshall, J.D., Traquina, P., *et al.*, 2007. Immunostimulatory DNA as a vaccine adjuvant. *Expert Rev Vaccines* **6**: 747–59.

Hoffmann, R., Popp, W. and van de Graaff, S. 1984. Atypical BKD predominantly causing ocular and skin lesions. *Bull Eur Assoc Fish Pathol* **4**: 7–9.

Holey, M.F., Elliott, R.F., Marcquenski, S.V., *et al.*, 1998. Chinook salmon epizootics in Lake Michigan: possible contributing factors and management implications. *J Aquat Anim Health* **10**: 202–10.

Jansson, E., Hongslo, T., Johannisson, A., *et al.*, 2003. Bacterial kidney disease as a model for studies of cell mediated immunity in rainbow trout (*Oncorhynchus mykiss*). *Fish Shellfish Immunol* **14**: 347–62.

Johnson, K.A., Flynn, J.K. and Amend, D.F. 1982. Duration of immunity in salmonids vaccinated by direct immersion with *Yersinia ruckeri* and *Vibrio anguillarum* bacterins. *J Fish Dis* **5**: 207–13.

Johnson, R.M., Bryden, C.A. and Heath, D.D. 2003. Utility of genetically based health indicators for selection purposes in captive-reared Chinook salmon, *Oncorhynchus tshawytscha*, Walbaum. *Aquacult Res* **34**: 1029–36.

Jones, D.T., Moffitt, C.M. and Peters, K.K. 2007. Temperature-mediated differences in bacterial kidney disease expression and survival in *Renibacterium salmoninarum*-challenged bull trout and other salmonids. *N Am J Fish Manag* **27**: 695–706.

Kaattari, S.L. and Piganelli, J.D. 1997. Immunization with bacterial antigens: bacterial kidney disease. *Dev Biol Stand* **90**: 145–52.

Kawamura, H., Awakura, T., Watanabe, K. and Matsumoto, H. 1977. Therapeutic effects of erythromycin and the sensitivity of four salmonid fishes to bacterial kidney disease. *Sci Rep Hokkaido Fish Hatch* **32**: 21–36.

Kent, M.L., Traxler, G.S., Kieser, D., *et al.*, 1998. Survey of salmonid pathogens in ocean-caught fishes in British Columbia, Canada. *J Aquat Anim Health* **10**: 211–19.

Kurath, G., Garver, K.A., Corbeil, S., *et al.*, 2006. Protective immunity and lack of histopathological damage two years after DNA vaccination against infectious hematopoietic necrosis virus in trout. *Vaccine* **24**: 345–54.

Lee, E.G.H. and Evelyn, T.P.T. 1994. Prevention of vertical transmission of the bacterial kidney disease agent *Renibacterium salmoninarum* by broodstock injection with erythromycin. *Dis Aquat Org* **18**: 1–4.

Lovely, J.E., Cabo, C., Griffiths, S.G. and Lynch, W.H. 1994. Detection of *Renibacterium salmoninarum* infection in asymptomatic Atlantic salmon. *J Aquat Anim Health* **6**: 126–32.

Lumsden, J.S., Russell, S., Huber, P., *et al.*, 2008. An immune-complex glomerulonephritis of Chinook salmon, *Oncorhynchus tshawytscha* (Walbaum). *J Fish Dis* **31**: 889–98.

MacLean, D.G. and Yoder, W.G. 1970. Kidney disease among Michigan salmon in 1967. *Prog Fish-Cult* **32**: 26–30.

Maresso, A.W. and Schneewind, O. 2008. Sortase as a target of anti-infective therapy. *Pharmacol Rev* **60**: 128–41.

Maule, A.G., Rondorf, D.W., Beeman, J. and Haner, P. 1996. Incidence of *Renibacterium salmoninarum* infections in juvenile hatchery spring Chinook salmon in the Columbia and Snake rivers. *J Aquat Anim Health* **8**: 37–46.

McCarthy, D.H., Croy, T.R. and Amend, D.F. 1984. Immunization of rainbow trout, *Salmo gairdneri* Richardson, against bacterial kidney disease: preliminary efficacy evaluation. *J Fish Dis* **7**: 65–71.

McIntosh, D., Austin, B., Flaño, E., *et al.*, 2000. Lack of uptake of *Renibacterium salmoninarum* by gill epithelia of rainbow trout. *J Fish Biol* **56**: 1053–61.

Mesa, M.G., Poe, T.P., Maule, A.G. and Schreck, C.B. 1998. Vulnerability to predation and physiological stress responses in juvenile Chinook salmon (*Oncorhynchus tshawytscha*) experimentally infected with *Renibacterium salmoninarum*. *Can J Fish Aquat Sci* **55**: 1599–606.

Mesa, M.G., Maule, A.G., Poe, T.P. and Schreck, C.B. 1999. Influence of bacterial kidney disease on smoltification in salmonids: is it a case of double jeopardy? *Aquaculture* **174**: 25–41.

Metzger, D.C., Elliott, D.G., Wargo, A., *et al*., 2010. Pathological and immunological responses associated with differential survival of Chinook salmon following *Renibacterium salmoninarum* challenge. *Dis Aquat Org* **90**: 31–41.

Meyers, T.R., Korn, D., Glass, K., *et al*., 2003. Retrospective analysis of antigen prevalences of *Renibacterium salmoninarum* (Rs) detected by enzyme-linked immunosorbent assay in Alaskan Pacific salmon and trout from 1988 to 2000 and management of Rs in hatchery Chinook and coho salmon. *J Aquat Anim Health* **15**: 101–10.

Midtlyng, P.J. 1996. A field study on intraperitoneal vaccination of Atlantic salmon (*Salmo salar* L.) against furunculosis. *Fish Shellfish Immunol* **6**: 553–65.

Midtlyng, P.J. and Lillehaug, A. 1998. Growth of Atlantic salmon *Salmo salar* after intraperitoneal administration of vaccines containing adjuvants. *Dis Aquat Org* **32**: 91–7.

Mitchum, D.L. and Sherman, L.E. 1981. Transmission of bacterial kidney disease from wild to stocked hatchery trout. *Can J Fish Aquat Sci* **38**: 547–51.

Mitchum, D.L., Sherman, L.E. and Baxter, G.T. 1979. Bacterial kidney disease in feral populations of brook trout (*Salvelinus fontinalis*), brown trout (*Salmo trutta*) and rainbow trout (*Salmo gairdneri*). *J Fish Res Board Can* **36**: 1370–76.

Moffitt, C.M. 1991. Oral and injectable applications of erythromycin in salmonid fish culture. *Vet Hum Toxicol* **33** (Suppl. 1): 49–53.

Moffitt, C.M. 1992. Survival of juvenile Chinook salmon challenged with *Renibacterium salmoninarum* and administered oral doses of erythromycin thiocyanate for different durations. *J Aquat Anim Health* **4**: 119–25.

Moffitt, C.M. and Kiryu, Y. 1999. Toxicity, teratogenesis, and efficacy of injectable erythromycin (Erythro-200) administered repeatedly to adult spring Chinook salmon. *J Aquat Anim Health* **11**: 1–11.

Munson, A.D., Elliott, D.G. and Johnson, K. 2010. Management of bacterial kidney disease in Chinook salmon hatcheries based on broodstock testing by enzyme-linked immunosorbent assay: a multiyear study. *N Am J Fish Manag* **30**: 940–55.

Murray, A.G., Hall, M., Munro, L.A. and Wallace, I.S. 2011. Modelling management strategies for a disease including undetected sub-clinical infection: Bacterial kidney disease in Scottish salmon and trout farms. *Epidemics* **3**: 171–82.

Murray, A.G., Munro, L.A. and Wallace, I.S., *et al*., 2012. Epidemiology of *Renibacterium salmoninarum* in Scotland and the potential for compartmentalised management of salmon and trout farming areas. *Aquaculture* **324–325**: 1–13.

Murray, C.B., Evelyn, T.P.T., Beacham, T.D., *et al*., 1992. Experimental induction of bacterial kidney disease in Chinook salmon by immersion and cohabitation challenges. *Dis Aquat Org* **12**: 91–6.

Mutoloki, S., Reite, O.B., Brudeseth, B., *et al*., 2006. A comparative immunopathological study of injection site reactions in salmonids following intraperitoneal injection with oil-adjuvanted vaccines. *Vaccine* **24**: 578–88.

O'Farrell, C.L., Elliott, D.G. and Landolt, M.L. 2000. Mortality and kidney histopathology of Chinook salmon *Oncorhynchus tshawytscha* exposed to virulent and attenuated *Renibacterium salmoninarum* strains. *Dis Aquat Org* **43**: 199–209.

Ordal, E.J. and Earp, B.J. 1956. Cultivation and transmission of the etiological agent of bacterial kidney disease. *Proc Soc Exp Biol Med* **92**: 85–8.

Pascho, R.J., Elliott, D.G. and Streufert, J.M. 1991. Brood stock segregation of spring Chinook salmon *Oncorhynchus tshawytscha* by use of the enzyme-linked immunosorbent assay (ELISA) and the fluorescent antibody technique (FAT) affects the prevalence and levels of *Renibacterium salmoninarum* infection in progeny. *Dis Aquat Org* **12**: 25–40.

Pascho, R.J., Goodrich, T.D. and McKibben, C.L. 1997. Evaluation by enzyme-linked immunosorbent assay (ELISA) of *Renibacterium salmoninarum* bacterins affected by persistence of bacterial antigens. *J Aquat Anim Health* **9**: 99–107.

Pascho, R.J., Elliott, D.G. and Chase, D.M. 2002. Comparison of traditional and molecular methods for detection of *Renibacterium salmoninarum*, in *Molecular Diagnosis of Salmonid Diseases* (ed. C.O. Cunningham). Dordrecht, Kluwer Academic Publishers, 157–209.

Paterson, W.D., Desautels, D. and Weber, J.M. 1981. Immune response of Atlantic salmon, *Salmo salar* L., to the causative agent of bacterial kidney disease, *Renibacterium salmoninarum*. *J Fish Dis* **4**: 99–111.

Pedersen, G.M., Johansen, A., Olsen, R.L. and Jørgensen, J.B. 2006. Stimulation of type I IFN activity in Atlantic salmon (*Salmo salar* L.) leukocytes: synergistic effects of cationic proteins and CpG ODN. *Fish Shellfish Immunol* **20**: 503–18.

Piganelli, J.D., Wiens, G.D. and Kaattari, S.L. 1999a. Elevated temperature treatment as a novel method for decreasing p57 on the cell surface of *Renibacterium salmoninarum*. *Dis Aquat Org* **36**: 29–35.

Piganelli, J.D., Wiens, G.D., Zhang, J.A., *et al*., 1999b. Evaluation of a whole cell, p57-vaccine against *Renibacterium salmoninarum*. *Dis Aquat Org* **36**: 37–44.

Pippy, J.H.C. 1969. Kidney disease in juvenile Atlantic salmon (*Salmo salar*) in the Margaree River. *J Fish Res Board Can* **26**: 2535–7.

Polinski, M.P., Fehringer, T.R., Johnson, K.A., *et al*., 2010. Characterization of susceptibility and carrier status of burbot, *Lota lota* (L.), to IHNV, IPNV, *Flavobacterium psychrophilum*, *Aeromonas salmonicida* and *Renibacterium salmoninarum*. *J Fish Dis* **33**: 559–70.

Purcell, M.K., Murray, A.L., Elz, A., *et al*., 2008. Decreased mortality of Lake Michigan Chinook salmon after bacterial kidney disease challenge: evidence for pathogen-driven selection? *J Aquat Anim Health* **20**: 225–35.

Rebl, A., Goldammer, T. and Seyfert, H.-M. 2010. Toll-like receptor signaling in bony fish. *Vet Immunol Immunopathol* **134**: 139–50.

Rhodes, L.D., Coady, A.M. and Deinhard, R.K. 2004a. Identification of a third msa gene in *Renibacterium salmoninarum* and the associated virulence phenotype. *Appl Environ Microbiol* **70**: 6488–94.

Rhodes, L.D., Rathbone, C.K., Corbett, S.C., *et al*., 2004b. Efficacy of cellular vaccines and genetic adjuvants against bacterial kidney disease in Chinook salmon (*Oncorhynchus tshawytscha*). *Fish Shellfish Immunol* **16**: 461–74.

Rhodes, L.D., Nguyen, O.T., Deinhard, R.K., *et al*., 2008. Characterization of *Renibacterium salmoninarum* with reduced susceptibility to macrolide antibiotics by a standard antibiotic susceptibility test. *Dis Aquat Org* **80**: 173–80.

Rhodes, L.D., Wallis, S. and Demlow, S.E. 2009. Genes associated with an effective host response by Chinook salmon to *Renibacterium salmoninarum*. *Dev Comp Immunol* **33**: 176–86.

Rhodes, L.D., Rice, C.A., Greene, C.M., *et al*., 2011. Nearshore ecosystem predictors of a bacterial infection in juvenile Chinook salmon. *Mar Ecol Prog Ser* **432**: 161–72.

Rockey, D.D., Turaga, P.S., Wiens, G.D., *et al*., 1991. Serine proteinase of *Renibacterium salmoninarum* digests a major autologous extracellular and cell-surface protein. *Can J Microbiol* **37**: 758–63.

Sakai, M. and Kobayashi, M. 1992. Detection of *Renibacterium salmoninarum*, the causative agent of bacterial kidney disease in salmonid fish, from pen-cultured coho salmon. *Appl Environ Microbiol* **58**: 1061–3.

Sakai, M., Ogasawara, F., Atsuta, S. and Kobayashi, M. 1989. Comparative sensitivity of carp *Cyprinus carpio* L and rainbow trout *Salmo gairdneri* Richardson, to *Renibacterium salmoninarum*. *J Fish Dis* **12**: 367–72.

Sakai, M., Atsuta, S. and Kobayashi, M. 1991. Susceptibility of five salmonid fishes to *Renibacterium salmoninarum*. *Fish Pathol* **26**: 159–60.

Sakai, M., Atsuta, S. and Kobayashi, M. 1993. The immune response of rainbow trout (*Oncorhynchus mykiss*) injected with five *Renibacterium salmoninarum* bacterins. *Aquaculture* **113**: 11–18.

Salonius, K., Siderakis, C., MacKinnon, A.M. and Griffiths, S.G. 2005. Use of *Arthrobacter davidanieli* as a live vaccine against *Renibacterium salmoninarum* and *Piscirickettsia salmonis* in salmonids. *Dev Biol (Basel)* **121**: 189–97.

Sami, S., Fischer-Scherl, T., Hoffmann, R.W. and Pfeil-Putzien, C. 1992. Immune complex-mediated glomerulonephritis associated with bacterial kidney disease in the rainbow trout (*Oncorhynchus mykiss*). *Vet Pathol* **29**: 169–74.

Sandell, T.A. and Jacobson, K.C. 2011. Comparison and evaluation of *Renibacterium salmoninarum* quantitative PCR diagnostic assays using field samples of Chinook and coho salmon. *Dis Aquat Org* **93**: 129–39.

Sanders, J.E. and Fryer, J.L. 1980. *Renibacterium salmoninarum* gen. nov., sp. nov., the causative agent of bacterial kidney disease in salmonid fishes. *Int J Syst Bacteriol* **30**: 496–502.

Sanders, J.E., Pilcher, K.S. and Fryer, J.L. 1978. Relation of water temperature to bacterial kidney disease in coho salmon (*Oncorhynchus kisutch*), sockeye salmon (*O. nerka*), and steelhead trout (*Salmo gairdneri*). *J Fish Res Board Can* **35**: 8–11.

Senson, P.R. and Stevenson, R.M. 1999. Production of the 57 kDa major surface antigen by a non-agglutinating strain of the fish pathogen *Renibacterium salmoninarum*. *Dis Aquat Org* **38**: 23–31.

Smith, I.W. 1964. The occurrence and pathology of Dee disease. *Freshw Salmon Fish Res* **34**: 1–12.
Sommerset, I., Krossøy, B., Biering, E. and Frost, P. 2005. Vaccines for fish in aquaculture. *Expert Rev Vaccines* **4**: 89–101.
Souter, B.W., Dwilow, A.G. and Knight, K. 1987. *Renibacterium salmoninarum* in wild Arctic charr *Salvelinus alpinus* and lake trout *S. namaycush* from the Northwest Territories, Canada. *Dis Aquat Org* **3**: 151–4.
Speare, D.J. 1997. Differences in patterns of meningoencephalitis due to bacterial kidney disease in farmed Atlantic and Chinook salmon. *Res Vet Sci* **62**: 79–80.
Starliper, C.E. and Morrison, P. 2000. Bacterial pathogen contagion studies among freshwater bivalves and salmonid fishes. *J Shellfish Res* **19**: 251–8.
Starliper, C.E., Smith, D.R. and Shatzer, T. 1997. Virulence of *Renibacterium salmoninarum* to salmonids. *J Aquat Anim Health* **9**: 1–7.
Stranger-Jones, Y.K., Bae, T. and Schneewind, O. 2006. Vaccine assembly from surface proteins of *Staphylococcus aureus*. *Proc Natl Acad Sci USA* **103**: 16942–7.
Sudheesh, P.S., Crane, S., Cain, K.D. and Strom, M.S. 2007. Sortase inhibitor phenyl vinyl sulfone inhibits *Renibacterium salmoninarum* adherence and invasion of host cells. *Dis Aquat Org* **78**: 115–27.
Suzuki, K. and Sakai, D.K. 2007. Real-time PCR for quantification of viable *Renibacterium salmoninarum* in chum salmon *Oncorhynchus keta*. *Dis Aquat Org* **74**: 209–23.
Suzumoto, B., Schreck, C. and McIntyre, J. 1977. Relative resistances of three transferrin genotypes of coho salmon (*Oncorhynchus kisutch*) and their hematological responses to bacterial kidney disease. *J Fish Res Board Can* **34**: 1–8.
Turaga, P., Wiens, G. and Kaattari, S. 1987. Bacterial kidney disease: the potential role of soluble protein antigen(s). *J Fish Biol* **31**: 191–4.
Wang, R., Neumann, N.F., Shen, Q. and Belosevic, M. 1995. Establishment and characterization of a macrophage cell line from goldfish. *Fish Shellfish Immunol* **5**: 329–46.
Wiens, G.D. and Vallejo, R.L. 2010. Temporal and pathogen-load dependent changes in rainbow trout (*Oncorhynchus mykiss*) immune response traits following challenge with biotype 2 *Yersinia ruckeri*. *Fish Shellfish Immunol* **29**: 639–47.
Wiens, G.D., Pascho, R. and Winton, J.R. 2002. A single Ala139-to-Glu substitution in the *Renibacterium salmoninarum* virulence-associated protein p57 results in antigenic variation and is associated with enhanced p57 binding to Chinook salmon leukocytes. *Appl Environ Microbiol* **68**: 3969–77.
Wiens, G.D., Rockey, D.D., Wu, Z., *et al*., 2008. Genome sequence of the fish pathogen *Renibacterium salmoninarum* suggests reductive evolution away from an environmental *Arthrobacter* ancestor. *J Bacteriol* **190**: 6970–82.
Wolf, K. and Dunbar, C.E. 1959. Test of 34 therapeutic agents for control of kidney disease in trout. *Trans Am Fish Soc* **88**: 117–24.
Wolke, R.E. 1975. Pathology of bacterial and fungal diseases affecting fish, in *The Pathology of Fishes* (ed. W.E. Ribelin and G. Migaki). Madison, University of Wisconsin Press, 33–116.
Wood, J.W. and Wallis, J. 1955. Kidney disease in adult Chinook salmon and its transmission by feeding to young Chinook salmon. *Oreg Fish Comm Res Brief* **6**: 32–40.
Wood, P.A. and Kaattari, S.L. 1996. Enhanced immunogenicity of *Renibacterium salmoninarum* in Chinook salmon after removal of the bacterial cell surface-associated 57 kDa protein. *Dis Aquat Org* **25**: 71–9.
Young, C.L. and Chapman, G.B. 1978. Ultrastructural aspects of the causative agent and renal histopathology of bacterial kidney disease in brook trout (*Salvelinus fontinalis*). *J Fish Res Board Can* **35**: 1234–48.

23 Vaccination against Diseases Caused by *Flavobacteriaceae* Species

Krister Sundell, Eva Högfors-Rönnholm and Tom Wiklund

Laboratory of Aquatic Pathobiology, Åbo Akademi University, Turku, Finland

ABSTRACT

In recent years, an increasing number of *Flavobacteriaceae* species have been associated with infections in fish. Still, diseases caused by *Flavobacterium branchiophilum* (bacterial gill disease), *F. columnare* (columnaris disease), *F. psychrophilum* (bacterial cold-water disease), and *Tenacibaculum maritimum* (tenacibaculosis) have been more extensively studied due to their significant economic impact on the aquaculture industry. Immunization with traditional bacterins against diseases caused by *Flavobacteriaceae* species has shown inconsistent results, and more research efforts have been placed on immunogenic evaluations of recombinant proteins and subunit vaccines. So far, commercial vaccines have been made available only against columnaris disease, while protection against bacterial cold-water disease has relied on autogenous vaccines. Since the launch of a live attenuated vaccine for use against columnaris disease in the US, the potential for similar vaccines against infections with *F. psychrophilum* has been under evaluation.

23.1 INTRODUCTION

The family *Flavobacteriaceae* contains several important fish pathogenic species, such as *Flavobacterium branchiophilum*, *F. columnare*, *F. psychrophilum*, and *Tenacibaculum maritimum* (see Bernardet *et al.*, 1996; Avendaño-Herrera *et al.*, 2006a; Barnes and Brown, 2011; Starliper and Schill, 2011). In addition, a number of bacterial species belonging to the *Flavobacteriaceae*, such as *Chryseobacterium scophthalmum* (Mudarris *et al.*, 1994; Vandamme *et al.*, 1994), *C. piscicola* (Ilardi *et al.*, 2009), *C. piscium* (de Beer *et al.*, 2006), *Flavobacterium johnsoniae* (Bernardet and Bowman, 2006; Flemming *et al.*, 2007), and *Flexibacter ovolyticus* (Hansen *et al.*, 1992) have been associated with occasional mortality in fish. The number of *Flavobacteriaceae* species affecting fish is continuously expanding, and recently three new species were described, *Flavobacterium chilense* and *F. araucananum*

twiklund@abo.fi

Fish Vaccination, First Edition. Edited by Roar Gudding, Atle Lillehaug and Øystein Evensen.

from diseased salmonids in Chile, and *F. oncorhynchi* from rainbow trout (*Oncorhynchus mykiss*) in Spain (Kämpfer *et al.*, 2012; Zamora *et al.*, 2012).

In this chapter the main focus will be on immunization against diseases caused by *F. branchiophilum*, *F. columnare*, *F. psychrophilum* and *T. maritimum*. These microorganisms are infecting a large number of fish species worldwide, causing significant problems in both marine and freshwater aquaculture.

23.2 BACTERIAL GILL DISEASE (*Flavobacterium branchiophilum*)

Flavobacterium branchiophilum was initially described as a pathogen causing gill infections in salmonids and other freshwater fish like sheatfish (*Silurus glanis*) and silver carp (*Hypophthalmichtys molitrix*) (Wakabayashi *et al.*, 1980; Farkas, 1985; Ostland *et al.*, 1994). Brook trout (*Salvelinus fontinalis*) and rainbow trout in hatcheries seem to be particularly vulnerable (Starliper and Schill, 2011). The pathogen has been reported from Canada, Hungary, Japan, South Korea and the US (Farkas, 1985; Wakabayashi *et al.*, 1989; Ferguson *et al.*, 1991; Ostland *et al.*, 1994; Ko and Heo, 1997) and possibly also in fish from the Netherlands (Farkas, 1985).

F. branchiophilum is mainly associated with gills of fish and it can produce extensive cellular colonization on the gill surfaces (Wakabayashi *et al.*, 1980; Speare *et al.*, 1991). The disease caused by this pathogen has thus been called bacterial gill disease (BGD). Although other pigmented *Cytophaga*-like bacteria and pathogens including *F. columnare* (Farkas and Oláh, 1986) have been isolated from affected gill tissue, *F. branchiophilum* is regarded as the most important agent of BGD (Speare *et al.*, 1995). The pathogen has seldom, if ever (Bernardet, 1997), been isolated from internal organs of fish, and *F. branchiophilum* is consequently considered not to cause systemic infections in fish (Ototake and Wakabayashi, 1985; Starliper and Schill, 2011).

The disease signs initially include lamellar epithelial hydropic degeneration and necrosis, as well as lamellar oedema (Speare *et al.*, 1991). Fusion of gill filaments (Ototake and Wakabayashi, 1985) and epithelial hyperplasia occur later in the infection process as a subacute or chronic response to *F. branchiophilum* (Speare *et al.*, 1991).

Attachment and colonization of the gills by the bacterium occur rapidly after exposure. The virulence has been suggested to be associated with the presence of fimbriae on the bacterial cells (Heo *et al.*, 1990b) for the attachment, or with extracellular products showing hemagglutinating and bacterioagglutinating activities (Ototake and Wakabayashi, 1985). The mortality due to *F. branchiophilum* has been connected with insufficient gas exchange at the gills (Wakabayashi and Iwado, 1985) or with circulatory disturbances (Byrne *et al.*, 1991).

Horizontal transmission of the bacterium in salmonids has successfully been induced from the water (Ostland *et al.*, 1995) or through cohabitation with infected fish both within and between species (Ferguson *et al.*, 1991). Both virulent and avirulent isolates of *F. branchiophilum* seem to adhere to gill tissue, but only virulent ones (Ostland *et al.*, 1995) are able to cause BGD. The fimbriae (Heo *et al.*, 1990b) produced by the bacterium have been suggested to facilitate its attachment to the gill epithelium. Indeed, Ostland *et al.* (1997) reported that adherence of *F. branchiophilum* was reduced following immersion of fish in water containing crude fimbriae extracts. Unfortunately, total inhibition was not achieved and the adherence reduction was only 22–33%, suggesting that other adhesion structures than the fimbriae might also be present.

Isolates of different geographic origin share common antigens, but antigenic diversity has been reported among isolates from different geographic regions. For example, Japanese isolates are serologically distinct from North American and Hungarian isolates (Wakabayashi *et al.*, 1980; Huh and Wakabayashi, 1989). Antigenic variation has also been reported among isolates from the same geographical area (Ostland *et al.*, 1994). Heo *et al.* (1990a) concluded that fish naturally infected with *F. branchiophilum* did not produce circulating antibodies against the pathogen, most probably due to the lack of a systemic infection. In contrast, experimental exposure of brook trout to *F. branchiophilum* by horizontal infection and a subsequent bath challenge induced a slight response in both serum and gill antibodies (Lumsden *et al.*, 1993). Subsequently, Lumsden *et al.* (1994) reported that fish surviving an experimental challenge with *F. branchiophilum* showed increased survival in a following second challenge, compared with control fish not previously exposed to the pathogen.

In immunization trials, promising results have been obtained. Lumsden *et al.* (1994) immunized rainbow trout repeatedly by bath or intraperitoneal (IP) injection with acetone-killed *F. branchiophilum*. Fish that were bath-immunized three times showed good protection against an experimental challenge with *F. branchiophilum*. Similar results were obtained in another study with rainbow trout bath-immunized twice with acetone-killed *F. branchiophilum* (Lumsden *et al.*, 1995). IP-immunized fish also showed protection against *F. branchiophilum*, although not to the same extent as bath-immunized fish (Lumsden *et al.*, 1994, 1995), indicating a possible transfer of protecting circulating antibodies to the gill surfaces. In a subsequent study, it was indeed observed that antibodies against *F. branchiophilum* were present in the gill mucosa after IP vaccination with acetone-killed bacteria (Lumsden *et al.*, 1995). It was, however, concluded that fish exposed to *F. branchiophilum* by immersion are better protected than those IP-injected with the same antigen (Lumsden *et al.*, 1995). Immunized fish showed significantly decreased *F. branchiophilum* loads on the gills compared with non-vaccinated control fish after a bacterial challenge. The authors concluded that the local immune response was probably responsible for the significant reduction in *F. branchiophilum* measured on the gills of vaccinated fish. It was suggested that future studies should focus on measuring the effect of vaccination on protection from horizontal challenge with *F. branchiophilum* (Lumsden *et al.*, 1994).

23.3 COLUMNARIS DISEASE (*Flavobacterium columnare*)

Flavobacterium columnare is the bacterial pathogen associated with columnaris disease affecting several freshwater fish species. For decades *F. columnare* has been a noted fish pathogen because of its wide geographic distribution and host range. Today, columnaris disease constitutes a huge threat to several commercially important aquaculture species such as the channel catfish (*Ictalurus punctatus*), common carp (*Cyprinus carpio*), and Nile tilapia (*Oreochromis niloticus*). In recent years, *F. columnare* has also become a serious nuisance for the Atlantic salmon (*Salmo salar*), brown trout (*S. trutta*), and rainbow trout fingerling production in parts of Europe (Kubilay *et al.*, 2008; Pulkkinen *et al.*, 2010) and Chile (Avendaño-Herrera *et al.*, 2011). The economic impacts of *F. columnare* infections have been particularly severe for the US channel catfish industry, with an estimated annual loss of US$30 million (Wagner *et al.*, 2002).

Columnaris disease occurs throughout the year, but more typically in water temperatures above 20°C. The disease is associated with stressful conditions resulting from poor water quality, high temperature, crowding and excessive handling. Feed training and starvation have also been shown to increase the susceptibility of fish to *F. columnare* infections (Shoemaker *et al.*, 2003; Bebak *et al.*, 2009). Fish infected with *F. columnare* generally exhibit severe gill and skin necrosis, but occasionally systemic infections occur without visible external signs of infection. The bacterium can be spread directly from fish-to-fish contact or indirectly via the water column (Welker *et al.*, 2005). Although the gravity of columnaris disease outbreaks is usually determined by strain virulence, high water temperatures and high rearing densities can accelerate the progression of the disease (Suomalainen *et al.*, 2005; Noga, 2010).

Despite extensive research, much still remains unknown about the virulence mechanisms of *F. columnare*. Serological studies have revealed four major serotypes of the pathogen, but no apparent connection between serotype and virulence has been ascertained (Anacker and Ordal, 1959; Noga, 2010). Triyanto and Wakabayashi (1999) found three distinct genetic groups or genomovars of *F. columnare*, which have been shown to differ in virulence (Decostere *et al.*, 1998) and host specificity (Olivares-Fuster *et al.*, 2007). Tissue-degrading chondroitin AC lyase activity and positive chemotaxis to fish mucus have also shown a positive correlation with the virulence of *F. columnare* (Suomalainen *et al.*, 2006; Klesius *et al.*, 2008). *F. columnare* isolated from fish have, under laboratory conditions, been shown to express differences in cell (Thomas-Jinu and Goodwin, 2004) and colony morphology (Song *et al.*, 1988). Furthermore, this pathogen has been shown to dissociate into four different colony types with different adhesion capacities and tissue-degrading properties (Kunttu *et al.*, 2009, 2011). Although morphological changes have not directly been connected to the virulence of *F. columnare*, they might play an important part in the pathogenesis of columnaris disease.

Ever since the detection of humoral and cutaneous antibody responses against *F. columnare* in economically significant fish species (Fujihara and Nakatani, 1971; Schachte and Mora, 1973; Grabowski *et al.*, 2004; Shoemaker *et al.*, 2005), the way has been paved for the development of vaccines against columnaris disease. Now that standardized infection models have become available for determining vaccine efficacy, the development has further increased in speed. Today a reproducible immersion challenge protocol for catfish (Klesius *et al.*, 1999; Shoemaker *et al.*, 2003) and rainbow trout (LaFrentz *et al.*, 2012) is available. An alternative model using the common zebra fish (*Danio rerio*) has also been developed (Moyer and Hunnicutt, 2007).

Overall the control of columnaris disease through any type of vaccination is complicated by the high susceptibility of fish to *F. columnare* infections during early life stages. At a time when the immunological memory of fish is not fully developed for long-term immunity, it is probable that disease resistance mainly relies upon non-specific immune responses. Passive immunization trials with antiserum have demonstrated only partial protection against *F. columnare* in juvenile channel catfish, suggesting that cell-mediated responses might play an important role in the acquired immunity to columnaris disease (Shelby *et al.*, 2007). Accordingly, Leal *et al.* (2010) found no correlation between immunoglobulin titers and disease protection after injection vaccination of Nile tilapia fingerlings against *F. columnare*. Since problems with *F. columnare* infections have been more oriented towards juvenile fish than adult fish, parenteral vaccination has not been considered the optimal strategy for controlling columnaris disease.

Therefore, the effort has been placed on the development of more practically deliverable vaccines. Although oral vaccination has provided protection against *F. columnare* in coho salmon (*Oncorhynchus kisutch*) (Fujihara and Nakatani, 1971; Ransom, 1975), this administration route is considered to be rather ineffective because of possible antigen degradation in the gastrointestinal tract. In one of few reported oral vaccination attempts against columnaris disease, Leal *et al.* (2010) obtained no protection in Nile tilapia despite embedding bacterins in alginate microparticles protecting the antigens from degradation.

Immersion vaccination attempts with formalin-inactivated bacterins have also resulted in limited effectiveness (Moore *et al.*, 1990; Mano *et al.*, 1996). Therefore, it has been suggested that formalin is responsible for the destruction of important bacterial antigens and is consequently not suitable for the inactivation of *F. columnare* for vaccine production (Bader *et al.*, 1997). Nevertheless, a few commercial bacterin-based vaccines against columnaris disease have already become available in North America and Chile. The unadjuvanted bacterin-based immersion vaccine Fryvacc 1 is available for use in salmonids in the US and Canada. In addition to Fryvacc 1, the bivalent Fryvacc 2, containing *F. columnare* and *Yersinia ruckeri* bacterins, has been available for immersion vaccination of salmonids in Chile since 1999 (Bravo and Midtlyng, 2007).

To overcome problems associated with antigen destruction during vaccine preparation and administration, the development and use of live attenuated immersion vaccines has become more attractive, despite concerns raised about their biosafety. As an aid in the prevention of columnaris disease in catfish species, a live attenuated vaccine Aquavac-Col® was released in the US in 2005. The live vaccine can be used for controlling columnaris disease even in other fish species under the direction of a licensed veterinarian (Yanong, 2008). Even though Aquavac-Col® has been shown to improve survival of eyed channel catfish eggs and fry against *F. columnare* infections under laboratory conditions (Shoemaker *et al.*, 2007, 2011), limited information is available of its effectiveness in fish farm environments. In a field trial with feed-trained largemouth bass fry (*Micropterus salmoides floridanus*), immunization with Aquavac-Col®, however, significantly reduced the risk of mortality from columnaris disease (Bebak *et al.*, 2009). Still, the effectiveness of Aquavac-Col® in salmonids is not known.

The mechanisms by which immunization with the live Aquavac-Col® vaccine results in disease protection in fish is not yet fully understood. However, immunization with the live vaccine has been shown to stimulate the production of antibodies that recognize lipopolysaccharide and protein antigens of *F. columnare* (Shoemaker *et al.*, 2007). In an immune gene expression study in channel catfish, up to 28 different genes were upregulated 10 minutes post-vaccination with Aquavac-Col®. Almost half of these genes represented immune response genes mostly involved in either innate or protective immunity following infection (Pridgeon and Klesius, 2010). The vaccine Aquavac-Col® is derived from an avirulent rifampicin-resistant *F. columnare* mutant originally belonging to the genomovar I. As genomovar II has been proven to be more virulent to channel catfish than genomovar I, the development of a live *F. columnare* vaccine from a genomovar II isolate has already begun (Olivares-Fuster and Arias, 2011).

To avoid potential risks associated with the use of modified live bacterins, second-generation recombinant vaccines would be preferable for a more widespread application. To date, several *F. columnare* proteins have been identified as potential vaccine targets for novel recombinant vaccines (Olivares-Fuster *et al.*, 2010; Liu *et al.*, 2012). Some of the proteins, however, show significant sequence variation between genomovars, which could translate into differences in their immunogenic properties (Olivares-Fuster *et al.*, 2010). In the first, and thus far only, reported attempt to immunize channel catfish with a subunit vaccine against *F. columnare*, the highly immunogenic heat-shock protein DnaJ failed to elicit protection against columnaris disease (Olivares-Fuster *et al.*, 2010). Since the identification of protective antigens is critical in the process of developing efficient subunit vaccines, a deeper knowledge of the immunogenic properties of *F. columnare* is needed.

23.4 BACTERIAL COLD-WATER DISEASE (*Flavobacterium psychrophilum*)

Flavobacterium psychrophilum (Bernardet *et al.*, 1996), the etiological agent of bacterial cold-water disease (BCWD) (Holt *et al.*, 1993), infects a variety of cold-water fish species. In addition to most farmed and wild salmonids, a wide range of non-salmonids are seriously affected by this fish pathogen (see Starliper, 2011). Since the first isolation of *F. psychrophilum* in the US in 1948, the pathogen has spread dramatically over the world and is now causing significant economic losses to the freshwater salmonid aquaculture industry worldwide (see Barnes and Brown, 2011; Starliper, 2011).

Outbreaks of BCWD usually occur at temperatures below 15°C and the clinical signs differ between fish of different sizes. Infections in fry appear to develop rapidly and sometimes even without clinical signs, and result in an acute systemic infection with spleen hypertrophy and high mortality as a consequence (see Dalsgaard, 1993; Nematollahi *et al.*, 2003b). *F. psychrophilum* infections in rainbow trout fry are also called rainbow trout fry syndrome (RTFS) (Lorenzen, 1994), but since the etiological agent is identical, BCWD has become the more established name for the disease. Infected fingerlings can appear lethargic or anemic and show exophthalmia, dark skin pigmentation and sometimes skin lesions as the first signs of infection. Clinical signs in juveniles are usually anemia, exophthalmia and larger necrotic skin lesions and ulcers. In fingerling and juvenile populations, infections are less acute and the mortalities are not as high as in fry populations (see Dalsgaard, 1993; Nematollahi *et al.*, 2003b).

In spite of extensive studies on BCDW, it is still not known how *F. psychrophilum* infects fish. A vertical transmission from brood fish to offspring has been proposed (see Starliper, 2011), but horizontal transmission of the bacterium from the water into the fish through gills, skin and/or the intestinal tract is, however, most likely (see Dalsgaard, 1993; Starliper, 2011).

In 2007 the complete genome sequence of a virulent isolate of *F. psychrophilum* was reported, describing several potential genes encoding for virulence factors (Duchaud *et al.*, 2007). Some of these virulence mechanisms are, for example, secreted proteases important for host tissue breakdown (Bertolini *et al.*, 1994) and nutrient acquirement (Pérez-Pascual *et al.*, 2011), hemolysins for cell destruction and nutrient acquisition (Högfors-Rönnholm and Wiklund, 2010b), adhesins for attachment to host tissues (Kondo *et al.*, 2002; Nematollahi *et al.*, 2003a) and cells (Møller *et al.*, 2003; Wiklund and Dalsgaard, 2003; Högfors-Rönnholm and Wiklund, 2010b) and proteins involved in biofilm formation (Álvarez *et al.*, 2006). Since *F. psychrophilum* expresses both antigenic (Wakabayashi *et al.*, 1994; Lorenzen and Olesen, 1997) and phase variation (Högfors-Rönnholm and Wiklund, 2010a), it is challenging to determine the overall virulence mechanisms for this pathogen as different types probably express diverse virulence mechanisms. It has been shown that even though all

F. psychrophilum isolates share some antigens, they can be divided into three (Wakabayashi *et al.*, 1994; Lorenzen and Olesen, 1997) or seven (Mata *et al.*, 2002) distinct serotypes. While the two phase variants share similar metabolic characteristics and are both virulent in rainbow trout, they show distinct physiological characteristics and differences in enzymatic, hemagglutinating and hemolytic activity (Högfors-Rönnholm and Wiklund, 2010a,b). Hence, for a vaccine to be efficient against *F. psychrophilum*, it could be necessary to include antigens from different serotypes and variants.

To this date, there is no general vaccine against *F. psychrophilum* commercially available due to several difficulties. One of the major problems is the fact that *F. psychrophilum* infections are most severe in fry populations. Newly-hatched fry have an undeveloped adaptive immune system and are both impractical and uneconomic to vaccinate by injection. The ideal vaccine delivery method, regarding any affected fish species or size, would therefore be an oral or immersion administration. Another problem is the lack of natural and reproducible challenge models to test the efficacy of vaccines. An immersion-based challenge model has been reported for ayu (*Plecoglossus altivelis*) (Kondo *et al.*, 2003), but for other salmonid species only injection-based challenge models with *F. psychrophilum* induce mortality (Lorenzen *et al.*, 2010).

Nevertheless, experimental vaccination trials have shown that a specific antibody response and a good protection against *F. psychrophilum* can be achieved in rainbow trout (LaFrentz *et al.*, 2002; Madetoja *et al.*, 2006; Högfors *et al.*, 2008) and in ayu (Rahman *et al.*, 2000, 2003) after IP immunization with whole inactivated cell preparations both with and without adjuvants. Although the specific antibody response in immunized fish often correlates with protection against experimental challenge with *F. psychrophilum*, other immune mechanisms are suggested to be necessary for complete protection against BCWD (LaFrentz *et al.*, 2002, 2003).

Attempts to immunize fish against *F. psychrophilum* by bath or immersion have so far been scarce. Immersion immunization trials with rainbow trout using inactivated whole cell preparations have failed to generate a specific antibody response and to protect the immunized fish against *F. psychrophilum* (LaFrentz *et al.*, 2002; Lorenzen *et al.*, 2010). Experimental trials on oral vaccination of ayu (Kondo *et al.*, 2003) and rainbow trout (Aoki *et al.*, 2007) with *F. psychrophilum* antigen preparations have been more successful, and high survival rates following immersion challenge have been reported in both species. However, both the antigen preparation and the challenge with rainbow trout were performed with the *F. psychrophilum* type strain NCIMB 1947^T isolated from coho salmon and previously shown to be non-virulent in rainbow trout (Madsen and Dalsgaard, 2000).

Because *F. psychrophilum* is a slow-growing fastidious bacterium, a whole cell vaccine might not be the best cost-effective alternative for a commercial vaccine. In recent years the focus has been on identification of immunogenic cell surface molecules, proteins or fractions that could be used as antigens in a recombinant subunit vaccine (LaFrentz *et al.*, 2004; Crump *et al.*, 2005; Gliniewicz *et al.*, 2012). Subunit vaccines also have the potential to be delivered orally or by immersion of fish in their early life stages when no oil-based adjuvants can be used. To date, most immunization trials with subunit vaccines have resulted in low protection against *F. psychrophilum* without the use of conventional adjuvants (Rahman *et al.*, 2000; Högfors *et al.*, 2008; Plant *et al.*, 2011). Through IP immunization of rainbow trout fry with a recombinant protein combined with an adjuvant, Crump *et al.* (2007) were able to obtain a relative percent survival of 82% after an injection challenge with *F. psychrophilum*. LaFrentz *et al.* (2004) observed that IP immunization of rainbow trout with a 70–100 kDa fraction combined with an adjuvant resulted in high specific antibody titers with high survival rates after subcutaneous injection with *F. psychrophilum*. Plant *et al.* (2009) used two highly immunogenic heat shock proteins, Hsp 60 and Hsp 70, derived from within the 70–100 kDa fraction in an immunization trial with rainbow trout. The recombinant heat-shock proteins elicited an antibody response when IP-injected, but failed to confer protection against challenge with *F. psychrophilum* both individually and in combination. When cloned and delivered intramuscularly (IM) as a DNA vaccine into rainbow trout, neither Hsp 60 nor Hsp 70 protected the fish against challenge with *F. psychrophilum* and only low specific antibody titers were detected (Plant *et al.*, 2009). Three other recombinant high molecular protein antigens (i.e., elongation factor-Tu, SufB Fe-S assembly protein and ATP synthaseβ) were tested in another immunization trial with rainbow trout, but these antigens also failed to elicit an antibody response or to confer protection against BCWD (Plant *et al.*, 2011).

Outer membrane fractions or proteins isolated from *F. psychrophilum* have been reported to be good candidates for a subunit vaccine (Rahman *et al.*, 2002; Dumetz *et al.*, 2006, 2007). Rahman *et al.* (2002) showed that IP immunization with an outer membrane fraction without an adjuvant resulted in high survival rates in both juvenile rainbow trout (93–95%) and in ayu (64–71%) after challenge with *F. psychrophilum*. Rainbow trout IP-immunized with an OmpH-like protein, the P18-enriched fraction, combined with an oil adjuvant also showed high survival rates (89%) after challenge with *F. psychrophilum*, which correlated with high specific serum antibody titers. While the P18-enriched fraction alone did not elicit a significant decrease in mortality, an increase in specific antibody titers was observed (Dumetz *et al.*, 2006), which is promising for future immersion vaccine development.

More recently, the potential of live attenuated vaccines against *F. psychrophilum* infections has been investigated (Álvarez *et al.*, 2008; LaFrentz *et al.*, 2008). Álvarez *et al.* (2008) showed that IM immunization with a *F. psychrophilum* mutant, deficient in growth under iron-limited conditions, resulted in a high survival rate (82%) in rainbow trout after challenge with the parent virulent *F. psychrophilum* strain. In an IP immunization trial using a rifampicin attenuated *F. psychrophilum* vaccine (patented in 2010), rainbow trout showed only a moderate survival rate (45%) after an injection challenge with the parent unattenuated strain, despite significantly elevated specific antibody titers (LaFrentz *et al.*, 2008). In the corresponding immersion trial, survival rates of 28% and 45% were reported for fish treated with or without adipose fin removal before immunization, respectively (LaFrentz *et al.*, 2008). Lorenzen *et al.* (2010) discovered that immersion exposure of rainbow trout fry to a live virulent wild-type *F. psychrophilum* isolate induced no mortality, but resulted in high survival rates (60–88%) after injection challenge with *F. psychrophilum*. Although high survival rates and an increase in specific antibody titers were reported in the immunized fish, the authors found it unlikely that a virulent wild-type *F. psychrophilum* isolate would be utilized for vaccination of fish under field conditions. These reports demonstrate the potential of a live *F. psychrophilum* immersion vaccine for fry, since attenuated bacterial cells can stimulate the fish immune system without causing disease.

Even though no commercial *F. psychrophilum* vaccines are available today, autogenous vaccines have been employed in some countries to prevent or clearly reduce BCWD outbreaks (Fredriksen *et al.*, 2013). Autogenous vaccines against *F. psychrophilum* have been used on salmon in Chile (Bravo and Midtlyng, 2007), on rainbow trout in Norway (Johansen *et al.*, 2011) and on both salmon and rainbow trout in the UK, where the vaccination has largely reduced BCDW outbreaks in a salmon and rainbow trout hatchery (Wallis *et al.*, 2009).

23.5 TENACIBACULOSIS (*Tenacibaculum maritimum*)

Tenacibaculum maritimum (Suzuki *et al.*, 2001), previously *Cytophaga marina*, *Flexibacter marinus* and *F. maritimus*, is the disease agent of tenacibaculosis in anadromous and marine fish. The disease caused by *T. maritimum* is known under several different names like "black patch necrosis", "saltwater columnaris disease", "marine flexibacteriosis", "eroded mouth syndrome" and "gliding bacterial disease of sea fish" (Bernardet *et al.*, 1990; Santos *et al.*, 1999). Affected fish show skin ulcers, eroded skin lesions, scale loss, frayed fins, necrotic gill lesions, mouth lesions (mouth rot), and occasionally corneal lesions and eye rupture (Chen *et al.*, 1995; Handlinger *et al.*, 1997; Ostland *et al.*, 1999). The pathogen can be isolated from ulcers and lesions of infected fish (Chen *et al.*, 1995; Handlinger *et al.*, 1997; Ostland *et al.*, 1999) and a systemic infection has also been suggested, involving different internal organs (Alsina and Blanch, 1993; Romalde *et al.*, 2005). *T. maritimum* seems to lack a strict host specificity, and the pathogen has been isolated from a number of cultured fish species in Australia, Europe, Japan, North and South America (see Avendaño-Herrera *et al.*, 2006a; Plumb and Hanson, 2011).

At least three major host-associated serogroups (O1, O2 and O3) occur among *T. maritimum*. Isolates from gilthead sea bream (*Sparus aurata*) have been suggested to belong to serotype O1, isolates from turbot (*Scophthalmus maximus*) have been defined as serotype O2 or O3, and isolates from Senegalese sole (*Solea senegalensis*) as serotype O1 or O3 (Avendaño-Herrera *et al.*, 2004; 2005; Castro *et al.*, 2007). These serotyping studies were done on isolates from a restricted geographic area around the Iberian Peninsula, and it is assumed that additional serotypes may be described if *T. maritimum* from other hosts and/or geographical areas were studied (Avendaño-Herrera *et al.*, 2006a; van Gelderen *et al.*, 2010a).

Different experimental infection studies with *T. maritimum* have shown a large variation in the results depending on the examined fish species, routes of infection and bacterial concentration. IP and subcutaneous injection of *T. maritimum* has often failed to produce infection in the experimental fish (Wakabayashi *et al.*, 1984; Alsina and Blanch, 1993; Avendaño-Herrera *et al.*, 2006b). Initially, bath challenge, with red sea bream (*Pagrus major*) and black sea bream (*Acanthopagrus schlegeli*), was tested and concluded not to be a reliable infection method either (Wakabayashi *et al.*, 1984; Baxa *et al.*, 1987). However, Avendaño-Herrera *et al.* (2006b) described a successful prolonged (18 h) immersion challenge model on turbot for *T. maritimum* serotype O2 and O3. Van Gelderen *et al.* (2010b) recently reported a reproducible infection model for the Atlantic salmon using a virulent strain of *T. maritimum* and a challenge time of 1 h. Both suggested models may be used for measuring the efficacy of future vaccination programs.

Rather fewer studies are available on the antibody response in fish after immunization with *T. maritimum*. Salati *et al.* (2005) showed that sea bass (*Dicentrarchus labrax*) immunized with formalin-killed cells and LPS preparations from *T. maritimum* produced an increased antibody response compared with non-immunized fish.

Both immersion and IP-administered vaccines against *T. maritimum* have been tested for different fish species. An immersion vaccine containing formalin-killed cells induced a significant protection ($P < 0.05$) in red sea bream compared with a non-vaccinated control group (Kato *et al.*, 2007). A vaccine for turbot against *T. maritimum* has also been tested and patented. This vaccine was applied by bath immersion when the fish were 1–2 g, and a booster was subsequently injected at the size of 20–30 g. An RPS value of 85% after bacterial challenge was obtained (Toranzo *et al.*, 2009). An IP-administered vaccine has been tested for the Senegalese sole giving good protection (RPS = 94%) under laboratory conditions (Romalde *et al.*, 2005). The efficacy of a polyvalent vaccine containing five whole cell antigens, including *T. maritimum*, for cultured olive flounder (*Paralichthys olivaceus*) was examined by IP administration. An RPS of 85% was obtained after a challenge with *T. maritimum* (Kang, 2011). A vaccine against tenacibaculosis in the Atlantic salmon was tested in the early 1990s with inconsistent results (Carson *et al.*, 1994). In a recent study, efficient protection (RPS = 80%) after IP immunization of Atlantic salmon was achieved using an adjuvanted vaccine (van Gelderen *et al.*, 2009).

The importance of tenacibaculosis for the fish-farming industry is probably underestimated due to difficulties in isolation of the pathogen (Labrie *et al.*, 2005). *T. maritimum* has been considered a potentially limiting factor for the culture of many marine fish species (Santos *et al.*, 1999), but there are indications that the importance of *T. maritimum* for the aquaculture industry can be reduced by introducing changes in husbandry practices (J. Carson, personal communication).

REFERENCES

Alsina, M. and Blanch, A.R. 1993. First isolation of *Flexibacter maritimus* from cultivated turbot (*Scophthalmus maximus*). *Bull Eur Assoc Fish Pathol* **13**: 157–60.

Álvarez, B., Secades, P., Prieto, M., *et al.*, 2006. A mutation in *Flavobacterium psychrophilum tlpB* inhibits gliding motility and induces biofilm formation. *Appl Environ Microbiol* **72**: 4044–53.

Álvarez, B., Álvarez, J., Menéndez, A. and Guijarro, J.A. 2008. A mutant in one of two *exbD* loci of a TonB system in *Flavobacterium psychrophilum* shows attenuated virulence and confers protection against cold water disease. *Microbiology* **154**: 1144–51.

Anacker, R.L. and Ordal, E.J. 1959. Studies on the myxobacterium *Chondrococcus columnaris*. I. Serological typing. *J Bacteriol* **78**: 25–32.

Aoki, M., Kondo, M., Nakatsuka, Y., *et al.*, 2007. Stationary phase culture supernatant containing membrane vesicles induced immunity to rainbow trout *Oncorhynchus mykiss* fry syndrome. *Vaccine* **25**: 561–9.

Avendaño-Herrera, R., Magariños, B., López-Romalde, S., *et al.*, 2004. Phenotypic characterization and description of two major O-serotypes in *Tenacibaculum maritimum* strains from marine fishes. *Dis Aquat Org* **58**: 1–8.

Avendaño-Herrera, R., Magariños, B., Moriñigo, M.A., *et al.*, 2005. A novel O-serotype in *Tenacibaculum maritimum* strains isolated from cultured sole (*Solea senegalensis*). *Bull Eur Assoc Fish Pathol* **25**: 70–74.

Avendaño-Herrera, R., Toranzo, A.E. and Magariños, B. 2006a. Tenacibaculosis infection in marine fish caused by *Tenacibaculum maritimum*: a review. *Dis Aquat Org* **71**: 255–66.

Avendaño-Herrera, R., Toranzo, A.E. and Magariños, B. 2006b. A challenge model for *Tenacibaculum maritimum* infection in turbot, *Scophthalmus maximus* (L.) *J Fish Dis* **29**: 371–4.

Avendaño-Herrera, R., Gherardelli, V., Olmos, P., *et al.*, 2011. *Flavobacterium columnare* associated with mortality of salmonids farmed in Chile: a case report of two outbreaks. *Bull Eur Assoc Fish Pathol* **31**: 36–44.

Bader, J.A., Klesius, P.H. and Vinitnantharat, S. 1997. Comparison of whole-cell antigens of pressure and formalin-killed *Flexibacter columnaris* from channel catfish (*Ictalurus punctatus*). *Am J Vet Res* **58**: 185–8.

Barnes, M.E. and Brown, M.L. 2011. A review of *Flavobacterium psychrophilum* biology, clinical signs, and bacterial cold water disease prevention and treatment. *Open Fish Sci J* **4**: 40–48.

Baxa, D.V., Kawai, K. and Kusuda, R. 1987. Experimental infection of *Flexibacter maritimus* in black sea bream (*Acanthopagrus schlegeli*) fry. *Fish Pathol* **22**: 105–9.

Bebak, J., Matthews, M. and Shoemaker, C. 2009. Survival of vaccinated, feed-trained largemouth bass fry (*Micropterus salmoides floridanus*) during natural exposure to *Flavobacterium columnare*. *Vaccine* **27**: 4297–301.

Bernardet, J.-F. 1997. Immunization with bacterial antigens. *Flavobacterium* and *Flexibacter* infections. *Biol Stand (Basel)* **90**: 179–88.

Bernardet, J.-F. and Bowman, J.P. 2006. The genus *Flavobacterium*, in *The Prokaryotes* (eds M. Dworkin, S. Falkow, E. Rosenberg, *et al*.,), Vol. **7**, 3rd edn. New York, Springer, 481–531.

Bernardet, J.-F., Campbell, A.C. and Buswell, J.A. 1990. *Flexibacter maritimus* is the agent of "black patch necrosis" in Dover sole in Scotland. *Dis Aquat Org* **8**: 233–7.

Bernardet, J.-F., Segers, P., Vancanneyt, M., *et al*., 1996. Cutting a Gordian knot: emended classification and description of the genus *Flavobacterium*, emended description of the family *Flavobacteriaceae*, and proposal of *Flavobacterium hydatis* nom. nov. (Basonym, *Cytophaga aquatilis* Strohl and Tait 1978). *Int J Syst Bacteriol* **46**: 128–48.

Bertolini, J.M., Wakabayashi, H., Watral, V.G., *et al*., 1994. Electrophoretic detection of proteases from selected strains of *Flexibacter psychrophilus* and assessment of their variability. *J Aquat Anim Health* **6**: 224–33.

Bravo, S. and Midtlyng, P.J. 2007. The use of fish vaccines in the Chilean salmon industry 1999–2003. *Aquaculture* **270**: 36–42.

Byrne, P., Ferguson, H.W., Lumsden, J.S. and Ostland, V.E. 1991. Blood chemistry of bacterial gill disease in brook trout *Salvelinus fontinalis*. *Dis Aquat Org* **10**: 1–6.

Carson, J., Schmidtke, L. and Lewis, T. 1994. Development of a vaccine against disease: results of efficacy testing of three types of vaccine, in *Proceedings of the SALTAS Research Review Seminar* (ed. P. Valentine). Hobart, Tasmania, SALTAS, 149–58.

Castro, N., Magariños, B., Núñez, S. and Toranzo, A.E. 2007. Reassessment of the *Tenacibaculum maritimum* serotypes causing mortalities in cultured marine fish. *Bull Eur Assoc Fish Pathol* **27**: 229–33.

Chen, M.F., Henry-Ford, D. and Groff, J.M. 1995. Isolation and characterization of *Flexibacter maritimus* from marine fishes of California. *J Aquat Anim Health* **7**: 318–26.

Crump, E.M., Burian, J., Allen, P.D. and Kay, W.W. 2005. Identification and expression of a host-recognized antigen, FspA, from *Flavobacterium psychrophilum*. *Microbiology* **151**: 3127–35.

Crump, E.M., Burian, J., Allen, P.D., *et al*., 2007. Identification of a ribosomal L10-like protein from *Flavobacterium psychrophilum* as a recombinant vaccine candidate for rainbow trout fry syndrome. *J Mol Microbiol Biotechnol* **13**: 55–64.

Dalsgaard, I. 1993. Virulence mechanisms in *Cytophaga psychrophila* and other *Cytophaga*-like bacteria pathogenic for fish. *Annu Rev Fish Dis* **3**: 127–44.

De Beer, H., Hugo, C.J., Jooste, P.J., *et al*., 2006. *Chryseobacterium piscium* sp. nov., isolated from fish of the South Atlantic Ocean off South Africa. *Int J Syst Evol Microbiol* **56**: 1317–22.

Decostere, A., Haesebrouck, F. and Devriese, L.A. 1998. Characterization of four *Flavobacterium columnare* (*Flexibacter columnaris*) strains isolated from tropical fish. *Vet Microbiol* **62**: 35–45.

Duchaud, E., Boussaha, M., Loux, V., *et al*., 2007. Complete genome sequence of the fish pathogen *Flavobacterium psychrophilum*. *Nat Biotechnol* **25**: 763–9.

Dumetz, F., Duchaud, E., LaPatra, S.E., *et al*., 2006. A protective immune response is generated in rainbow trout by an OmpH-like surface antigen (P18) of *Flavobacterium psychrophilum*. *Appl Environ Microbiol* **72**: 4845–52.

Dumetz, F., LaPatra, S.E., Duchaud, E., *et al*., 2007. The *Flavobacterium psychrophilum* OmpA, an outer membrane glycoprotein, induces humoral response in rainbow trout. *J Appl Microbiol* **103**: 1461–70.

Farkas, J. 1985. Filamentous *Flavobacterium* sp. isolated from fish with gill diseases in cold water. *Aquaculture* **44**: 1–10.

Farkas, J. and Oláh, J. 1986. Gill necrosis – a complex disease of carp. *Aquaculture* **58**: 17–26.

Ferguson, H.W., Ostland, V.E., Byrne, P. and Lumsden, J.S. 1991. Experimental production of bacterial gill disease in trout by horizontal transmission and by bath challenge. *J Aquat Anim Health* **3**: 118–23.

Flemming, L., Rawlings, D. and Chenia, H. 2007. Phenotypic and molecular characterisation of fish-borne *Flavobacterium johnsoniae*-like isolates from aquaculture systems in South Africa. *Res Microbiol* **158**: 18–30.

Fredriksen, N.B., Olsen, R.H., Furevik, A., *et al*., 2013. Efficacy of a divalent and a multivalent water-in-oil formulated vaccine against a highly virulent strain of *Flavobacterium psychrophilum* after intramuscular challenge of rainbow trout (*Oncorhynchus mykiss*). *Vaccine* **31**: 1994–8.

Fujihara, M.P. and Nakatani, R.E. 1971. Antibody production and immune responses of rainbow trout and coho salmon to *Chondrococcus columnaris*. *J Fish Res Board Can* **28**: 1253–8.

Gliniewicz, K., LaPatra, S.E., LaFrentz, B.R., *et al*., 2012. Comparative proteomic analysis of virulent and rifampicin-attenuated *Flavobacterium psychrophilum*. *J Fish Dis* **35**: 529–39.

Grabowski, L.D., LaPatra, S.E. and Cain, K.D. 2004. Systemic and mucosal antibody response in tilapia, *Oreochromis niloticus* (L.) following immunization with *Flavobacterium columnare*. *J Fish Dis* **27**: 573–81.

Handlinger, J., Soltani, M. and Percival, S. 1997. The pathology of *Flexibacter maritimus* in aquaculture species in Tasmania, Australia. *J Fish Dis* **20**: 159–68.
Hansen, G.H., Bergh, Ø., Michaelsen, J. and Knappskog, D. 1992. *Flexibacter ovolyticus* sp. nov., a pathogen of eggs and larvae of Atlantic halibut, *Hippoglossus hippoglossus* L. *Int J Syst Bacteriol* **42**: 451–8.
Heo, G.-J., Kasai, K. and Wakabayashi, H. 1990a. Occurrence of *Flavobacterium branchiophila* associated with bacterial gill disease at a trout hatchery. *Fish Pathol* **25**: 99–105.
Heo, G.-J., Wakabayashi, H. and Watabe, S. 1990b. Purification and characterization of pili from *Flavobacterium branchiophila*. *Fish Pathol* **25**: 21–7.
Högfors, E., Pullinen, K.R., Madetoja, J. and Wiklund, T. 2008. Immunization of rainbow trout, *Oncorhynchus mykiss* (Walbaum), with a low molecular mass fraction isolated from *Flavobacterium psychrophilum*. *J Fish Dis* **31**: 899–911.
Högfors-Rönnholm, E. and Wiklund, T. 2010a. Phase variation in *Flavobacterium psychrophilum*: characterization of two distinct colony phenotypes. *Dis Aquat Org* **90**: 43–53.
Högfors-Rönnholm, E. and Wiklund, T. 2010b. Hemolytic activity in *Flavobacterium psychrophilum* is a contact-dependent two-step mechanism and differently expressed in smooth and rough phenotypes. *Microb Pathogen* **49**: 369–75.
Holt, R.A., Rohovec, J.S. and Fryer, J.L. 1993. Bacterial cold-water disease, in Bacterial Diseases of Fish (eds V. Inglis, R.J. Roberts, N.R. Bromage). Oxford, Blackwell Scientific Publications, 3–23.
Huh, G.-J. and Wakabayashi, H. 1989. Serological characteristics of *Flavobacterium branchiophila* isolated from gill diseases of freshwater fishes in Japan, USA and Hungary. *J Aquat Anim Health* **1**: 142–7.
Ilardi, P., Fernández, J. and Avendaño-Herrera, R. 2009. *Chryseobacterium piscicola* sp. nov., isolated from diseased salmonid fish. *Int J Syst Evol Microbiol* **59**: 3001–5.
Johansen, L.H., Jensen, I., Mikkelsen, H., *et al.*, 2011. Disease interaction and pathogens exchange between wild and farmed fish populations with special reference to Norway. *Aquaculture* **315**: 167–86.
Kämpfer, P., Lodders, N., Martin, K. and Avendaño-Herrera, R. 2012. *Flavobacterium chilense* sp. nov. and *Flavobacterium araucananum* sp. nov., isolated from farmed salmonid fish. *Int J Syst Evol Microbiol* **62**: 1402–8.
Kang, B. 2011. Efficacy of *Edwardsiella tarda*, *Streptococcus iniae*, *Streptococcus parauberis*, *Vibrio anguillarum*, and *Tenacibaculum maritimum*. International Conference & Exhibition on Vaccines & Vaccination. Philadelphia, US (abstract).
Kato, F., Ishimaru, K., Murata, O and Kumai, H. 2007. The efficacy of immersion-vaccination against gliding bacterial disease in red sea bream *Pagrus major*. *Nippon Suisan Gakkaishi* **73**: 51–4.
Klesius, P., Lim, C. and Shoemaker, C. 1999. Effect of feed deprivation on innate resistance and antibody response to *Flavobacterium columnare* in channel catfish, *Ictalurus punctatus*. *Bull Eur Assoc Fish Pathol* **19**: 156–8.
Klesius, P.H., Shoemaker, C.A. and Evans, J.J. 2008. *Flavobacterium columnare* chemotaxis to channel catfish mucus. *FEMS Microbiol Lett* **288**: 216–20.
Ko, Y.-M. and Heo, G.-J. 1997. Characteristics of *Flavobacterium branchiophilum* isolated from rainbow trout in Korea. *Fish Pathol* **32**: 97–102.
Kondo, M., Kawai, K., Kurohara, K. and Oshima, S. 2002. Adherence of *Flavobacterium psychrophilum* on the body surface of the ayu *Plecoglossus altivelis*. *Microbes Infect* **4**: 279–83.
Kondo, M., Kawai, K., Okabe, M., *et al.*, 2003. Efficacy of oral vaccine against bacterial coldwater disease in ayu *Plecoglossus altivelis*. *Dis Aquat Org* **55**: 261–4.
Kubilay, A., Altun, S., Diler, Ö. and Ekici, S. 2008. Isolation of *Flavobacterium columnare* from cultured rainbow trout (*Oncorhynchus mykiss*) fry in Turkey. *Turkish J Fish Aquat Sci* **8**: 165–9.
Kunttu, H.M., Suomalainen, L.R., Jokinen, E.I. and Valtonen, E.T. 2009. *Flavobacterium columnare* colony types: connection to adhesion and virulence. *Microb Pathog* **46**: 21–7.
Kunttu, H.M., Jokinen, E.I., Valtonen, E.T. and Sundberg, L.R. 2011. Virulent and nonvirulent *Flavobacterium columnare* colony morphologies: characterization of chondroitin AC lyase activity and adhesion to polystyrene. *J Appl Microbiol* **111**: 1319–26.
Labrie, L., Grisez, L., Komar, C. and Tan, Z. 2005. *Tenacibaculum maritimum* an underestimated fish pathogen in Asian marine fish culture, in *International Peace and Development through Aquaculture*. World Aquaculture Society, Bali, Indonesia (abstract).
LaFrentz, B.R., LaPatra, S.E., Jones, G.R., *et al.*, 2002. Characterization of serum and mucosal antibody responses and relative per cent survival in rainbow trout, *Oncorhynchus mykiss* (Walbaum), following immunization and challenge with *Flavobacterium psychrophilum*. *J Fish Dis* **25**: 703–13.

LaFrentz, B.R., LaPatra, S.E., Jones, G.R. and Cain, K.D. 2003. Passive immunization of rainbow trout, *Oncorhynchus mykiss* (Walbaum), against *Flavobacterium psychrophilum*, the causative agent of bacterial coldwater disease and rainbow trout fry syndrome. *J Fish Dis* **26**: 377–84.

LaFrentz, B.R., LaPatra, S.E., Jones, G.R. and Cain, K.D. 2004. Protective immunity in rainbow trout *Oncorhynchus mykiss* following immunization with distinct molecular mass fractions isolated from *Flavobacterium psychrophilum*. *Dis Aquat Org* **59**: 17–26.

LaFrentz, B.R., LaPatra, S.E., Call, D.R. and Cain, K.D. 2008. Isolation of rifampicin resistant *Flavobacterium psychrophilum* strains and their potential as live attenuated vaccine candidates. *Vaccine* **26**: 5582–9.

LaFrentz, B.R., LaPatra, S.E., Shoemaker, C.A. and Klesius, P.H. 2012. Reproducible challenge model to investigate the virulence of *Flavobacterium columnare* genomovars in rainbow trout (*Oncorhynchus mykiss*). *Dis Aquat Org* **101**: 115–22.

Leal, C.A.G., Carvalho-Castro, G.A., Sacchetin, P.S.C., *et al.*, 2010. Oral and parenteral vaccines against *Flavobacterium columnare*: evaluation of humoral immune response by ELISA and *in vivo* efficiency in Nile tilapia (*Oreochromis niloticus*). *Aquac Int* **18**: 657–66.

Liu, Z.X., Liu, G.Y., Li, N., *et al.*, 2012. Identification of immunogenic proteins of *Flavobacterium columnare* by two-dimensional electrophoresis immunoblotting with antibacterial sera from grass carp, *Ctenopharyngodon idella* (Valenciennes). *J Fish Dis* **35**: 255–63.

Lorenzen, E. 1994. *Studies on Flexibacter psychrophilus in relation to rainbow trout fry syndrome*. PhD thesis, Royal Veterinary and Agricultural School, Copenhagen.

Lorenzen, E. and Olesen, N.J. 1997. Characterization of isolates of *Flavobacterium psychrophilum* associated with coldwater disease or rainbow trout fry syndrome II: serological studies. *Dis Aquat Org* **31**: 209–20.

Lorenzen, E., Brudeseth, B.E., Wiklund, T. and Lorenzen, N. 2010. Immersion exposure of rainbow trout (*Oncorhynchus mykiss*) fry to wildtype *Flavobacterium psychrophilum* induces no mortality, but protects against later intraperitoneal challenge. *Fish Shellfish Immunol* **28**: 440–4.

Lumsden, J.S., Ostland, V.E., Byrne, P.J. and Ferguson, H.W. 1993. Detection of a distinct gill-surface antibody response following horizontal infection and bath challenge of brook trout *Salvelinus fontinalis* with *Flavobacterium branchiophilum*, the causative agent of bacterial gill disease. *Dis Aquat Org* **16**: 21–7.

Lumsden, J.S., Ostland, V.E., MacPhee, D.D., *et al.*, 1994. Protection of rainbow trout from experimentally induced bacterial gill disease caused by *Flavobacterium branchiophilum*. *J Aquatic Anim Health* **6**: 292–302.

Lumsden, J.S., Ostland, V.E., MacPhee, D.D. and Ferguson, H.W. 1995. Production of gill-associated and serum antibody by rainbow trout (*Oncorhynchus mykiss*) following immersion immunization with acetone-killed *Flavobacterium branchiophilum* and the relationship to protection from experimental challenge. *Fish Shellfish Immunol* **5**: 151–65.

Madetoja, J., Lönnström, L.G., Björkblom, C., *et al.*, 2006. Efficacy of injection vaccines against *Flavobacterium psychrophilum* in rainbow trout, *Oncorhynchus mykiss* (Walbaum). *J Fish Dis* **29**: 9–20.

Madsen, L. and Dalsgaard, I. 2000. Comparative studies of Danish *Flavobacterium psychrophilum* isolates: ribotypes, plasmid profiles, serotypes and virulence. *J Fish Dis* **23**: 211–18.

Mano, N., Inui, T., Arai, D., *et al.*, 1996. Immune response in the skin of eel against *Cytophaga columnaris*. *Fish Pathol* **31**: 65–70.

Mata, M., Skarmeta, A. and Santos, Y. 2002. A proposed serotyping system for *Flavobacterium psychrophilum*. *Lett Appl Microbiol* **35**: 166–70.

Møller, D.M., Larsen, J.L., Madsen, L. and Dalsgaard, I. 2003. Involvement of sialic acid-binding lectin with hemagglutination and hydrophobicity of *Flavobacterium psychrophilum*. *Appl Environ Microbiol* **69**: 5275–80.

Moore, A.A., Eimers, M.E. and Cardella, N.A. 1990. Attempts to control *Flexibacter columnaris* epizootics in pond-reared channel catfish by vaccination. *J Aquat Anim Health* **2**: 109–11.

Moyer, T.R. and Hunnicutt, D.W. 2007. Susceptibility of zebra fish *Danio rerio* to infection by *Flavobacterium columnare* and *F. johnsoniae*. *Dis Aquat Org* **76**: 39–44.

Mudarris, M., Austin, B., Segers, P., *et al.*, 1994. *Flavobacterium scophthalmum* sp. nov., a pathogen of turbot (*Scophthalmus maximus* L.). *Int J Syst Bacteriol* **44**: 447–53.

Nematollahi, A., Decostere, A., Pasmans, F., *et al.*, 2003a. Adhesion of high and low virulence *Flavobacterium psychrophilum* strains to isolated gill arches of rainbow trout *Oncorhynchus mykiss*. *Dis Aquat Org* **55**: 101–7.

Nematollahi, A., Decostere, A., Pasmans, F. and Haesebrouck, F. 2003b. *Flavobacterium psychrophilum* infections in salmonid fish. *J Fish Dis* **26**: 563–74.

Noga, E.J. 2010. Problem 37. Columnaris infection (myxobacterial disease, saddleback, fin rot, cotton wool disease, black patch necrosis), in *Fish Disease: Diagnosis and Treatment*, 2nd edn. Ames, Iowa, Wiley-Blackwell, 166–9.

Olivares-Fuster, O. and Arias, C.R. 2011. Development and characterization of rifampicin-resistant mutants from high virulent strains of *Flavobacterium columnare*. *J Fish Dis* **34**: 385–94.

Olivares-Fuster, O., Baker, J.L., Terhune, J.S., *et al.*, 2007. Host-specific association between *Flavobacterium columnare* genomovars and fish species. *Syst Appl Microbiol* **30**: 624–33.

Olivares-Fuster, O., Terhune, J.S., Shoemaker, C.A. and Arias, C.R. 2010. Cloning, expression, and immunogenicity of *Flavobacterium columnare* heat shock protein DnaJ. *J Aquat Anim Health* **22**: 78–86.

Ostland, V.E., Lumsden, J.S., MacPhee, D.D. and Ferguson, H.W. 1994. Characteristics of *Flavobacterium branchiophilum*, the cause of salmonid bacterial gill disease in Ontario. *J Aquat Anim Health* **6**: 13–26.

Ostland, V.E., MacPhee, D.D., Lumsden, J.S. and Ferguson, H.W. 1995. Virulence of *Flavobacterium branchiophilum* in experimentally infected salmonids. *J Fish Dis* **18**: 249–62.

Ostland, V.E., Lumsden, J.S., MacPhee, D.D., *et al.*, 1997. Inhibition of the attachment of *Flavobacterium branchiophilum* to the gills of rainbow trout, *Oncorhynchus mykiss* (Walbaum). *J Fish Dis* **20**: 109–17.

Ostland, V.E., LaTrace, C., Morrison, D. and Ferguson, H.W. 1999. *Flexibacter maritimus* associated with a bacterial stomatitis in Atlantic salmon smolts reared in net-pens in British Columbia. *J Aquat Anim Health* **11**: 35–44.

Ototake, M. and Wakabayashi, H. 1985. Characteristics of extracellular products of *Flavobacterium* sp., a pathogen of bacterial gill disease. *Fish Pathol* **20**: 167–71.

Pérez-Pascual, D., Gómez, E., Álvarez, B., *et al.*, 2011. Comparative analysis and mutation effects of fpp2-fpp1 tandem genes encoding proteolytic extracellular enzymes of *Flavobacterium psychrophilum*. *Microbiology* **157**: 1196–204.

Plant, K.P., LaPatra, S.E. and Cain, K.D. 2009. Vaccination of rainbow trout, *Oncorhynchus mykiss* (Walbaum), with recombinant and DNA vaccines produced to *Flavobacterium psychrophilum* heat shock proteins 60 and 70. *J Fish Dis* **32**: 521–34.

Plant, K.P., LaPatra, S.E., Call, D.R. and Cain, K.D. 2011. Immunization of rainbow trout, *Oncorhynchus mykiss* (Walbaum), with *Flavobacterium psychrophilum* proteins elongation factor-Tu, SufB Fe-S assembly protein and ATP synthaseβ. *J Fish Dis* **34**: 247–50.

Plumb, J.A. and Hanson, L.A. 2011. *Health Maintenance and Principal Microbial Diseases of Cultured Fishes* (3rd edn). Ames, Iowa, Wiley-Blackwell.

Pridgeon, J.W. and Klesius, P.H. 2010. Identification and expression profile of multiple genes in channel catfish fry 10 min after modified live *Flavobacterium columnare* vaccination. *Vet Immunol Immunopathol* **138**: 25–33.

Pulkkinen, K., Suomalainen, L.R., Read, A.F., *et al.*, 2010. Intensive fish farming and the evolution of pathogen virulence: the case of columnaris disease in Finland. *Proc Biol Sci* **277**: 593–600.

Rahman, M.H., Ototake, M., Iida, Y., *et al.*, 2000. Efficacy of oil-adjuvanted vaccine for coldwater disease in ayu *Plecoglossus altivelis*. *Fish Pathol* **35**: 199–203.

Rahman, M.H., Kuroda, A., Dijkstra, J.M., *et al.*, 2002. The outer membrane fraction of *Flavobacterium psychrophilum* induces protective immunity in rainbow trout and ayu. *Fish Shellfish Immunol* **12**: 169–79.

Rahman, M.H., Ototake, M. and Nakanishi, T. 2003. Water-soluble adjuvants enhance the protective effect of *Flavobacterium psychrophilum* vaccines in ayu *Plecoglossus altivelis*. *Fish Pathol* **38**: 171–6.

Ransom, D.P. 1975. *Immune responses of salmonids: A) Oral immunization against Flexibacter columnaris. B) Effects of combining antigens in parenterally administered polyvalent vaccines*. MA thesis, Oregon State University, Corvallis.

Romalde, J.L., Ravelo, C., López-Romalde, S., *et al.*, 2005. Vaccination strategies to prevent emerging diseases for Spanish aquaculture. *Dev Biol (Basel)* **121**: 85–95.

Salati, F., Cubadda, C., Viale, I. and Kusuda, R. 2005. Immune response of sea bass *Dicentrarchus labrax* to *Tenacibaculum maritimum* antigens. *Fish Sci* **71**: 563–7.

Santos, Y., Pazos, F. and Barja, J.L. 1999. *Flexibacter maritimus*, causal agent of flexibacteriosis in marine fish. *ICES identification leaflets for diseases and parasites of fish and shellfish*. Copenhagen, ICES, Leaflet No. 55.

Schachte, J.H. Jr and Mora, E.C. 1973. Production of agglutinating antibodies in the channel catfish (*Ictalurus punctatus*) against *Chondrococcus columnaris*. *J Fish Res Board Can* **30**: 116–18.

Shelby, R.A., Shoemaker, C.A. and Klesius, P.H. 2007. Passive immunization of channel catfish *Ictalurus punctatus* with anti-*Flavobacterium columnare* sera. *Dis Aquat Org* **77**: 143–7.

Shoemaker, C.A., Klesius, P.H., Lim, C. and Yildirim, M. 2003. Feed deprivation of channel catfish, *Ictalurus punctatus* (Rafinesque), influences organosomatic indices, chemical composition and susceptibility to *Flavobacterium columnare*. *J Fish Dis* **26**: 553–61.

Shoemaker, C.A., Xu, D., Shelby, R.A. and Klesius, P.H. 2005. Detection of cutaneous antibodies against *Flavobacterium columnare* in channel catfish, *Ictalurus punctatus* (Rafinesque). *Aquac Res* **36**: 813–18.

Shoemaker, C.A., Klesius, P.H. and Evans, J.J. 2007. Immunization of eyed channel catfish, *Ictalurus punctatus*, eggs with monovalent *Flavobacterium columnare* vaccine and bivalent *F. columnare* and *Edwardsiella ictaluri* vaccine. *Vaccine* **25**: 1126–31.

Shoemaker, C.A., Klesius, P.H., Drennan, J.D. and Evans, J.J. 2011. Efficacy of a modified live *Flavobacterium columnare* vaccine in fish. *Fish Shellfish Immunol* **30**: 304–8.

Song, Y.L., Fryer, J.L. and Rohovec, J.S. 1988. Comparison of gliding bacteria isolated from fish in North America and other areas of the Pacific Rim. *Fish Pathol* **23**: 197–202.

Speare, D.J., Ferguson, H.W., Beamish, F.W.M., *et al.*, 1991. Pathology of bacterial gill disease: sequential development of lesions during natural outbreaks of disease. *J Fish Dis* **14**: 21–32.

Speare, D.J., Markham, R.J.F., Despres, B., *et al.*, 1995. Examination of gills from salmonids with bacterial gill disease using monoclonal antibody probes for *Flavobacterium branchiophilum* and *Cytophaga columnaris*. *J Vet Diagn Invest* **7**: 500–5.

Starliper, C.E. 2011. Bacterial coldwater disease of fishes caused by *Flavobacterium psychrophilum*. *J Adv Res* **2**: 97–108.

Starliper, C.E. and Schill, W.B. 2011. Flavobacterial diseases: Columnaris disease, coldwater disease and bacterial gill disease, in *Fish Diseases and Disorders, Vol. 3: Viral, Bacterial and Fungal Infections* (eds P.T.K. Woo and D.W. Bruno). 2nd edn. Wallingford, CABI, 606–31.

Suomalainen, L.R., Tiirola, M. and Valtonen, E.T. 2005. Influence of rearing conditions on *Flavobacterium columnare* infection of rainbow trout, *Oncorhynchus mykiss* (Walbaum). *J Fish Dis* **28**: 271–7.

Suomalainen, L.R., Tiirola, M. and Valtonen, E.T. 2006. Chondroitin AC lyase activity is related to virulence in fish pathogenic *Flavobacterium columnare*. *J Fish Dis* **29**: 757–63.

Suzuki, M., Nakagawa, Y., Harayama, S. and Yamamoto, S. 2001. Phylogenetic analysis and taxonomic study of marine *Cytophaga*-like bacteria: proposal for *Tenacibaculum* gen. nov. with *Tenacibaculum maritimum* comb. nov. and *Tenacibaculum ovolyticum* comb. nov., and description of *Tenacibaculum mesophilum* sp. nov. and *Tenacibaculum amylolyticum* sp. nov. *Int J Syst Evol Microbiol* **51**: 1639–52.

Thomas-Jinu, S. and Goodwin, A.E. 2004. Morphologic and genetic characteristics of *Flavobacterium columnare* isolates: Correlations with virulence in fish. *J Fish Dis* **27**: 29–35.

Toranzo, A.E., Romalde, J.L., Magariños, B. and Barja, J.L. 2009. Present and future of aquaculture vaccines against fish bacterial diseases, in *The Use of Veterinary Drugs and Vaccines in Mediterranean Aquaculture* (eds C. Rodgers and B. Basurko). Op Méditerr, A/No 86, 155–76.

Triyanto, K. and Wakabayashi, H. 1999. Genotypic diversity of strains of *Flavobacterium columnare* from diseased fishes. *Fish Pathol* **34**: 65–71.

Vandamme, P., Bernardet, J.-F., Segers, P., *et al.*, 1994. New perspectives in the classification of the Flavobacteria: description of *Chryseobacterium* gen. nov., *Bergeyella* gen. nov., and *Empedobacter* nom. rev. *Int J Syst Bacteriol* **44**: 827–31.

Van Gelderen, R., Carson, J. and Nowak, B. 2009. Experimental vaccination of Atlantic salmon (*Salmo salar* L.) against marine flexibacteriosis. *Aquaculture* **288**: 7–13.

Van Gelderen, R., Carson, J., Gudkovs, N. and Nowak, B. 2010a. Physical characterisation of *Tenacibaculum maritimum* for vaccine development. *J Appl Microbiol* **109**: 1668–76.

Van Gelderen, R., Carson, J. and Nowak, B. 2010b. Experimentally induced marine flexibacteriosis in Atlantic salmon smolts *Salmo salar*. I. Pathogenicity. *Dis Aquat Org* **91**: 121–8.

Wagner, B.A., Wise, D.J., Khoo, L.H. and Terhune, J.S. 2002. The epidemiology of bacterial diseases in food-size channel catfish. *J Aquat Anim Health* **14**: 263–72.

Wakabayashi, H. and Iwado, T. 1985. Changes in glycogen, pyruvate and lactate in rainbow trout with bacterial gill disease. *Fish Pathol* **20**: 161–5.

Wakabayashi, H., Egusa, S. and Fryer, J.L. 1980. Characteristics of filamentous bacteria isolated from a gill disease of salmonids. *Can J Fish Aquat Sci* **37**: 1499–504.

Wakabayashi, H., Hikida, M. and Masumura, K. 1984. *Flexibacter* infection in cultured marine fish in Japan. *Helgoländer Meeresunters* **37**: 587–93.
Wakabayashi, H., Huh, G.J. and Kimura, N. 1989. *Flavobacterium branchiophila* sp. nov., a causative agent of bacterial gill disease of freshwater fishes. *Int J System Bacteriol* **39**: 213–16.
Wakabayashi, H., Toyama, T. and Iida, T. 1994. A study on serotyping of *Cytophaga psychrophila* isolated from fishes in Japan. *Fish Pathol* **29**: 101–4.
Wallis, T., Dalsgaard, I., Hopewell, R. and Kardos, G. 2009. The potential of autogenous vaccines based on *Flavobacterium psychrophilum* for the control of rainbow trout fry syndrome and red mark syndrome in salmonids: Typing of *F. psychrophilum* isolates from salmon and trout in the UK. *Proceedings of the 2nd Conference on Members of the Genus Flavobacterium*, MGEN, Paris.
Welker, T.L., Shoemaker, C.A., Arias, C.R. and Klesius, P.H. 2005. Transmission and detection of *Flavobacterium columnare* in channel catfish, *Ictalurus punctatus*. *Dis Aquat Org* **63**: 129–38.
Wiklund, T. and Dalsgaard, I. 2003. Association of *Flavobacterium psychrophilum* with rainbow trout (*Oncorhynchus mykiss*) kidney phagocytosis *in vitro*. *Fish Shellfish Immunol* **15**: 387–95.
Yanong, R.P.E. 2008. *Use of vaccines in finfish aquaculture*. Gainesville: University of Florida. Available at http://edis.ifas.ufl.edu/fa156
Zamora, L., Fernández-Garayzábal, J.F., Svensson-Stadler, L.A., *et al.*, 2012. *Flavobacterium oncorhynchi* sp. nov., new species isolated from rainbow trout (*Oncorhynchus mykiss*). *System Appl Microbiol* **35**: 86–91.

24 Vaccination against Viral Hemorrhagic Septicemia and Infectious Hematopoietic Necrosis

Stéphane Biacchesi and Michel Brémont

National Institute for Agricultural Research (INRA), Jouy en Josas, France

ABSTRACT

Viral hemorrhagic septicemia (VHS) and infectious hematopoietic necrosis (IHN) are very contagious viral diseases leading to high mortality mainly, but not exclusively, in young salmonid fish. Although research on vaccine development has been ongoing for more than four decades, no mass delivery vaccine against these two important pathogens is yet available. Several candidate vaccines, based on inactivated virus, recombinant G protein, attenuated virus strains, and DNA vectors have been proved to be efficient to induce specific and long-lasting protective immunity in fish. A DNA vaccine against IHNV has recently been licensed for commercial use in Atlantic salmon in Canada. Nevertheless, the commercialization of this vaccine in Europe is not approved and a mass delivery system for vaccination of fish fry is required. In parallel, reverse genetics systems have allowed the generation of promising multivalent live attenuated vaccines. Additional work is needed to improve the safety of such vaccines.

24.1 OCCURRENCE AND SIGNIFICANCE

Viral hemorrhagic septicemia (VHS) and infectious hematopoietic necrosis (IHN) are very contagious viral diseases leading to high mortality in young cultured and wild fish worldwide and are listed as notifiable by the World Organization for Animal Health (OIE) (Skall *et al.*, 2005; Walker and Winton, 2010). VHS and IHN are two of the seven fish viral diseases considered by the OIE as serious economic and social threats for fish farms with significant environmental impacts on natural resources and endangered fish species (OIE, 2013). For example, the cost of rhabdoviral diseases in 2001–2004 to Canadian aquaculture was CAD$ 200 million (Salonius *et al.*, 2007).

stephane.biacchesi@jouy.inra.fr

Fish Vaccination, First Edition. Edited by Roar Gudding, Atle Lillehaug and Øystein Evensen.

Concerning the epidemiological data of prevalence of VHS and IHN in Europe, there is still a severe underreporting since the infection status is known for only 36% and 38% of farms, for VHS and IHN respectively (Olesen and Nicolajsen, 2011). For both diseases, virus reservoirs are infected domestic or wild fish and survivor fish of epizootics that could become long-term carriers (Bootland and Leong, 2011). Transmission primarily occurs horizontally through contaminated water by direct excretion of virus from infected fish. Consequently, all infected batches have to be destroyed and surface disinfection of fertilized eggs with an iodophor solution may aid to reduce vertical transmission (OIE, 2013). Fish living in endemic regions for IHNV and VHSV are likely to be coinfected by both viruses, as previously observed during experimental coinfection (Brudeseth *et al.*, 2002; Biacchesi *et al.*, 2010). Since no cross-protection exists between these two viruses, an efficient vaccine against both VHSV and IHNV is required (Hattenberger-Baudouy *et al.*, 1995). Nevertheless, Denmark, through a permanent surveillance and control program, has been declared VHS-free and no new outbreak was recorded for more than two years (Mellergaard, 2011). In other countries, control of VHSV and IHNV in the absence of any treatment is achieved by prevention of introduction and eradication by stamping-out in case of disease outbreaks.

VHS is primarily a disease of farmed rainbow trout (*Oncorhynchus mykiss*), turbot (*Scophthalmus maximus*) and Japanese flounder (*Paralichthys olivaceus*), as well as a broad range of freshwater and marine species, caused by infection with *Viral hemorrhagic septicemia virus* (VHSV, also called Egtved virus). To date, VHSV has been isolated from more than 82 different freshwater and marine species throughout the Northern Hemisphere, including North America, Asia and Europe (Skall *et al.*, 2005; Jonstrup *et al.*, 2009; Kim and Faisal, 2011; OIE, 2013). Although the disease caused by VHSV was known since 1938 as an exclusive threat for rainbow trout aquaculture in continental Europe (Wolf, 1988; Bootland and Leong, 2011), it has become clear since the 1980s that the virus spread throughout the Northern Hemisphere and that VHSV causes significant losses in a large host range of both freshwater and marine fish species (Skall *et al.*, 2005). The recovery of VHSV from an increasing number of free-living asymptomatic marine fish, representing an extensive reservoir, causes problems for VHS disease control and could lead to the emergence of new, highly virulent strains for domestic fish (Snow, 2011; Kurath and Winton, 2011).

Two recent events nicely illustrate these concerns. In a recent Norwegian VHS outbreak in marine rainbow trout farms that occurred in 2007, the marine origin of the VHSV isolate was clearly suspected (Dale *et al.*, 2009). This isolate is closely related to marine isolates that were not considered to be pathogenic for rainbow trout, thus indicating a high capability of VHSV adaptation. Another example of the highly adaptable nature of VHSV was given by mass mortalities observed in the 2000s in the Great Lakes region of North America and involving at least 31 freshwater fish species (Kim and Faisal, 2011). Indeed, after the first VHSV isolation from muskellunge (*Esox masquinongy*) caught from Lake St Clair in 2003 (Elsayed *et al.*, 2006), this initial discovery was followed by the virus spreading into the five Great Lakes where no rhabdoviruses were previously observed.

IHN is a viral disease affecting essentially all species of salmonid fish and is caused by infection with *Infectious hematopoietic necrosis virus* (IHNV) (OIE, 2013). However, losses due to IHNV are principally observed among Pacific salmon including sockeye salmon (*Oncorhynchus nerka*), chinook salmon (*O. tshawytscha*), pink salmon (*O. gurbuscha*), chum salmon (*O. keta*), masou salmon (*O. masou*), Atlantic salmon (*Salmo salar*), and rainbow trout. Originally isolated from dying sockeye salmons in farms located in the western portion of North America in the 1950s, IHNV emerged in the 1970s to become an important pathogen of farmed rainbow trout. IHNV has been spread by the historically common practice of salmon transplantations and the widespread use of raw or unpasteurized fish products as feed for salmon fry in hatcheries throughout the western US during the 1950s to 1960s. The virus, originally absent from other continents, is thought to have been disseminated by the movement of fish and/or fish eggs to Europe and Asia (Wolf, 1988; Bootland and Leong, 2011). To date, 23 different freshwater and marine species throughout the Northern Hemisphere have been found to be infected by IHNV or shown to be susceptible by experimental infection (OIE, 2013). The isolation of IHNV from wild and domestic fish in both seawater and freshwater indicates the highly adaptable nature of IHNV with regard to host specificities and host environments during its infectious cycle. Moreover, the non-salmonid marine and freshwater fish species could represent potential reservoirs that may play a role in the lifecycle of IHNV and its host. Indeed, when anadromous fish return to spawn as adults, the animals are initially negative for infectious virus, and as they mature to spawning age, the prevalence of virus-positive animals increases. But, we cannot exclude the possibility of fish carrying undetectable amounts of IHNV until they are immunosuppressed by the stress of the migration, and infectious virus is then produced (Meyers, 1998; Kim *et al.*, 1999).

24.2 ETIOLOGY

IHNV and VHSV belong to the family *Rhabdoviridae* within the order *Mononegavirales* (Hoffmann *et al.*, 2005; Tordo *et al.*, 2005). These viruses are both enveloped within a typical bullet-shaped morphology (about 180 nm long and 70 nm in diameter). Their genomes consist of a non-segmented negative-sense single-stranded RNA molecule of about 11 kilobases which encodes six proteins in the order 3'-N-P-M-G-NV-L-5' (Morzunov *et al.*, 1995; Schutze *et al.*, 1995, 1999). The viral RNA is tightly encapsulated with a nucleoprotein (N), a polymerase-associated phosphoprotein (P) and the large RNA-dependent RNA polymerase (L) to form the helical ribonucleoprotein complex (RNP). The matrix protein (M) interacts with the RNP and the viral envelope and is involved in the budding step. Finally, the viral surface glycoprotein (G) is implicated in the entry step and thus represents the unique target for neutralizing and protective antibodies (Lorenzen *et al.*, 1990, 2000; Bearzotti *et al.*, 1995). In contrast to other rhabdoviruses, IHNV and VHSV genomes possess an additional gene, localized between the G and L genes, that encodes a small non-structural NV (non-virion) protein (Kurath *et al.*, 1985; Kurath and Leong, 1985; Schutze *et al.*, 1996). Due to the presence of the NV gene, IHNV and VHSV were classified together in the genus *Novirhabdovirus* (Tordo *et al.*, 2005). Using reverse genetics systems, NV protein was shown to be dispensable, but necessary for efficient virus replication in cell culture (Biacchesi *et al.*, 2000, 2010; Ammayappan *et al.*, 2011; Kim *et al.*, 2011), and essential for virus pathogenicity in rainbow trout (Thoulouze *et al.*, 2004; Harmache *et al.*, 2006a), yellow perch (*Perca flavescens*) (Ammayappan *et al.*, 2011) and Japanese olive flounder (Kim and Kim, 2011).

Molecular epidemiology has been largely used to compare VHSV and IHNV isolated worldwide and from a wide range of farmed and wild fish species. These studies have contributed to improving isolate genotyping, giving a better understanding of the natural distribution, origins and host range of both VHSV and IHNV (Bandin and Dopazo, 2011; Snow, 2011). To date, four major genotypes of VHSV (I–IV) have been identified based on

N-gene and G-gene sequences (Einer-Jensen *et al.*, 2004; Snow *et al.*, 2004). The phylogenetic analyses reflect a geographic rather than a species-specific distribution. Moreover, VHSV isolates originating from marine fish show low pathogenicity to rainbow trout and Atlantic salmon, although some of these isolates are pathogenic for turbot. The analysis of several nearly complete genome sequences from marine and freshwater isolates displaying variable levels of virulence in rainbow trout have suggested that only a limited number of amino-acid residues might be involved in the level of virulence between isolates (Betts and Stone, 2000; Campbell *et al.*, 2009). Interestingly, molecular analysis provides evidence that the marine environment is the original reservoir of VHSV and that species barrier jumps may have occurred several times, mainly from marine fish to trout (Kurath and Winton, 2011). Finally, it is still not clear whether VHSV isolates represent three serotypes or subtypes within a single serotype (Olesen *et al.*, 1993). Thus, VHSV isolates share several antigenic epitopes, although serogrouping does not correlate with genotypes. Concerning IHNV, three major genogroups (U, M and L) have been described based on phylogenetic analyses of partial nucleotide sequences of the G gene of several North American isolates (Kurath *et al.*, 2003), which correspond to only one major serotype (Engelking *et al.*, 1991). European isolates seem to be of a monophyletic origin and closely related to the genogroup M (Enzmann *et al.*, 2005). In contrast, Asian isolates are closely related to the genogroup U but have diverged somewhat independently (Nishizawa *et al.*, 2006). The phylogenetic relationship mainly correlates with the geographic origin of virus isolates, although certain strains belonging to the U and M types differ in host-specific virulence: the U strain is virulent in sockeye salmon but not rainbow trout, and the M strain is virulent in rainbow trout but not sockeye salmon (Penaranda *et al.*, 2009, 2011b).

24.3 PATHOGENESIS

VHS and IHN are acute systemic diseases (Wolf, 1988; Bootland and Leong, 2011). Fish of any age are susceptible to infection, although fry and juveniles are the most sensitive. Mortality varies depending on a variety of environmental and physiological factors such as fish age, rearing conditions, stress, fish species, virus strain, water temperature, and so on. The disease is most severe at 10 °C and rare at temperatures above 15 °C. The virus is transmitted by contaminated water, direct contact with infected fish, or by feeding contaminated food. The use of a non-invasive bioluminescence imaging device and recombinant viruses expressing the luciferase gene have provided evidence that the fins are the portal of entry of IHNV into rainbow trout (Harmache *et al.*, 2006a). Oral transmission as another route of infection for both viruses has been demonstrated (Helmick *et al.*, 1995; Schonherz *et al.*, 2012). In trout fry (0.3–2 g) experimentally infected with either VHSV or IHNV, mortality is characterized by a rapid onset starting at 4 to 6 days post-infection and reaching 80 to 100% of cumulative mortality 15 to 20 days post-infection. The clinical signs and lesions are not clearly specific and are common to other systemic viral diseases (for more details, see Wolf, 1988). Infected fish are lethargic with hyperactivity periods and erratic swimming behavior such as spiraling. Fish display exophthalmia due to the impairment of the osmotic balance and are anemic, which is characterized by pale gills. Punctiform hemorrhages are evident in periocular tissues, skeletal muscle and viscera. The kidney is dark red in the acute phase, the spleen is swollen, and the liver is often pale. The hematopoietic tissues of the kidney and spleen of young fish are the most severely affected and are the first tissues to show extensive necrosis.

Two forms of VHS can be observed. The acute disease is characterized by high mortality. Endothelial cells of the anterior kidney and spleen are the primary targets of the virus. The liver sinusoids are engorged with blood, and hepatocytes show focal to extensive degeneration and necrosis. Similar changes occur in the spleen and in the hematopoietic and renal elements of the kidneys. High virus titer is found in kidney and spleen tissues. In contrast, the chronic disease is characterized by a slower and prolonged mortality, with high virus titer isolated from the brain.

Two forms of IHN can also be observed: a "hematopoietic" form and a "neurotropic" form (LaPatra *et al.*, 1995). Rainbow trout with "hematopoietic" IHN exhibit typical disease signs, with highest virus titers in kidney and spleen tissues. Histopathological examination of this acute IHNV infection reveals prominent necrosis of hematopoietic tissue including melanomacrophages of the kidney, red pulp of the spleen and hepatic parenchyma. Necrosis of the submucosal eosinophilic granular cells in the intestinal tract is considered pathognomonic for IHN. Intranuclear and intracytoplasmic inclusions are occasionally observed in acinar and islet cells of pancreas. In contrast, fish with the "neurotropic" form of IHN display abnormal behavior, very slow and prolonged mortality, and highest virus titer in the brain tissue. The basis of this altered virus tropism is still unknown, although mutations in the glycoprotein G have been proposed to be responsible (Kim *et al.*, 1994).

24.4 VACCINES

Although research on vaccine development against VHSV and IHNV has been ongoing for more than four decades, and a DNA vaccine against IHNV has recently been licensed for commercial use in Atlantic salmon in Canada, no mass-delivery vaccine against these two important pathogens is yet available. Several candidate vaccines, based on inactivated virus, recombinant G protein expressed from prokaryotic and eukaryotic systems, attenuated virus strains, and DNA vectors have been proved to be efficient in inducing specific and long-lasting protective immunity in fish, but no one candidate met the full list of requirements: immunogenicity, protective immunity, efficacy for a broad number of fish species, easy and low-cost production, safety, and mass delivery in young fish. The following paragraphs review the work related to VHSV and IHNV vaccine development.

24.4.1 Non-replicating vaccines

Initially, vaccination against VHSV and IHNV was attempted with inactivated virus. Inactivation of virus can be easily achieved either by chemical or physical treatment, the major constraints being the mass production of the virus and the complete inactivation (absence of residual infectivity) without altering the immunogenicity and antigenicity of the virion. Vaccines based upon inactivated virus, especially obtained by β-propiolactone treatment, were proved to be very efficient in inducing long-term protection when delivered by intraperitoneal injection (Amend, 1976; de Kinkelin *et al.*, 1995; Anderson *et al.*, 2008). In contrast, vaccine delivery by bath immersion was not sufficient to significantly protect fish against virus challenge. For this reason, non-replicating vaccines are not suitable for mass delivery in young fish, but still represent potential vaccines for high-value fish, such as salmon, before transfer to an open aquatic environment. Moreover, a high degree of protection can be achieved even in the absence of adjuvant, thus limiting the appearance of vaccine-induced side-effects (Anderson *et al.*, 2008).

24.4.2 Subunit vaccines

The glycoprotein G is the unique target of neutralizing and protective antibodies, and thus recombinant subunit vaccines were based on this protein. Several prokaryotic and eukaryotic systems were tested to produce full-length or a portion of the G protein. The recombinant G proteins of VHSV and IHNV produced in *Escherichia coli* (Gilmore *et al.*, 1988; Xu *et al.*, 1991; Lorenzen *et al.*, 1993), *Caulobacter crescentus* (Simon *et al.*, 2001), *Yersina ruckeri* (Estepa *et al.*, 1994), yeast (Estepa *et al.*, 1994) and baculovirus/insect cells (Lecocq-Xhonneux *et al.*, 1994; Cain *et al.*, 1999; Biering *et al.*, 2005) did not elicit high levels of protection against homologous virus challenge, although in some cases neutralizing antibodies could be detected in sera of immunized animals. Moreover, these low levels of protection were only achieved when recombinant G was administrated by intraperitoneal injection in combination with an adjuvant (Biering *et al.*, 2005; Lecocq-Xhonneux *et al.*, 1994). Similarly, synthetic peptides, representing putative antigenic determinants of the IHNV G protein, were also poorly immunogenic (Emmenegger *et al.*, 1997). Due to its cost of production and route of delivery, recombinant G protein does not appear to be suitable for mass delivery to fish fry. To circumvent this problem, attenuated *Aeromonas salmonicida* was tested as a vector for the expression of VHSV and IHNV G protein fragments (Noonan *et al.*, 1995). Fish immunized by bath immersion or spray were moderately protected against homologous challenge. Together, these results reflect the complexity of expressing a G protein with the correct antigenic structure to be able to induce protective immunity.

24.4.3 DNA vaccines

Anderson and colleagues (1996) were the first to report the successful use of DNA vaccines to protect rainbow trout against IHNV challenge. A similar approach was then described to immunize rainbow trout against VHSV (Lorenzen *et al.*, 1998). The vaccines consisted of naked DNA plasmids expressing IHNV or VHSV G proteins under the control of a strong constitutive promoter derived from the human cytomegalovirus, and were administered by intramuscular injection. Since these first descriptions, DNA vaccines against both viruses have been extensively tested by several laboratories and shown to be highly efficacious in inducing specific and protective immunity under a wide range of conditions and in several marine and freshwater fish species (for review, see Chapter 5). Moreover, dual vaccination assays with a single dose containing both VHSV and IHNV DNA vaccines have been shown to induce neutralizing antibodies specific to both viruses (Boudinot *et al.*, 1998) and protect fish against coinfection (Einer-Jensen *et al.*, 2009). A single intramuscular injection of as little as 1–10 ng of vaccine can significantly protect rainbow trout fry (Corbeil *et al.*, 2000b; McLauchlan *et al.*, 2003). In practice, vaccine doses of 0.1–1 μg reproducibly induce high levels of protection in juvenile animals (between 1 to 10 g in weight), and 0.5–1 μg of vaccine dose are required for bigger animals (body weight >100 g). Intramuscular injection and gene gun immunization induce protective immunity in fry, while intraperitoneal injection provides lower levels of protection (Corbeil *et al.*, 2000a; McLauchlan *et al.*, 2003). In most of the studies, DNA vaccines have been shown to elicit an extremely rapid onset of innate immunity that is sufficient to cross-protect fish against any virus infection during the first four to seven days post-vaccination (LaPatra *et al.*, 2001; Lorenzen *et al.*, 2002). This early antiviral immunity is a consequence of the upregulation of the type-I interferon system and is followed by the development of the specific immune response leading to the production of detectable amounts of neutralizing antibodies (Purcell *et al.*, 2006). This specific immune response settled a long-lasting immunity that could protect fish up to two years (Kurath *et al.*, 2006). Finally, DNA vaccines were found to be capable of inducing broad, significant cross-protection between heterologous virus strains, but the efficacy was reduced when the G gene and the challenge virus were from different genotypes (Lorenzen *et al.*, 1999; Penaranda *et al.*, 2011a).

In 2005, the efficacy of these vaccines led to the licensing and commercialization of a DNA vaccine against IHNV for Atlantic salmon (APEX-IHN; Novartis Animal Health Canada Inc.) in Canada (for review, see Chapter 5 and Salonius *et al.*, 2007). Nevertheless, the commercialization of this vaccine in Europe is not approved, mainly because of the possible consideration of DNA-vaccinated fish as genetically modified organisms (GMOs) as long as the injected DNA is present in the fish. This might have significant economic consequences. Moreover, several aspects of this DNA vaccine have to be improved. First, the intramuscular injection of the DNA vaccine is labour-intensive and does not allow mass immunization of fish fry. Other routes of delivery including scarification of the skin, oral administration of encapsulated DNA, immersion in DNA-coated microsphere, and ultrasound-enhanced immersion delivery, which have been investigated but with limited success (Corbeil *et al.*, 2000a; Fernandez-Alonso *et al.*, 2001; Adomako *et al.*, 2012). More studies are also needed to clearly define the level of cross-protection between isolates belonging to different genotypes, and the necessity (or not) to use a mixture of DNA plasmids encoding distantly-related G proteins in the goal to induce as broad a protection as possible. Although DNA vaccines seem to be well tolerated and safe for fish (Kurath *et al.*, 2006), certain safety concerns need to be addressed, including plasmid DNA persistence and/or integration in the genome of immunized animals, the use of the human cytomegalovirus promoter, and the environmental release of DNA vaccines. Indeed, relatively long-term persistence of plasmid DNA has been reported (up to 728 days post-vaccination) (Salonius *et al.*, 2007; Tonheim *et al.*, 2007). This could be overcome by the use of suicidal DNA vectors that encode a cell-death factor under the control of an inducible promoter (Alonso *et al.*, 2011). Moreover, the human cytomegalovirus promoter could easily be replaced by another promoter of fish origin (Alonso *et al.*, 2003; Chico *et al.*, 2009).

24.4.4 Replicating vaccines

Live attenuated viruses were first developed by conventional methods: multiple passages on cell culture (Jørgensen, 1982; Ristow *et al.*, 2000; Adelmann *et al.*, 2008), neutralization escape mutants (Kim *et al.*, 1994; Roberti *et al.*, 1998 Gaudin *et al.*, 1999), and thermoresistant viruses (de Kinkelin *et al.*, 1980; Bernard *et al.*, 1983). In these studies, high levels of protection were obtained by bath immersion and oral delivery against lethal virus challenges. However, residual virulence was observed in most cases. Recent advances in reverse genetics make it possible to manipulate VHSV and IHNV RNA genomes and thus to introduce targeted mutations including nucleotide substitution, gene deletion, heterologous gene exchange and additional gene insertion, with the goal to attenuate the virus and use it as a gene vector (Biacchesi, 2011). This technique simplifies the random and uncertain selection of fully attenuated viruses obtained by conventional methods. Moreover, recombinant viruses recovered by reverse genetics can be engineered as "DIVA" (differentiating between infected and vaccinated animals) vaccines, thus allowing easy discrimination between vaccinated and naturally-infected fish in the field (Meeusen *et al.*, 2007). Several approaches have already been tested to get fully attenuated viruses that could be used as safe live-attenuated vaccines.

Recombinant IHNV and VHSV containing a deletion of the NV gene (ΔNV) resulted in irreversible attenuation of virus pathogenicity in rainbow trout (Thoulouze *et al.*, 2004; Harmache *et al.*, 2006a), yellow perch (Ammayappan *et al.*, 2011) and Japanese olive flounder (Kim and Kim, 2011). These viruses were highly attenuated, and low levels of mortality could only be recorded when the viruses were IP-injected (20–25% of total cumulative mortality versus 90–100% with the recombinant wild-type virus 4 weeks post-infection). ΔNV-immunized fish were fully protected against a subsequent virus challenge with a highly pathogenic virus at 30 days post-immunization (Thoulouze *et al.*, 2004), but mortalities could be recorded for challenge performed at a later period post-immunization (A. Harmache and M. Brémont, unpublished data). Using a non-invasive bioluminescence imaging device and a virus, in which the NV gene was replaced by the luciferase gene, Harmache and colleagues demonstrated that limited virus replication exclusively occurred in the fins, and that virus could persist in the fins up to 3 weeks post-infection without any further spread into the infected fish (Harmache *et al.*, 2006a). These observations could explain why IHNV-ΔNV could not be detected by RT-PCR in internal organs, and in part the absence of induced-antibody expression (Thoulouze *et al.*, 2004; Romero *et al.*, 2008). These results suggest that the short-term protection was the consequence of an interference phenomenon in the fins between the deletion mutant and the wild-type virus. ΔNV-viruses were also tested as vaccine vectors (Novoa *et al.*, 2006; Romero *et al.*, 2008; Kim and Kim, 2012a; A. Harmache and M. Brémont, unpublished data). Although these viruses were highly attenuated, they were all able to efficiently express detectable amounts of the foreign protein in cell cultures and to induce neutralizing antibodies when injected into fish. By bath immersion, these viruses were non-pathogenic, but too attenuated to be used as vaccine vectors.

Harmache and colleagues investigated the potential of IHNV as a vaccine vehicle against other fish viral diseases (Harmache *et al.*, 2006b; A. Harmache and M. Brémont, unpublished data). They engineered recombinant IHNV vectors that carry three expression cassettes of foreign antigens derived from four of the most devastating fish viral pathogens: VHSV G glycoprotein, infectious pancreatic necrosis virus VP2, sleeping disease virus C-E3-E2, and infectious salmon anemia virus (ISAV) hemagglutinin-esterase glycoprotein and fusion protein. They found that these three foreign antigens were efficiently and stably expressed by the recombinant virus, although its genome was increased in size by more than 50% compared with the wild-type genome (about 5.5 kb of foreign sequences). These IHNV vectors were highly attenuated in trout, leading to only 10% of cumulative mortality. Nevertheless, surviving trout were protected against subsequent challenges not only by the pathogenic IHNV but also by the targeted viruses. Thus, genome size increase has an effective attenuation effect and can be assumed to be relatively stable due to the low rate of recombination observed in rhabdovirus genomes. The introduction of additional targeted mutations in the genome of these IHNV vectors could fully attenuate and make them safer. Such mutations have already been described. Indeed, the presence of four incidental mutations in the IHNV genome was enough to highly attenuate the recombinant virus. There were two amino-acid substitutions in N, one in P and one in M, leading to less than 10% cumulative mortality in trout by bath immersion and strong induction of IHNV-specific antibodies (Biacchesi, 2002; Romero *et al.*, 2005).

Finally, recombinant viruses have been generated by exchanging the unique surface glycoprotein with different, distantly related and antigenically distinct fish rhabdoviruses (Biacchesi *et al.*, 2002; Kim and Kim, 2012b). The IHNV genome was engineered such that the IHNV G gene was replaced by those of VHSV (51% homology between both proteins) and spring viremia of carp virus (SVCV; a fish vesiculovirus, 29% homology between both G). Similarly, the VHSV G gene was replaced with that of the hirame rhabdovirus (another fish *Novirhabdovirus*, 51% homology between both G). Chimeric recombinant viruses were successfully recovered and were found to be as efficient as parental viruses for multicycle replication in cell culture. Moreover, IHNV-Gvhsv was as virulent as its biological parents (IHNV and VHSV) in rainbow trout (Biacchesi, 2002; Romero *et al.*, 2005). Interestingly, although SVCV is not pathogenic in rainbow trout, a high cumulative mortality could be observed with IHNV-Gsvcv by bath immersion (93% of cumulative mortality with IHNV-Gsvcv versus 95% with IHNV), demonstrating that SVCV G is fully functional in the IHNV background and that another SVCV protein should be involved in the host restriction (S. Biacchesi and M. Brémont, unpublished data). Thus, the G exchange is an attractive property to enable the use of these chimeric viruses as vaccine vectors for re-immunization.

24.5 CONCLUDING REMARKS

In conclusion, no efficient vaccine against VHSV and IHNV combining high immunogenicity, long-term protection and ease of delivery is yet available, in spite of the considerable amount of work published these last four decades. Reverse genetics systems for VHSV and IHNV have allowed the genomic manipulation of these viruses and thus the generation of promising multivalent live attenuated vaccines. Replicating vaccines could be one of the optimal fish vaccines in term of cost, protective efficacy and ease of administration, in contrast to other efficacious vaccines including killed virus and DNA vaccines which are not yet suitable for mass delivery in young fish. Additional work is needed to remove residual virulence, control the absence of any virus persistence, and avoid reversion to a wild-type phenotype. Regulatory constraints are the main obstacle for this kind of vaccine, even if they have been proved to be an effective means for preventing many human and animal viral diseases (Lauring *et al.*, 2010). A remarkable feature of aquaculture is the culture of fish in ponds or nets with no physical barriers to wild stocks. So, even if non-pathogenic for the targeted animal, the attenuated virus has to be safe for all other species in the aquatic environment. An alternative would be the use of these live virus vaccines in a confined environment during the immunization protocol before housing the immunized fish in an open aquatic environment. Reverse genetics systems could also be used to generate single-replication cycle, virus-based vaccine vectors such as replicons (Biacchesi, 2011). Although this kind of vaccine was found to be safe and protective in mammals after injection, the immunogenicity in fish of such vaccines should be demonstrated when administered by bath immersion. Finally, genetic immunization appears to be highly efficient for vaccination against both VHSV and IHNV. However, an improved delivery system is required before this method can gain widespread use. Several groups are working actively on novel oral and immersion delivery (Plant and Lapatra, 2011). Even if these potential delivery strategies do not yet elicit the levels of protection seen when DNA vaccines are delivered by intramuscular injection, some of them have great potential.

24.6 ACKNOWLEDGEMENTS

The authors received financial support from the French National Institute for Agricultural Research (INRA). The authors thank all the members of the Fish Molecular Virology Group (INRA) who contributed to this work.

REFERENCES

Adelmann, M., Kollner, B., Bergmann, S.M., *et al.*, 2008. Development of an oral vaccine for immunisation of rainbow trout (*Oncorhynchus mykiss*) against viral hemorrhagic septicaemia. *Vaccine* **26**: 837–44.

Adomako, M., St-Hilaire, S., Zheng, Y., *et al.*, 2012. Oral DNA vaccination of rainbow trout, *Oncorhynchus mykiss* (Walbaum), against infectious hematopoietic necrosis virus using PLGA [Poly(D,L-Lactic-Co-Glycolic Acid)] nanoparticles. *J Fish Dis* **35**: 203–14.

Alonso, M., Johnson, M., Simon, B. and Leong, J.A. 2003. A fish specific expression vector containing the interferon regulatory factor 1A (IRF1A) promoter for genetic immunization of fish. *Vaccine* **21**: 1591–1600.

Alonso, M., Chiou, P.P. and Leong, J.A. 2011. Development of a suicidal DNA vaccine for infectious hematopoietic necrosis virus (IHNV). *Fish Shellfish Immunol* **30**: 815–23.

Amend, D.F. 1976. Prevention and control of viral disease of salmonids. *J Fish Res Board Can* **33**: 1059–66.

Ammayappan, A., Kurath, G., Thompson, T.M. and Vakharia, V.N. 2011. A reverse genetics system for the Great Lakes strain of viral hemorrhagic septicemia virus: the NV gene is required for pathogenicity. *Mar Biotechnol (NY)* **13**: 672–83.

Anderson, E.D., Mourich, D.V., Fahrenkrug, S.C., *et al.*, 1996. Genetic immunization of rainbow trout (*Oncorhynchus mykiss*) against infectious hematopoietic necrosis virus. *Mol Mar Biol Biotechnol* **5**: 114–22.

Anderson, E., Clouthier, S., Shewmaker, W., *et al.*, 2008. Inactivated infectious hematopoietic necrosis virus (IHNV) vaccines. *J Fish Dis* **31**: 729–45.

Bandin, I. and Dopazo, C.P. 2011. Host range, host specificity and hypothesized host shift events among viruses of lower vertebrates. *Vet Res* **42**: 67.

Bearzotti, M., Monnier, A.F., Vende, P., *et al.*, 1995. The glycoprotein of viral hemorrhagic septicemia virus (VHSV): antigenicity and role in virulence. *Vet Res* **26**: 413–22.

Bernard, J., de Kinkelin, P. and Bearzotti-LeBerre, M. 1983. Viral hemorrhagic septicemia of rainbow trout: relation between the G polypeptide and antibody production in protection of the fish after infection with the F25 attenuated variant. *Infect Immun* **39**: 7–14.

Betts, A.M. and Stone, D.M. 2000. Nucleotide sequence analysis of the entire coding regions of virulent and avirulent strains of viral hemorrhagic septicaemia virus. *Virus Genes* **20**: 259–62.

Biacchesi, S. 2002. *Recovery of recombinant piscine rhabdovirus by reverse genetics*. Paris XI Orsay, Orsay.

Biacchesi, S. 2011. The reverse genetics applied to fish RNA viruses. *Vet Res* **42**: 12.

Biacchesi, S., Thoulouze, M.I., Bearzotti, M., *et al.*, 2000. Recovery of NV knockout infectious hematopoietic necrosis virus expressing foreign genes. *J Virol* **74**: 11247–53.

Biacchesi, S., Bearzotti, M., Bouguyon, E. and Brémont, M. 2002. Heterologous exchanges of the glycoprotein and the matrix protein in a *Novirhabdovirus*. *J Virol* **76**: 2881–9.

Biacchesi, S., Lamoureux, A., Mérour, E., *et al.*, 2010. Limited interference at the early stage of infection between two recombinant novirhabdoviruses: viral hemorrhagic septicemia virus and infectious hematopoietic necrosis virus. *J Virol* **84**: 10038–50.

Biering, E., Villoing, S., Sommerset, I. and Christie, K.E. 2005. Update on viral vaccines for fish. *Dev Biol (Basel)* **121**: 97–113.

Bootland, L.M. and Leong, J.C. 2011. Infectious haematopoietic necrosis virus, in *Fish Diseases and Disorders, Vol. 3: Viral, Bacterial and Fungal Infections*, 2nd edn (eds P.T.K. Woo and D.W. Bruno). Wallingford, CABI, 66–109.

Boudinot, P., Blanco, M., de Kinkelin, P. and Benmansour, A. 1998. Combined DNA immunization with the glycoprotein gene of viral hemorrhagic septicemia virus and infectious hematopoietic necrosis virus induces double-specific protective immunity and nonspecific response in rainbow trout. *Virology* **249**: 297–306.

Brudeseth, B.E., Castric, J. and Evensen, Ø. 2002. Studies on pathogenesis following single and double infection with viral hemorrhagic septicemia virus and infectious hematopoietic necrosis virus in rainbow trout (*Oncorhynchus mykiss*). *Vet Pathol* **39**: 180–89.

Cain, K.D., LaPatra, S.E., Shewmaker, B., *et al.*, 1999. Immunogenicity of a recombinant infectious hematopoietic necrosis virus glycoprotein produced in insect cells. *Dis Aquat Org* **36**: 67–72.

Campbell, S., Collet, B., Einer-Jensen, K., *et al.*, 2009. Identifying potential virulence determinants in viral haemorrhagic septicaemia virus (VHSV) for rainbow trout. *Dis Aquat Org* **86**: 205–12.

Chico, V., Ortega-Villaizan, M., Falco, A., *et al.*, 2009. The immunogenicity of viral haemorragic septicaemia rhabdovirus (VHSV) DNA vaccines can depend on plasmid regulatory sequences. *Vaccine* **27**: 1938–48.

Corbeil, S., Kurath, G. and LaPatra, S.E. 2000a. Fish DNA vaccine against infectious hematopoietic necrosis virus: efficacy of various routes of immunisation. *Fish Shellfish Immunol* **10**: 711–23.

Corbeil, S., LaPatra, S.E., Anderson, E.D. and Kurath, G. 2000b. Nanogram quantities of a DNA vaccine protect rainbow trout fry against heterologous strains of infectious hematopoietic necrosis virus. *Vaccine* **18**: 2817–24.

Dale, O.B., Ørpetveit, I., Lyngstad, T.M., *et al.*, 2009. Outbreak of viral haemorrhagic septicaemia (VHS) in seawater-farmed rainbow trout in Norway caused by VHS virus Genotype III. *Dis Aquat Org* **85**: 93–103.

de Kinkelin, P., Bearzotti-LeBerre, M. and Bernard, J. 1980. Viral hemorrhagic septicemia of rainbow trout: selection of a thermoresistant virus variant and comparison of polypeptide synthesis with the wild-type virus strain. *J Virol* **36**: 652–8.

de Kinkelin, P., Bearzotti, M., Castric, J., *et al.*, 1995. Eighteen years of vaccination against viral haemorrhagic septicaemia in France. *Vet Res* **26**: 379–87.

Einer-Jensen, K., Ahrens, P., Forsberg, R. and Lorenzen, N. 2004. Evolution of the fish rhabdovirus viral haemorrhagic septicaemia virus. *J Gen Virol* **85**: 1167–79.

Einer-Jensen, K., Delgado, L., Lorenzen, E., *et al.*, 2009. Dual DNA vaccination of rainbow trout (*Oncorhynchus mykiss*) against two different rhabdoviruses, VHSV and IHNV, induces specific divalent protection. *Vaccine* **27**: 1248–53.

Elsayed, E., Faisal, M., Thomas, M., *et al.*, 2006. Isolation of viral haemorrhagic septicaemia virus from muskellunge, *Esox masquinongy* (Mitchill), in Lake St Clair, Michigan, USA reveals a new sublineage of the North American genotype. *J Fish Dis* **29**: 611–19.

Emmenegger, E., Landolt, M., LaPatra, S. and Winton, J. 1997. Immunogenicity of synthetic peptides representing antigenic determinants on the infectious hematopoietic necrosis virus glycoprotein. *Dis Aquat Org* **28**: 175–84.

Engelking, H.M., Harry, J.B. and Leong, J.A. 1991. Comparison of representative strains of infectious hematopoietic necrosis virus by serological neutralization and cross-protection assays. *Appl Environ Microbiol* **57**: 1372–8.

Enzmann, P.J., Kurath, G., Fichtner, D. and Bergmann, S.M. 2005. Infectious hematopoietic necrosis virus: monophyletic origin of European isolates from North American genogroup M. *Dis Aquat Org* **66**: 187–95.

Estepa, A., Thiry, M. and Coll, J.M. 1994. Recombinant protein fragments from haemorrhagic septicaemia rhabdovirus stimulate trout leukocyte anamnestic responses *in vitro*. *J Gen Virol* **75**: 1329–38.

Fernandez-Alonso, M., Rocha, A. and Coll, J.M. 2001. DNA vaccination by immersion and ultrasound to trout viral haemorrhagic septicaemia virus. *Vaccine* **19**: 3067–75.

Gaudin, Y., de Kinkelin, P. and Benmansour, A. 1999. Mutations in the glycoprotein of viral haemorrhagic septicaemia virus that affect virulence for fish and the pH threshold for membrane fusion. *J Gen Virol* **80**: 1221–9.

Gilmore, R.D., Engelking, H.M., Manning, D.S. and Leong, J.A. 1988. Expression in *Escherichia coli* of an epitope of the glycoprotein of infectious hematopoietic necrosis virus protects against viral challenge. *Bio/Technology* **6**: 295–300.

Harmache, A., LeBerre, M., Droineau, S., *et al.*, 2006a. Bioluminescence imaging of live infected salmonids reveals that the fin bases are the major portal of entry for *Novirhabdovirus*. *J Virol* **80**: 3655–9.

Harmache, A., LeBerre, M., Lamoureux, A. and Bremont, M. 2006b. Recombinant IHNV expressing three foreign expression units an efficient bath immersion vaccine in salmonids, in *XIII International Conference on Negative Strand Viruses*. Salamanca, Spain.

Hattenberger-Baudouy, A.M., Danton, M., Merle, G. and de Kinkelin, P. 1995. Serum neutralization test for epidemiological studies of salmonid rhabdoviroses in France. *Vet Res* **26**: 512–20.

Helmick, C.M., Bailey, J.F., LaPatra, S. and Ristow, S. 1995. The esophagus/cardiac stomach region: site of attachment and internalization of infectious hematopoietic necrosis virus in challenged juvenile rainbow trout *Oncorhynchus mykiss* and coho salmon *O. kisutch*. *Dis Aquat Org* **23**: 189–99.

Hoffmann, B., Beer, M., Schutze, H. and Mettenleiter, T.C. 2005. Fish rhabdoviruses: molecular epidemiology and evolution. *Curr Top Microbiol Immunol* **292**: 81–117.

Jonstrup, S.P., Gray, T., Kahns, S., *et al.*, 2009. FishPathogens.eu/vhsv: a user-friendly viral haemorrhagic septicaemia virus isolate and sequence database. *J Fish Dis* **32**: 925–9.

Jørgensen, P.E.V. 1982. Egtved virus: temperature-dependent immune response of trout to infection with low-virulence virus. *J Fish Dis* **5**: 47–55.

Kim, C.H., Winton, J.R. and Leong, J.C. 1994. Neutralization-resistant variants of infectious hematopoietic necrosis virus have altered virulence and tissue tropism. *J Virol* **68**: 8447–53.

Kim, C.H., Dummer, D.M., Chiou, P.P. and Leong, J.A. 1999. Truncated particles produced in fish surviving infectious hematopoietic necrosis virus infection: mediators of persistence? *J Virol* **73**: 843–9.

Kim, M.S. and Kim, K.H. 2011. Protection of olive flounder, *Paralichthys olivaceus*, against viral hemorrhagic septicemia virus (VHSV) by immunization with NV gene-knockout recombinant VHSV. *Aquaculture* **314**: 39–43.

Kim, M.S. and Kim, K.H. 2012a. Effects of NV gene knock-out recombinant viral hemorrhagic septicemia virus (VHSV) on Mx gene expression in *Epithelioma papulosum cyprini* (EPC) cells and olive flounder (*Paralichthys olivaceus*). *Fish Shellfish Immunol* **32**: 459–63.

Kim, M.S. and Kim, K.H. 2012b. Generation of recombinant viral hemorrhagic septicemia viruses (VHSVs) harboring G gene of hirame rhabdovirus (HIRRV) and their ability to induce serum neutralization activity in olive flounder (*Paralichthys olivaceus*). *Aquaculture* **330–333**: 37-41.

Kim, M.S., Kim, D.S. and Kim, K.H. 2011. Generation and characterization of NV gene-knockout recombinant viral hemorrhagic septicemia virus (VHSV) genotype IVa. *Dis Aquat Org* **97**: 25–35.

Kim, R. and Faisal, M. 2011. Emergence and resurgence of the viral hemorrhagic septicemia virus (*Novirhabdovirus, Rhabdoviridae, Mononegavirales*). *J Adv Res* **2**: 9–21.

Kurath, G. and Leong, J.C. 1985. Characterization of infectious hematopoietic necrosis virus mRNA species reveals a nonvirion rhabdovirus protein. *J Virol* **53**: 462–8.

Kurath, G. and Winton, J. 2011. Complex dynamics at the interface between wild and domestic viruses of finfish. *Curr Opin Virol* **1**: 73–80.

Kurath, G., Ahern, K.G., Pearson, G.D. and Leong, J.C. 1985. Molecular cloning of the six mRNA species of infectious hematopoietic necrosis virus, a fish rhabdovirus, and gene order determination by R-loop mapping. *J Virol* **53**: 469–76.

Kurath, G., Garver, K.A., Troyer, R.M., *et al.*, 2003. Phylogeography of infectious haematopoietic necrosis virus in North America. *J Gen Virol* **84**: 803–14.

Kurath, G., Garver, K.A., Corbeil, S., *et al.*, 2006. Protective immunity and lack of histopathological damage two years after DNA vaccination against infectious hematopoietic necrosis virus in trout. *Vaccine* **24**: 345–54.

LaPatra, S.E., Lauda, K.A., Jones, G.R., *et al.*, 1995. Characterization of IHNV isolates associated with neurotropism. *Vet Res* **26**: 433–7.

LaPatra, S.E., Corbeil, S., Jones, G.R., *et al.*, 2001. Protection of rainbow trout against infectious hematopoietic necrosis virus four days after specific or semi-specific DNA vaccination. *Vaccine* **19**: 4011–19.

Lauring, A.S., Jones, J.O. and Andino, R. 2010. Rationalizing the development of live attenuated virus vaccines. *Nat Biotechnol* **28**: 573–9.

Lecocq-Xhonneux, F., Thiry, M., Dheur, I., *et al.*, 1994. A recombinant viral haemorrhagic septicaemia virus glycoprotein expressed in insect cells induces protective immunity in rainbow trout. *J Gen Virol* **75**: 1579–87.

Lorenzen, N., Olesen, N.J. and Jørgensen, P.E. 1990. Neutralization of Egtved virus pathogenicity to cell cultures and fish by monoclonal antibodies to the viral G protein. *J Gen Virol* **71**: 561–7.

Lorenzen, N., Olesen, N.J., Vestergård-Jørgensen, P.E., *et al.*, 1993. Molecular cloning and expression in *Escherichia coli* of the glycoprotein gene of VHS virus, and immunization of rainbow trout with the recombinant protein. *J Gen Virol* **74**: 623–30.

Lorenzen, N., Lorenzen, E., Einer-Jensen, K., *et al.*, 1998. Protective immunity to VHS in rainbow trout (*Oncorhynchus mykiss*, Walbaum) following DNA vaccination. *Fish Shellfish Immunol* **8**: 261–70.

Lorenzen, N., Lorenzen, E., Einer-Jensen, K., *et al.*, 1999. Genetic vaccination of rainbow trout against viral haemorrhagic septicaemia virus: small amounts of plasmid DNA protect against a heterologous serotype. *Virus Res* **63**: 19–25.

Lorenzen, N., Cupit, P.M., Einer-Jensen, K., *et al.*, 2000. Immunoprophylaxis in fish by injection of mouse antibody genes. *Nat Biotechnol* **18**: 1177–80.

Lorenzen, N., Lorenzen, E., Einer-Jensen, K. and LaPatra, S.E. 2002. Immunity induced shortly after DNA vaccination of rainbow trout against rhabdoviruses protects against heterologous virus but not against bacterial pathogens. *Dev Comp Immunol* **26**: 173–9.

McLauchlan, P.E., Collet, B., Ingerslev, E., *et al.*, 2003. DNA vaccination against viral haemorrhagic septicaemia (VHS) in rainbow trout: size, dose, route of injection and duration of protection: early protection correlates with Mx expression. *Fish Shellfish Immunol* **15**: 39–50.

Meeusen, E.N., Walker, J., Peters, A., *et al.*, 2007. Current status of veterinary vaccines. *Clin Microbiol Rev* **20**: 489–510.

Mellergaard S. 2011. Surveillance and eradication of VHS in Denmark, in *Report on the 15th Annual Meeting of the National Reference Laboratories for Fish Diseases*, Copenhagen: 18. Available at http://www.crl-fish.eu/upload/sites/eurl-fish/activities/annual_meetings/15_am_report.pdf

Meyers, T.R. 1998. Healthy juvenile sockeye salmon reared in virus-free hatchery water return as adults infected with infectious hematopoietic necrosis virus (IHNV): a case report and review of controversial issues in the epizootiology of IHNV. *J Aquat Anim Health* **10**: 172–81.

Morzunov, S.P., Winton, J.R. and Nichol, S.T. 1995. The complete genome structure and phylogenetic relationship of infectious hematopoietic necrosis virus. *Virus Res* **38**: 175–92.

Nishizawa, T., Kinoshita, S., Kim, W.S., *et al.*, 2006. Nucleotide diversity of Japanese isolates of infectious hematopoietic necrosis virus (IHNV) based on the glycoprotein gene. *Dis Aquat Org* **71**: 267–72.

Noonan, B., Enzmann, P.J. and Trust, T.J. 1995. Recombinant infectious hematopoietic necrosis virus and viral hemorrhagic septicemia virus glycoprotein epitopes expressed in *Aeromonas salmonicida* induce protective immunity in rainbow trout (*Oncorhynchus mykiss*). *Appl Environ Microbiol* **61**: 3586–91.

Novoa, B., Romero, A., Mulero, V., *et al.*, 2006. Zebrafish (*Danio rerio*) as a model for the study of vaccination against viral haemorrhagic septicemia virus (VHSV). *Vaccine* **24**: 5806–16.

OIE. 2013. *Manual of diagnostic tests for aquatic animals.* Available at http://www.oie.int/en/international-standard-setting/aquatic-manual/access-online/.

Olesen, N.J. and Nicolajsen, N. 2011. Overview of the disease situation and surveillance in Europe in 2010, in *Report on the 15th Annual Meeting of the National Reference Laboratories for Fish Diseases*, Copenhagen: 9–11. Available at http://www.crl-fish.eu/upload/sites/eurl-fish/activities/annual_meetings /15_am_report.pdf

Olesen, N.J., Lorenzen, N. and Jørgensen, P.E. 1993. Serological differences among isolates of viral haemorrhagic septicaemia virus detected by neutralizing monoclonal and polyclonal antibodies. *Dis Aquat Org* **16**: 163–70.

Penaranda, M.M., Purcell, M.K. and Kurath, G. 2009. Differential virulence mechanisms of infectious hematopoietic necrosis virus in rainbow trout (*Oncorhynchus mykiss*) include host entry and virus replication kinetics. *J Gen Virol* **90**: 2172–82.

Penaranda, M.M., LaPatra, S.E. and Kurath, G. 2011a. Specificity of DNA vaccines against the U and M genogroups of infectious hematopoietic necrosis virus (IHNV) in rainbow trout (*Oncorhynchus mykiss*). *Fish Shellfish Immunol* **31**: 43–51.

Penaranda, M.M., Wargo, A.R. and Kurath, G. 2011b. *In vivo* fitness correlates with host-specific virulence of *Infectious hematopoietic necrosis virus* (IHNV) in sockeye salmon and rainbow trout. *Virology* **417**: 312–19.

Plant, K.P. and LaPatra, S.E. 2011. Advances in fish vaccine delivery. *Dev Comp Immunol* **35**: 1256–62.

Purcell, M.K., Nichols, K.M., Winton, J.R., *et al.*, 2006. Comprehensive gene expression profiling following DNA vaccination of rainbow trout against infectious hematopoietic necrosis virus. *Mol Immunol* **43**: 2089–2106.

Ristow, S.S., LaPatra, S.E., Dixon, R., *et al.*, 2000. Responses of cloned rainbow trout *Oncorhynchus mykiss* to an attenuated strain of infectious hematopoietic necrosis virus. *Dis Aquat Org* **42**: 163–72.

Roberti, K.A., Rohovec, J.S. and Winton, J.R. 1998. Vaccination of rainbow trout against infectious hematopoietic necrosis (IHN) by using attenuated mutants selected by neutralizing monoclonal antibodies. *J Aquat Anim Health* **10**: 328–37.

Romero, A., Figueras, A., Tafalla, C., *et al.*, 2005. Histological, serological and virulence studies on rainbow trout experimentally infected with recombinant infectious hematopoietic necrosis viruses. *Dis Aquat Org* **68**: 17–28.

Romero, A., Figueras, A., Thoulouze, M.I., *et al.*, 2008. Recombinant infectious hematopoietic necrosis viruses induce protection for rainbow trout *Oncorhynchus mykiss*. *Dis Aquat Organ* **80**: 123–35.

Salonius, K., Simard, N., Harland, R. and Ulmer, J.B. 2007. The road to licensure of a DNA vaccine. *Curr Opin Investig Drugs* **8**: 635–41.

Schonherz, A.A., Hansen, M.H., Jørgensen, H.B., *et al.*, 2012. Oral transmission as a route of infection for viral haemorrhagic septicaemia virus in rainbow trout, *Oncorhynchus mykiss* (Walbaum). *J Fish Dis* **35**: 395–406.

Schutze, H., Enzmann, P.J., Kuchling, R., *et al.*, 1995. Complete genomic sequence of the fish rhabdovirus infectious haematopoietic necrosis virus. *J Gen Virol* **76**: 2519–27.

Schutze, H., Enzmann, P.J., Mundt, E. and Mettenleiter, T.C. 1996. Identification of the non-virion (NV) protein of fish rhabdoviruses viral haemorrhagic septicaemia virus and infectious haematopoietic necrosis virus. *J Gen Virol* **77**: 1259–63.

Schutze, H., Mundt, E. and Mettenleiter, T.C. 1999. Complete genomic sequence of viral hemorrhagic septicemia virus, a fish rhabdovirus. *Virus Genes* **19**: 59–65.

Simon, B., Nomellini, J., Chiou, P., *et al.*, 2001. Recombinant vaccines against infectious hematopoietic necrosis virus: production by the *Caulobacter crescentus* S-layer protein secretion system and evaluation in laboratory trials. *Dis Aquat Org* **44**: 17–27.

Skall, H.F., Olesen, N.J. and Mellergaard, S. 2005. Viral haemorrhagic septicaemia virus in marine fish and its implications for fish farming: a review. *J Fish Dis* **28**: 509–29.

Snow, M. 2011. The contribution of molecular epidemiology to the understanding and control of viral diseases of salmonid aquaculture. *Vet Res* **42**: 56.

Snow, M., Bain, N., Black, J., *et al.*, 2004. Genetic population structure of marine viral haemorrhagic septicaemia virus (VHSV). *Dis Aquat Org* **61**: 11–21.

Thoulouze, M.I., Bouguyon, E., Carpentier, C. and Bremont, M. 2004. Essential role of the NV protein of *Novirhabdovirus* for pathogenicity in rainbow trout. *J Virol* **78**: 4098–4107.

Tonheim, T.C., Leirvik, J., Løvoll, M., *et al.*, 2007. Detection of supercoiled plasmid DNA and luciferase expression in Atlantic salmon (*Salmo salar* L.) 535 days after injection. *Fish Shellfish Immunol* **23**: 867–76.

Tordo, N., Benmansour, A., Calisher, C., *et al.*, 2005. Rhabdovidae, in *Virus Taxonomy: Classification and Nomenclature of Viruses* (eds C.M. Fauquet, M.A. Mayo, J. Maniloff, *et al.*,). 8th Report of the International Committee on the Taxonomy of Viruses. London, Elsevier, 623–44.

Walker, P.J. and Winton, J.R. 2010. Emerging viral diseases of fish and shrimp. *Vet Res* **41**: 51.

Wolf, K. 1988. *Fish Viruses and Fish Viral Diseases*. Ithaca, NY, Comstock.

Xu, L., Mourich, D.V., Engelking, H.M., *et al.*, 1991. Epitope mapping and characterization of the infectious hematopoietic necrosis virus glycoprotein, using fusion proteins synthesized in *Escherichia coli*. *J Virol* **65**: 1611–15.

25 Vaccination against Infectious Pancreatic Necrosis

Espen Rimstad

Norwegian School of Veterinary Science, Oslo, Norway

ABSTRACT

Vaccination against infectious pancreatic necrosis (IPN) has so far not been a success story in countries with salmonid fish farming. Disease outbreaks are still prevalent in farms vaccinating against IPN. The disease was classically observed in fry, but after sea-farming of salmonids became popular, the disease has been found in different life stages, including post-smolts. IPN vaccines contain various antigen components, obtained from cell-culture propagated virus or recombinantly-produced viral antigens. Although different oral and bathing vaccination procedures have been described, IPN vaccines are usually administered by intraperitoneal injection and aim to protect salmonid fish in the seawater stage. The induction of specific antibody response after vaccination has not been found to correlate with protection against IPN.

25.1 OCCURRENCE AND SIGNIFICANCE

Infectious pancreatic necrosis virus (IPNV) was the first virus isolated from fish when it was isolated from brook trout (*Salvelinus fontinalis*) in 1957 (Wolf *et al.*, 1960). Already in the 1940s there were reports describing a disease called acute catarrhal enteritis of salmonid fingerlings, which later became known as infectious pancreatic necrosis (IPN) (M'Gonigle, 1940). IPN was characterized as a highly contagious viral disease of young, farmed salmonid fish (Wolf *et al.*, 1960).

Viruses with more or less close antigenic and genetic similarities to IPNV from salmonids have been isolated worldwide from numerous other species of non-salmonid fish families. The disease characteristics seen in other species may be different from that of IPN in salmonids (Castric *et al.*, 1987; Nakajima and Sorimachi, 1994), for example, nephritis and lamellar gill disease in Japanese eels (*Anguilla japonica*) (Hsu *et al.*, 1993; Lee *et al.*, 1999), ascites and cranial hemorrhage in yellowtail fingerlings (*Seriola quinqueradiata*) (Nakajima and Sorimachi,

espen.rimstad@nmbu.no

Fish Vaccination, First Edition. Edited by Roar Gudding, Atle Lillehaug and Øystein Evensen.

1994), and hematopoietic and renal necrosis in turbot (*Scophthalmus maximus*) (Castric *et al.*, 1987). The global presence of these viruses provides significant potential for disease outbreaks and economic damage.

Clinical signs of IPN in salmonid fish are dark pigmentation, distended abdomen and spiral swimming (Wolf *et al.*, 1960). Cumulative mortalities may vary from less than 10% to more than 90%, depending on virus strain (McAllister and Owens, 1995), infectious dose (Bebak and McAllister, 2009), and host and management and environmental factors such as water temperature (Bebak-Williams *et al.*, 2002).

IPN in salmonids has a wide geographic distribution, occurring in most major salmonid-farming countries of North and South America, Europe, Asia and Oceania (Ahne, 1980). Economic losses due to IPN are also related to the occurrence of other diseases appearing as a sequel to the IPN disease. After an IPN outbreak, surviving fish may become persistently infected (Yamamoto, 1975a).

IPNV can be introduced to a hatchery by eggs, equipment, different species of animals, and influx water. The impacts of these introductory alternatives may vary. When Atlantic salmon (*Salmo salar*) are moved to seawater, increased risk of IPN outbreaks is associated with mixing populations from several hatcheries, mode of transportation, and small size of smolts (Jarp, 1999).

IPNV is transmitted horizontally via the water route, and by movement of fish and eggs. Horizontal transmission is efficient when the virus shedding is high, such as during an outbreak. Subclinically infected fish may be important sources of virus, and it has been shown that such fish may be intermittent virus shedders (Urquhart *et al.*, 2008).

Vertical transmission from one generation to the next, through the gametes, has been demonstrated for brook trout (Wolf *et al.*, 1968; Bullock *et al.*, 1976), rainbow trout (*Oncorhynchus mykiss*) (Dorson and Torchy, 1985), and arctic char (*Salvelinus alpinus*) (Ahne and Negele, 1985), and there is circumstantial evidence that vertical transmission occurs in Atlantic salmon (Smail and Munro, 1989). The probability of vertical transmission of IPNV through the gametes is dependent upon the virus load in the ovarian fluid or milt (Bootland *et al.*, 1991, 1995). In brook trout it was found that virus titres of over 10^4 $TCID_{50}$/ml in ovarian fluid correlated with the isolation of IPN virus from egg homogenates (Wolf *et al.*, 1968). Even though the virus is not considered to cause infection of the gametes, IPNV can adhere to sperm (Mulcahy and Pascho, 1984; Dorson and Torchy, 1985) and egg shell of uninfected eggs (Ahne and Negele, 1985), and thereby cause transmission. Surface iodophore disinfection of eggs is not entirely effective in preventing vertical transmission (Bullock *et al.*, 1976).

IPNV has been isolated from a multitude of marine fish species close to marine Atlantic salmon farms with ongoing IPN outbreaks (Wallace *et al.*, 2008), so it seems the virus is rather promiscuous regarding its ability to infect different fish species. In the same study they also found that the number of IPNV-positive fish declined with increasing distance and time from the outbreak (Wallace *et al.*, 2008).

It has been estimated that a relatively large part of the variation seen in resistance to IPN in Atlantic salmon is caused by the genetic outfit of the host, and that major quantitative trait loci (QTL) affect IPN resistance at both the freshwater and seawater stages (Wetten *et al.*, 2007; Moen *et al.*, 2009; Houston *et al.*, 2010). This may provide general protective benefits through reduced infection pressure, reduced numbers of carrier fish, and less vertical transmission. Nevertheless, this is not a question of looking at *either* selective breeding or vaccination, but rather yes to both options.

25.2 ETIOLOGY

Infectious pancreatic necrosis virus is the type species of the genus *Aquabirnavirus* of the family *Birnaviridae* (Delmas *et al.*, 2011). Aquabirnaviruses have a very wide occurrence, and often there is no direct association with virus isolation and disease, which have led to difficulties in assigning nomenclature of the genus *Aquabirnavirus*. There are currently three approved species of the genus *Aquabirnavirus*: *Infectious pancreatic necrosis virus, Tellina virus*, and *Yellowtail ascites virus*, while Marine birnavirus has not been approved as a separate species (Delmas *et al.*, 2011). There is very close genetic relationship between the species in genus *Aquabirnavirus*, but they display considerable antigenic diversity (Okamoto *et al.*, 1983; Melby *et al.*, 1994; Hill and Way, 1995), and there are two serogroups that do not cross-react in neutralization tests (Underwood *et al.*, 1977; Olesen *et al.*, 1988). Most strains belong to serogroup A. Nine cross-reactive serotypes in serogroup A have been described, and the amino-acid sequences of the capsid protein (VP2) correlate well with serological classification, but also with geographical distribution (Hill and Way, 1995). Based on nucleotide sequence similarities, six genogroups can be defined. This number can be anticipated to increase when aquabirnaviruses from different species of fish at diverse geographical locations are described (Blake *et al.*, 2001).

Birnaviruses have a bi-segmented (segments A and B), double-stranded (ds) RNA genome. The genome is contained in a medium-sized, single-shelled icosahedral capsid. IPNV is a naked virus, that is, there is no envelope.

The genomic segment A has two open-reading frames (ORFs). The larger of these encodes a polyprotein. The order of the virus proteins in the polyprotein is NH2-pVP2-VP4-VP3-COOH. The polyprotein is self-cleaved at the pVP2-VP4 and the VP4-VP3 junctions by the viral protease VP4, which happens during the translation process (Duncan *et al.*, 1987). The pVP2 is further trimmed to mature VP2 by several cleavages of pVP2 at the carboxy-terminal end. The pVP2 to VP2 conversion is a slow process and is probably performed by host cell proteases rather than the proteolytic action of the VP4 (Dobos, 1995). VP2 may contain O-linked carbohydrates (Estay *et al.*, 1990, Hjalmarsson *et al.*, 1999). The second major structural protein, VP3, is an internal dsRNA binding protein (Pedersen *et al.*, 2007) inducing apoptosis (Chiu *et al.*, 2010), and is absent in empty capsids, making virus-like particles (VLPs) that lack viral RNA (Dobos, 1995). The lack of presence of VP3 in empty capsids demonstrates that VP2 is capable of making virus-like particles (VLPs) alone.

Genome segment A contains an additional small open-reading frame (ORF), which overlaps the amino terminal end of the polyprotein ORF. This small ORF encodes a polypeptide called VP5, an auxiliary non-structural viral protein with functions that are not entirely determined (Hong *et al.*, 2002; Santi *et al.*, 2005a, b; Chiu *et al.*, 2010). The product of genome segment B is VP1, the virion-associated RNA-dependent RNA polymerase (RdRp) (Duncan *et al.*, 1991).

The stability of IPNV in the aquatic environment is important for transmission. In general, a low temperature is beneficial for survival of viruses in the environment. An inactivation profile of approximately 3 $\log_{10}$ per three weeks was reported for IPNV in untreated fresh-, estuarine- and seawater at 15 °C (Toranzo and Hetrick, 1982), which approximates to a weekly 10-fold reduction. Survival of IPNV infectivity will ultimately depend upon local conditions.

25.3 PATHOGENESIS

It was observed early on that the susceptibility of salmonids to IPN is age-dependent (Snieszko *et al.*, 1959; Dorson and Torchy, 1981), and susceptibility to IPN generally decreases with age (Wolf and Quimby, 1971). But after marine farming of salmonids became widespread, IPN was not only observed in fry, but also in post-smolts after sea transfer (Smail *et al.*, 1992; Jarp *et al.*, 1995; Bowden *et al.*, 2002). Mortality is highest at temperatures between 10–16 °C (Dorson and Torchy, 1981). After a challenge experiment of fry with IPNV and subsequent testing for the presence of neutralizing antibodies, none of the survivors could be considered as immunologically tolerant (Dorson and Torchy, 1981). Covertly infected fish shed virus through seminal and ovarian fluids (Bootland *et al.*, 1995). Stress has been shown to increase shedding of virus in the feces (Yamamoto, 1975b; Reno *et al.*, 1978; Yamamoto and Kilistoff, 1979). The peak shedding rate for IPNV following intraperitoneal challenge in post-smolts occurred 11 days post-challenge and was estimated to be 6.8×10^3 $TCID_{50}/h^{-1}\ kg^{-1}$ (Urquhart *et al.*, 2008). Thus, IPNV carriers are a risk factor for other fish either in the same population or in other stocks of fish, for instance when smolts from different hatcheries are mixed at the sea production site.

Anti-IPNV antibodies have not been found to have a protective function in viral persistence, and circulating neutralizing antibodies do not clear off an IPNV infection (Bootland *et al.*, 1991, 1995). In Atlantic salmon, IPNV carriers demonstrate large variation in the level of anti-IPNV antibodies with no correlation between the level of IPNV in tissue and antibody level in plasma (Melby and Falk, 1995). When adult brook trout were vaccinated with inactivated IPNV in Freund's complete adjuvant, a strong humoral immune response was raised but the fish still became IPNV carriers, and the presence of neutralizing anti-IPNV antibody titres did not influence the rate of infection of leukocytes (Bootland *et al.*, 1995).

The minimum dose required to obtain IPNV infection in Atlantic salmon post-smolts by bath immersion for 4 h has been estimated to be less than 10^{-1} $TCID_{50}$/ml of IPNV in the immersed water (Urquhart *et al.*, 2008). These findings indicate that neither the carrier state nor virus shedding is prevented by humoral immune response to the virus, and that the infectious dose is low.

25.4 VACCINES AND VACCINE EFFECT

Commercial vaccines against IPNV have been marketed in Norway since 1995, usually in multivalent formulations together with bacterial vaccines. The vaccines contain various IPNV antigen components, including the most immunogenic protein, VP2, as part of inactivated virus particles obtained from cell cultures or in recombinant form (rVP2) obtained from different expressing systems. There are a limited number of publications demonstrating the efficacy of the vaccines. Four companies currently offer IPNV vaccines with oil-adjuvant for IP injection. Pharmaq AS, Novartis Animal Health and Centrovet produce vaccines containing inactivated IPNV, whereas MSD Animal Health uses a VP2 protein fragment expressed in *E. coli*.

The majority of commercial IPNV vaccines aim to protect salmonid fish in the post-smolt stage in seawater. However, even if the vaccines were efficient this would still leave the fish vulnerable to IPN at a young age prior to vaccination. The majority of registered IPN outbreaks in Norwegian fish farming occurs in seawater at an age where most of the fish population is vaccinated, but for the period up to 2010 there was still no downward trend in number of IPN outbreaks. The downward trend seen in 2011 can be assumed to have been caused by the introduction of QTL selective bred fish (Hjeltnes *et al.*, 2012). This could indicate that current vaccines against IPNV have limited efficacy under field conditions (i.e. commercial farming of Atlantic salmon).

Limited field efficacy and undesirable side-effects such as tissue adhesions and melanization caused by intraperitoneal injection of the oil adjuvants, which is present primarily because of positive effects for protection to certain bacterial pathogens, demonstrate the need for alternative antigens and different antigen delivery systems.

Development of suitable experimental models for IPN with high mortality of non-vaccinated controls has been challenging (Bowden *et al.*, 2002; Ramstad *et al.*, 2007). The lack of challenge models that correlate well with field efficacy has hampered the development of efficient vaccines against IPN.

Nevertheless, in experimental challenge models the vaccines may perform reasonably well. The inoculation of inactivated IPNV in adjuvant in fish will induce a specific neutralizing antibody response, but the level of circulating antibodies is not necessarily linked to the ability to protect against IPN. In a field study, two IPN-vaccinated groups of Atlantic salmon showed relative percent survival (RPS) in approximately the same range, 50.6% and 53.2% respectively, in a natural outbreak of IPN appearing six weeks after sea transfer. One of these groups displayed significantly elevated specific antibody levels to IPNV 6 weeks after vaccination, whereas the other group did not (Erdal *et al.*, 2003).

25.4.1 Antigen vaccines

Atlantic salmon parr immunized with multivalent, oil-adjuvanted vaccine containing recombinant VP2 (rVP2) IPNV expressed in *E. coli* were found to have lower probability of being IPNV-infected when sampled 12 weeks post-challenge (Frost and Ness, 1997). Immunization with a commercially vaccine containing rVP2 antigen, and challenged by subsequent bath and cohabitation, induced approximately 70% protection compared with a vaccine without this antigen (Ramstad *et al.*, 2007).

When rabbits were immunized with rVP2 from *E. coli* or with purified VP2 obtained from IPNV-infected cell cultures, only serum from the purified VP2 immunized rabbits was able to neutralize IPNV infection in a cell culture. This could indicate that differences in conformational epitopes between rVP2 and native VP2, or lack of sugar moieties on bacterial expressed rVP2, could be of importance in eliciting a neutralizing immune response, at least in the way these antigens are recognised by the rabbit immune system (Fridholm *et al.*, 2007).

In a comparative test in Atlantic salmon, vaccines with either whole virus antigens, whole virus antigens entrapped in nanoparticles, *E. coli*-expressed subunit antigens fused with putative translocating domains of *Pseudomonas aeruginosa* exotoxin, or plasmid DNA encoding segment A were used. Although the differences in performance between the antigen groups were moderate, the whole-virus antigen vaccines conferred highest protection (Munang'andu *et al.*, 2012). A complicating factor in the design of such comparative experiments is that it is difficult to determine whether an equal dose of antigen was administered in the different groups; for example, the whole virus antigen was measured in $TCID_{50}$/ml, while recombinant antigen is measured in μg/ml purified protein. Nevertheless, the results indicate that whole-virus antigen vaccines are currently the most protective vaccines. The same group found that when IPNV containing virulent or non-virulent associated motifs of the VP2 protein were used for vaccine preparation, they were equally protective in a challenge experiment when the antigen and delivery parameters were kept equal, thus indicating that there is strong cross-protection within isolates of the same serotype of IPNV (Munang'andu *et al.*, 2012).

Many different expression systems have been utilized for VP2 expression. *E. coli* has been mentioned above, and another bacterial system that has been used is the expression of VP2-VP3 fusion protein in *Lactobacillus casei*. After immunizing rainbow trout through oral dosing of antigen, a 10-fold reduction in viral load compared with the control group was obtained (Zhao *et al.*, 2012). Expression of VP2 in yeast yielded rVP2-VLPs, and when such particles were used to vaccinate rainbow trout either by injection or by feeding, induction of anti-IPNV antibodies was achieved. Challenge of immunized trout with a heterologous IPNV strain and subsequent viral load determination demonstrated that both injection and orally vaccinated fish had lower IPNV loads than naïve or sham-vaccinated fish (Allnutt *et al.*, 2007). Expression of all structural IPNV protein genes in insect cells and in larvae through a baculovirus expression system also gave VLPs, but when rainbow trout fry were vaccinated by immersion in this antigen, no protection was achieved, and similar intraperitoneal immunization of Atlantic salmon pre-smolts with an oil-adjuvant formulation gave a very modest protective response (Shivappa *et al.*, 2005). Production of VLPs has also been demonstrated by expression of the entire segment A of IPNV in mammalian cell cultures using an expression system based upon the alphavirus Semliki Forest virus. Correct processing of the polyprotein was assumed to occur based upon recognition of the expressed antigen by conformation-dependent monoclonal antibodies to IPNV, but vaccination-challenge experiments were not reported (McKenna *et al.*, 2001).

25.4.2 DNA vaccines

DNA vaccines relocate the expression of the antigen from *in vitro* systems to the cells of the vaccinated fish, and this endogenously produced antigen triggers different components of the host immune system. The DNA vaccines have been found to be very efficient against novirhabdovirus diseases in salmonids and induce rapid and long-lasting protection. DNA vaccines against IPN, however, have so far not been found to be similarly successful. The oil adjuvant that is a necessary part of the IP-injected multivalented salmonid antigen vaccines is not a component of DNA vaccines.

In an experiment with intramuscular injection of a DNA vaccine consisting of plasmids, in which expression was under the control of the cytomegalovirus immediate early promoter, an RPS of 84% was obtained for fish immunized with plasmids expressing the polyprotein ORF of genome segment A. However, the mortality in the control group was only 33%. Vaccine constructs containing only VP2 or part of VP2 did not induce similar protection (Mikalsen *et al.*, 2004).

When a DNA vaccine expressing the VP2 gene was encapsulated in alginate microspheres and orally administered, neutralizing antibodies could be detected after 15 days and an RPS of around 80% was achieved in both brown trout (*Salmo trutta*) and rainbow trout when challenged at 15 and 30 days after vaccine delivery. The viral loads detected in the surviving vaccinated fish were much lower than those in the control fish (de Las Heras *et al.*, 2009, 2010).

25.5 VACCINE-INDUCED IMMUNE RESPONSES

Antibody response in teleost fish does not show isotype switching (Kaattari *et al.*, 2002), and has a relatively low affinity maturation. The induction of specific antibody titre or neutralizing antibodies after vaccination has not been found to correlate with protection against IPN (Shivappa *et al.*, 2005; Cuesta *et al.*, 2010). It is tempting, but speculative, to assume that the nature of the humoral response and lack of protection is correlated; however, the lack of humoral protection could also be related to specific properties of the viral propagation. The findings suggest that a humoral response is not sufficient to prevent the IPNV from causing disease, and it is not clear whether the humoral response can prevent virus infection, or reduce dissemination of virus within the infected host. Therefore, measurement of humoral response is of limited value in visualizing the efficacy of IPN vaccines. The uses of functional measurements, that is, the ability to resist highly virulent viral challenges (expressed as RPS), changes in histopathological scoring, or the capacity to eliminate the carrier state of IPNV, are improvements that would better show protection against IPN. An ideal vaccine would prevent the establishment of infection. However, it has been found that the consistency and outcome of protection of IPN vaccination is highly dependent upon the genetic constitution of the experimental fish (Ramstad and Midtlyng, 2008). Furthermore, differences in virulence of viruses have been found not to be the main reason for the lack of protection in the field outbreaks in Atlantic salmon. Both findings indicate that there are strong non-virus components of the development of the disease in Atlantic salmon post-smolts (Julin *et al.*, 2013).

In a recently study where attenuated, replication-competent subviral particles were used to vaccinate rainbow trout fry, it was proposed that the efficacy of the vaccine was better predicted by measuring both the titre of neutralizing antibodies and non-specific cytotoxic activity than by the humoral immune response alone (Rivas-Aravena *et al.*, 2012).

25.6 REGULATIONS

In general there are regulatory concerns related to fish DNA vaccines, and these concerns are not specifically directed to vaccines against IPN. But inherently, the risks with DNA vaccines should not be any greater than with the fish vaccines that are currently used. The concerns are related to the persistence of the DNA vaccine in the fish, long-term safety issues related to both the environment and the consumer, and the acceptance of the consumers (Lorenzen and LaPatra, 2005).

Similarly, general environmental safety concerns currently hinder the development and use of live virus vaccines in fish.

REFERENCES

Ahne, W. 1980. Occurrence of infectious pancreatic necrosis virus (IPN) in different fish species. *Berliner Munch Tierarztl Wochenschr* **93**: 14–16.

Ahne, W. and Negele, R. 1985. Studies on the transmission of infectious pancreatic necrosis virus via eyed eggs and sexual products of salmonid fish, in *Fish and Shellfish Pathology* (ed. A. Ellis). London, Academic Press, 262–70.

Allnutt, F.C.T., Bowers, R.M., Rowe, C.G., *et al.*, 2007. Antigenicity of infectious pancreatic necrosis virus VP2 subviral particles expressed in yeast. *Vaccine* **25**: 4880–88.

Bebak, J. and McAllister, P.E. 2009. Continuous exposure to infectious pancreatic necrosis virus during early life stages of rainbow trout, *Oncorhynchus mykiss* (Walbaum). *J Fish Dis* **32**: 173–81.

Bebak-Williams, J., McAllister, P.E., Smith, G. and Boston, R. 2002. Effect of fish density and number of infectious fish on the survival of rainbow trout fry, *Oncorhynchus mykiss* (Walbaum), during epidemics of infectious pancreatic necrosis. *J Fish Dis* **25**: 715–26.

Blake, S., Ma, J.Y., Caporale, D.A., *et al.*, 2001. Phylogenetic relationships of aquatic birnaviruses based on deduced amino acid sequences of genome segment A cDNA. *Dis Aquat Org* **45**: 89–102.

Bootland, L.M., Dobos, P. and Stevenson, R.M.W. 1991. The IPNV carrier state and demonstration of vertical transmission in experimentally infected brook trout. *Dis Aquat Org* **10**: 13–21.

Bootland, L.M., Dobos, P. and Stevenson, R.M.W. 1995. Immunization of adult brook trout, *Salvelinus fontinalis* (Mitchill), fails to prevent the infectious pancreatic necrosis virus (IPNV) carrier state. *J Fish Dis* **18**: 449–58.

Bowden, T.J., Smail, D.A. and Ellis, A.E. 2002. Development of a reproducible infectious pancreatic necrosis virus challenge model for Atlantic salmon, *Salmo salar* L. *J Fish Dis* **25**: 555–63.

Bullock, G.L., Rucker, R.R., Amend, D., *et al.*, 1976. Infectious pancreatic necrosis – transmission with iodine-treated and nontreated eggs of brook trout (*Salvelinus fontinalis*). *J Fish Res Board Can* **33**: 1197–8.

Castric, J., Baudin-Laurencin, F., Coustans, M.F. and Auffret, M. 1987. Isolation of infectious pancreatic necrosis virus, Ab serotype, from an epizootic in farmed turbot, *Scophthalmus maximus*. *Aquaculture* **67**: 117–26.

Chiu, C.L., Wu, J.L., Her, G.M., *et al.*, 2010. Aquatic birnavirus capsid protein, VP3, induces apoptosis via the Bad-mediated mitochondria pathway in fish and mouse cells. *Apoptosis* **15**: 653–68.

Cuesta, A., Chaves-Pozo, E., de Las Heras, A.I., *et al.*, 2010. An active DNA vaccine against infectious pancreatic necrosis virus (IPNV) with a different mode of action than fish *Rhabdovirus* DNA vaccines. *Vaccine* **28**: 3291–3300.

de Las Heras, A.I., Prieto, S.I.P. and Saint-Jean, S.R. 2009. *In vitro* and *in vivo* immune responses induced by a DNA vaccine encoding the VP2 gene of the infectious pancreatic necrosis virus. *Fish Shellfish Immunol* **27**: 120–29.

de Las Heras, A.I., Saint-Jean, S.R. and Perez-Prieto, S.I. 2010. Immunogenic and protective effects of an oral DNA vaccine against infectious pancreatic necrosis virus in fish. *Fish Shellfish Immunol* **28**: 562–70.

Delmas, B., Mundt, E., Vakharia, V.N. and Wu, J.L. 2011. Birnaviridae, in *Virus Taxonomy Classification and Nomenclature of Viruses* (eds A.M.Q. King, M.J. Adams. E.B. Carstens and E.J. Lefkowitz). Amsterdam, Elsevier, 499–507.

Dobos, P. 1995. The molecular biology of infectious pancreatic necrosis virus. *Annu Review Fish Dis* **5**: 25–54.

Dorson, M. and Torchy, C. 1981. The influence of fish age and water temperature on mortalities of rainbow trout, *Salmo gairdneri* Richardson, caused by a European strain of infectious Pancreatic Necrosis Virus. *J Fish Dis* **4**: 213–21.

Dorson, M. and Torchy, C. 1985. Experimental transmission of infectious pancreatic necrosis virus via the sexual products, in *Fish and Shellfish Pathology* (ed. A. Ellis). London, Academic Press, 251–61.

Duncan, R., Nagy, E., Krell, P.J. and Dobos, P. 1987. Synthesis of the infectious pancreatic necrosis virus polyprotein, detection of a virus-encoded protease, and fine-structure mapping of genome segment-a coding regions. *J Virol* **61**: 3655–64.

Duncan, R., Mason, C.L., Nagy, E., *et al.*, 1991. Sequence analysis of infectious pancreatic necrosis virus genome segment-B and its encoded VP1 protein: a putative RNA-dependent RNA polymerase lacking the Gly-Asp-Asp Motif. *Virology* **181**: 541–52.

Erdal, J.I., Skjelstad, B. and Soleim, K.B. 2003. Evaluation of protection from vaccination against infectious pancreatic necrosis (IPN) in a GCP field trial in Norway, in *Abstracts from the 11th International Conference of EAFP: Diseases of Fish and Shellfish*. Saint Julians, Malta, 2003.

Estay, A., Farias, G., Soler, M. and Kuznar, J. 1990. Further analysis on the structural proteins of infectious Pancreatic Necrosis Virus. *Virus Res* **15**: 85–96.

Fridholm, H., Eliasson, L. and Everitt, E. 2007. Immunogenicity properties of authentic and heterologously synthesized structural protein VP2 of infectious pancreatic necrosis virus. *Viral Immunol* **20**: 635–48.

Frost, P. and Ness, A. 1997. Vaccination of Atlantic salmon with recombinant VP2 of infectious pancreatic necrosis virus (IPNV), added to a multivalent vaccine, suppresses viral replication following IPNV challenge. *Fish Shellfish Immunol* **7**: 609–19.

Hill, B.J. and Way, K. 1995. Serological classification of infectious pancreatic necrosis (IPN) virus and other aquatic birnaviruses. *Annu Rev Fish Dis* **5**: 55–77.

Hjalmarsson, A., Carlemalm, E. and Everitt, E. 1999. Infectious pancreatic necrosis virus: Identification of a VP3-containing ribonucleoprotein core structure and evidence for O-linked glycosylation of the capsid protein VP2. *J Virol* **73**: 3484–90.

Hjeltnes, B., Olsen, A.B. and Hellberg, H. (eds) 2012. *Fiskehelserapporten 2011* [Farmed fish health report 2011]. Oslo, Norwegian Veterinary Institute.

Hong, J.R., Gong, H.Y. and Wu, J.L. 2002. IPNV VP5, a novel anti-apoptosis gene of the Bcl-2 family, regulates Mcl-1 and viral protein expression. *Virology* **295**: 217–29.

Houston, R.D., Haley, C.S., Hamilton, A., *et al.*, 2010. The susceptibility of Atlantic salmon fry to freshwater infectious pancreatic necrosis is largely explained by a major QTL. *Heredity* **105**: 318–27.

Hsu, Y.L., Chen, B.S. and Wu, J.L. 1993. Demonstration of infectious pancreatic necrosis virus-Strain Vr-299 in Japanese eel, *Anguilla japonica* Temminck and Schlegel. *J Fish Dis* **16**: 123–9.

Jarp, J. 1999. Epidemiological aspects of viral diseases in the Norwegian farmed Atlantic salmon (*Salmo salar* L.). *Bull Eur Assoc Fish Pathol* **19**: 240–44.

Jarp, J., Gjevre, A.G., Olsen, A.B. and Bruheim, T. 1995. Risk-factors for furunculosis, infectious pancreatic necrosis and mortality in post-smolt of Atlantic salmon, *Salmo salar* L. *J Fish Dis* **18**: 67–78.

Julin, K., Mennen, S. and Sommer, A.I. 2013. Study of virulence in field isolates of infectious pancreatic necrosis virus obtained from the northern part of Norway. *J Fish Dis* **36**: 89–102.

Kaattari, S.L., Zhang, H.L.L., Khor, I.W., *et al.*, 2002. Affinity maturation in trout: clonal dominance of high affinity antibodies late in the immune response. *Dev Comp Immunol* **26**: 191–200.

Lee, N.S., Nomura, Y. and Miyazaki, T. 1999. Gill lamellar pillar cell necrosis, a new birnavirus disease in Japanese eels. *Dis Aquat Org* **37**: 13–21.

Lorenzen, N. and LaPatra, S.E. 2005. DNA vaccines for aquacultured fish. *Rev Sci Tech* **24**: 201–13.

McAllister, P.E. and Owens, W.J. 1995. Assessment of the virulence of fish and molluscan isolates of infectious pancreatic necrosis virus for salmonid fish by challenge of brook trout, *Salvelinus fontinalis* (Mitchill). *J Fish Dis* **18**: 97–103.

McKenna, B.M., Fitzpatrick, R.M., Phenix, K.V., *et al.*, 2001. Formation of infectious pancreatic necrosis virus-like particles following expression of segment A by recombinant semliki forest virus. *Mar Biotechnol (NY)* **3**: 103–10.

Melby, H.P., Caswell-Reno, P. and Falk, K. 1994. Antigenic analysis of Norwegian aquatic birnavirus isolates using monoclonal antibodies – with special reference to fish species, age and health status. *J Fish Dis* **17**: 85–91.

Melby, H.P. and Falk, K. 1995. Study of the interaction between a persistent infectious pancreatic necrosis virus (IPNV) infection and experimental infectious salmon anaemia (ISA) in Atlantic salmon, *Salmo salar* L. *J Fish Dis* **18**: 579–86.

M'Gonigle, R.H. 1940. Acute catarrhal enteritis of salmonid fingerlings. *Trans Am Fish Soc* **70**: 297–302.

Mikalsen, A.B., Torgersen, J., Aleström, P., *et al.*, 2004. Protection of Atlantic salmon *Salmo salar* against infectious pancreatic necrosis after DNA vaccination. *Dis Aquat Org* **60**: 11–20.

Moen, T., Baranski, M., Sonesson, A.K. and Kjøglum, S. 2009. Confirmation and fine-mapping of a major QTL for resistance to infectious pancreatic necrosis in Atlantic salmon (*Salmo salar*): population-level associations between markers and trait. *BMC Genomics* **10**: 368

Mulcahy, D. and Pascho, R.J. 1984. Adsorption to fish sperm of vertically transmitted fish viruses. *Science* **225**: 333–5.

Munang'andu, H.M., Fredriksen, B.N., Mutoloki, S., *et al.*, 2012. Comparison of vaccine efficacy for different antigen delivery systems for infectious pancreatic necrosis virus vaccines in Atlantic salmon (*Salmo salar* L.) in a cohabitation challenge model. *Vaccine* **30**: 4007–16.

Nakajima, K. and Sorimachi, M. 1994. Serological and biochemical characterization of 2 birnaviruses – Vdv and Yav isolated from cultured yellowtail. *Fish Pathol* **29**: 183–6.

Okamoto, N., Sano, T., Hedrick, R.P. and Fryer, J.L. 1983. Antigenic relationships of selected strains of infectious pancreatic necrosis virus and European eel virus. *J Fish Dis* **6**: 19–25.

Olesen, N.J., Jørgensen, P.E.V., Bloch, B. and Mellergaard, S. 1988. Isolation of an IPN-like virus belonging to the serogroup II of the aquatic birnaviruses from dab, *Limanda limanda* L. *J Fish Dis* **11**: 449–51.

Pedersen, T., Skjesol, A. and Jørgensen, J.B. 2007. VP3, a structural protein of infectious pancreatic necrosis virus, interacts with RNA-dependent RNA polymerase VP1 and with double-stranded RNA. *J Virol* **81**: 6652–63.

Ramstad, A. and Midtlyng, P.J. 2008. Strong genetic influence on IPN vaccination-and-challenge trials in Atlantic salmon, *Salmo salar* L. *J Fish Dis* **31**: 567–78.

Ramstad, A., Romstad, A.B., Knappskog, D.H. and Midtlyng, P.J. 2007. Field validation of experimental challenge models for IPN vaccines. *J Fish Dis* **30**: 723–31.

Reno, P.W., Darley, S. and Savan, M. 1978. Infectious pancreatic necrosis – experimental induction of a carrier state in trout. *J Fish Res Board Can* **35**: 1451–6.

Rivas-Aravena, A., Martin, M.C.S., Galaz, J., *et al.*, 2012. Evaluation of the immune response against immature viral particles of infectious pancreatic necrosis virus (IPNV): a new model to develop an attenuated vaccine. *Vaccine* **30**: 5110–17.

Santi, N., Sandtrø, A., Sindre, H., *et al.*, 2005a. Infectious pancreatic necrosis virus induces apoptosis *in vitro* and *in vivo* independent of VP5 expression. *Virology* **342**: 13–25.

Santi, N., Song, H., Vakharia, V.N. and Evensen, Ø. 2005b. Infectious pancreatic necrosis virus VP5 is dispensable for virulence and persistence. *J Virol* **79**: 9206–16.

Shivappa, R.B., McAllister, P.E., Edwards, G.H., *et al.*, 2005. Development of a subunit vaccine for Infectious pancreatic necrosis virus using a baculovirus insect/larvae system. *Dev Biol (Basel)* **121**: 165–74.

Smail, D.A. and Munro, A.L.S. 1989. Infectious pancreatic necrosis virus in Atlantic salmon: transmission via the sexual products?, in *Viruses of Lower Vertebrates* (eds W. Ahne and E. Kurstak). Berlin, Springer Verlag, 292–301.

Smail, D.A., Bruno, D.W., Dear, G., *et al.*, 1992. Infectious pancreatic necrosis (IPN) virus Sp serotype in farmed Atlantic salmon, *Salmo salar* L, post-smolts associated with mortality and clinical disease. *J Fish Dis* **15**: 77–83.

Snieszko, S.F., Wolf, K., Amper, J.E. and Pettijohn, L.L. 1959. Infectious nature of pancreatic necrosis. *Trans Am Fish Soc* **88**: 289–93.

Toranzo, A.E. and Hetrick, F.M. 1982. Comparative stability of 2 salmonid viruses and poliovirus in fresh, estuarine and marine waters. *J Fish Dis* **5**: 223–31.

Underwood, B.O., Smale, C.J., Brown, F. and Hill, B.J. 1977. Relationship of a virus from *Tellina tenuis* to infectious pancreatic necrosis virus. *J Gen Virol* **36**: 93–109.

Urquhart, K., Murray, A.G., Gregory, A., *et al.*, 2008. Estimation of infectious dose and viral shedding rates for infectious pancreatic necrosis virus in Atlantic salmon, *Salmo salar* L., post-smolts. *J Fish Dis* **31**: 879–87.

Wallace, I.S., Gregory, A., Murray, A.G., *et al.*, 2008. Distribution of infectious pancreatic necrosis virus (IPNV) in wild marine fish from Scottish waters with respect to clinically infected aquaculture sites producing Atlantic salmon, *Salmo salar* L. *J Fish Dis* **31**: 177–86.

Wetten, M., Aasmundstad, T., Kjøglum, S. and Storset, A. 2007. Genetic analysis of resistance to infectious pancreatic necrosis in Atlantic salmon (*Salmo salar* L.). *Aquaculture* **272**: 111–17.

Wolf, K. and Quimby, M.C. 1971. Salmonid viruses – infectious pancreatic necrosis virus – morphology, pathology, and serology of first European isolations. *Arch Gesamte Virusforsch* **34**: 144–56.

Wolf, K., Snieszko, S.F., Dunbar, C.E. and Pyle, E. 1960. Virus nature of infectious pancreatic necrosis in trout. *Proc Soc Exp Biol Med* **104**: 105–8.

Wolf, K., Bradford, A.D. and Quimby, M.C. 1968. Egg-associated transmission of IPN virus of trouts. *Virology* **21**: 317–21.

Yamamoto, T. 1975a. Frequency of detection and survival of infectious pancreatic necrosis virus in a carrier population of brook trout (*Salvelinus fontinalis*) in a lake. *J Fish Res Board Canada* **32**: 568–70.

Yamamoto, T. 1975b. Infectious pancreatic necrosis (IPN) virus carriers and antibody-production in a population of rainbow-trout (*Salmo gairdneri*). *Can J Microbiol* **21**: 1343–7.

Yamamoto, T. and Kilistoff, J. 1979. Infectious pancreatic necrosis virus – quantification of carriers in lake populations during a 6-year period. *J Fish Res Board Canada* **36**: 562–7.

Zhao, L.L., Liu, M., Ge, J.W., *et al.*, 2012. Expression of infectious pancreatic necrosis virus (IPNV) VP2-VP3 fusion protein in *Lactobacillus casei* and immunogenicity in rainbow trouts. *Vaccine* **30**: 1823–9.

26 Vaccination against Infectious Salmon Anemia

Knut Falk

Norwegian Veterinary Institute, Oslo, Norway

ABSTRACT

Infectious salmon anemia (ISA) is a serious disease in marine farming of Atlantic salmon, caused by the ISA-virus, an orthomyxovirus. Vaccines against ISA are most commonly inactivated ISA-virus cell culture preparations with adjuvants, administered by intraperitoneal injection of smolts before transfer to seawater netpens. Such vaccines have been reported to provide a RPS of 84–95% during experimental trials. As several ISA outbreaks have been observed in vaccinated populations, the field effects of the vaccines have been questioned. Recently, a Chilean company has marketed vaccines based on a recombinantly expressed ISAV protein, both for injection and oral administration. However, studies demonstrating the effect of these vaccines have not been published. Vaccination against ISA has been included in ISAV control programs in Canada since 1999, in the Faroe Islands since 2005, and in Chile since 2010. In Norway, vaccination was part of a control program implemented in 2009 in a region with several ISA outbreaks.

26.1 OCCURRENCE AND SIGNIFICANCE

Infectious salmon anemia (ISA) is a significant infectious viral disease of farmed Atlantic salmon, and was first reported in Norway in 1984 (Thorud and Djupvik, 1988). ISA is a World Organization for Animal Health (OIE) notifiable disease, and is categorized as a list 2 disease within the European Union. The disease has now been reported in farmed Atlantic salmon in Canada, the US, Scotland, the Faroe Islands and in Chile (Rimstad *et al.*, 2011).

ISA spread rapidly throughout the Norwegian aquaculture industry, resulting in a peak of more than 90 outbreaks in 1990 (Håstein *et al.*, 1999). Although the virus causing ISA was not identified until 1995 (Dannevig *et al.*, 1995), a number of biosecurity measures were introduced to combat and control the disease. The measures were based on general hygienic principles focusing on lowering infection pressure and interrupting

knut.falk@vetinst.no

Fish Vaccination, First Edition. Edited by Roar Gudding, Atle Lillehaug and Øystein Evensen.

the spread of infection. This included early detection and slaughter of diseased populations, regulations on transport, disinfection of offal and waste from slaughter-houses, year class separation at farming sites, and improved health control and certification. The effect was remarkable, and in 1994 only two new outbreaks were recorded, demonstrating that ISA can be controlled without the use of drugs and vaccines, and even without knowing the etiological agent or the epidemiology and pathogenesis of the disease. ISA still occurs at a low prevalence in Norway, while the other previously affected countries seem to have controlled the disease with only a few sporadically occurring disease outbreaks. Epidemiological disease information may be found in the World Animal Health Information Database – WAHID (available at http://www.oie.int/wahis_2/public/wahid.php/Wahidhome/Home).

Farmed Atlantic salmon is the only species in which ISA occurs naturally, and the majority of cases have occurred during the seawater stage. However, virus replication without disease development has been demonstrated experimentally in a range of other fish species, including brown trout, rainbow trout, Arctic char, chum salmon, coho salmon, herring, and Atlantic cod (Rimstad *et al.*, 2011). ISA virus has also been detected in healthy wild Atlantic salmon and sea trout (Raynard *et al.*, 2001a; Plarre *et al.*, 2005), thus these species may potentially act as carriers or a reservoir of the virus.

At farm level, ISA is a slowly developing, systemic disease. Usually, diseased fish are only found in a few netpens in a farm, and daily mortality is typically 0.05% to 0.1%. However, if nothing is done to limit disease development, spread to other cages will occur and accumulated mortality in a farm may reach more than 80% during a period of several months.

26.2 ETIOLOGY

The *Infectious salmon anemia virus* (ISAV) belongs to the genus *Isavirus* of the family *Orthomyxoviridae*, and possesses the major functional, biochemical and morphological characteristics of this virus family (Palese *et al.*, 2007; Rimstad *et al.*, 2011). This includes a single stranded, segmented, negative-sense RNA genome encoding ten proteins (Mjaaland *et al.*, 1997; Clouthier *et al.*, 2002; Falk *et al.*, 2004). The viral particles contain four major structural proteins: the nucleoprotein (NP), the matrix protein (M), the hemagglutinin-esterase (HE) protein, and the fusion (F) protein (Falk *et al.*, 1997, 2004; Krossøy *et al.*, 2001; Rimstad *et al.*, 2001, 2011; Aspehaug *et al.*, 2004, 2005). The two latter are glycoproteins embedded in the viral envelope, forming the characteristic spikes of the virion (Falk *et al.*, 1997). Both these proteins are supposed to be important for virulence and as targets for immune protection. ISAV gene segment 6 encodes the HE protein, which is responsible for both receptor binding and the release (receptor-destroying enzyme activity; RDE) of newly formed viral particles from the host cell (Falk *et al.*, 2004; Hellebø *et al.*, 2004).

The ISAV genome is highly conserved, and the two gene segments with the highest variability are those coding for the HE- and the F-proteins (i.e. segment 6 and 5, respectively). Phylogenetic analyses of ISAV isolates, based on the HE-gene, have revealed two major clades, one European and one North American (Devold *et al.*, 2001). In addition, ISAV have been characterized and typed based on amino-acid patterns of a highly polymorphic region (HPR), consisting of 11–35 amino acids, just upstream of the transmembrane domain of the HE-protein (Rimstad *et al.*, 2011). The HPR variants can be explained as various deletions (Mjaaland *et al.*,

2002) from a putative full-length ancestral sequence (HPR0), first identified in a wild salmon in Scotland (Cunningham *et al.*, 2002). Whereas all ISAV isolates from ISA disease outbreaks have deletions in the HPR region, the HPR0 subtype has not been associated with clinical or pathological signs of ISA (Cunningham *et al.*, 2002; Cook-Versloot *et al.*, 2004; Nylund *et al.*, 2006; McBeath *et al.*, 2009; Christiansen *et al.*, 2011) and is frequently detected in gills during RT-PCR surveys (Christiansen *et al.*, 2011; Lyngstad *et al.*, 2012). As opposed to HPR-deleted ISAV, which is readily isolated in susceptible cell cultures (Dannevig *et al.*, 1995; Devold *et al.*, 2001), cultivation of the HPR0 type has so far not been reported, which has hampered the characterization of this virus type.

ISA-virus isolates vary in virulence, as observed by differences in disease development, mortality and clinical signs in field outbreaks, as well as in experimental trials (Mjaaland *et al.*, 2005; Kibenge *et al.*, 2006; Ritchie *et al.*, 2009). At the molecular level, virus virulence is thought to be a polygenic trait, both generally and in relation to other orthomyxoviruses. This is exemplified by the investigation of influenza H7N7 viruses isolated from human conjunctivitis and a human fatal case during a highly pathogenic avian influenza (HPAI) H7N7 virus outbreak in the Netherlands in 2003. The two HPAI H7N7 viruses differed in 15 amino-acid positions in five gene segments (de Witt *et al.*, 2010). However, only two putative ISA-virus virulence markers have been identified so far. One is the above-mentioned HPR0 type, and the other, also found associated with HPR0 virus, is a leucine to glutamine amino-acid substitution at position 266 in the F-protein, close to the putative proteolytic activation site (Markussen *et al.*, 2008).

26.3 PATHOGENESIS

The disease ISA is a systemic and lethal condition, and clinical signs suggest circulatory failure with severe anemia, ascites, congestion, and enlargement of the liver and spleen (Evensen *et al.*, 1991). By autopsy, a variable set of hemorrhages and necrosis in several organs are usually observed. ISA-virus mainly affects the circulatory system, and the major target cells for infection are endothelial cells lining blood vessels of all organs, including sinusoids, endocardium and scavenger endothelial cells (Aamelfot *et al.*, 2012), which may at least partly explain the clinical and pathological findings.

The incubation time in natural outbreaks is difficult to determine, but has been estimated to be from a few weeks to several months (Vågsholm *et al.*, 1994; Jarp and Karlsen, 1997). ISA can be experimentally reproduced in Atlantic salmon by intraperitoneal injection, through infected cohabitants (Trojans), or through immersion challenge (Raynard *et al.*, 2001b). The incubation period in experimental infection is usually 10-20 days (Rimstad *et al.*, 2011).

Both innate and adaptive cellular and humoral immune responses against ISAV have been experimentally demonstrated in Atlantic salmon (Falk *et al.*, 1995; Jørgensen *et al.*, 2007; Ritchie *et al.*, 2009; LeBlanc *et al.*, 2010; Lauscher *et al.*, 2011). Part-protection against experimental ISAV infection was demonstrated in fish injected with serum from fish that had previously survived an ISAV infection (i.e., passive immunization), suggesting the significance of humoral factors for immunity (Falk *et al.*, 1995). Experiments with DNA vaccines expressing the HE-protein have also demonstrated the importance of this antigen for a protective immune response (Mikalsen *et al.*, 2005; Wolf *et al.*, 2013). On the other hand, field observations in four farms where ISAV HPR0 infection was detected in gills by qPCR, 1–4 months prior to clinical ISA outbreaks, did not suggest a significant protection due to infection with this ISAV biotype (Lyngstad *et al.*, 2011).

26.4 VACCINES

Reports on ISA vaccines and their effects in the scientific literature are scanty, although several non-peer-reviewed conference abstracts and internet publications support findings by Jones *et al.* (1999), who reported a RPS of 84–95% in experimental trials using an adjuvanted, inactivated ISA-virus cell culture preparation. A recent publication by Lauscher *et al.* (2011) also tested a virus cell culture preparation against experimental infections, and found a RPS of 86%. They also found protection to be dependent upon the amount of vaccine antigen injected, and also to correlate with detectable anti-ISAV antibodies.

Although commercial vaccine development has mainly concentrated on inactivated ISAV cell culture preparations, research using molecular biological principles has been reported. Mikalsen *et al.* (2005) injected plasmids coding for the HE protein three times at three-week intervals, but were only able to demonstrate a very modest protection with RPS of 40–60% in parallel groups. In this experiment, fish were challenged by IP injection, which may partly explain the results of rather poor protection. In a recent publication, Wolf *et al.* (2013) vaccinated fish by IM injection of an ISAV hemagglutinin-esterase-expressing salmonid alphavirus replicon, followed by an experimental cohabitation challenge. The observed RPS ranged from 65–69%, contrasted with 80% in controls immunized with an inactivated ISAV cell culture antigen (Wolf *et al.*, 2013).

At present, there are two commercial ISAV vaccines available, based on injection of oil-adjuvanted, inactivated ISAV cell culture antigens, produced by Novartis Animal Health and Pharmaq (Finne-Fridell *et al.*, 2011) respectively. These vaccine preparations are either delivered as monovalent vaccines, or as one of the components of multivalent vaccines, and are typically injected in smolts prior to seawater transfer (Table 26.1). In addition to this, the Chilean pharmaceutical company Centrovet is now marketing an oil-adjuvanted injection vaccine, as well as an oral vaccine, both based on ISAV HE-protein expressed in yeast. In the oral vaccine, a proprietary MicroMatrix technology for encapsulation of expressed protein from Advanced BioNutrition Corporation is used. Neither of these vaccines from Centrovet have been documented in peer-reviewed journals. However, the oral Centrovet vaccine has been described in a conference abstract, reporting encouraging effects (Tobar *et al.*, 2010).

Vaccination against ISAV was first attempted on the east coast of Canada in 1999. During the first years of vaccination in Canada, ISA outbreaks were recorded in vaccinated populations, thus the vaccine efficacy was questioned. To date, there are no reports in the scientific literature documenting the field performance of ISAV vaccines. In Canada, vaccination was combined with control programs including preventive measures related to farming and transport, continuous surveillance of health status, and control measures when disease or infection occurred. In this way, ISA was controlled with no ISA outbreaks between 2006 and 2012. In 2012, however, one ISA outbreak was reported in Nova Scotia. Further examples of the use of ISA vaccination include the successful control program following serious problems with multiple ISA outbreaks in the Faroe Islands during the years 2000–2005. Vaccination with an oil-adjuvanted inactivated, cell culture grown virus vaccine preparation was combined with a very strict control regime, based on general hygienic principles, as outlined by Håstein *et al.*

Table 26.1 Commercially available vaccines against infectious salmon anemia.

Product Name	Vaccine Type	Antigen	Adjuvant	Delivery Route	Vaccine Company
ILAvacc	Inactivated cell culture preparation, monovalent	ISAV, North American biotype	Mineral oil	IP injection	Novartis Animal Health, Canada
Pentium Forte Plus ILA Pentium V II	Inactivated cell culture preparation, multivalent	ISAV, North American biotype	Mineral oil	IP injection	Novartis Animal Health, Canada
Alpha Ject micro 1 ISA	Inactivated cell culture preparation, monovalent	ISAV, European biotype	Mineral oil	IP injection	Pharmaq, Norway
Alpha Ject micro 7 ILA Alpha Ject 5-1	Inactivated cell culture preparation, multivalent	ISAV, European biotype	Mineral oil	IP injection	Pharmaq, Norway
Subunit vaccine against infectious salmon anemia, monovalent, or multivalent with *P. salmonis*, IPNV and *Vibrio ordalii*	Recombinant protein expressed in yeast	ISAV HE	Mineral oil	IP injection	Centrovet, Chile
Subunit vaccine against infectious salmon anemia, monovalent, or divalent with *Piscirickettsia salmonis*	Recombinant protein expressed in yeast	ISAV HE expressed in yeast		Oral	Centrovet, Chile

(1999). No ISA outbreaks have been recorded on the Faroe Islands since 2005, although an extensive surveillance program has demonstrated frequent findings of the ISAV HPR0 type (Christiansen *et al.*, 2011). A similar approach, including vaccination, has also been implemented in Chile, where no ISA outbreaks have been recorded since September 2010, with the exception of one reported case in 2012, where ISAV was detected using RT-PCR. In Norway, vaccination was introduced to combat a local ISA epidemic; however, three ISA outbreaks were recorded in the region in 2010 in vaccinated populations.

26.5 REGULATORY ISSUES

Vaccination against ISA has been included in ISA-virus control programs in Canada since 1999, in the Faroe Islands since 2005, and in Chile since 2010. In the European Union (EU), including Norway, ISA was a "list 1" disease until 2006, implying a ban of the use of vaccines. In spite of this, Scotland was able to control ISA by implementing preventive measures without vaccination. From 2006, ISA was downgraded to list 2, which allowed ISA vaccines to be used as an integrated part of a specific control program in areas with undetermined ISA status (i.e. "category 3" areas). Because of this change, ISA vaccination was allowed in attempts to control a serious local ISA epidemic in northern Norway in the years 2007–2010. During the last year of the epidemic, three ISA disease outbreaks were registered in ISA-vaccinated Atlantic salmon. Thus, the field performance of ISAV vaccines is still an open question, although a beneficial effect when combined with good management and biosecurity, and other control measures, may be anticipated.

REFERENCES

Aamelfot, M., Dale, O.B., Weli, S.C., *et al.*, 2012. Expression of the infectious salmon anemia virus receptor on Atlantic salmon endothelial cells correlates with the cell tropism of the virus. *J Virol* **86**: 10571–8.

Aspehaug, V., Falk, K., Krossøy, B, *et al.*, 2004. Infectious salmon anemia virus (ISAV) genomic segment 3 encodes the viral nucleoprotein (NP), an RNA-binding protein with two monopartite nuclear localization signals (NLS). *Virus Res* **106**: 51–60.

Aspehaug, V., Mikalsen, A.B., Snow, M., *et al.*, 2005. Characterization of the infectious salmon anemia virus fusion protein. *J Virol* **79**: 12544–53.

Christiansen, D.H., Østergaard, P.S., Snow, M., *et al.*, 2011. A low-pathogenic variant of infectious salmon anemia virus (ISAV-HPR0) is highly prevalent and causes a non-clinical transient infection in farmed Atlantic salmon (*Salmo salar* L.) in the Faroe Islands. *J Gen Virol* **92**: 909–18.

Clouthier, S.C., Rector, T., Brown, N.E.C. and Anderson, E.D. 2002. Genomic organization of infectious salmon anaemia virus. *J Gen Virol* **83**: 421–8.

Cook-Versloot, M., Griffiths, S., Cusack, R., *et al.*, 2004. Identification and characterization of infectious salmon anaemia virus (ISAV) haemagglutinin gene highly polymorphic region (HPR) type 0 in North America. *Bull Eur Assoc Fish Pathol* **24**: 203–8.

Cunningham, C.O., Gregory, A., Black, J., *et al.*, 2002. A novel variant of the infectious salmon anaemia virus (ISAV) haemagglutinin gene suggests mechanisms for virus diversity. *Bull Eur Assoc Fish Pathol* **22**: 366–74.

Dannevig, B.H., Falk, K. and Namork, E. 1995. Isolation of the causal virus of infectious salmon anaemia (ISA) in a long-term cell line from Atlantic salmon head kidney. *J Gen Virol* **76**: 1353–9.

Devold, M., Falk, K., Dale, O.B., *et al.*, 2001. Strain variation, based on the hemagglutinin gene, in Norwegian ISA virus isolates collected from 1987 to 2001: indications of recombination. *Dis Aquat Org* **47**: 119–28.

de Witt, E., Munster, V.J., van Riel, D., *et al.*, 2010. Molecular determinants of adaptation of highly pathogenic avian influenza H7N7 viruses to efficient replication in the human host. *J Virol* **84**: 1597–1606.

Evensen, Ø., Thorud, K.E. and Olsen, Y.A. 1991. A morphological study of the gross and light microscopic lesions of infectious anaemia in Atlantic salmon (*Salmo salar*). *Res Vet Sci* **51**: 215–22.

Falk, K. and Dannevig, B.H. 1995. Demonstration of infectious salmon anaemia (ISA) viral antigens in cell cultures and tissue sections. *Vet Res* **26**: 499–504.

Falk, K., Namork, E., Rimstad, E., *et al.*, 1997. Characterization of infectious salmon anemia virus, an orthomyxo-like virus isolated from Atlantic salmon (*Salmo salar* L.). *J Virol* **71**: 9016–23.

Falk, K., Aspehaug, V., Vlasak, R. and Endresen, C. 2004. Identification and characterization of viral structural proteins of infectious salmon anemia virus. *J Virol* **78**: 3063–71.

Finne-Fridell, F., Aas-Eng, A., Fyrand, K., *et al.*, 2011. Infeksiøs lakseanemi – vaksineutvikling. *Nor Fiskeoppdr* **36**(5): 54–6.

Håstein, T., Hill, B.J. and Winton, J.R. 1999. Successful aquatic animal disease emergency programmes. *Rev Sci Tech* **18**: 214–27.

Hellebø, A., Vilas, U., Falk, K. and Vlasak, R. 2004. Infectious salmon anemia virus specifically binds to and hydrolyzes 4-*O*-acetylated sialic acids. *J Virol* **78**: 3055–62.

Jarp, J. and Karlsen, E. 1997. Infectious salmon anaemia (ISA) risk factors in sea-cultured Atlantic salmon *Salmo salar*. *Dis Aquat Org* **28**: 79–86.

Jones, S.R.M., MacKinnon, A.M. and Salonius, K. 1999. Vaccination of fresh-water-reared Atlantic salmon reduces mortality associated with infectious salmon anaemia virus. *Bull Eur Assoc Fish Pathol* **19**: 98–101.

Jørgensen, S.M., Hetland, D.L., Press, C.McL., *et al.*, 2007. Effect of early infectious salmon anaemia virus (ISAV) infection on expression of MHC pathway genes and type I and II interferon in Atlantic salmon (*Salmo salar* L.) tissues. *Fish Shellfish Immunol* **23**: 576–88.

Kibenge, F.S.B., Kibenge, M.J.T., Groman, D. and McGeachy, S. 2006. *In vivo* correlates of infectious salmon anemia virus pathogenesis in fish. *J Gen Virol* **87**: 2645–52.

Krossøy, B., Devold, M., Sanders, L., *et al.*, 2001. Cloning and identification of the infectious salmon anaemia virus haemagglutinin. *J Gen Virol* **82**: 1757–65.

Lauscher, A., Krossøy, B., Frost, P., *et al.*, 2011. Immune responses in Atlantic salmon (*Salmo salar*) following protective vaccination against infectious salmon anemia (ISA) and subsequent ISA virus infection. *Vaccine* **29**: 6392–401.

LeBlanc, F., Laflamme, M. and Gagné, N. 2010. Genetic markers of the immune response of Atlantic salmon (*Salmo salar*) to infectious salmon anemia virus (ISAV). *Fish Shellfish Immunol* **29**: 217–32.

Lyngstad, T.M., Hjortaas, M.J., Kristoffersen, A.B., *et al.*, 2011. Use of molecular epidemiology to trace transmission pathways for infectious salmon anaemia virus (ISAV) in Norwegian salmon farming. *Epidemics* **3**: 1–11.

Lyngstad, T.M., Kristoffersen, A.B., Hjortaas, M.J., *et al.*, 2012. Low virulent infectious salmon anaemia virus (ISAV-HPR0) is prevalent and geographically structured in Norwegian salmon farming. *Dis Aquat Org* **101**: 197–206.

Markussen, T., Jonassen, C.M., Numanovic, S., *et al.*, 2008. Evolutionary mechanisms involved in the virulence of infectious salmon anaemia virus (ISAV), a piscine orthomyxovirus. *Virology* **374**: 515–27.

McBeath, A.J.A., Bain, N. and Snow, M. 2009. Surveillance for infectious salmon anaemia virus HPR0 in marine Atlantic salmon farms across Scotland. *Dis Aquat Org* **87**: 161–9.

Mikalsen, A.B., Sindre, H., Mjaaland, S., Rimstad, E. 2005. Expression, antigenicity and studies on cell receptor binding of the hemagglutinin of infectious salmon anemia virus. *Arch Virol* **150**: 1621–37.

Mjaaland, S., Rimstad, E., Falk, K. and Dannevig, B.H. 1997. Genomic characterization of the virus causing infectious salmon anemia in Atlantic salmon (*Salmo salar* L.): an orthomyxo-like virus in a teleost. *J Virol* **71**: 7681–6.

Mjaaland, S., Hungnes, O., Teig, A., *et al.*, 2002. Polymorphism in the infectious salmon anemia virus hemagglutinin gene: importance and possible implications for evolution and ecology of infectious salmon anemia disease. *Virology* **304**: 379–91.

Mjaaland, S., Markussen, T., Sindre, H., *et al.*, 2005. Susceptibility and immune responses following experimental infection of MHC compatible Atlantic salmon (*Salmo salar* L.) with different infectious salmon anaemia virus isolates. *Arch Virol* **8**: 1621–37.

Nylund, A., Plarre, H., Karlsen, M., *et al.*, 2006. Transmission of infectious salmon anaemia virus (ISAV) in farmed populations of Atlantic salmon (*Salmo salar*). *Arch Virol* **152**: 151–79.

Palese, P. and Shaw, M.L. 2007. Orthomyxoviridae: the viruses and their replication, in *Fields Virology* (5th edn) (eds D.M. Knipe and P.M. Howley). Philadelphia, Lippincott Williams & Wilkins, 1647–89.

Plarre, H., Devold, M., Snow, M. and Nylund, A. 2005. Prevalence of infectious salmon anaemia virus (ISAV) in wild salmonids in western Norway. *Dis Aquat Org* **66**: 71–9.

Raynard, R.S., Murray, A.G. and Gregory, A. 2001a. Infectious salmon anaemia virus in wild fish from Scotland. *Dis Aquat Org* **46**: 93–100.

Raynard, R.S., Snow, M. and Bruno, D.W. 2001b. Experimental infection models and susceptibility of Atlantic salmon *Salmo salar* to a Scottish isolate of infectious salmon anaemia virus. *Dis Aquat Org* **47**: 169–74.

Rimstad, E., Mjaaland, S., Snow, M., *et al.*, 2001. Characterization of the infectious salmon anemia virus genomic segment that encodes the putative hemagglutinin. *J Virol* **75**: 5352–6.

Rimstad, E., Dale, O.B., Dannevig, B.H. and Falk, K. 2011. Infectious salmon anaemia, in *Fish Diseases and Disorders: Volume 3: Viral, Bacterial and Fungal Infections* (2nd edn) (eds P.T.K. Woo and D.W. Bruno). Oxfordshire, CAB International, 143–65.

Ritchie, R.J., McDonald, J.T., Glebe, B., *et al.*, 2009. Comparative virulence of infectious salmon anaemia virus isolates in Atlantic salmon, *Salmo salar* L. *J Fish Dis* **32**: 157–71.

Thorud, K. and Djupvik, H.O. 1988. Infectious salmon anaemia in Atlantic salmon (*Salmo salar*). *Bull Eur Assoc Fish Pathol* **8**: 109–11.

Tobar, J.A., Caruffo, M., Betz, Y., *et al.*, 2010. Oral immunity against infectious salmon anaemia in Atlantic salmon (*Salmo salar*). *XVIII International Conference on Bioencapsulation*, Porto, Portugal. Available at http://impascience.eu/bioencapsulation/340_contribution_texts/2010-10-01_P-088.pdf?PHPSESSID=9ae917c5d25114d8dd4a81ebbfddac16

Vågsholm, I., Djupvik, H.O., Willumsen, F.V., *et al.*, 1994. Infectious salmon anemia (ISA) epidemiology in Norway. *Prev Vet Med* **19**: 277–90.

Wolf, A., Hodneland, K., Frost, P., *et al.*, 2013. A hemagglutinin-esterase-expressing salmonid alphavirus replicon protects Atlantic salmon (*Salmo salar*) against infectious salmon anemia (ISA). *Vaccine* **31**: 661–9.

27 Vaccination against Koi Herpesvirus Disease

Arnon Dishon[1], Ofer Ashoulin[2], E. Scott Weber III[3] and Moshe Kotler[4]

[1]KoVax Ltd, Jerusalem, Israel
[2]Dagon, Maagan Michael Fish Farm, Israel
[3]University of California, Davis, California, USA
[4]The Hebrew University–Hadassah Medical School, Jerusalem, Israel

ABSTRACT

For over a decade, koi herpesvirus disease has posed a threat to the common carp and ornamental koi industries. The agent causing the disease was identified as a large double-stranded DNA virus named *Cyprinid herpesvirus 3*. Outbreaks of the disease are characterized by very high mortality rates reaching up to 100% of the infected fish population. The intense farming, highly infectious nature of the virus, and the extensive global trade of koi fish, resulted in rapid spread of the disease. Efforts to control the spread of the disease by imposing restrictions on importation and culling of infected populations have resulted in limited success as the disease has become endemic in both wild and domestic carp populations in several countries and has spread worldwide. A live attenuated vaccine has been used in Israel since 2005. The vaccine has played an important role in the recovery and sustainability of the koi- and carp-rearing industries in Israel. More recently the vaccine was licensed in Indonesia and the US where it can serve as a prophylactic treatment to prevent this deadly disease.

27.1 OCCURRENCE AND SIGNIFICANCE

Common carp (*Cyprinus carpio carpio*) is a fish species that is widely cultivated for human consumption, with 3.7 million tons harvested annually, principally by China, other Asian and eastern European countries (FAO, 2013). The common carp is an economically important fish and serves as a major protein source and traditional food item. In contrast to common carp, the subspecies koi (*Cyprinus carpio koi*) is an ornamental pet, the focus of a hobby whose enthusiasts keep koi in backyard ponds and large display aquaria for personal pleasure or competitive showing.

arnon.dishon@kovax.co.il

Fish Vaccination, First Edition. Edited by Roar Gudding, Atle Lillehaug and Øystein Evensen.

Since the mid 1990s the sustainability of the common carp and koi-rearing industries has been compromised by a lethal disease known as koi herpesvirus disease (KHVD). Initial reports of KHVD came in 1998 following mass mortalities of koi and common carp in Israeli coastal farms and in the mid-Atlantic region of the US (Ariav *et al.*, 1999; Hedrick *et al.*, 2000). A herpesvirus was isolated by Hedrick *et al.* (2000) associated with these epizootics, named *koi herpesvirus* (KHV). The magnitude of the disease for the Israeli aquaculture industry was devastating, spreading to 90% of the carp farms within a few years and costing an estimated US$3 million annually (Perelberg *et al.*, 2003). Subsequently similar mortalities of koi were reported in Germany (Bretzinger *et al.*, 1999) and from the UK (Walster, 1999). KHV was isolated by others in Germany (Neukirch and Kunz, 2001) and Israel (Perelberg *et al.*, 2003; Ronen *et al.*, 2003). Retrospective PCR analysis of unexplained mass mortalities of koi, collected in 1996 in the UK, identified KHV DNA in archived samples from these outbreaks (Haenen *et al.*, 2004). In Europe KHV is confirmed to be present in over 15 countries and has posed a threat not only to the koi market but to the large edible carp industry as well (Haenen *et al.*, 2004; Haenen and Olesen, 2009).

Indonesia experienced a devastating outbreak of KHVD starting in March 2002 (Sunarto *et al.*, 2005). Following importation of fish from China via Hong Kong, the first episode of mass mortality of cultured koi was recorded in East Java. From this entry point the virus rapidly spread through movement of sick fish to West Java, and, early in 2003, outbreaks had occurred as far as South Sumatra. The socio-economic impact of KHVD in Indonesia was and still is substantial. The Directorate of Fish Health and Environment (DFHE) estimated that as of December 2002 and 2003, losses due to KHV were US$10 million and $15 million, respectively (Bondad-Reantaso *et al.*, 2007).

In Japan, the first outbreak of KHVD was reported in 2003, followed by a nationwide mass mortality in 2004 and 2005 (Sano *et al.*, 2004), threatening the US$75 million Japanese ornamental koi industry (Haenen *et al.*, 2004). Japanese authorities introduced new legislation in efforts to control the spread of the disease. Despite these efforts, nationwide surveys indicate that the virus is endemic in natural waters throughout Japan (Minamoto *et al.*, 2009, 2012; Uchii *et al.*, 2009).

In April 2002, an outbreak of disease in imported koi occurred in a farm in Guangdong Province, China, with high levels of mortality; PCR analysis confirmed the presence of KHV (Lih *et al.*, 2002). Since then disease occurrence and isolation of KHV in China has been reported (Dong *et al.*, 2011, 2013). Other Asian countries reporting high mortality events associated with KHVD include Thailand (Pikulkaew *et al.*, 2009), the Philippines (Somga *et al.*, 2010), Singapore (Lio-Po, 2011), South Korea (Oh *et al.*, 2001), Malaysia (Haenen *et al.*, 2004; Rathore *et al.*, 2012), and Taiwan (Tu *et al.*, 2004). With the exceptions of South America, northern Africa and Australia, KHV has been identified on all continents and has caused severe economic losses.

27.2 ETIOLOGY

Koi herpesvirus was initially named as such due to its morphological similarity to viruses of the order *Herpesvirales* (Hedrick *et al.*, 2000). The virus is enveloped and has a typical icosahedral capsid which contains the double-stranded DNA genome, surrounded by a proteinaceous tegumet (Hedrick *et al.*, 2000; Hutoran *et al.*, 2005). The virus was also referred to as carp interstitial nephritis and gill necrosis virus (CNGV) due to the pathology manifested by the disease (Pikarsky *et al.*, 2004; Ronen *et al.*, 2005). Genomic sequencing of the virus revealed a very large genome of 295 kbp with little sequence homology to known mammalian, avian and reptilian herpes viruses (Hutoran *et al.*, 2005; Waltzek *et al.*, 2005; Aoki *et al.*, 2007). Following the recent revision of herpesvirus taxonomy by the International Committee on the Taxonomy of Viruses (ICTV) and on the basis of homology to other cyprinid herpesviruses the virus was assigned to the family *Alloherpesviridae*, genus *Cyprinivirus*, species *Cyprinid herpesvirus 3* (CyHV-3) (King *et al.*, 2012).

The 295 kbp genome of CyHV-3 is the largest genome recorded to date within the order *Herpesvirales*, and consists of a large central portion flanked by two 22 kbp repeats designated as left and right repeats. Comparison of the full sequences of three isolates (from Japan, the US and Israel) revealed more than 99% identity (Aoki *et al.*, 2007). The virus isolates from Israel and the US (U/I) are more closely related than the Japanese isolate (J). DNA comparison of virus extracted from sick common carp and koi, both cultured and wild, collected from mostly Asian and European origin (a single sample from the US and Israel), revealed ten variable areas in three regions within the CyHV-3 genome. Based on the polymorphism observed in three loci analyzed, two genotypes were identified as an Asian genotype and a European genotype, containing 7 and 2 variants, respectively (Kurita *et al.*, 2009). Genomic comparison based on the difference between the variable numbers of tandem repeats (VNTR) identified Indonesian isolates as distant from the Japanese isolate (Avarre *et al.*, 2011). Moreover, it has been shown that the Indonesian isolates may be an intermediate between the European and Asian genotypes (Sunarto *et al.*, 2011).

The genome encodes 156 potential protein open-reading frames (Aoki *et al.*, 2007). A total of 40 structural proteins were characterized including 3 capsid, 13 envelope, 2 tegument and 22 unclassified proteins (Rosenkranz *et al.*, 2008; Michel *et al.*, 2010b). All 156 ORFs have been shown to be transcribed *in vitro* and were classified, as other herpesviruses, into immediate early (IE or α), early (E or β) and late (L or γ) classes (Ilouze *et al.*, 2012a). Replication and transcription of the CyHV-3 genome has been shown to be regulated by temperature and has given insight to the potential mechanisms of viral latency evolution in poikilotherms (Dishon *et al.*, 2007; Ilouze *et al.*, 2012b).

27.3 PATHOGENESIS

The disease caused by CyHV-3 is seasonal, appearing in spring and autumn when the water temperature in open-air ponds is 18–28 °C. It is highly contagious, spreads horizontally from infected to healthy fish sharing the same pond, and is lethal in 80–100% of the fish in infected open-air ponds. Mortality occurs within 6 to 22 days post-infection, peaking at 8 to 12 d.p.i. and afflicting fish of all ages and sizes. Although the disease is highly contagious and extremely virulent, morbidity and mortality are restricted to koi and common carp (*Cyprinus carpio*) populations (Bretzinger *et al.*, 1999; Walster, 1999; Perelberg *et al.*, 2003). The virus does not induce the disease in fish other than *Cyprinus carpio*, yet recent findings suggest that cyprinids such as goldfish (*Carrassius auratus*) may serve as carriers of CyHV-3 (Soliman and El-Matbouli, 2005; Davidovich *et al.*, 2007; Sadler *et al.*, 2008). Sick fish become anorexic, lethargic and gather close to the water surface or near waterfalls/water outlets, as they are unable to get adequate oxygenation. Gill necrosis appears as early as 3 d.p.i., coupled with an increase in the levels of external parasites and bacteria (Ariav *et al.*, 1999). The skin shows a lack of luster, with pale, slightly raised patches of epidermis, and increased mucus secretions (Hedrick *et al.*, 2000; Perelberg *et al.*, 2003, 2005; Haenen *et al.*, 2004).

The skin is the major portal of entry for CyHV-3 into the fish body (Costes *et al.*, 2009b). Once replicating in the epidermis, the virus disseminates rapidly and causes a systemic infection. At 24 hours post-infection the virus is detected in high numbers by qPCR from almost all internal organs, including liver, gastrointestinal tract, kidney, brain and spleen (Gilad *et al.*, 2004).

Outbreaks of the disease occur when water temperatures are within the "permissive range" of 18–28 °C. Exposure of naïve carp to sick fish, or to a virus harvested from infected cultured cells within the permissive range, resulted in a high mortality of 75–95% (Hedrick *et al.*, 2000; Gilad *et al.*, 2002, 2003; Perelberg *et al.*, 2003, 2005; Hutoran *et al.*, 2005). However, infected fish kept at a temperature of 29 °C or 15 °C survived during the entire duration of the experiment without manifesting any clinical signs of the disease (Gilad *et al.*, 2003; Ronen *et al.*, 2003). These experiments indicate that the progression of the disease, similar to other fish viruses, is temperature-dependent (Gilad *et al.*, 2003; Ronen *et al.*, 2003).

In vitro studies show that infectious virus is preserved in cultured cells maintained for 30 days at 30 °C. CyHV-3-infected vacuolated cells with deformed morphology converted to normal, and plaques disappeared following an upwards shift in temperature and reappeared after transfer to the permissive temperature. These results imply that CyHV-3 could persist for long periods in fish, enabling re-infection and development of clinical signs upon a shift to a permissive temperature (Dishon *et al.*, 2007).

Temperature reactivation and its association with persistence and latency of CyHV-3 have been also demonstrated *in vivo*. Following infection, surviving fish were positive for CyHV-3 DNA by qPCR at 65 days post-infection (Gilad *et al.*, 2004). After undergoing temperature stress, some researchers were able to induce disease from clinically healthy fish previously exposed to CyHV-3 (St-Hilaire *et al.*, 2005; Eide *et al.*, 2011), while others performing similar manipulations could not reactivate disease (Gilad *et al.*, 2003).

27.4 VACCINE AND VACCINATION

An inactivated CyHV-3 vaccine candidate has been described by Yasumoto *et al.* (2006). Formalin-inactivated virus was trapped within a liposome compartment and fed to fish over a three-day period. Efficacy was determined by challenge 21 days later, showing ~70% protection through feed (Yasumoto *et al.*, 2006). A TK-deficient recombinant virus was generated through bacterial artificial cloning (BAC) of the CyHV-3 virus. The recombinant virus was only partially attenuated as a substantial residual lethality was apparent, although surviving fish were protected against a challenge infection (Costes *et al.*, 2009a). No further studies on field testing or commercialization of the above vaccines were reported.

Live attenuated vaccines potentially have many advantages in aquaculture and appear to be the most appropriate for mass vaccination of carp (Benmansour and de Kinkelin, 1997; Shoemaker and Klesius, 2014). In general, live vaccine stimulates all phases of the immune system, resulting in balanced systemic and local responses involving both humoral and cellular branches of the immune system. The advantages of using live attenuated virus vaccine are especially evident in fish, where heat-inactivated virus is poorly immunogenic and large amounts of proteins are required for achieving appropriate efficacy and duration of the immune response (Marsden *et al.*, 1996, 1998). Moreover, the chance that a reverted mutated DNA virus will appear and threaten immunized populations is small.

Experiments to achieve a non-pathogenic attenuated form of CyHV-3 have been carried out in Israel since 2003 (Ronen *et al.*, 2003, 2005; Perelberg *et al.*, 2005). The attenuated virus was isolated following serial transfer of the Israeli CyHV-3 isolate in koi fin cells. Viruses harvested after 20 passages in culture induced the disease in a small percentage of naïve fingerlings following injection or bathing (Figure 27.1) (Ronen *et al.*, 2003, 2005; Perelberg *et al.*, 2005). The lack of an immune system *in vitro* generates genetic alterations that accumulated in the virus genome through passage in cell culture. The accumulated mutations create a virus population that is better adapted for growth in cultured cells, yet as it has not gone through the selection of the fish immune system, it is less competent *in vivo*. Following passage, physically cloned viruses were UV-irradiated and then re-cloned in order to insert additional mutations into the viral genome (Figure 27.2) (Freese, 1963; Drake, 1969, 1976; Ronen *et al.*, 2003). Sequence

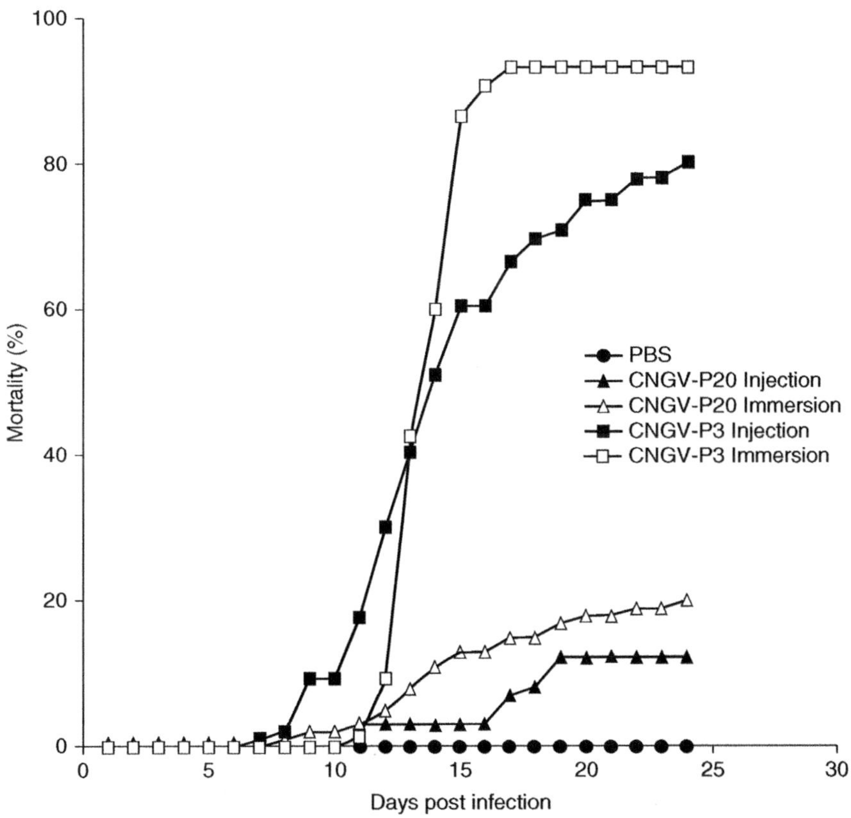

Fig. 27.1 Mortality rate among fish exposed to CNGV-P20 or CNGV-P3. Fish (n = 100 fish in each group, average weight = 50 g) were exposed to the viruses either by intraperitoneal injection or by immersion. Fish injected with PBS were used as negative controls. (Source: Ronen *et al.* 2003. Reproduced with permission from Elsevier.)

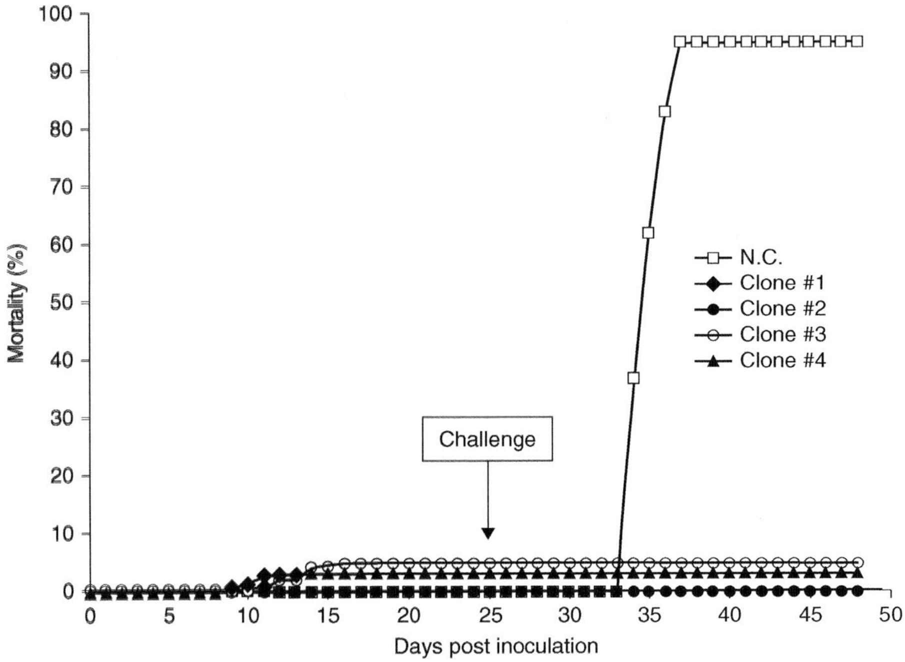

Fig. 27.2 Mortality rate in vaccinated fish following a challenge infection. Fish (n = 100 fish in each group, average weight = 50 g) were vaccinated by intraperitoneal injection of four cloned viruses derived from CNGV-P26. Fish injected with PBS were used as negative control (NC). Twenty-five days post-infection, fish were re-challenged by cohabitation with sick fish. (Source: Ronen *et al.* 2003. Reproduced with permission from Elsevier.)

analysis of over 60% of the attenuated clone has revealed several mutations within the vaccine genome, including four deletions and insertion within putative open-reading frames (Ilouze *et al.*, 2008). Based on the identified deletions, a PCR-based assay was generated to differentiate the vaccine strain virus from the wild-type CyHV-3 (unpublished).

The selected attenuated virus clone does not induce the lethal disease and efficiently protects the immunized fish against challenge infection for quite long periods (Ronen *et al.*, 2003; Perelberg *et al.*, 2005). Carp are very sensitive to pathogenic and attenuated viruses, and a short immersion of fish in water containing the virus is sufficient for infection. Vaccination with the attenuated viruses is temperature-dependent; fish held at the non-permissive temperature immediately following vaccination were not protected against the disease. The attenuated virus must propagate in the host fish in order to induce resistance against viral infections. Like the pathogenic virus, which induces the disease only at the permissive temperature, the attenuated virus requires the appropriate temperature to confer protection. Efficient protection is achieved by immersing fish in water containing the attenuated virus for 40–60 min, followed by maintaining the fish within the permissive temperature range (18–28 °C) for an additional 5 days (Perelberg *et al.*, 2005).

In Israel, field vaccination is performed by immersion (Lillehaug, 2014) of tens of thousands of juvenile fish at a minimal age of 3 months for optimal performance (Ashoulin, 2008). Fish are collected from ponds, weighed and introduced to large vaccination tanks. In the tanks,

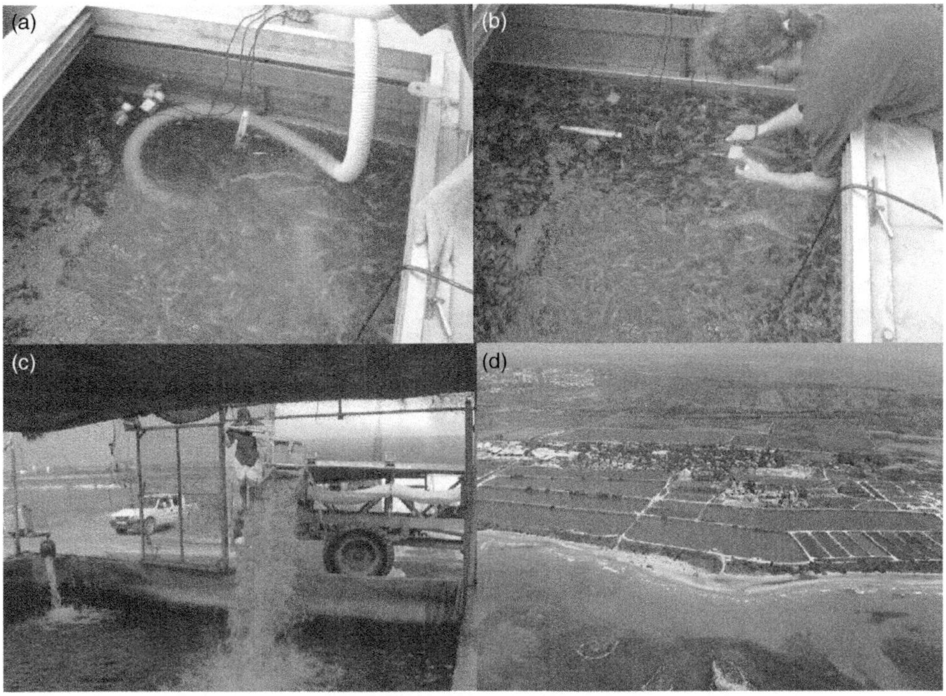

Fig. 27.3 Vaccination of koi at the Maagan Michael Fish Farm on the Mediteranean coast. (a) Fish are acclimated in a vaccination tank, temperature is monitored and water is supplemented with oxygen. (b) Vaccine bottles are thawed and poured into the vaccination tank. (c) Following exposure for 45–60 min, fish are transferred to a "virus-free" environment for at least 5 days. (d) Fish are returned to earthen ponds. (Source: Photos courtesy of Dagon Fish Farm. Reproduced with permission of Madan-Ma'agan Michael.)

fish are held at a density 20–30% w/v and are supplemented with oxygen. Vaccine is poured into the tanks as per the biomass of fish and allowed to incubate for 40–60 min. Fish are then transferred to ponds where the water temperature is within the permissive range, for at least 5 days, and then they are placed back in the earthen ponds (Figure 27.3).

27.5 EFFICACY

When the temperature regimen and proper vaccination protocol is observed, the attenuated vaccine is efficacious and generates a durable protection both in controlled studies and in the field, with RPS values >80% (Perelberg *et al.*, 2005, 2008; Ronen *et al.*, 2005; Zak *et al.*, 2007; Ashoulin, 2008; Weber *et al.*, 2011). Protection against disease caused by CyHV-3 is associated with elevation of specific antibodies against the wild-type virus. On primary exposure to the vaccine, CyHV-3-specific antibody titer rises after 7 d.p.i. and peaks at 20–40 d.p.i. (Figure 27.4). In the absence of re-exposure, the level of anti-CyHV-3 antibodies gradually decreases in vaccinated fish over a period of 6–9 months to a level slightly higher than that of naïve fish. Although at primary infection a correlation between the survival rate and increased titers of anti-CyHV-3 antibodies in the infected fish is observed, in long-term

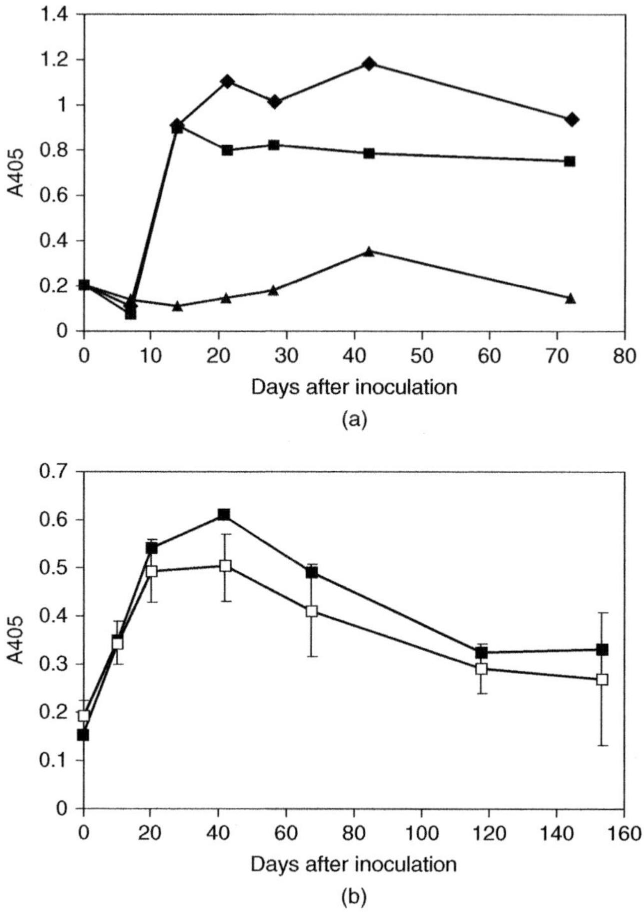

Fig. 27.4 Anti-virus antibodies in CyHV-3 inoculated fish. (a) Anti-virus ELISA performed with 1/150-diluted pooled sera of wt (♦) and attenuated virus (■) inoculated fish. PBS-injected fish served as the negative control (▲). At each time point the pooled sera were made from 5–7 fish. (b) Kinetics of anti-virus antibodies in fish inoculated with attenuated virus. (■) ELISA of pooled sera derived from 5–7 fish. (□) Calculated average of ELISA values of anti-virus antibody of separate fish. The $OD4_{05}$ value of the sera of virus non-inoculated fish at each time point was subtracted from the corresponding values of the virus-inoculated fish. The results, presented with their standard deviation, refer to 1/150-diluted serum samples. (Source: Perelberg *et al.* 2008. Reproduced with permission from Elsevier.)

protection studies immunized fish are significantly protected against a challenge infection in the absence of detectable antibodies. This is probably due to the fact that protection was accomplished by virus-induced activation of memory cells, which engender a rapid humoral and cellular protective response (Figure 27.5) (Perelberg *et al.*, 2008). Although significant, protection at 13 months post-vaccination to a challenge with wild-type virus is not as efficacious as at 9 months post-vaccination, and therefore an annual booster should be considered (Perelberg *et al.*, 2008).

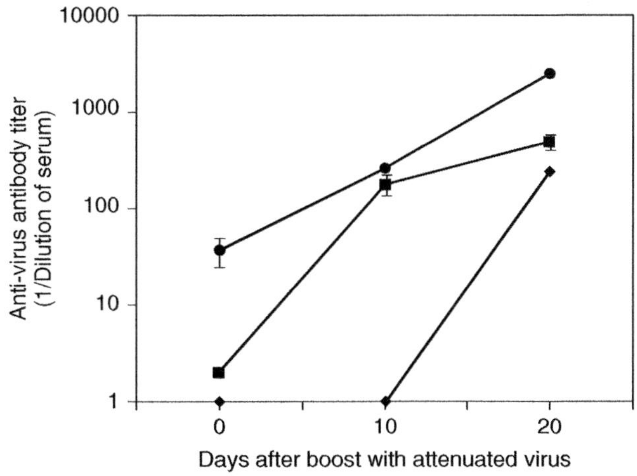

Fig. 27.5 Induction of anti-virus antibodies in attenuated virus-boosted fish. Fish with a variable history of exposure to CyHV-3 were boosted with attenuated virus and anti-virus antibodies in serially diluted serum samples were measured by ELISA. Antibody activity is presented as the reciprocal dilution corresponding to an optical absorption of 0.8 at 405 nm. (●) Four-year-old fish with 3–5 exposures to wt CyHV-3 before the final boost. (■) Fish that were inoculated with attenuated virus 6 months before the final boost. (◆) Naïve fish never before confronted with the virus. The sera of three fish were pooled for each time point. (Source: Perelberg *et al.* 2008. Reproduced with permission from Elsevier.)

27.6 SAFETY

A favorable safety profile of the vaccine has been established in field studies conducted for regulatory purposes in Israel, Indonesia, and the US. Proper fish management with good hygiene and limited stress are key factors in the prophylaxis of infectious diseases (Sommerset *et al.*, 2005). Adverse events observed in vaccinated fish have been associated with the health status of the fish prior to their vaccination (Perelberg *et al.*, 2008). Poor water quality, overcrowding of fish, and low dissolved oxygen levels coupled with the stress of vaccination may lead to undesired side-effects, which if untreated may prove lethal to a portion of the vaccinated fish population. Stressed fish are prone to infections from common endemic parasites (i.e. *Ichthyobodo sp*, *Gyrodactylus sp.*) and opportunistic bacteria (i.e. *Aeromonas sp.*). The vaccination process and immune stress imposed on the fish can in some cases lead to an elevated presence of such pathogens. In US-reared koi, a better tolerance to the vaccine was observed in larger koi (>80 g) than small fingerlings (Weber *et al.*, 2011).

Tolerance to the attenuated vaccine may vary in some carp strains. Testing on Hungarian carp (Szarvas-22 and Dinnyes) imported to Israel showed a higher level of post-vaccination mortality when compared with local strains or Hungarian crossbred strains (Zak *et al.*, 2007). The authors attributed the mortality observed to the poor acclimation of the Hungarian species to a new climate and water quality conditions, as other physical problems unassociated with the vaccine were apparent in this population of fish.

One of the primary safety concerns regarding the use of live attenuated vaccines is their reversion through mutation to a pathogenic phenotype (Michel *et al.*, 2010a; Rathore *et al.*, 2012). The attenuated virus used as the vaccine was cloned twice in cultured cells in order to avoid undesired recombination and complementation. Furthermore, in a "Backpassage assay" (VICH-GL41, 2007; VS-MEMO800.201, 2008), a process in which the vaccine strain is administered to susceptible host animals, and after an appropriate incubation time recovered from these animals and directly administered to a second group of susceptible host animals, the vaccine virus did not revert to the virulent phenotype following five passages *in vivo* (Dishon, 2009).

Ecological safety concerns are also raised when dealing with live vaccines. The potential of a live agent causing disease in unrelated, more susceptible species than the vaccinated target has hindered the use of such vaccines. Yet unlike aquatic RNA viruses that are pathogenic to a wide variety of fish species, there is wide consensus that the only species affected by koi herpesvirus disease are common carp and koi (Ilouze *et al.*, 2006; Michel *et al.*, 2010a). Pathogenic wild-type virus is shed in the environment through feces (Dishon *et al.*, 2005) and mucus secretion of viral particles into water (Perelberg *et al.*, 2003). Following vaccination the attenuated vaccine strain has a minimal shedding time and is undetectable in fish excrements at 2–3 weeks post-vaccination both by PCR and ELISA (Dishon *et al.*, 2005; Dishon, 2009). QPCR analysis of vaccinated fish organ extracts reveals no presence of vaccine virus at 28 days post-vaccination in 60% of the fish tested, and a very low detectable viral load in the remaining vaccinated population (Weber *et al.*, 2011). Moreover, post-challenge CyHV-3 copy numbers suggest that wild-type virus is unable to consistently establish infection in vaccinates, as 21 days post-challenge vaccinates were negative for CyHV-3 by qPCR (O'Connor *et al.*, unpublished).

27.7 REGULATORY ISSUES

Currently the live attenuated strain of CyHV- 3 (produced by Kovax Ltd.) is the only licensed vaccine available. The vaccine has been licensed in Israel since 2005 and has been widely used in both ornamental and edible carp. Following field studies performed in Indonesia, the vaccine has been licensed for use in carp fingerlings since 2010. In early 2012 the US Department of Agriculture issued a full license for sales and distribution of the vaccine in the US.

REFERENCES

Aoki, T., Hirono, I., Kurokawa, K., *et al.*, 2007. Genome sequences of three koi herpesvirus isolates representing the expanding distribution of an emerging disease threatening koi and common carp worldwide. *J Virol* **81**: 5058–65.

Ariav, R., Tinman, S., Paperna, I. and Bejerano, I. 1999. First report of newly emerging viral disease of *Cyprinus carpio* species in Israel, in *Proceedings of the 9th International Conference of the EAFP*, Rhodes, Greece.

Ashoulin, O. 2008. *KV3 In Practice – A Clinician Perspective*. International Workshop on CyHV-3 (KHV) Cyprinid Herpes Viruses – basic and applied aspects, Caesaria, Israel.

Avarre, J.C., Madeira, J.P., Santika, A., *et al.*, 2011. Investigation of Cyprinid herpesvirus-3 genetic diversity by a multi-locus variable number of tandem repeats analysis. *J Virol Methods* **173**: 320–27.

Benmansour, A. and de Kinkelin, P. 1997. Live fish vaccines: history and perspectives. *Dev Biol Stand* **90**: 279–89.

Bondad-Reantaso, M.G., Sunarto, A. and Subasinghe, R.P. 2007. Managing the koi herpesvirus disease outbreak in Indonesia and the lessons learned. *Dev Biol (Basel)* **129**: 21–8.

Bretzinger, A., Fischer-Scherl, T., Oumouma, M., *et al.*, 1999. Mass mortalities in koi, *Cyprinus carpio*, associated with gill and skin disease. *Bull Eur Assoc Fish Pathol* **19**: 182–5.

Costes, B., Lieffrig, F. and Vanderplasschen, A. 2009a. A recombinant koi herpesvirus (KHV) or Cyprinid herpesvirus 3 (CyHV-3) and a vaccine for the prevention of a disease caused by KHV/CyHV-3 in *Cyprinus carpio carpio* or *Cyprinus carpio koi*. European Patent 2195021 A1.

Costes, B., Raj, V.S., Michel, B., *et al.*, 2009b. The major portal of entry of koi herpesvirus in *Cyprinus carpio* is the skin. *J Virol* **83**: 2819–30.

Davidovich, M., Dishon, A., Ilouze, M. and Kotler, M. 2007. Susceptibility of cyprinid cultured cells to cyprinid herpesvirus 3. *Arch Virol* **152**: 1541–6.

Dishon, A. 2009. *Back passage/shed assay for Cyprinid Herpes Virus Type 3 modified live virus according to VS Memorandum No. 800.201*. Kovax Ltd.

Dishon, A., Perelberg, A., Bishara-Shieban, J., *et al.*, 2005. Detection of carp interstitial nephritis and gill necrosis virus in fish droppings. *Appl Environment Microbiol* **71**: 7285–91.

Dishon, A., Davidovich, M., Ilouze, M. and Kotler, M. 2007. Persistence of cyprinid herpesvirus 3 in infected cultured carp cells. *J Virol* **81**: 4828–36.

Dong, C., Li, X., Weng, S., *et al.*, 2013. Emergence of fatal European genotype CyHV-3/KHV in mainland China. *Vet Microbiol* **162**: 239–44.

Dong, C., Weng, S., Li, X., *et al.*, 2011. Characterization of a new cell line from caudal fin of koi, *Cyprinus carpio koi*, and first isolation of cyprinid herpesvirus 3 in China. *Virus Res* **161**: 140–49

Drake, J.W. 1969. Mutagenic mechanisms. *Annu Rev Genetics* **3**: 247–68.

Drake, J.W. 1976. The biochemistry of mutagenesis. *Annu Rev Biochem* **45**: 11–37.

Eide, K.E., Miller-Morgan, T., Heidel, J.R., *et al.*, 2011. Investigation of koi herpesvirus (KHV) latency in koi. *J Virol* **85**: 4954–62.

FAO. 2013. FAO – Fisheries and Aquaculture Information and Statistics Service 10/04/2013.

Freese, E. 1963. Molecular mechanisms of mutations, in *Molecular Genetics* (ed. J.H. Taylor). New York, Academic Press, p.207.

Gilad, O., Yun, S., Andree, K.B., *et al.*, 2002. Initial characteristics of koi herpesvirus and development of a polymerase chain reaction assay to detect the virus in koi, *Cyprinus carpio koi*. *Dis Aquat Org* **48**: 101–8.

Gilad, O., Yun, S., Adkison, M.A., *et al.*, 2003. Molecular comparison of isolates of an emerging fish pathogen, koi herpesvirus, and the effect of water temperature on mortality of experimentally infected koi. *J Gen Virol* **84**: 2661–8.

Gilad, O., Yun, S., Zagmutt-Vergara, F.J., *et al.*, 2004. Concentrations of a Koi herpesvirus (KHV) in tissues of experimentally infected *Cyprinus carpio koi* as assessed by real-time TaqMan PCR. *Dis Aquat Org* **60**: 179–87.

Haenen, O. and Olesen, N.J. 2009. Koi herpes virus world wide: results on global koi herpesvirus questionnaire, in *14th EAFP International Conference on Diseases of Fish and Shellfish*, Prague, Czech Republic (poster).

Haenen, O.L.M., Way, K., Bergmann, S.M. and Ariel, E. 2004. The emergence of koi herpesvirus and its significance to European aquaculture. *Bull Eur Ass Fish Pathol* **24**: 293–307.

Hedrick, R.P., Gilad, O., Yun, S., *et al.*, 2000. A herpesvirus associated with mass mortality of juvenile and adult koi, a strain of common carp. *J Aquat Animal Health* **12**: 44–55.

Hutoran, M., Ronen, A., Perelberg, A., *et al.*, 2005. Description of an as yet unclassified DNA virus from diseased *Cyprinus carpio* species. *J Virol* **79**: 1983–91.

Ilouze, M., Dishon, A. and Kotler, M. 2006. Characterization of a novel virus causing a lethal disease in carp and koi. *Microbiol Mol Biol Rev* **70**: 147–56.

Ilouze, M., Dishon, A., Davidovich, M., *et al.*, 2008. Characterization of attenuated CyHV-3 genes essential for virus multiplication and for inducing a mortal disease in carp, in *International Workshop on CyHV-3 (KHV) Cyprinid Herpes Viruses – Basic and Applied Aspects*. Caesarea, Israel.

Ilouze, M., Dishon, A. and Kotler, M. 2012a. Coordinated and sequential transcription of the cyprinid herpesvirus-3 annotated genes. *Virus Res* **169**: 98–106.

Ilouze, M., Dishon, A. and Kotler, M. 2012b. Down-regulation of the cyprinid herpesvirus-3 annotated genes in cultured cells maintained at restrictive high temperature. *Virus Res* **169**: 289–95.

King, A.M.Q., Lefkowitz, E., Adams, M.J. and Carstens, E.B. (eds) 2012. *Virus Taxonomy. Ninth Report of the International Committee on Taxonomy of Viruses*. San Diego, Elsevier Academic Press.

Kurita, J., Yuasa, K., Ito, T., *et al.*, 2009. Molecular epidemiology of Koi herpesvirus. *Fish Pathol* **44**: 59–66.

Lih, H., Shi, X., Gao, L. and Jiang, Y. 2002. Study on the aetiology of koi epizootic disease using method of nested-polymerase chain reaction assay (nested-PCR). *J Huazhong Agricult Univ* **21**: 414–18.

Lillehaug, A. 2014. Vaccination strategies and procedures, in *Fish Vaccination* (eds R. Gudding, A. Lillehaug and Ø. Evensen). Oxford, John Wiley & Sons, Ltd., 140–152.

Lio-Po, G.D. 2011. Recent developments in the study and surveillance of koi herpesvirus (KHV) in Asia, in *Diseases in Asian Aquaculture VII. Taipei 2008*. (eds M.G. Bondad-Reantaso, J.B. Jones, F. Corsin and T. Aoki). Selangor, Malaysia, 13–28.

Marsden, M.J., Vaughan, L.M., Foster, T.J. and Secombes, C.J. 1996. A live (delta aroA) *Aeromonas salmonicida* vaccine for furunculosis preferentially stimulates T-cell responses relative to B-cell responses in rainbow trout (*Oncorhynchus mykiss*). *Infect Immun* **64**: 3863–9.

Marsden, M.J., Vaughan, L.M., Fitzpatrick, R.M., *et al*., 1998. Potency testing of a live, genetically attenuated vaccine for salmonids. *Vaccine* **16**: 1087–94.

Michel, B., Fournier, G., Lieffrig, F., *et al*., 2010a. Cyprinid herpesvirus 3. *Emerging Infect Dis* **16**: 1835–43.

Michel, B., Leroy, B., Stalin Raj, V., *et al*., 2010b. The genome of cyprinid herpesvirus 3 encodes 40 proteins incorporated in mature virions. *J Gen Virol* **91**: 452–62.

Minamoto, T., Honjo, M.N., Uchii, K., *et al*., 2009. Detection of cyprinid herpesvirus 3 DNA in river water during and after an outbreak. *Vet Microbiol* **135**: 261–6.

Minamoto, T., Honjo, M.N., Yamanaka, H., *et al*., 2012. Nationwide Cyprinid herpesvirus 3 contamination in natural rivers of Japan. *Res Vet Sci* **93**: 508–14.

Neukirch, M. and Kunz, U. 2001. Isolation and preliminary characterization of several viruses from koi (*Cyprinus carpio*) suffering gill necrosis and mortality. *Dis Aquat Org* **21**: 125–35.

Oh, M.J., Jung, S.J., Choi, T.J., *et al*., 2001. A viral disease occurring in cultured carp *Cyprinus carpio* in Korea. *Fish Pathol* **36**: 147–51.

Perelberg, A., Smirnov, M., Hutoran, M., *et al*., 2003. Epidemiological description of a new viral disease afflicting cultured *Cyprinus carpio* in Israel. *Isr J Aquac – Bamidgeh* **55**: 5–12.

Perelberg, A., Ronen, A., Hutoran, M., *et al*., 2005. Protection of cultured *Cyprinus carpio* against a lethal viral disease by an attenuated virus vaccine. *Vaccine* **23**: 3396–3403.

Perelberg, A., Ilouze, M., Kotler, M. and Steinitz, M. 2008. Antibody response and resistance of *Cyprinus carpio* immunized with cyprinid herpes virus 3 (CyHV-3). *Vaccine* **26**: 3750–56.

Pikarsky, E., Ronen, A., Abramowitz, J., *et al*., 2004. Pathogenesis of acute viral disease induced in fish by carp interstitial nephritis and gill necrosis virus. *J Virol* **78**: 9544–51.

Pikulkaew, S., Meeyam, T. and Banlunara, W. 2009. The outbreak of koi herpesvirus (KHV) in koi (*Cyprinus carpio koi*) from Chiang Mai Province, Thailand. *Thai J Vet Med* **39**: 53–8.

Rathore, G., Kumar, G., Raja Swaminathan, T. and Swain, P. 2012. Koi herpes virus: a review and risk assessment of Indian aquaculture. *Indian J Virol* **23**: 124–33.

Ronen, A., Perelberg, A., Abramowitz, J., *et al*., 2003. Efficient vaccine against the virus causing a lethal disease in cultured *Cyprinus carpio*. *Vaccine* **21**: 4677–84.

Ronen, A., Perelberg, A., Hutoran, M., *et al*., 2005. Prevention of a mortal disease of carps induced by the carp interstitial and gill necrosis virus (CNGV) in Israel. *Bull Fish Res Agency Suppl* **2**: 9–11.

Rosenkranz, D., Klupp, B.G., Teifke, J.P., *et al*., 2008. Identification of envelope protein pORF81 of koi herpesvirus. *J Gen Virol* **89**: 896–900.

Sadler, J., Marecaux, E. and Goodwin, A.E. 2008. Detection of koi herpes virus (CyHV-3) in goldfish, *Carassius auratus* (L.), exposed to infected koi. *J Fish Dis* **31**: 71–2.

Sano, M., Takafumi, I., Kurita, J., *et al*., 2004. First detection of Koi herpesvirus in cultured common carp *Cyprinus carpio* in Japan. *Fish Pathol* **39**: 165–76.

Shoemaker, C. and Klesius, P. 2014. Replicating vaccines, in *Fish Vaccination* (eds R. Gudding, A. Lillehaug and Ø. Evensen). Oxford, John Wiley & Sons, Ltd., 33–46

Soliman, H. and El-Matbouli, M. 2005. An inexpensive and rapid diagnostic method of Koi herpesvirus (KHV) infection by loop-mediated isothermal amplification. *Virol J* **2**: 83.

Somga, J., de la Pena, L.D. and Sombito, C.D. 2010. Koi herpesvirus associated mortalities in quarantined koi carp in the Philippines. *Bull Eur Assoc Fish Pathol* **30**: 2–7.

Sommerset, I., Krossøy, B., Biering, E. and Frost, P. 2005. Vaccines for fish in aquaculture. *Exp Rev Vaccines* **4**: 89–101.

St-Hilaire, S., Beevers, N., Way, K., *et al*., 2005. Reactivation of koi herpesvirus infections in common carp *Cyprinus carpio*. *Dis Aquat Org* **67**: 15–23.

Sunarto, A., Rukyani, A. and Itami, T. 2005. Indonesian experience on the outbreak of koi herpesvirus in koi and carp (*Cyprinus carpio*). *Bull Fish Res Agency Suppl* **2**: 15–21.

Sunarto, A., McColl, K.A., Crane, M.S., *et al*., 2011. Isolation and characterization of koi herpesvirus (KHV) from Indonesia: identification of a new genetic lineage. *J Fish Dis* **34**: 87–101.

Tu, C., Weng, M., Shiau, J. and Lin. S. 2004. Detection of Koi herpesvirus in koi *Cyprinus carpio* in Taiwan. *Fish Pathol* **39**: 109–10.

Uchii, K., Matsui, K., Iida, T. and Kawabata, Z. 2009. Distribution of the introduced cyprinid herpesvirus 3 in a wild population of common carp, *Cyprinus carpio* L. *J Fish Dis* **32**: 857–64.

VICH-GL41. 2007. Target animal safety: examination of live veterinary vaccines in target animals for absence of reversion to virulence, in *International Cooperation on Harmonisation of Technical Requirements for Registration of Veterinary Medicinal Products*, Bruxelles, Belgium.

VS-MEMO800.201. 2008. *Veterinary Services Memorandum 800.201*. Washington, DC.

Walster, C. 1999. Clinical observations of severe mortalities in koi carp, *Cyprinus carpio*, with gill disease. *Fish Vet J* **3**: 54–8.

Waltzek, T.B., Kelley, G.O., Stone, D.M., *et al.*, 2005. Koi herpesvirus represents a third cyprinid herpesvirus (CyHV-3) in the family Herpesviridae. *J Gen Virol* **86**: 1659–67.

Weber, E.S., Hedrick, R., Dishon, A. and Salonius, K. 2011. Detailed study of the kinetics of infection following vaccination with a modified live CyHV3 vaccine and challenge with wild-type CyHV3 virus in koi carp (*Cyprinis carpio koi*). *Proceedings of the Eastern Fish Health Conference*, Lake Placid, New York.

Yasumoto, S., Kuzuya, Y., Yasuda, M., *et al.*, 2006. Oral immunization of common carp with a liposome vaccine fusing koi herpesvirus antigen. *Fish Pathol* **41**: 141–5.

Zak, T., Perelberg, A., Magen, Y., *et al.*, 2007. Heterosis in the growth rate of Hungarian-Israeli common carp crossbreeds and evaluation of their sensitivity to Koi herpes virus (KHV) disease. *Isr J Aquac – Bamidgeh* **59**: 63–72.

28 Vaccination against Diseases Caused by *Salmonid alphavirus*

Emilie Mérour and Michel Brémont

National Institute for Agricultural Research (INRA), Jouy en Josas, France

ABSTRACT

The first salmonid alphaviruses, *Salmon pancreas disease virus* (SPDV) and *Sleeping disease virus* (SDV), were discovered and molecularly characterized more than 15 years ago, and since then few studies have really focused on vaccine development. However, these viruses are now becoming a real threat for farmed fish and wild fish populations. Pancreas disease has recently been listed as a notifiable disease in Norway, and there is renewed interest in developing strategies to protect fish from these pathogens. In this chapter we will present an update on what is known of the molecular biology of these viruses, the diagnostics tools that have been developed, the more recent epidemiological studies, and the existing and possible future vaccines to fight against these emerging viruses.

28.1 OCCURRENCE AND SIGNIFICANCE

The so-called pancreas disease (PD) in Atlantic salmon was first observed in 1976 in Scotland (Munro *et al.*, 1984) and has subsequently been followed by several other descriptions. The disease has been reported in Ireland, Norway, France, the US, and Spain (Kent and Elston 1987; Raynard *et al.*, 1992), with the most serious impacts reported in Ireland, Norway, and Scotland. The clinical signs associated with pancreas disease in salmon may be a sudden loss of appetite, lethargy, an increased number of fecal casts in the enclosures, and increased mortality. The affected fish may have difficulty maintaining position in the water due to muscle damage.

Sleeping disease in trout was first observed in France in 1985. Disease in rainbow trout is characterized by the abnormal behavior of the fish, which stay on their side at the bottom of the tanks, reminiscent of a "sleeping state", and thus giving the terminology of sleeping disease (Boucher and Baudin-Laurencin, 1994). The lesion responsible for this behavior was presumed to be extensive necrosis of the skeletal red muscle. This chronic stage follows

michel.bremont@jouy.inra.fr

Fish Vaccination, First Edition. Edited by Roar Gudding, Atle Lillehaug and Øystein Evensen.

characteristic sequential histological lesions of the exocrine pancreas and heart (Boucher and Baudin-Laurencin, 1996). Rainbow trout at all stages of production may be affected by this disease.

Salmonid alphavirus (SAV) is now classified into three subtypes: SAV1 is the *Salmon pancreas disease virus* causing pancreas disease in salmon in Ireland and Scotland; SAV2 is the *Sleeping disease virus* causing sleeping disease in freshwater rainbow trout; and SAV3 is the *Salmon pancreas disease virus* causing pancreas disease in salmon and marine rainbow trout in Norway. The geographic distribution of these viruses in Europe is presented in Figure 28.2. SAV is becoming more and more predominant in recent years, and now represents a real challenge for eradication in most fish farms. These viruses have been shown to efficiently transmit horizontally via direct water-borne transmission (McLoughlin, 1996). The Norwegian subtype 3 (SAV3) is present in production systems for Atlantic salmon *Salmo salar* and rainbow trout *Oncorhynchus mykiss* in western Norway. SAV3 is also present at smolt production sites in Norway. Thus it has been suggested and demonstrated a few years ago that SAV3 is transmitted through smolt transport from the main area for SAV disease in western Norway, at freshwater production sites for Atlantic salmon smolts, to as far as northern Norway (Bratland and Nylund, 2009). Moreover it has been shown that there is a lack of evidence for vertical transmission of Norwegian salmonid alphavirus (SAV3) using gametes of Atlantic salmon, *Salmo salar* L., exposed by natural and experimental routes (Kongtorp *et al.*, 2010). Whether a fish reservoir for SAV exists is not yet clear. The observation that a unique SAV subtype, SAV2, is found in freshwater rainbow trout in France may be explained by the dissemination in trout farms from a single infection at the origin (Snow, 2011). However, recently the screening of marine fish species by real-time PCR in areas remote from aquaculture has indicated the presence of SAV RNA in marine species including common dab (*Limanda limanda*) and plaice (*Pleuronectes platessa*) (Snow *et al.*, 2010). Thus it cannot be excluded that the origins of SAV in freshwater rainbow trout may have been from a marine source.

28.2 ETIOLOGY

The viral etiology of this disease has been suspected (Boucher *et al.*, 1994; Castric *et al.*, 1997) and further confirmed in our laboratory as being alphavirus-like (Villoing *et al.*, 2000). Genome sequences of the *Sleeping disease virus* (SDV) and the *Salmon pancreas disease virus* (SPDV) have now been entirely determined (Villoing *et al.*, 2000; Weston *et al.*, 2002). SAV genomes consist of a single positive-strand RNA molecule of 11 900 and 11 919 nt long, respectively, encoding, as for all alphaviruses, two polyproteins (Figure 28.1), which after processing through proteolytic cleavages produce the viral mature products, the non-structural proteins nsP1, nsP2, nsP3 and nsP4, altogether constituting the replicase complex and the major structural proteins capsid (C) and the two external glycoproteins (E2 and E1).

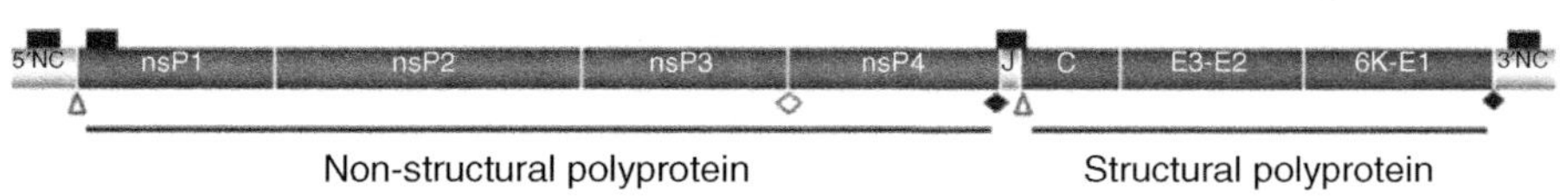

Fig. 28.1 Schematic representation of SAV RNA genome encoding the two non-structural and structural polyproteins.

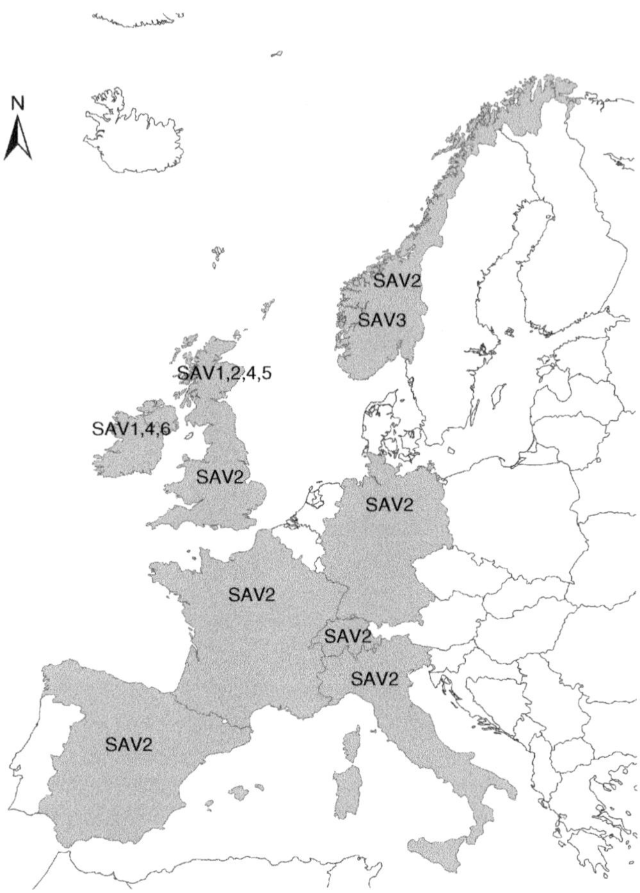

Fig. 28.2 Geographic distribution of SAVs in European countries.

The amino-acid identity between SDV and SPDV is 95% and 93.6% for non-structural and structural proteins, respectively. Moreover, both viruses have been shown to serologically cross-react (Boucher and Baudin-Laurencin, 1996). This close relationship allows the classification of SDV and SPDV (as already mentioned above) as salmonid alphavirus (SAV) (Weston *et al.*, 2002). This new classification is based upon at least three main features: (i) SDV and SPDV are closely related together, but differ from the other alphaviruses; (ii) non-structural and structural proteins are larger than those of mammalian alphaviruses; and (iii) arthropod-independent virus transmission to the host has been demonstrated in cohabitation experiments (Boucher, 1995), a phenomenon that has never been documented for mammalian alphaviruses. Some studies now suggest that there may be up to six different subtypes of the virus (Fringuelli *et al.*, 2008), but SAV2 only infects trout.

As already mentioned, SAVs are atypical compared with mammalian alphavirus, and indeed although the SAVs' genome organization is similar to that of the other alphaviruses, the 5' and

3' non-coding regions of the genome are much smaller than that of "classical" alphaviruses (approximately 20, versus 60 to 80 nucleotides for the 5' end) and the size of most of the mature proteins is larger than that of other alphaviruses. The amino-acid sequences of the SAV proteins are only distantly related to those of mammalian alphaviruses, roughly 30–35% of identity for the non-structural proteins and 40–45% for the structural proteins. In addition, a remarkable feature of SAVs is that, to date, no intermediate hosts (e.g., arthropods) have been identified, and thus it is assumed that direct transmission of the SAVs occurs. The recent description of an alphavirus from lice (*Lepidophthirus macrorhini*) isolated on elephant seals has added to speculation that sea lice could act as vectors or transmitters of alphavirus to salmonids (Linn *et al.*, 2001) and to be a potential reservoir in the field. There is as yet no clear evidence for that, and in contrast, it has been clearly established that under controlled conditions, such as in experimental fish facilities, virus can be transmitted from infected fish to naïve fish by cohabitation.

As for most viruses infecting salmonids, SAV is adapted to replicate at low temperatures ranging from 10–14 °C. Classical fish-derived cell lines like CHSE-214 (Chinook salmon embryos), BF2 (bluegill fry), RTG (rainbow-trout gonads) and even EPC (epithelial papulosum cyprinid) cells have been used to grow SAV, the virus-induced cytopathic effect being limited to refractive rounded cells 7–10 days post-infection. Titer of the produced virus may reach 10^8 pfu/ml. SDV has successfully been purified and analyzed on a Coomassie blue-stained SDS-polyacrylamide gel electrophoresis and visualized by electron-microscopy observation (Merour and Lepault, unpublished data; Figure 28.3).

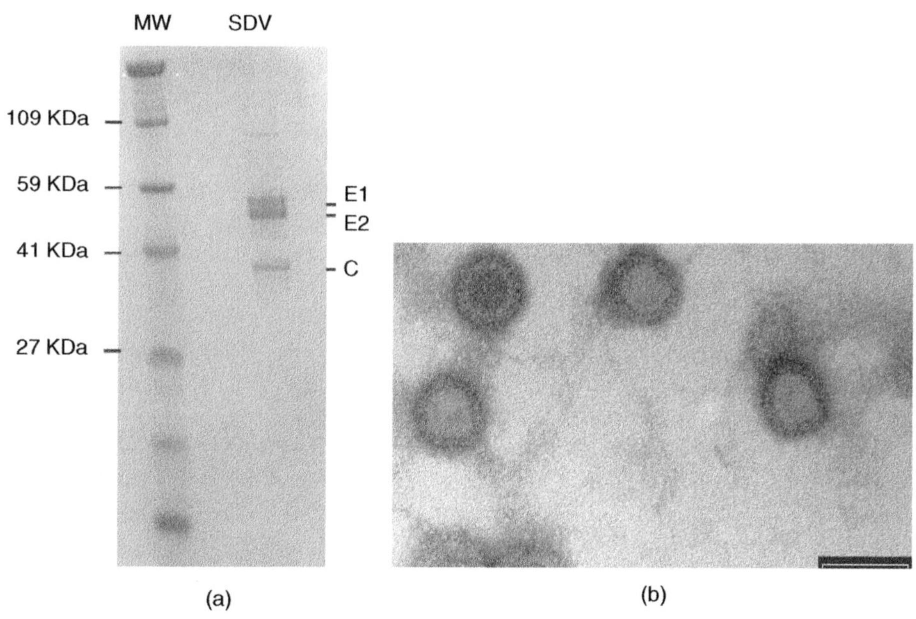

Fig. 28.3 (a) SDS-PAGE of sucrose-gradient purified SDV. MW, molecular weight marker; SDV, purified sleeping disease virus. (b) Electron-microscopy observation of purified SDV.

28.3 PATHOGENESIS

Early studies confirmed that plasma, blood leucocytes, and kidney extracts could transmit salmonid alphavirus diseases, and that the time course of the disease was temperature-dependent, with afaster progression at 14 °C than at 9 °C (McLoughlin, unpublished data). Both SAV1 and 2 cause lesions in the pancreas, heart and muscle in salmon or trout, although the severity of lesions in salmon is fish-strain dependent. The initial histological lesion noted for salmonid pancreatic disease, logically, was necrosis of the pancreas. However, subsequent studies also showed profound cardiomyopathy and skeletal myopathy (for a review, see McLoughlin and Graham, 2007). Time course studies confirmed pancreatic necrosis during the very acute phase of the disease, with destruction of the acinar tissue with little or no inflammatory responses, whereas development of lesions in cardiac muscle was somewhat slower. The skeletal muscle lesions only appeared rather late in the course of infection, some 3–4 weeks after the pancreatic and heart lesions. Involvement of muscle accounts for the abnormal behavior of affected fish.

28.4 IMMUNITY AND VACCINE DEVELOPMENT

The humoral immune response of fish is a major factor helping fish to survive SAV infection. That has been clearly demonstrated by passive transfer of serum from SAV-infected to naïve fish (Houghton and Ellis, 1996). Also, type-I interferon response has been shown to play a major role in the fish protection against SAV *in vitro* (Gahlawat *et al.*, 2009; Xu *et al.*, 2010). Fish that recover from primary salmonid alphavirus infection are resistant to infection for at least 9 months, and the disease does not recur in naturally exposed fish that survive the infection. Neutralizing antibodies can be detected in the majority of infected fish by 14–16 days after infection, and in 100% of fish by 28 days (McLoughlin *et al.*, 1996).

To date, most of the available virus vaccines for aquaculture are based on inactivated virus or recombinant subunit proteins. Currently a unique licensed vaccine is being used in the field (Bang Jensen *et al.*, 2012). NORVAX® Compact PD, developed by Intervet-Norbio (now MSD), is an inactivated virus vaccine against pancreas disease for intraperitoneal injection in Atlantic salmon (*Salmo salar*). A cross-protection against different salmonid alphavirus subtypes has been shown. The main features of this vaccine are a long-term protection, up to 80 weeks post-vaccination in field trials, and 12 months even in laboratory trials. The benefits of vaccination are the reduction in the mortality rate caused by SAV, a reduction in virus replication of SAV, and a reduction in lesions caused by SAV.

Recently, a new inactivated vaccine based on a strain of SAV subtype 3 – ALV405 – has been developed (Karlsen *et al.*, 2012). The efficacy and safety of this new vaccine have been evaluated in the laboratory and the field, demonstrating that it could be an attractive new tool for controlling SAV epizootics. Efficacy of the vaccine was tested in three fundamentally different challenge models. The ALV405-based vaccine was shown to (a) protect salmon against SAV-induced mortality and disease following intraperitoneal challenge; (b) induce protection against the development of pancreas disease in a cohabitation challenge model; and finally (c) reduce SAV-induced mortality in a field outbreak.

The immunogenicity and protective ability of subunit and DNA vaccines based on E1 and E2 spike proteins of salmonid alphavirus subtype 3 (SAV3) have also been investigated and compared with the inactivated, whole-virus vaccine in Atlantic salmon (Xu *et al.*, 2012). DNA vaccination is a promising strategy for the control of infection with intracellular pathogens including teleost fish, in which such an approach has been shown to be very efficient against fish rhabdovirus (Boudinot *et al.*, 1998). However, for SAV it was observed that the E1 and E2 SAV-derived DNA vaccine did not elicit a significant antibody response after immunization and challenge, and fish were not protected against mortality when compared with mock-immunized fish. Subunit vaccines, composed of E1 or E2 recombinant proteins, appear to be more promising as future potential vaccines. Indeed, the comparison of the efficiency of the E2 subunit vaccine and SAV-inactivated vaccine showed the induction of SAV-directed neutralizing antibodies at the time of challenge, which is the main mechanism mediating protection against infection and mortality. In contrast, in fish immunized with E1 subunit vaccine, no neutralizing antibody response was recorded.

Live attenuated vaccines could be the most promising option, since in contrast to all the other vaccines, live vaccines present the great advantage of being administered by bath immersion. This is the easiest method of administration, and also there is no need for additional adjuvant and thus no adverse effect due to the oil contained in the adjuvant formulation. For SAV, the first and only fully attenuated live vaccine has been generated from the trout sleeping disease virus (SDV, SAV2) using a reverse genetics system allowing rescue of a replicating recombinant SDV virus from infectious cDNA (a full-length cDNA copy of SDV RNA genome) (Moriette *et al.*, 2006). That recombinant rSDV was in fact shown to be totally attenuated in rainbow trout when administered by either immersion in a water bath or injection. A long-lasting (at least 7 months) and complete protection was induced in the rSDV-vaccinated trout challenged with the wild-type SDV by immersion in a water bath and also by injection. In addition, rSDV vaccinated fish were also protected from a challenge with the wild-type *Salmon pancreas disease virus* (SAV1). Recently it has been shown that the phenotype attenuated was mainly due to the change of a single amino-acid residue in the E2 glycoprotein (Mérour *et al.*, 2013). Although it has been demonstrated that recombinant live virus may be a powerful tool for the development of live attenuated vaccines, some safety constraints still exist and need to be overcome before a generalization of the use in the aquaculture field of such live attenuated vaccines. Main limitations are safety concerns for consumers and the environment (Shoemaker and Klesius, 2014). For the future, a possible alternative is to find a way to generate recombinant live attenuated virus, which can be administered by bath immersion, and which is defective in its replication cycle following fish immunization to prevent shedding and dissemination in the environment. To reach this objective, undoubtedly it will take many years of research.

REFERENCES

Bang Jensen, B., Kristoffersen, A.B., Myr, C. and Brun, E. 2012. Cohort study of effect of vaccination on pancreas disease in Norwegian salmon aquaculture. *Dis Aquat Org* **102**: 23–31.

Boucher, P. 1995. *Etiologie et pathogénie de la maladie du pancréas et de la maladie du sommeil chez les salmonidés d'élevage*. PhD thesis, University of Rennes 1.

Boucher, P. and Baudin-Laurencin, F. 1994. Sleeping disease of salmonids. *Bull Eur Assoc Fish Pathol* **14**: 179–80.

Boucher, P. and Baudin-Laurencin, F. 1996. Sleeping disease and pancreas disease comparative histopathology and acquired cross-protection. *J Fish Dis* **19**: 303–10.

Boucher, P., Castric, J. and Baudin-Laurencin F. 1994. Observation of virus-like particles in rainbow trout *Oncorhyncus mykiss* infected with sleeping disease. *Bull Eur Assoc Fish Pathol* **14**: 215–16.

Boudinot, P., Blanco, M., de Kinkelin, P. and Benmansour, A. 1998. Combined DNA immunization with the glycoprotein gene of viral hemorrhagic septicemia virus and infectious hematopoietic necrosis virus induces double-specific protective immunity and nonspecific response in rainbow trout. *Virology* **249**: 297–306.

Bratland, A. and Nylund, A. 2009. Studies on the possibility of vertical transmission of Norwegian salmonid alphavirus in production of Atlantic salmon in Norway. *J Aquat Anim Health* **21**: 173–8.

Castric, J., Baudin-Laurencin, F., Brémont, M., *et al.*, 1997. Isolation of the virus responsible for sleeping disease in experimentally infected rainbow trout (*Oncorhynchus mykiss*). *Bull Eur Assoc Fish Pathol* **17**: 27–30.

Fringuelli, E., Rowley, H.M., Wilson, J.C., *et al.*, 2008. Phylogenetic analyses and molecular epidemiology of European salmonid alphaviruses (SAV) based on partial E2 and nsP3 gene nucleotide sequences. *J Fish Dis* **31**: 811–23.

Gahlawat, S.K., Ellis, A.E. and Collet, B. 2009. Expression of interferon and interferon–induced genes in Atlantic salmon *Salmo salar* cell lines SHK-1 and TO following infection with salmon alphavirus SAV. *Fish Shellfish Immunol* **26**: 672–5.

Houghton, G. and Ellis, A.E. 1996. Pancreas disease in Atlantic salmon: serum neutralisation and passive immunisation. *Fish Shellfish Immunol* **6**: 465–72.

Karlsen, M., Tingbø, T., Solbakk, I.T., *et al.*, 2012. Efficacy and safety of an inactivated vaccine against salmonid alphavirus (family *Togaviridae*). *Vaccine* **30**: 5688–94.

Kent, M.L. and Elston, R.A. 1987. Pancreas disease in pen-reared Atlantic salmon in North America. *Bull Europ Assoc Fish Pathol* **7**: 29–31.

Kongtorp, R.T., Stene, A., Andreassen, P.A., *et al.*, 2010. Lack of evidence for vertical transmission of SAV 3 using gametes of Atlantic salmon, *Salmo salar* L., exposed by natural and experimental routes. *J Fish Dis* **33**: 879–88.

Linn, M.L., Gardner, J., Warrilow, D., *et al.*, 2001. Arbovirus of marine mammals: a new alphavirus isolated from the elephant seal louse, *Lepidophthirus macrorhini*. *J Virol* **75**: 4103–9.

McLoughlin, M.F. and Graham, D.A. 2007. Alphavirus infections in salmonids – a review. *J Fish Dis* **30**: 511–31.

McLoughlin, M.F., Nelson, R.T., Rowley, H.M., *et al.*, 1996. Experimental pancreas disease in Atlantic salmon *Salmo salar* post-smolts induced by salmon pancreas disease virus (SPDV). *Dis Aquat Org* **26**: 117–24.

Mérour, E., Lamoureux, A., Bernard, J., *et al.*, 2013. A fully attenuated recombinant salmonid alphavirus becomes pathogenic through a single amino acid change in the E2 glycoprotein. *J Virol* **87**: 6027–30.

Moriette, C., Leberre, M., Lamoureux, A., *et al.*, 2006. Recovery of a recombinant salmonid alphavirus fully attenuated and protective for rainbow trout. *J Virol* **80**: 4088–98.

Munro, A.L.S., Ellis, A.E., McVicar, A.H., *et al.*, 1984. An exocrine pancreas disease of farmed Atlantic salmon in Scotland. *Helgol Meeresunters* **37**: 571–86.

Raynard, R., Houghton, G., Munro, A.L.S. 1992. *Pancreas Disease of Atlantic Salmon: Proceedings of a European Commission Workshop*. Edinburgh, Scottish Office Agriculture and Fisheries Department (Scottish Aquaculture Research Report No. 1).

Shoemaker, C.A. and Klesius, P.H. 2014. Replicating vaccines, in *Fish Vaccination* (eds R. Gudding, A. Lillehaug and Ø. Evensen). Oxford, John Wiley & Sons, Ltd., 33–46.

Snow, M. 2011. The contribution of molecular epidemiology to the understanding and control of viral diseases of salmonid aquaculture. *Vet Res* **42**: 56.

Snow, M., Black, J.A., Matejusova, I., *et al.*, 2010. Evidence for the detection of salmonid alphavirus (SAV) RNA in wild marine fish in areas remote from aquaculture activity: Implications for the origins of salmon pancreas disease (SPD) in aquaculture. *Dis Aquat Org* **91**: 189–200.

Villoing, S., Béarzotti, M., Chilmonczyk, S., *et al.*, 2000. Rainbow trout sleeping disease virus is an atypical alphavirus. *J Virol* **74**: 173–83.

Weston, J., Villoing, S., Brémont, M., *et al.*, 2002. Comparison of two aquatic alphaviruses, salmon pancreas disease virus and sleeping disease virus, by genome sequence analysis, monoclonal reactivity, and cross-infection. *J Virol* **76**: 6155–63.

Xu, C., Guo, T.C., Mutoloki, S., *et al.*, 2010. Alpha interferon and not gamma interferon inhibits salmonid alphavirus subtype 3 replication *in vitro*. *J Virol* **84**: 8903–12.

Xu, C., Mutoloki, S. and Evensen, Ø. 2012. Superior protection conferred by inactivated whole virus vaccine over subunit and DNA vaccines against salmonid alphavirus infection in Atlantic salmon (*Salmo salar* L). *Vaccine* **30**: 3918–28.

29 Vaccination against Diseases Caused by *Betanodavirus*

Sonal Patel[1] and Audun H. Nerland[2]

[1]Institute of Marine Research, Bergen, Norway
[2]University of Bergen, Bergen, Norway

ABSTRACT

Betanodavirus infects several fish species around the world, causing the disease viral encephalopathy and retinopathy (VER), with mortalities up to 100%. Disease caused by *Betanodavirus* has also been named viral nervous necrosis (VNN). Vaccine development against *Betanodavirus*, as with other intracellular pathogens, has been challenging, and to date commercial vaccines against *Betanodavirus* are not available. Several approaches have been considered in experimental settings both in laboratory and field trials, and the use of recombinant viral proteins combined with effective adjuvants has given promising results. However, the fact that the disease outbreaks are mainly observed during early larval and juvenile stages, when the immune system is not fully developed, makes developing vaccines against this virus especially challenging. Some work on broodstock immunization has been carried out, and this needs to be further explored. We suggest that administration of immunostimulants during the larval and juvenile stages, and then vaccinating the juveniles once the adaptive immune system is developed, would be the best way to overcome major mortalities seen with VER.

29.1 VIRAL ENCEPHALOPATHY AND RETINOPATHY (VER)

Around 1990 a disease affecting the nervous system of various fish species was reported. In these reports a viral etiology was suggested, as large amounts of virus-like particles could be observed in the lesions. The disease was thus referred to as viral nervous necrosis (VNN) (Yoshikoshi and Inoue, 1990), encephalomyelitis (Bloch *et al.*, 1991), or viral encephalopathy and retinopathy (VER) (Munday *et al.*, 1992). In this chapter we will use the latter term.

The causal virus was characterized (Mori *et al.*, 1992) and found to have an architecture similar to a virus that had previously been isolated from insects. The insect virus had been

sonal.patel@imr.no

Fish Vaccination, First Edition. Edited by Roar Gudding, Atle Lillehaug and Øystein Evensen.

named *Nodavirus* after the village Nodamura in Japan where the virus was first found. Later the insect virus was designated *Alphanodavirus* and the piscine virus as *Betanodavirus*. However, *Betanodavirus* is also referred to as NNV (*Nervous necrosis virus*), a term we for simplicity will use in the remaining of this chapter.

29.2 OCCURRENCE AND SIGNIFICANCE

VER has been diagnosed in more than 30 different fish species all over the world, often in larval and juvenile stages, and mainly in marine fish (Munday *et al.*, 2002). Mass mortalities reaching 100% mostly occur during acute infections at larval and juvenile stages, while several fish species susceptible at grow-out phases may reach mortalities up to 50%. In some cases the disease is subacute and a percentage of the population might become persistently infected, giving rise to asymptomatic carriers where no disease symptoms are detectable. NNV has been a big problem for farming of warm-water marine fish at various geographic localities, such as sea bass and sea bream in the Mediterranean sea (Bovo *et al.*, 1999; Ucko *et al.*, 2004), parrotfish in Japan (Yoshikoshi and Inoue, 1990), turbot in Norway (Bloch *et al.*, 1991), and barramundi in Australia (Glazebrook *et al.*, 1990). Infection by NNV has been one of the main factors preventing farming of the cold water species Atlantic halibut from becoming a big industry (Grotmol *et al.*, 1997), and the virus has also been problematic for farming of Atlantic cod (Patel *et al.*, 2007). Although NNV mainly affects marine fish, the disease has also been detected in a few freshwater species. Since the year 2002, the freshwater species affected by NNV are increasing (Munday *et al.*, 2002; Athanassopoulou *et al.*, 2004; Bigarré *et al.*, 2009), the latest being a hybrid between striped bass and white bass *(Morone saxatilis* × *Morone chrysops)* and largemouth bass *Micropterus salmoides* (Bovo *et al.*, 2011).

In general, fish are more susceptible to NNV at the early stages of the lifecycle, with exceptions in a few fish species. For example, NNV gives high mortality in larvae of Atlantic halibut, but when halibuts have gone through metamorphosis (around 2 g) they seem to be highly resistant against the virus.

29.3 ETIOLOGY

NNV belongs to the family *Nodaviridae*, which consist of small (25–35 nm), non-enveloped viruses with a very simple architecture. As mentioned, members of this family were first isolated from insects, then from fish, but later similar viruses have also been isolated from crustaceans (Bonami and Widada, 2011) and nematodes (Félix *et al.*, 2011). The simple organization of the virus may explain why viruses from this family are able to replicate in cells from a variety of species. The NNV genome consists of two positive-sense, single-stranded RNA segments: RNA1 (3100 nucleotides) encoding the catalytic part of the RNA-dependent RNA polymerase (RdRp) responsible for replication of the genome, and RNA2 (1400 nt) encoding the capsid protein that builds up the icosahedral capsid into which the genome is packaged. In addition, there is a third RNA segment, RNA3, generated sub-genomically from RNA1 and encoding the polypeptide B2. RNA3 is present only in the infected cells and is not packaged into the viral particles. There are indications that B2 interacts with and inhibits an RNA interference system used by the fish to protect against virus infections.

Several viral strains of the NNV identified so far can be classified into four major genotypes based on a variable region (called the T4-region) of the RNA2 segment (Nishizawa *et al.*, 1997): *Striped jack nervous necrosis virus* (SJNNV), *Red spotted grouper nervous necrosis virus* (RGNNV), *Tiger puffer nervous necrosis virus* (TPNNV) and *Barfin flounder nervous necrosis virus* (BFNNV). A fifth genotype for the NNV isolate from turbot has been suggested (Johansen *et al.*, 2004b). The genotypes were named after the fish species from which they were first isolated. Later findings indicated that the strains are not very species-specific, but seem to be geographically distributed, and that water temperature is an important factor in the geographic distribution (Hata *et al.*, 2010). NNV has been shown to be very stable under extreme environmental conditions (Frerichs *et al.*, 2000).

29.4 PATHOGENESIS

The main target organ of the NNV is the central nervous system (CNS) and the retina, where microscopic lesions characterized by cellular vacuolization and neuronal degeneration are found. Small foci with positive immunostaining can be seen during early infection phase, while later, aggregates with immunopositive macrophage-like cells and intra- or extracellular vacuoles can be seen in brain. In retina, the photoreceptor contains degenerated cones, and clumping of melanin can be seen. Destroyed architecture and infiltration of cells can often be seen both in brain and sensory retina of the diseased fish, resulting in major necrosis of the tissue.

The entry of NNV into the cells has been suggested to be dependent upon the endocytotic pathway (Adachi *et al.*, 2007; Liu *et al.*, 2005), and sialic acid on the surface of SSN-1 cells has been suggested to be involved in the initial binding of the virus particle (Liu *et al.*, 2005). The NNV is believed to escape the host cell by the induction of apoptosis and secondary necrosis (Guo *et al.*, 2003; Chen *et al.*, 2007; Su *et al.*, 2009).

The observations from affected fish species around the world confirm that salinity is not a limiting factor, and thus raises the possibility that other economically important freshwater and saltwater fish may be susceptible to the disease.

Clinical signs such as abnormal swimming patterns with uncoordinated darting, rolling and pitching, loss of appetite and change in pigmentation are frequently observed associated with this disease (Munday *et al.*, 2002). Occasionally, tonic spasms of the myotomal musculature resulting in temporary flexion of the body can be observed. Little is known about the clinical signs of VER reported from freshwater species, but mostly they are consistent with the typical signs observed in marine species and include listlessness and emaciation.

The transmission route of NNV is yet not fully understood. The virus can be transmitted vertically from the brood fish via the eggs or sperm, or may enter the rearing unit through the inlet water, or from the feed, and then spread horizontally. Recent reports have shown that the virus can persist for a long time in subclinically infected fish and still be infectious (Johansen *et al.*, 2004a). The virus has been detected in gonads and in association with eggs. Moreover, experimental vertical transmission has been demonstrated in sea bass (Breuil *et al.*, 2002; Kai *et al.*, 2010). High concentrations of NNV in rearing units in which infected halibut larvae were held have been detected (Nerland *et al.*, 2007), indicating that horizontal transmission may take place. It is therefore tempting to speculate that normal transmission is vertical, from subclinically infected parents to the larvae, and if a few of these acquire the disease the virus is shed into the water and then spread horizontally. Once the virus has entered a farm or rearing unit, it may be very difficult to exterminate.

29.5 IMMUNE STATUS AND RESPONSE TO NNV

Several factors such as life stage of the fish, co-infection status, environmental and physiological stress levels, and genetic variations of the virus and the host, influences disease outcome and also the effect of vaccines.

Challenge experiments with turbot show an age-dependent trend, although differing a little, as high mortality of fish up to 10 g, moderate mortality of around 20 g fish, and low mortality of fish larger than 40 g has been observed. In contrast, there are examples of fish species, like spotted coralgroupers (*Plectropomus maculatus*), where adults are much more susceptible to NNV (Nopadon *et al.*, 2009).

The differences between the immune system and response of different fish species to a specific pathogen gives an extra challenge in the understanding of the uptake and removal of the virus from the various fish species that NNV infects. These differences in immune response are not only due to the environmental and physiological stress, but rather due to fluctuations in these parameters. Both humoral and cellular responses are important to achieve good protection against the virus, whether it is during infection or through vaccination. During the early life-stages, larvae/fry are protected by maternally transferred components like lectins and antibodies, and the larvae are dependent upon the innate defense mechanisms, many of which are already present during early egg stages. The development of the adaptive immune system may take from days to months, as seen in Atlantic halibut. Temperature plays a vital role in all these processes. The fact that NNV infects such a wide range of fish species, cultured at varying temperatures, means that it is difficult to compare and transfer knowledge about the progress of infection, immune response and disease outcome from one species and one NNV genotype to other combinations of fish species and viral genotypes without further validation. This is important to bear in mind when working with vaccine strategies against NNV.

29.6 VACCINES

Commercial vaccines against NNV are currently unavailable, although experimental vaccination using several approaches has shown high protection. The experimental vaccines have been tried out on fish that have passed the larval stage, and thus not the most common stage when the fish are infected. Vaccination at the larval stage is difficult for two reasons: (1) the immune system is not well developed; and (2) the small size of the fish at that point makes injections impractical, and mass vaccination protocols employing bath or oral administration are not well developed. One possibility could be to immunize the brood fish before spawning, in order to prevent vertical transmission.

Being an intracellular pathogen, an effective protection against NNV is probably dependent upon proper stimulation of B- and T-cells. Specific antibodies produced by B-cells will bind to virus particles at the time of infection and later when the virus particles are released from infected cells to spread in the fish body. However, inside the cells the virus particle cannot be reached by the antibodies unless the cells are lysed by means of cytotoxic T-cells (T_c-cells).

This is especially important for pathogens like NNV, where the pathogen can hide inside cells and persist for a long time. Both B- and T_c-cells are dependent upon signals from helper T-cells (T_h-cells) to get the necessary stimulation for propagation and action. To develop a protective vaccine, presentation of the antigens in a way that stimulates both B-cells and T-cells is required.

In addition to specific immunity, the innate immune system will also give protection against viral infections. The innate immune system gives high protection soon after stimulation, but the protection is not very long-lasting. However, for vaccine design an innate immune response is interesting for two reasons. Firstly, an innate immune response will be part of the inflammation that normally is necessary to get a specific immune response. Secondly, the innate immune response will protect the fish during the lag period required for the specific immunity to be effective.

Several different administration routes such as injection (intraperitoneal or intramuscular) or mass delivery (immersion or oral administration) have been applied for vaccinating fish in experimental vaccination trials against NNV. These alternatives have different advantages and disadvantages with respect to their level of protection, side-effects, practicality and cost-efficiency. Often the chosen route depends upon the size of the fish to be vaccinated, the specific virus and formulation of the vaccine. When it concerns vaccines against NNV, the main target size are larvae and small fingerlings, and thus, mass delivery methods such as immersion or oral deliveries are practical and easy. One has more flexibility in choosing the delivery method when working with juveniles and bigger fish, which is also the case for some of the fish species like sea bass and Atlantic cod affected by NNV. Vertical transmission of NNV may occur where the virus is packed into the eggs during egg development, or it may be delivered into the eggs by the sperm during fertilization. This is supported by the findings in farmed grouper where NNV was not on the surface of the eggs but present in the embryo, and that the virus could continue to replicate during the embryo development (Kuo *et al.*, 2012). Thus, considering broodstock vaccination is very important for NNV.

In the following sections, and Table 29.1, we will give an overview and examples of various approaches used to date to prepare experimental vaccines against some of the genotypes of NNV. Commercial vaccines against NNV are not yet available, and thus established methods for formulation, delivery and study of the effects and side-effects cannot be discussed. However, testing of experimental vaccines in the laboratory, and some in field trials, will be considered here.

29.7 REPLICATING VACCINES

Fish infected with live virus are able to mount a specific protective immune response against the injected pathogenic virus. However, a relatively high dose of virus similar to that of a fatal dose must be administered for the fish to gain immunity to the infecting virus by either intramuscular injection or immersion. This method does not require relatively expensive vaccine development and preparation.

Live NNV immunization in combination with poly-IC immunization conferred protection in sevenband grouper, *Epinehelus septemfasciatus* (Thunberg) against RGNNV infection (Nishizawa *et al.*, 2009). In a field study, it was shown that the survival rate of immunized fish was 97.5–99.8%, compared with naïve fish with a 71–79.5% survival rate depending on the

Table 29.1 Selected examples illustrating various approaches for formulation of experimental vaccines against different genotypes of betanodaviruses, and their administration routes followed by challenge tests. There are several published papers on production of recombinant protein as an antigen formulation for vaccine design, and thus only selected examples representing different genotypes of NNV are shown here. Percent survival for negative control and vaccinated groups rather than relative percent survival for vaccinated groups has been shown for each experimental vaccine, and a range of survival has been presented, as most of these studies either had several trials, or several concentrations of vaccine, or experiments were carried out at differing conditions.

Fish Species	NNV Genotype	Antigen Type	Amount	Average Weight	Administration Route	Percent Survival		Reference
						Control	Vaccine	
Sevenband grouper	RGNNV	Live virus	0.1 ml of NNV $10^{4.3}$ $TCID_{50}$/ml per fish	52/80 g	IM	71–79.5	97.5–99.8	Oh *et al.* (2012)
Sevenband grouper	RGNNV	Formalin-inactivated	0.1 ml of NNV $10^{9.1}$ $TCID_{50}$/ml per fish	12.3 g	IP	4–40	67–96	Yamashita *et al.* (2005)
Sevenband grouper	RGNNV	Rec protein	2 × 60 µg/fish	28 g	IM	0–35	12–65	Tanaka *et al.* (2001)
Humpback grouper	RGNNV	Rec protein of 3 strains	3 × 0.21 mg (0.07 mg of each)	27 g	IM	0	60–77.5	Yuasa *et al.* (2002)
Turbot	BFNNV	Rec protein	10 µg/fish	2.2 g	IP	61	87	Sommerset *et al.* (2005)
	BFNNV	DNA vaccine	20 µg/fish	2.2 g	IM	57	57–59	
Turbot	SJNNV	Rec protein	15 µg/fish	1.8 g	IP	52–56	68–92	Husgård *et al.* (2001)
Grouper	RGNNV?	Rec protein	*	18–19 dph	Oral (*Artemia* encapsulation)	44–54	80–86	Lin *et al.* (2007)

RGNNV? – The NNV virus is isolated from grouper fish, but information about genotype is not clear.

*Formaldehyde-inactivated *E. coli* expressing NNV capsid protein were fed to *Artemia*, and *Artemia*-containing bacteria were used live for oral vaccination.

IM, intramuscular; IP, intraperitoneal; dph, days post-hatching.

Latin names of the fish species: Sevenband grouper, *Epinephelus septemfasciatus* (Thunberg); Humpback grouper, *Cromileptes altivelis* (Valenciennes); Turbot, *Scophthalmus maximus*; Grouper, *Epinephelus coioides*.

size of the fish at the time of vaccination and VER outbreak (Oh *et al.*, 2012). More importantly, it was demonstrated that poly-IC injection 20 days after VER outbreak could confer protection against NNV and improve the survival rate, and that the protection lasted for more than 10 months. Similarly, use of only immunostimulants without inclusion of a specific antigen, as an anti-pathogen immunostimulant and a new candidate to fight against NNV infection in fish, has been suggested (Kuan *et al.*, 2012).

By employing a low dose of live NNV ($10^{4.3}$ $TCID_{50}$ g^{-1} or less) for sevenband grouper it was demonstrated that the multiplication rate of NNV *in vivo* strongly correlated with NNV virulence and fish mortality (Nishizawa *et al.*, 2012). In the fish reared at 17 °C, NNV multiplied slowly compared with that at 26 °C. NNV titre at the peak was far below the critical level of NNV but greatly above the threshold level. This may explain the survival and mounting of a specific protective immune response against NNV of the fish reared at 17 °C. It could thus be concluded that downregulation of NNV multiplication by rearing fish at 17 °C enabled not only control of VER onset, but also live NNV vaccine, suggesting a strong potentiality for immunization with live NNV by rearing at lower temperatures. However, as this approach implies that infectious and pathogenic virus is released to the environment, it is doubtful that it will be approved.

29.8 INACTIVATED VIRUS

A few studies have been carried out using different approaches to inactivate NNV, giving promising results. When juvenile sevenband grouper were intraperitoneal (IP)-injected once with formalin-inactivated RGNNV, the vaccinated fish showed significantly lower mortalities than the control fish both in the laboratory and upon exposure to natural infection in net pens (Yamashita *et al.*, 2005). A field trial in which fish were exposed to natural infection in net pens also resulted in higher survival rates of 85% RPS in the vaccinated fish during the experimental period of 9 weeks. Comparing the efficacies of formalin-inactivated vaccines with or without encapsulation, through bath immunization in orange-spotted grouper (*Epinephelus coioides*) at early larval stage followed by bath challenge, revealed that the efficacy of formalin-inactivated vaccine could be significantly improved by nano-encapsulation (Kai and Chi, 2008). However, the processes used to inactivate the virus need to be closely followed, and often 100% quality assurance of inactivation is not possible to achieve due to drawbacks in the available analysis method for viruses compared with bacteria.

29.9 RECOMBINANT PROTEIN/PEPTIDE

Expression of recombinant protein corresponding to the capsid protein of NNV is the approach most commonly employed for development of experimental NNV vaccines. Vaccination with recombinant capsid protein (recCP), expressed in *E. coli*, has given good results in different fish species. Significant protection and virus-neutralizing activity in the sera was demonstrated in turbot juveniles and other fish species with an oil-adjuvanted IP-injected recombinant C fragment from SJNNV (Husgard *et al.*, 2001). An *Artemia*-encapsulated recCP was apparently found to induce a protective immune response in orange-spotted grouper, with adsorption of antigens into the hindgut and subsequent production of specific anti-recCP (Yang *et al.*, 2007).

Similar results were obtained by mixing recombinant C proteins from three Japanese isolates from the red-spotted grouper NNV, injected into humpback grouper, *Cromileptes altivelis* (Valenciennes), and later challenged with an Indonesian NNV isolate (Yuasa *et al.*, 2002). Comparing *E. coli* and *V. anguillarum* as systems to express NNV capsid open-reading frame and delivering this orally through *Artemia* to orange-spotted grouper (*Epinephelus coioids*) showed that the *V. anguillarum*-based vaccine gave a stronger and earlier immune response in addition to higher RPS (Chen *et al.*, 2011).

Vaccinating Atlantic halibut with recCP in combination with an oil adjuvant reduced the viral load so that 5 out of 8 fish were negative for NNV, thus confirming that the recCP is a promising candidate for vaccine development (Øvergård *et al.*, 2013). However, considering that the larval stages are mainly influenced by VER, oral vaccination of halibut using *Artemia*-encapsulated antigen is likely to be unsuccessful, as the adaptive immune system is still developing during the live feed larval stage. Although experiments initiated during the late live feed stage sometime after 94 dph may prove to be successful (Patel, 2009; Øvergård, 2012). A different approach, using a reverse genetics system for the efficient recovery of infectious virus particles, has been used to design possible experimental vaccines based on attenuated NNV (Takizawa *et al.*, 2008).

Synthetic peptides could be an alternative to traditional or recombinant vaccines. A preliminary approach to find synthetic peptides from NNV capsid protein demonstrated that heat-inactivated NNV protected sea bass, and that the N-terminal peptide is a potentially protective peptide (Coeurdacier *et al.*, 2003), but it needs further development. Up to now, synthetic peptides have mostly been used to investigate protein structure and very few experiments have looked at the possibility of using them as vaccines.

29.10 DNA VACCINES

A DNA vaccine is prepared by cloning the sequence encoding a protein antigen of the pathogen into a plasmid behind a strong eukaryotic promoter and injecting into the muscle tissue of the host. Inside the cells the antigen will be expressed from the plasmid, thus mimicking the infection by a replicating virus, and thereby processed and presented to the immune system that will stimulate the T_c-cells, which can kill virus infected cells. Encouraged by the success of the DNA vaccine against rhabdoviruses (Anderson *et al.*, 1996), the gene encoding NNV capsid protein was cloned into the same plasmid vector and behind the same eukaryotic promoter (Sommerset *et al.*, 2005). Unfortunately, injection of this plasmid did not give any protection of turbots against VER. The reason for this difference is unclear. Probably, the rabdoviral G-proteins, which are glycosylated membrane proteins, have unique immunological properties. One interesting observation was that the DNA vaccine encoding the VHSV G-protein also induced a high protection against VER, starting a short time post-vaccination but was not long-lasting, indicating an innate non-specific protection.

Some of the aspects to be considered when working with DNA vaccines are persistence of the introduced DNA in the fish, their possible impact on the aquatic environment, and the acceptance by potential consumers (Gomez-Casado *et al.*, 2011). Moreover, it is still controversial whether the vaccinated fish should be regarded as a genetically modified organisms (GMOs).

29.11 FUTURE PROSPECTS AND RECOMMENDATIONS

To control the VER disease through a practical vaccination regime, more detailed data on various parameters, such as the administration route, effective dose and duration of protection, will be required. To date, the efficacies of most vaccines have been evaluated on juvenile or young fish using injection as the administration route, while the highest mortality occurs at the larval stage, a size too small to be immunized by injection. Using immunostimulants to increase general immunity during the early larval stages may also provide the opportunity to pass through the critical window until the adaptive immune system is developed. Therefore, immunization of pre-spawning broodstock might be a potential means to protect larval stages. The studies on this subject are still scarce and the results are controversial. To cope with the critical situation with NNV infections, future research needs to focus on the challenging broodstock vaccination field, and multivalent vaccines that can give cross-protection against several NNV strains/genotypes. Taking into consideration the geographic distribution and range of genotypes of NNV, a combination of effective prophylaxis and vaccination at larval, juvenile and broodstock stages will be needed to circumvent VER.

REFERENCES

Adachi, K., Ichinose, T., Takizawa, N., *et al.*, 2007. Inhibition of betanodavirus infection by inhibitors of endosomal acidification. *Arch Virol* **152**: 2217–24.

Anderson, E.D., Mourich, D.V., Fahrenkrug, S.C., *et al.*, 1996. Genetic immunization of rainbow trout (*Onchorhynchus mykiss*) against infectious hematopoietic necrosis virus. *Mol Mar Biol Biotech* **5**: 114–22.

Athanassopoulou, F., Billinis, C. and Prapas, T. 2004. Important disease conditions of newly cultured species in intensive freshwater farms in Greece: first incidence of nodavirus infection in *Acipenser* sp. *Dis Aquat Org* **60**: 247–52.

Bigarré, L., Cabon, J., Baud, M., *et al.*, 2009. Outbreak of betanodavirus infection in tilapia, *Oreochromis niloticus* (L.), in fresh water. *J Fish Dis* **32**: 667–73.

Bloch, B., Gravningen, K. and Larsen, J.L. 1991. Encephalomyelitis among turbot associated with a picornavirus-like agent. *Dis Aquat Org* **10**: 65–70.

Bonami, J.R. and Widada, J.S. 2011. Viral diseases of the giant fresh water prawn *Macrobrachium rosenbergii*: a review. *J Invertebr Pathol* **106**: 131–42.

Bovo, G., Nishizawa, T., Maltese, C., *et al.*, 1999. Viral encephalopathy and retinopathy of farmed marine fish species in Italy. *Virus Research* **63**: 143–6.

Bovo, G., Gustinelli, A., Quaglio, F., *et al.*, 2011. Viral encephalopathy and retinopathy outbreak in freshwater fish farmed in Italy. *Dis Aquat Org* **96**: 45–54.

Breuil, G., Pepin, J.F.P., Boscher, S. and Thiery, R. 2002. Experimental vertical transmission of nodavirus from broodfish to eggs and larvae of the sea bass, *Dicentrarchus labrax* (L.). *J Fish Dis* **25**: 697–702.

Chen, S.P., Wu, J.L., Su, Y.C. and Hong, J.R. 2007. Anti-Bcl-2 family members, zfBcl-x(L) and zfMcl-1a, prevent cytochrome c release from cells undergoing betanodavirus-induced secondary necrotic cell death. *Apoptosis* **12**: 1043–60.

Chen, Y.M., Shih, C.H., Liu, H.C., *et al.*, 2011. An oral nervous necrosis virus vaccine using *Vibrio anguillarum* as an expression host provides early protection. *Aquaculture* **321**: 26–33.

Coeurdacier, J.L., Laporte, F. and Pepin, J.F. 2003. Preliminary approach to find synthetic peptides from nodavirus capsid potentially protective against sea bass viral encephalopathy and retinopathy. *Fish Shellfish Immunol* **14**: 435–47.

Félix, M.A., Ashe, A., Piffaretti, J., *et al.*, 2011. Natural and experimental infection of *Caenorhabditis* nematodes by novel viruses related to nodaviruses. *PloS Biol 9e*1000586.

Frerichs, G.N., Tweedie, A., Starkey, W.G. and Richards, R.H. 2000. Temperature, pH and electrolyte sensitivity, and heat, UV and disinfectant inactivation of sea bass (*Dicentrarchus labrax*) neuropathy nodavirus. *Aquaculture* **185**: 13–24.

Glazebrook, J.S., Heasman, M.P. and Debeer, S.W. 1990. Picorna-like viral particles associated with mass mortalities in larval barramundi, *Lates calcarifer* Bloch. *J Fish Dis* **13**: 245–9.

Gomez-Casado, E., Estepa, A. and Coll, J.M. 2011. A comparative review on European-farmed finfish RNA viruses and their vaccines. *Vaccine* **29**: 2657–71.

Grotmol, S., Totland, G.K., Thorud, K. and Hjeltnes, B.K. 1997. Vacuolating encephalopathy and retinopathy associated with a nodavirus-like agent: a probable cause of mass mortality of cultured larval and juvenile Atlantic halibut *Hippoglossus hippoglossus*. *Dis Aquat Org* **29**: 85–97.

Guo, Y.X., Wei, T., Dallmann, K. and Kwang, J. 2003. Induction of caspase-dependent apoptosis by betanodaviruses GGNNV and demonstration of protein alpha as an apoptosis inducer. *Virology* **308**: 74–82.

Hata, N., Okinaka, Y., Iwamoto, T., *et al.*, 2010. Identification of RNA regions that determine temperature sensitivities in betanodaviruses. *Arch Virol* **155**: 1597–1606.

Husgard, S., Grotmol, S., Hjeltnes, B.K., *et al.*, 2001. Immune response to a recombinant capsid protein of striped jack nervous necrosis virus (SJNNV) in turbot *Scophthalmus maximus* and Atlantic halibut *Hippoglossus hippoglossus*, and evaluation of a vaccine against SJNNV. *Dis Aquat Org* **45**: 33–44.

Johansen, R., Grove, S., Svendsen, A.K., *et al.*, 2004a. A sequential study of pathological findings in Atlantic halibut, *Hippoglossus hippoglossus* (L), throughout one year after an acute outbreak of viral encephalopathy and retinopathy. *J Fish Dis* **27**: 327–41.

Johansen, R., Sommerset, I., Tørud, B., *et al.*, 2004b. Characterization of nodavirus and viral encephalopathy and retinopathy in farmed turbot, *Scophthalmus maximus* (L.). *J Fish Dis* **27**: 591–601.

Kai, Y.H. and Chi, S.C. 2008. Efficacies of inactivated vaccines against betanodavirus in grouper larvae (*Epinephelus coioides*) by bath immunization. *Vaccine* **26**: 1450–57.

Kai, Y.H., Su, H.M., Tai, K.T. and Chi, S.C. 2010. Vaccination of grouper broodfish (*Epinephelus tukula*) reduces the risk of vertical transmission by nervous necrosis virus. *Vaccine* **28**: 996–1001.

Kuan, Y.C., Sheu, F., Lee, G.C., *et al.*, 2012. Administration of recombinant Reishi immunomodulatory protein (rLZ-8) diet enhances innate immune responses and elicits protection against nervous necrosis virus in grouper *Epinephelus coioides*. *Fish Shellfish Immunol* **32**: 986–93.

Kuo, H.C., Wang, T.Y., Hsu, H.H., *et al.*, 2012. Nervous necrosis virus replicates following the embryo development and dual infection with iridovirus at juvenile stage in grouper. *PloS One* **7**: e36183.

Lin, C.C., Liu, J.H.Y., Chen, M.S. and Yang, H.L. 2007. An oral nervous necrosis vaccine that induces protective immunity in larvae of grouper (*Epinephelus coioides*). *Aquaculture* **268**: 265–73.

Liu, W.T., Hsu, C.H., Hong, Y.R., *et al.*, 2005. Early endocytosis pathways in SSN-1 cells infected by dragon grouper nervous necrosis virus. *J Gen Virol* **86**: 2553–61.

Mori, K.I., Nakai, T., Muroga, K., *et al.*, 1992. Properties of a new virus belonging to nodaviridae found in larval striped jack (*Pseudocaranx dentex*) with nervous necrosis. *Virology* **187**: 368–71.

Munday, B.L., Langdon, J.S., Hyatt, A. and Humphrey, J.D. 1992. Mass mortality associated with a viral-induced vacuolating encephalopathy and retinopathy of larval and juvenile barramundi, *Lates calcarifer* Bloch. *Aquaculture* **103**: 197–211.

Munday, B.L., Kwang, J. and Moody, N. 2002. Betanodavirus infections of teleost fish: a review. *J Fish Dis* **25**: 127–42.

Nerland, A.H., Skår, C., Eriksen, T.B. and Bleie, H. 2007. Detection of nodavirus in seawater from rearing facilities for Atlantic halibut *Hippoglossus hippoglossus* larvae. *Dis Aquat Org* **73**: 201–5.

Nishizawa, T., Furuhashi, M., Nagai, T., *et al.*, 1997. Genomic classification of fish nodaviruses by molecular phylogenetic analysis of the coat protein gene. *Appl Environ Microb* **63**: 1633–6.

Nishizawa, T., Takami, I., Kokawa, Y. and Yoshimizu, M. 2009. Fish immunization using a synthetic double-stranded RNA Poly(I:C), an interferon inducer, offers protection against RGNNV, a fish nodavirus. *Dis Aquat Org* **83**: 115–22.

Nishizawa, T., Gye, H.J., Takami, I. and Oh, M.J. 2012. Potentiality of a live vaccine with nervous necrosis virus (NNV) for sevenband grouper *Epinephelus septemfasciatus* at a low rearing temperature. *Vaccine* **30**: 1056–63.

Nopadon, P., Aranya, P., Tipaporn, T., *et al.*, 2009. Nodavirus associated with pathological changes in adult spotted coralgroupers (*Plectropomus maculatus*) in Thailand with viral nervous necrosis. *Res Vet Sci* **87**: 97–101.

Oh, M.J., Takami, I., Nishizawa, T., *et al.*, 2012. Field tests of Poly(I:C) immunization with nervous necrosis virus (NNV) in sevenband grouper, *Epinephelus septemfasciatus* (Thunberg). *J Fish Dis* **35**: 187–91.

Patel, S. 2009. *Immune related genes in Atlantic halibut (Hippoglossus hippoglossus), Expression of B and T cell markers during ontogenesis*. PhD thesis, Molecular Biology Institute, University of Bergen.

Patel, S., Korsnes, K., Bergh, Ø., *et al.*, 2007. Nodavirus in farmed Atlantic cod *Gadus morhua* in Norway. *Dis Aquat Org* **77**: 169–73.

Sommerset, I., Skern, R., Biering, E., *et al.*, 2005. Protection against Atlantic halibut nodavirus in turbot is induced by recombinant capsid protein vaccination but not following DNA vaccination. *Fish Shellfish Immunol* **18**: 13–29.

Su, Y.C., Wu, J.L. and Hong, J.R. 2009. Betanodavirus non-structural protein B2: a novel necrotic death factor that induces mitochondria-mediated cell death in fish cells. *Virology* **385**: 143–54.

Takizawa, N., Adachi, K. and Kobayashi, N. 2008. Establishment of reverse genetics system of Betanodavirus for the efficient recovery of infectious particles. *J Virol Methods* **151**: 271–6.

Tanaka, S., Mori, K., Arimoto, M., *et al.*, 2001. Protective immunity of sevenband grouper *Epinephelus septemfasciatus* Thunberg, against experimental viral nervous necrosis. *J Fish Dis* **24**: 15–22.

Ucko, M., Colorni, A. and Diamant, A. 2004. Nodavirus infections in Israeli mariculture. *J Fish Dis* **27**: 459–69.

Yamashita, H., Fujita, Y., Kawakami, H. and Nakai, T. 2005. The efficacy of inactivated virus vaccine against viral nervous necrosis (VNN). *Fish Pathol* **40**: 15–21.

Yang, H.L., Lin, C.C., Lin, J.H.Y. and Chen, M.S. 2007. An oral nervous necrosis virus vaccine that induces protective immunity in larvae of grouper (*Epinephelus coioides*). *Aquaculture* **268**: 265–73.

Yoshikoshi, K. and Inoue, K. 1990. Viral nervous necrosis in hatchery-reared larvae and juveniles of Japanese parrotfish, *Oplegnathus fasciatus* (Temminck and Schlegel). *J Fish Dis* **13**: 69–77.

Yuasa, K., Koesharyani, I., Roza, D., *et al.*, 2002. Immune response of humpback grouper, *Cromileptes altivelis* (Valenciennes) injected with the recombinant coat protein of betanodavirus. *J Fish Dis* **25**: 53–6.

Øvergård, A.C. 2012. *T-cells and cytokines of Atlantic halibut (Hippoglossus hippoglossus L.). Gene expression levels during ontogenesis, vaccination and experimental nodavirus infection*. PhD thesis, University of Bergen.

Øvergård, A.C., Patel, S., Nøstbakken, O.J. and Nerland, A.H. 2013. Halibut T-cell and cytokine response upon vaccination and challenge with nodavirus. *Vaccine* **31**: 2395–402.

30 Immunostimulation of Crustaceans

Indrani Karunasagar, Singaiah NaveenKumar, Biswajit Maiti and Praveen Rai

Karnataka Veterinary, Animal and Fisheries Sciences University, College of Fisheries, Mangalore, India

ABSTRACT

In crustaceans, the mechanisms of defense against pathogens, although powerful, are poorly understood. Crustaceans depend heavily on the non-specific defense mechanisms, and therefore immunostimulants capable of stimulating these mechanisms may have an important role in protection against disease. The immunostimulatory effect of a few compounds such as β-1,3-glucans, bacterins, peptidoglycans, lipopolysaccharides, fucoidans, and so on, have been studied by various investigators. They have been reported to enhance both humoral and cell-mediated components of the non-specific defense system. Several modes of administration such as injection, immersion and oral delivery have been tried, and results show a significant enhancement of non-specific defense activities, a consequence of which is increased survival when challenged by microbial pathogens.

30.1 INTRODUCTION

The past decade has witnessed a booming aquaculture production which increased significantly to 59.9 million tonnes in 2010, with an average annual growth rate of 6.3% and an estimated value of US$119.4 billion (FAO, 2012). Crustaceans, which include shrimps, prawns, crabs, lobsters, and crayfish, contributed about 9.6% of aquaculture production at ~5.7 million tonnes (FAO, 2012). The last two decades have witnessed revolutionary changes in aquaculture. The shrimp industry in particular grew at an astounding pace in the 1990s, bringing huge areas under farming, intensification of existing farming practices, and high economic inputs for maximizing profits. However, the increase in production was not proportional to the expansion of the industry, both vertically and horizontally, resulting in a decline in the annual growth of the sector. The decline in overall production since the 1990s has mainly been attributed to the outbreak of microbial diseases, which exposed the risk associated with culture of invertebrates

karuna8sagar@yahoo.com

Fish Vaccination, First Edition. Edited by Roar Gudding, Atle Lillehaug and Øystein Evensen.

due to their vulnerability to infections by pathogenic microorganisms. Cumulative losses due to microbial infection during the last 15 years were about US$15.0 billion, with viral diseases accounting for approximately 60% of the total loss. Bacterial pathogens accounted for about 20%, and the remainder was attributed to other pathogens including parasites (Flegel, 2012). About 20 different shrimp viruses have been implicated in mass mortalities and diseases in cultured shrimp, and include some of the most dreaded ones such as white spot syndrome virus (WSSV), yellow head virus (YHV), infectious hypodermal and hematopoietic necrosis virus (IHHNV), and Taura syndrome virus (TSV) (Lightner, 2011). Gram-negative bacteria such as *Vibrio harveyi*, *Vibrio parahaemolyticus* and other vibrios also cause significant economic losses by affecting the larval forms in the hatchery as well as the juveniles in grow-out farms. Some gram-positive bacteria such as *Aerococcus* spp. have also been reported to cause mortality. Parasites, particularly protozoans such as ciliates, gregarians and microsporidians, affect shrimps during developmental stages, causing problems in shrimp aquaculture. Fungi are opportunistic pathogens of shrimp, with *Lagenidium* and *Sirolpidium* spp. being common aquatic fungi affecting the larval stages in the hatchery. It is apparent that the magnitude of loss to the shrimp industry due to various pathogens is enormous, and threatens the sustainability and viability of commercial aquaculture. Hence, intense research is being carried out worldwide to address issues related to management of the disease problems plaguing the industry.

Sensitive and specific diagnosis of causative agents by immunological and molecular methods helps in the early detection of disease agents. Antibiotics are not recommended in the aquaculture industry, since their indiscriminate use results in accumulation of residues in the animal as well as resistance among the pathogens and transfer to other bacteria, destruction of many useful/innocuous organisms in the environment responsible for biogeochemical cycles, and finally disturbing the delicate ecological balance (Karunasagar *et al.*, 1994). Development of specific pathogen-free broodstock and screening of larvae prior to stocking are some of the scientific management approaches implemented. Despite stocking pathogen-free larvae, disease outbreaks occur, proving that larvae may be infected through numerous routes during culture. The use of recirculation systems to exclude external contamination and entry of pathogens via carriers is seen as not economically viable for the extremely large areas of culture in several Asian countries. The use of disinfectants and sanitizers to treat the ponds prior to stocking, antiviral drugs, chemicals and other inputs such as probiotics, and bioremediators have met with variable success. Sustainability and management of crustacean aquaculture would be favored by an in-depth knowledge of the crustacean immune system and its modulation through the use of immunostimulants.

30.2 IMMUNE SYSTEM OF CRUSTACEANS

Crustaceans depend upon innate immunity, which is highly developed in these invertebrates. Their exoskeleton consists of multilayered chitinized material which covers their entire body and acts as a first line of defense against the invading pathogens. If the pathogens successfully breach this layer, they have an array of non-specific factors, both cellular as well as humoral, in the form of circulating hemocytes that include hyaline, semi-granular and granular cells, soluble factors in the hemolymph and the lymphoid organ (found exclusively in penaied shrimps), which are actively involved in host defense (Rusaini and Owens, 2010; Söderhäll and Cerenius,

1992). In recent years, the immune system of crustaceans has evinced much interest among researchers. A number of novel conserved proteins have been identified and characterized using expressed sequence tag (EST) libraries, microarray studies and proteomics approaches, most of which are summarized in Table 30.1. The antimicrobial peptides (AMPs), pattern recognition proteins (PRPs), agglutinins (lectins), cytokine-like factors, hydrolytic enzymes, and so on, constitute important molecules of the humoral defense. Commonly described cellular defense reactions that are active against invading microorganisms include phagocytosis, nodule formation, wound repair, cell-mediated cytotoxicity, encapsulation, clotting, melanization, and prophenoloxidase (proPO) activation (Aguirre-Guzman *et al.*, 2009).

30.2.1 Humoral defense system

30.2.1.1 Recognition

The activation of an innate immune response involves the specific recognition of microorganisms by host proteins called pattern recognition proteins (PRPs). Several PRPs like β-1,3-glucan binding protein (BGBP), C-type lectins, gram-negative binding protein (GNBP) or lipopolysaccharide (LPS)-binding protein (LBP), thioester-containing proteins (TEPs), peptidoglycan-binding protein (PGBP), galectins, scavenger receptors (SRs), fibrinogen-related proteins (FREPs), toll-like receptors (TLRs), and LPS and β-1,3-glucan binding protein (LGBP), recognize and respond to microbial intruders (Wang and Wang, 2013a). These PRPs are capable of binding to a variety of microbial cell-wall components referred to as pathogen-associated molecular patterns (PAMPs). PAMPs include structural components of bacterial and fungal cell wall such as peptidoglycan (PG), LPS, lipoteichoic acid (LTA) and β-1,3-glucans. Bacterial and viral unmethylated CpG DNA and single-stranded and double-stranded RNA from viruses can also act as PAMPs (Wang and Wang, 2013a). This recognition leads to rapid humoral and cellular responses.

30.2.1.2 Lectins

Lectins are glycoproteins that bind to specific carbohydrate moieties (glucose, mannose and fructose) found on the surface of pathogens, and are hence regarded as primary candidates for pattern recognition receptors (PRRs) in crustacean innate immunity. There are 13 different types of lectins found in animals, of which seven are reported in shrimp including calcium-dependent (C-type), L-type, M-type, P-type, fibrinogen-like domain lectins, galectins, and calnexin/calreticulin (Wang and Wang, 2013b). An important lectin type, C-type, has been well-studied and characterized in crustaceans. Carbohydrate recognition domain (CRD) is found in C-type lectins, which helps in pathogen recognition and also plays an important role in the clearance of microorganisms by promotion of phagocytosis, nodule formation, encapsulation, prophenoloxidase activation and melanization. In shrimps, C-type lectin exhibits activity mainly against bacteria and fungi, and studies of its effect on shrimp viruses are limited.

30.2.1.3 Toll

Toll or TLRs play a key role in recognizing the cleaved form of the cytokine Spätzle. Toll and TLRs are evolutionarily highly conserved transmembrane glycoproteins with extra- and intracellular domains. These domains are composed of various numbers of leucine-rich repeat

Table 30.1 Important proteins of the crustacean immune system that have been identified and characterized.

Sl. No.	Protein Name	Species	Accession number(s)	Reference(s)
1.	α2 macroglobulin	*Penaeus monodon*	DQ355145	Lin *et al.* (2007)
2.	β-Actin	*Penaeus monodon, Fenneropenaeus chinensis, Litopenaeus vannamei*	DQ205426, JN808449, JF288784	Zhang *et al.* (2006); Ponprateep *et al.* (2012)
3.	Antiviral-like c-type lectin	*Fenneropenaeus indicus*	HM034320	Unpublished
4.	Anti-lipopolysaccharide factor	*Pacifastacus leniusculus*	EF523760	Liu *et al.* (2006)
5.	Argonuate 1 isoform A and B	*Penaeus monodon*	DQ663629, DQ663630	Dechklar *et al.* (2008)
6.	Astakine	*Penaeus monodon, Pacifastacus leniusculus*	AY787657, AY787656	Söderhäll *et al.* (2005)
7.	C-type lectin	*Penaeus monodon*	DQ078266	Luo *et al.* (2006)
8.	Caspase	*Penaeus monodon*	DQ846887	Wongprasert *et al.* (2007)
9.	Caspase 3	*Penaeus monodon*	HM034317	Unpublished
10.	Chitinase	*Penaeus monodon*	AF157503.1	Tan *et al.* (2000)
11.	Clip domain serine protease homolog (c-SPH)	*Penaeus monodon*	-	Lin *et al.* (2006)
12.	Crustin	*Litopenaeus schmitti*	EF182748	Rosa *et al.* (2007)
13.	Crustin 1, 2 & 3	*Fenneropenaeus chinensis, Pacifastacus leniusculus*	FJ853146 to FJ853148, EF523612 to EF523614	Sun *et al.* (2010); Jiravanichpaisal *et al.* (2007)
14.	Cyclophilin A	*Penaeus monodon*	EU164775	Qiu *et al.* (2009)
15.	Eukaryotic translation initiation factor 5A (eIF5A)	*Penaeus monodon*	DQ851145	Phongdara *et al.* (2007)
16.	Ferritin	*Penaeus monodon, Fenneropenaeus chinensis, Litopenaeus vannamei*	EF523241, DQ205422, AY955373	Maiti *et al.* (2010); Zhang *et al.* (2006); Hsieh *et al.* (2006)
17.	Glutathione peroxidase	*Litopenaeus vannamei*	AY973252	Liu *et al.* (2007)
18.	Hemocyanin	*Penaeus monodon, Pacifastacus leniusculus*	AF431737, AF522504	and Johnson (2002); Söderhäll *et al.* (2005)
19.	Heat shock cognate 70	*Penaeus monodon*	EF472918	Chuang *et al.* (2007)
20.	IFA-14 intracellular fatty acid binding protein	*Penaeus monodon*	EU287463	Unpublished

(*continued*)

Table 30.1 *(continued)*

Sl. No.	Protein Name	Species	Accession number(s)	Reference(s)
21.	Lipopolysaccharide and β-1,3-glucan binding protein	*Penaeus monodon* , *Pacifastacus leniusculus*, *Eriocheir sinensis*	JN415536, AJ250128, FJ605172	Amparyup *et al.* (2012); Lee *et al.* (2000); Zhao *et al.* (2009)
22.	Lysozyme	*Penaeus monodon*	EU095851	Tyagi *et al.* (2007)
23	Mannose-binding protein	*Pacifastacus leniusculus*	AY861653	Sricharoen *et al.* (2005)
24.	Melanization interactin protein	*Pacifastacus leniusculus*	EU308499	Söderhäll *et al.* (2009)
25	Pacifastin	*Pacifastacus leniusculus*	U81825	Liang *et al.* (1997)
26.	Penaeidin classes (2a -2d; 3a-3n, 4a; 4c & 4d	*Litopenaeus setiferus*, *Litopenaeus vannamei*	Y14925-Y14928, AF390140-AF390147, AF390149, AF387660, AY039202-AY039207	Destoumieux *et al.* (1997); Cuthbertson *et al.* (2002)
27.	Penaeidin-3	*Penaeus monodon*, *Fenneropenaeus indicus*	BI784459, HM535650	Supungul *et al.* (2004); Shanthi and Vaseeharan (2012)
28.	Penaeidin 5	*Penaeus monodon*	FJ686018	Tassanakajon *et al.* (2010)
29.	Peroxinectin	*Penaeus monodon*, *Pacifastacus leniusculus*	AF188840, X91409	Sritunyalucksana *et al.* (2001); Johansson (1999)
30.	Phagocytosis activating protein (PAP)	*Penaeus monodon*	-	Deachamag *et al.* (2006)
31.	PmAV	*Penaeus monodon*	DQ641258	Luo *et al.* (2007)
32.	Prophenol oxidase (proPO)	*Penaeus monodon*, *Pacifastacus leniusculus*	AF099741, X83494	Sritunyalucksana *et al.* (1999); Aspan *et al.* (1995)
33.	Rab7	*Penaeus monodon*	DQ231062.1	Sritunyalucksana *et al.* (2006)
34.	Receptor for activated protein kinase c1(RACK1)	*Penaeus monodon*	EF569136	Tonganunt *et al.* (2009)
35.	Ribosomal protein L26		EF523242	Unpublished
36.	Single whey acidic protein domain-containing protein isoforms 1, 2 & 3	*Penaeus monodon*	EU623979, EU623980, EU623981	Amparyup *et al.* (2008)
37.	Serine protease	*Fenneropenaeus chinensis*, *Pacifastacus leniusculus*	FJ770383, AJ007668	Ren *et al.* (2009); Wang *et al.* (2001b)
38.	Syntenin	*Penaeus monodon*	AF335106	Unpublished
39.	Transglutaminase	*Penaeus monodon*, *Marsupenaeus japonicus*, *Pacifastacus leniusculus*	AF469484, AF336805	Yeh *et al.* (2006); Wang *et al.* (2001a)
40.	Tropomyosin II	*Penaeus monodon*	-	Tan *et al.* (2000)

(LRR) motifs and a cytoplasmic signaling domain homologous to that of the interleukin-1 receptor (IL-1R) (Bowie and O'Neill, 2000). Recent studies show that tolls are more involved in innate immune response to bacterial rather than viral infection (Assavalapsakul and Panyim, 2012).

30.2.2 Prophenoloxidase system (proPO)

The prophenoloxidase (proPO) system affords a highly efficient innate immune response against foreign materials in the hemolymph of invertebrates. The proPO system in crustaceans is involved in phagocytosis, melanization, cytotoxic reactant production, cell adhesion, encapsulation and formation of nodules and capsules. The first primary structure of proPO cDNA was reported in crayfish (Aspan *et al.*, 1995). Several proPOs have been subsequently characterized from different invertebrates, such as echinoderms, bivalves, mollusks, insects, ascidians, millipedes, and brachiopods (Cerenius *et al.*, 2008).

30.2.2.1 Activation of proPO system

In shrimp, the activation of the proPO system is a stepwise process with the recognition of microbial cell-wall components (PAMPs) (i.e., LPS, BG or PG) by PRPs (PGBP, LGBP and βGBP), resulting in the formation of melanin (Figure 30.1). This process initiates the activation of several serine proteinases (SPs) through a cascade that leads to the conversion of the proPO-activating enzyme (PPAE) to an active proteinase that converts the inactive enzyme precursor proPO to phenoloxidase (PO). PO, the main enzyme involved in melanin synthesis, is a bifunctional copper-containing enzyme, tyrosinase, which catalyses hydroxylation of monophenols and oxidation of o-diphenols to o-quinones (Sugumaran, 1996; Söderhäll and Cerenius, 1998). These quinones and other short-lived reaction intermediates lead to the formation of polymeric melanin around the invading microorganisms and increase the adhesion of hemocytes to bacteria, thus accelerating their removal by nodule formation (da Silva, 2002; Cerenius *et al.*, 2008). In shrimp, proPO is synthesized in the hemocytes and localized in the

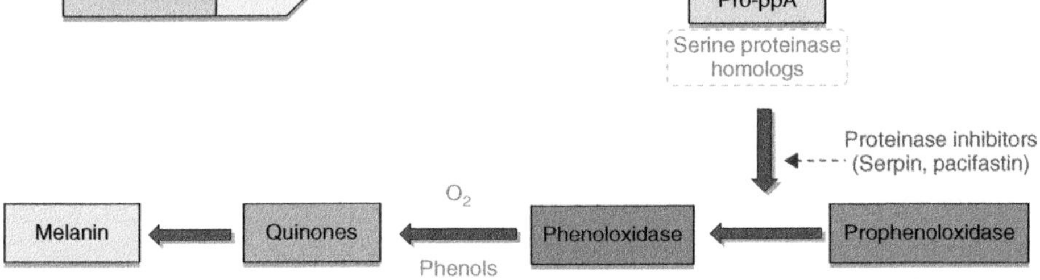

Fig. 30.1 An overview of the prophenoloxidase (proPO)-activating system.

semigranular cells (SGCs) and the granular cells (GCs) (Perazzolo and Barracco, 1997). The mRNA of proPO was shown to be expressed only in hemocytes (Sritunyalucksana *et al.*, 1999). While in most crustaceans only a single proPO gene has been found, in *Penaeus monodon* and *Litopenaeus vannamei*, two proPOs, PmproPO1 and PmproPO2, have been reported in the hemocytes. Two proPO-activating enzymes, namely PmPPAE1 and PmPPAE2, that carry out the proteolysis of the proPO precursor have also been recorded (Amparyup *et al.*, 2013).

30.2.2.2 Regulation of proPO system

The proPO system needs to be carefully regulated to prevent excessive activation of endogenous cascades and to avoid the deleterious effects of active components of the system, such as the active PO, which can produce highly reactive and toxic quinone intermediates that can cause damage and death of the host cells. Therefore, positive and negative regulators of the proPO system that control melanin synthesis are essential. Melanin formation is controlled and regulated at multiple levels by several melanization-inhibitory molecules, including proteinase inhibitors (inhibition of the SP cascade), phenoloxidase inhibitors (POI), and melanization-inhibiting protein (MIP) (Daquing *et al.*, 1999; Sugumaran and Nellaiappan, 2000). However, most of them belong to the well-established families of proteinase inhibitors such as Kazal, Kunitz, serpins, α-macroglobulins and metalloproteinase inhibitors (Wedde *et al.*, 1998; Kanost, 1999). Host proteinase inhibitors also inhibit proteases of invading pathogens. There are three families of serine protease inhibitors that have been reported in penaeid shrimp, namely Kazal-type serine proteinase inhibitors (KPIs), serpins, and α_2-macroglobulins (A2Ms).

The KPI is a cysteine-rich protein and contains one or more Kazal domains of 50–60 amino-acid residues. Each domain contains six cysteine residues forming three intra-domain disulfide bridges (Rimphanitchayakit and Tassanakajon, 2010). Since KPIs contain more than one Kazal domain, it is predicted that each KPI may inhibit more than one proteinase. The SPIPm2 is a Kazal-type serine proteinase expressed in hemocytes of *P. monodon*, which possesses bacteriostatic and antiviral activities in addition to the proteinase inhibitory activity (Ponprateep *et al.*, 2011).

The serpins are known to be inhibitors of proteinase and act as suicide substrates, inserting the reactive center loop (RCL) into the active site of the proteinase, thus inducing a conformational change to form a covalent serpin–proteinase complex. Serpins have been reported in *Fenneropenaeus chinensis* and *P. monodon* and found to be localized in hemocytes and expressed in response to pathogens (Somnuk *et al.*, 2012; Amparyup *et al.*, 2013).

The A2Ms are non-specific, broad-spectrum protease inhibitors that belong to the thioester-containing protein superfamily and have been highly conserved throughout evolution. They react by a unique mechanism involving the physical entrapment of target protease within the folds of a molecule of A2M. This entrapment process involves a reorganization of the A2M molecule mediated by proteolytic cleavage by the target protease. This results in entrapment of the proteinase molecule within an internal pocket in the molecule of A2M. Recently, A2Ms have been identified and characterized from hemocytes of *P. monodon*, *L. vannamei*, *F. chinensis* and *F. paulensis* (Wang and Wang, 2013a). In shrimps, A2Ms are homodimers and are located in the vesicles of the granular hemocytes. The expression levels of A2M are increased on microbial infection. In *P. monodon*, functional analysis of A2M revealed that it can bind to syntenin, a cytosolic protein with diverse biological function, possibly facilitate the entry of the phagocytosis activating protein (PAP) into phagocytic cells, and increase the survival rate of the shrimp after being infected by white spot syndrome virus (WSSV) (Tonganunt *et al.*, 2005; Chotigeat *et al.*, 2007).

30.2.3 Antimicrobial peptides

Antimicrobial peptides (AMPs) are important defense molecules of crustaceans that are produced at a very early stage of life and help to protect them against various infections. AMPs are low molecular weight (<10 kDa) peptides which are catatonic and amphipathic in nature, possessing antimicrobial properties (Boman, 1995). Based on the amino-acid sequence, structure and function, these AMPs are categorized as: (i) α-helices; (ii) β-sheet and small proteins; (iii) peptides with thio-ether rings; (iv) peptides with an over-representation of one or two amino acids; (v) lipopeptides; and (vi) macrocyclic cystine knot peptides (Epand and Vogel, 1999). Most of the AMPs act by forming pores in microbial membranes or otherwise disrupting membrane integrity (Tam *et al.*, 2000). Some AMPs such as penaeidins, crustins, and anti-lipopolysaccharide factors (ALFs) have strong antibacterial and antifungal activities and comprise multiple classes or isoforms. For example, penaeidins have PEN2, PEN3, PEN4 and PEN5 isoforms and crustins have three, crustin 1, crustin 2 and crustin 3 (Table 30.1). Penaeidins belong to a unique family of AMPs that were originally isolated from plasma and hemocytes of *L. vannamei* (Destoumieux *et al.*, 1997; Tassanakajon *et al.*, 2010). They are typically very short, low molecular weight peptides (5.5–6.5 kDa) and mainly act on gram-positive bacteria with either bactericidal or bacteriostatic effects. These peptides do not show any activity against gram-negative shrimp pathogens such as *Vibrio* spp. Interestingly, they can inhibit the growth of filamentous fungi such as *Fusarium oxysporum*. Crustins previously reported in *Carcinus maenas* as an 11.5 kDa protein with several isoforms have also been recorded in a variety of shrimps such as *L. vannamei*, *L. setiferus*, *F. chinensis*, *P. monodon*, and *Pandalopsis japonica*. The expression of lysosomal enzyme (lysozyme) in invertebrates in response to bacterial challenge has been well documented. Lysozyme has antibacterial activity against both gram-negative as well as gram-positive bacteria (Tyagi *et al.*, 2007). Another important AMP, the ALFs, show a broad spectrum of antimicrobial activity which includes activity against bacteria, fungi, parasites and viruses (Tassanakajon *et al.*, 2010). ALFs have also been cloned, expressed and characterized from the giant freshwater prawn, *Macrobrachium rosenbergii*, and possessed broad-spectrum antimicrobial activity (Ren *et al.*, 2012). Histone proteins (H2A, H2B, H3, and H4) from *L. vannamei* showed antimicrobial activity against several gram-positive bacteria (Patat *et al.*, 2004).

30.2.4 Cellular defense factors

30.2.4.1 Hemocytes

Crustaceans possess a large number of circulating blood cells called hemocytes, as they are derived from hemocoel. Hemocytes are important in removing foreign entities that gain entry into the crustacean body cavity. There are different types of hemocyte found in crustaceans which can be distinguished by their morphology and by staining techniques. They are functionally differentiated into semigranular cells (SGs), granular cells (GCs) and hyaline cells (Söderhäll and Cerenius, 1992). Hyaline cells lack granules, may have cytoplasmic inclusions, and are capable of phagocytosis and initiating coagulation. SG cells contain variable numbers of small granules and are rapidly lysed in the presence of microbial polysaccharides like β-1,3-glucans or LPS. It is the major cell type involved in encapsulation reactions. GCs are filled with comparatively large granules and are a repository of a number of molecules like proPO, serine protease zymogens, cell adhesion molecules and AMPs.

30.2.4.2 Phagocytosis

Phagocytosis is the most common of the cellular defense reactions, and together with humoral components constitutes the first line of defense once the pathogens have overcome the physiochemical barrier of the cuticle. All hemocyte types are capable of phagocytosis, but hyalinocytes and SG cells are more actively phagocytic than GCs and have been experimentally demonstrated with gram-negative bacteria. Efficient phagocytosis of bacteria depends upon various factors present in the hemolymph plasma (Albores *et al.*, 1998). There is evidence to prove that the proPO system provides factors that behave as opsonins (Smith and Söderhäll, 1983).

30.2.4.3 Nodule formation

Nodule formation is the entrapment of microorganisms in several layers of hemocytes, and occurs when the numbers of microorganisms are higher than can be removed by phagocytosis. The nodule is melanized due to the host PO activity. The first phase is initiated by the contact between GCs and bacteria, resulting in degranulation and release of a "sticky coagulum" within a minute of exposure to bacteria. This happens in the presence of the endogenous proteins, peroxinectin and BGBP. Thereafter proPO activation leads to melanin deposition around the bacteria (Söderhäll and Smith, 1986). The second phase is marked by the attachment and spreading of the hemocytes which form an outer sheath around the developing nodule. The microbes in the nodule are rapidly removed from circulation and localized in hemocyte clumps, usually present in the gills and sinuses between the hepatopancreatic tubules.

30.2.4.4 Encapsulation

Encapsulation is a readily observed defense mechanism that occurs when the size of the pathogen to be engulfed is large; several hemocytes collaborate by sealing off the foreign particles from circulation and becoming flattened and melanized. SGs are the first cell type to react to foreign molecules. It has been shown that peroxinectin, a multifunctional protein released by hemocytes upon degranulation, promotes encapsulation and nodulation. To encapsulate, hemocytes first need to recognize the foreign targets as non-self and change from non-adhesion cells to adhesive flattened cells that adhere to the foreign targets and one another (Johansson, 1999).

30.2.4.5 Cytotoxicity

GCs and SGs are capable of secreting cytotoxic molecules which are capable of destroying both tumor and non-tumor cells. Even though the cytotoxic mechanism is not clearly understood in the crustaceans, it is believed that once the GCs recognize the foreign substance, they attach to the target and secrete cytotoxic molecules which disrupt the foreign particles or tumor cells.

30.2.5 Primitive specific immunity of crustaceans

Invertebrates including crustaceans were assumed to have only innate immunity with no specific memory (Janeway and Medzhitov, 2002). The earliest studies came from the copepod *Macrocyclops albidus*, wherein it was shown that prior exposure of the copepods to related parasites protected them, and they had less secondary infection with the specific parasites than unrelated parasites, suggesting the possible involvement of some kind of adaptive immunity (Kurtz and Franz, 2003). A "quasi-immune system" protected *P. japonicus* that had survived a WSSV outbreak when the animals were subsequently challenged with the virus (Venegas *et al.*, 2000). Transgenerational transfer of immunity in invertebrates including shrimps has also been demonstrated (Little *et al.*, 2003). All of the above studies provided evidence of alternative adaptive immunity in invertebrates, were based only on qualitative research observations (mortality rate, relative percent survival, etc.) in a few species of invertebrates, and failed to explain the molecular mechanisms involved. However, studies on Down's syndrome cell adhesion molecule (DSCAM) belonging to immunoglobulin superfamily (IgSF) in *Drosophila melanogaster* and *Anopheles gambiae* (*AgDscam*) have attempted to explain the molecular basis that may be involved in specific immunity in invertebrates by documenting challenge-specific isoform expression of the gene in immunologically important cells. Further, silencing of the *Dscam* gene compromised the resistance of the host animal against infection (Dong *et al.*, 2006). It is noteworthy that the *Dscam* gene has been identified and reported in the cultured invertebrates *L. vannamei* (*LvDscam*) and *P. monodon* (*PmDscam*) (Chou *et al.*, 2009, 2011).

More studies on the specific immunity in invertebrates are required for a better understanding of the immune system. Some of the classical experimental studies mentioned above have motivated researchers to look at vaccination as a possibility for control of disease in cultured crustaceans. It is still premature to use the term "vaccination" as studies involving "vaccine" administration for specific protection have yielded variable results, especially in prophylaxis of shrimps against WSSV, which includes the whole virus vaccines, subunit recombinant vaccines and oral (subunit) recombinant vaccines. Owing to the practical difficulties involved with injection vaccination, studies are focusing on oral vaccination (Mustaq and Kwang, 2011) and use of various delivery strategies for optimum benefit.

30.3 IMMUNOSTIMULANTS OF CRUSTACEANS

Nearly 40 years ago, Snieszko (1974) proposed that disease in aquatic animal systems was due to the breakdown of the delicate balance between the host, the pathogen and environmental factors, and one of the strategies to minimize the disease problem would be to improve host factors through the use of vaccines and immunostimulants. As invertebrates depend heavily on innate immunity to combat infectious diseases, an in-depth knowledge of innate immune response parameters and their protective role in response to administration of immunostimulants is worthwhile considering, as this would keep animals in a state of alert by upregulation of humoral and cellular processes against invaders and affording resistance. Various studies on the non-specific immune system of crustaceans revealed that these defense mechanisms can be stimulated by molecules such as glucans, peptidoglycans, bacterin, nucleotides, and so on to impart resistance to bacterial and viral infections. An immunostimulant has been defined as a chemical, drug, stressor or action that elevates the non-specific defense mechanisms or the specific immune response (Anderson, 1992). Subsequently, due to the discovery of PRRs of the phagocytic cells, Bricknell and Dalmo (2005) redefined immunostimulants as "*naturally occurring compounds that modulate the immune system by increasing the host's resistance against diseases that in most circumstances are caused by pathogens*". It has been suggested that immunostimulants may be used in anticipation of disease outbreaks to prevent losses, in cases where such events are cyclic and can be predicted (Anderson, 1992).

The encouraging results achieved in fish systems with immunostimulants have led to similar studies in crustaceans, including shrimp. Immunostimulants and adjuvants have shown remarkable results in enhancing the disease resistance of shrimps in captivity. The use of immunostimulants in shrimp culture for prevention of diseases is a promising development, and several products/molecules with immunostimulatory properties are reported. They can be classified depending on their origin and mode of action: bacterial products, algae-derived, animal- and plant-derived, nutritional factors and enzymes/hormones/cytokines (Sakai, 1999). Several products have been derived from bacteria (*Bacillus* spp.), fungi (*Saccharomyces cerevisiae*, *Schizophyllum commune*), algae (*Sargassum polycystum*), and herbs (Chang *et al*., 2003; Liu *et al*., 2006; Yogeeswaran *et al*., 2012) that find application in shrimp aquaculture.

30.3.1 Induction of hemolymph factors by immunostimulants

A number of hemolymph factors are associated with defense systems in crustaceans. These include agglutinins, precipitins, bactericidins, lysins, lysozyme, phosphatase, phospholipase, peroxidase, protease, and other bacteriostatic and cidal molecules. Induction of such hemolymph factors in crustaceans including shrimp has been reported. Evans *et al*. (1969) reported induction of bactericidins following injection of killed bacteria in spiny lobster, *Panulirus argus*. Likewise, agglutinins and bactericidal substances were induced following injection of *Vibrio* bacterin in *Squilla mantis* (Danielli *et al*., 1989). A natural agglutinin was isolated and characterized from the white shrimp (*F. indicus*) which could recognize acetyl groups and showed the ability to selectively agglutinate various bacterial pathogens of shrimps (Maheswari *et al*., 2002). Injection of heat-killed *V. alginolyticus* to black tiger shrimp, *P. monodon*, induced bactericidins and other humoral factors within day one which peaked at day two and persisted until day five (Adams, 1991). A practical method for routine administration through oral delivery was tested by feeding shrimp with diet containing *Vibrio* bacterin which was found to be beneficial as seen through the enhanced immune parameters as well as improved survival (Devaraja *et al*., 1998). Enhancement of bactericidal activity in hemolymph of *P. monodon* treated with immunostimulants such as β-1,3-glucan, zymosan or *Vibrio* bacterin was demonstrated by Sung *et al*. (1996). Devaraja *et al*. (1998) also reported induction of vibriocidal activity in the hemolymph of *P. monodon* fed with a diet containing yeast β-1,3-glucan. Interestingly, they also observed that when *Vibrio* bacterin and yeast β-1,3-glucans were incorporated together in the diet, much higher vibriocidal activity was induced compared with either component alone, suggesting synergistic effects of these immunostimulants in *P. monodon*. The possibility of induction of other humoral factors by injection or spray application of *Vibrio* bacterin was studied by Itami *et al*. (1989), who showed that hemolymph from immunized prawns had chemokinetic factor(s) that activated hemocytes to migrate through a membrane in a Boyden chamber.

In freshwater crayfish, *Pacifastacus leniusculus*, purification and characterization of a βGBP has been done, and the hemocyte receptor to which it binds after reacting with β-1,3-glucan has also been partially characterized (Amparyup *et al.*, 2013; Lee *et al.*, 2000). Zhao *et al.* (2009) cloned and characterized the LPS and βGBP from Chinese mitten crab (*Eriocheir sinensis*) and noticed upregulation at 1.5 h post-injection of bacteria, followed by a step-by-step recovery at 12 and 24 h. BGBP of Chinese shrimp, *F. chinensis*, was studied by Lai *et al.* (2011), who observed differential expression of this protein in different tissues when the shrimp was challenged with WSSV. In the white shrimp, *L. vannamei*, LGBP showed increased levels of expression at 3 and 6 h after *V. alginolyticus* injection (Cheng *et al.*, 2005). Proteins binding to β-1,3-glucan have also been purified and characterized in other shrimps such as *P. californiensis*, *L. vannamei* and *L. stylirostris* (Amparyup *et al.*, 2013). BGBP enhanced the activity of PPAE, which then induced activation of PO (Aspan and Söderhäll 1991; Amparyup *et al.*, 2012). Enhanced PO activity has been observed in *P. monodon* treated with immunostimulants such as β-1,3-glucans by immersion (Sung *et al.*, 1996) and through feed (Devaraja *et al.*, 1998).

Several studies have been carried out on the regulation of AMPs upon immunostimulation. Significant upregulation of the crustin gene was observed when fed with probiotic bacteria and peptidoglycan, followed by challenge with *V. harveyi* (Antony *et al.*, 2011). However, down-regulation of the same gene was recorded when fed with immunostimulants such as yeasts, LPS and glucan (Antony *et al.*, 2011). Babu *et al.* (2013) studied the potential application of marine yeast (*Candida aquaetextoris* S527) incorporated into diet given once in seven days as an immunostimulant, and observed the differential expression of AMP genes in *P. monodon* challenged with WSSV. There was upregulation of important AMPs such as crustin 1, 2, and 3, penaeidin-3 and penaeidin-5 genes. Wang *et al.* (2008) also reported the differential expression of important AMPs in *L. vannamei* fed with β-1,3 glucan and noted upregulation of lysozyme and cytosolic manganese superoxide dismutase though the mRNA expression of the AMP, while PEN3 was significantly down-regulated.

30.3.2 Induction of cellular activities by immunostimulants

Hemocytes play a very important role in defense of crustaceans against pathogens, and phagocytosis by hyaline cells is a very important process. Foreign particles such as bacterial cells can be removed by phagocytosis or by hemocyte encapsulation, which is initiated by the proPO system (Söderhäll and Cerenius, 1992). Sung *et al.* (1996) noted that cells of *Vibrio* spp. are largely eliminated from shrimp hemolymph within 12 h following invasion and are completely undetectable at 24 h. Both oxygen-dependent reactions such as generation of reactive oxygen species like superoxide anions, hydrogen peroxide, hydroxide ions, singlet oxygen, and myeloperoxidase-catalyzed hypochlorite, and non-oxygen dependent substances such as digestive enzymes, are involved in the destruction of phagocytized microorganisms. Using nitroblue tetrazolium (NBT) staining to detect the presence of superoxide anions, Song and Hsieh (1994) showed that while in normal *P. monodon*, 5% of cells took up the stain, in animals treated with β-1,3-glucans, 41% of cells were stained. Treatment with zymosan and phorbol 12-myristate 13-acetate (PMA) resulted in staining of 31% and 9% of the cells respectively. On the basis of these results, they suggested that β-1,3-glucan and zymosan could be good immunostimulants for shrimp. Sung *et al.* (1996) treated *P. monodon* with β-1,3-glucan, zymosan and *Vibrio* bacterin by immersion, and noted that production of reactive oxygen species (ROS) was significantly greater in β-1,3-glucan and zymosan-treated shrimp compared with control shrimp at 3–6 h following immersion, while in the case of shrimp treated with *Vibrio* bacterin, enhanced ROS production was noted at 6 h following immersion. Devaraja *et al.* (1998), on the other hand, observed enhanced ROS production in shrimp treated with β-1,3-glucan and *Vibrio* bacterin through feed, and in these treatments, peak activity was recorded at 48 h after feeding. They further noted that treatment with β-1,3-glucan and *Vibrio* together resulted in much higher activity compared with the two components given individually. These results suggest the possible enhancement of antimicrobial activity in shrimp hemocytes due to immunostimulants. Itami *et al.* (1994) observed enhanced phagocytic activity in hemocytes of *P. japonicus* fed with β-1,3-glucan at the rate of 50 mg per kg body weight for 10 days, or 100 mg per kg body weight for 3 days. Feeding *P. japonicus* with PG derived from *Bifidobacterium thermophilum* also resulted in enhanced phagocytic activity (Itami *et al.*, 1998a). The proPO system is an important component of crustacean defense which participates in the activation and expression of functionally important microbiocidal compounds such as quinones and melanin (Bachere *et al.*, 1995; Smith *et al.*, 2003). Enhanced PO activity following treatment with immunostimulants has been recorded in crustaceans by several workers. *In vitro* studies by Sung *et al.* (1994) showed enhanced PO in shrimp hemocytes following β-1,3-glucan treatment, and they also found that when *P. monodon* was treated with β-1,3-glucan by immersion, enhanced PO activity was observed from 5 min to 24 h after treatment, with peak activity at 3 h and returning to basal levels on day 3 (Sung *et al.*, 1996). Devaraja *et al.* (1998) studied PO activity in hemocytes of *P. monodon* orally administered with feed including *Vibrio* bacterin and β-1,3-glucan. They noted peak activity at 48 h after feeding and observed that the enhancement was greater when β-1,3-glucan was given along with *Vibrio* bacterin, suggesting a synergistic effect between the two immunostimulants. These reports indicate that immunostimulation using microbial cell wall components enhances the cellular component of non-specific defense in shrimp.

30.3.3 Higher survival rates of shrimp treated with immunostimulants

A few workers have reported enhanced survival rates for shrimp treated with immunostimulants when challenged with bacterial or viral pathogens (Table 30.2). Itami *et al.* (1989) observed that cultured kuruma prawns treated with *Vibrio* bacterin by injection, immersion or spray showed reduced mortalities compared with untreated controls upon challenge by *Vibrio* injection 30 days after treatment. *P. monodon* treated with β-1,3-glucan by immersion showed better survival when challenged with *V. vulnificus* cells, and the protective effect lasted until day 18 (Sung *et al.*, 1994). In a survival study on the kuruma prawn *P. japonicus* fed with β-1,3-glucan from *S. commune* challenged by *Vibrio*, the treated animals showed higher survival than untreated controls (Itami *et al.*, 1994), and although mortality was observed in the treated batch, it was delayed. There was no statistical difference in the final mortality rates. This could be attributed to the short-lived nature of the immunostimulatory effect. A similar study on kuruma prawns fed with PG derived from *B. thermophilum* for 7 consecutive days followed by 7 days without PG showed better survival when challenged with *V. penaeicida* or WSSV (Itami *et al.*, 1998a). Takahashi *et al.* (1998) performed studies on treatment of kuruma prawn with fucoidan, a sulphated polysaccharide and observed improved survival upon challenge with WSSV. Improved survival of *P. monodon* fed on a diet containing a combination of β-1,3-glucan and *Vibrio* bacterin was seen upon challenge with WSSV (Karunasagar and Karunasagar, 1999). Similar results were reported by Itami *et al.* (1998b), who also noted that

Table 30.2 Immunostimulants and their reported effects in crustaceans.

Sl. No.	Immunostimulants	Method of Application	Effects	Reference
1.	β-1,3-glucan	Oral	Improved immunity and significant survival challenged with WSSV	Chang *et al.* (2003)
2.	β-1,3-glucan	Immersion	Improved survival on challenge with *Vibrio alginolyticus* up to day 18	Sung *et al.* (1994)
3.	β-1,3-glucan	Oral	Increased phagocytic index, improved survival on challenge with *Vibrio*	Itami *et al.* (1994)
4.	β-glucan	Immersion	Increased total hemocyte counts and soluble hemocyte protein after 48–120 h	Campa-Cordova *et al.* (2002)
5.	β-glucan	Oral	Increased proPO and reactive oxygen intermediate activity	Anas *et al.* (2009)
6.	β-glucan	Oral	Increased total hemocyte counts, phenoloxidase, superoxide anion and superoxide dismutase until day 27	Bai *et al.* (2010)
7.	β-1,3-glucan, Zymosan, *Vibrio* bacterin	Immersion	Enhanced PO activity, oxygen burst activity	Sung *et al.* (1996)
8.	β-1,3-glucan, *Schizophyllum commune*	Oral	Enhanced survival, hemocyte activity, cell adhesion and superoxide anion production	Chang *et al.* (2000)
9.	β-1,3-glucan, *vibrio* bacterin	Oral	Enhanced bactericidal, oxygen burst, PO activity, improved survival on challenge with WSSV	Devaraja *et al.* (1998) Karunasagar and Karunasagar (1999)
10.	Herbal immunostimulants	Oral	Significant survival on challenge with WSSV	Yogeeswaran *et al.* (2012)
11.	Fucoidan	Oral	Improved survival on challenge with WSSV	Takahashi *et al.* (1998)
12.	Peptidoglycan	Oral	Enhanced phagocytic index, improved survival on challenge with WSSV	Itami *et al.* (1998a,b)
13.	*Vibrio* bacterin	Injection, immersion spray	Improved survival on challenge on day 30	Itami *et al.* (1989)
14.	*Vibrio alginolyticus* bacterin	Injection	Induction of bactericidines lasting until day 5	Adams (1991)
15.	Yeast glucan	Oral	Increased phenoloxidase, number of hemocytes and bacterial killing activity against *Vibrio harveyi*	Thanardkit *et al.* (2002)
16.	Yeast glucan	Oral	Increased total hemocyte and granular hemocyte counts	Chotikachinda *et al.* (2008)
17.	Zingerone	Oral	Increased level of phenoloxidase, lysozyme and phagocytic activities, higher survival on challenge of *Vibrio alginolyticus*	Chang *et al.* (2012)

PG-fed kuruma prawns survived better than controls even though they harboured the virus. Post-larvae and juveniles of *P. monodon* fed with a β-1,3-glucan-containing diet for 20 days showed improved immunity and higher rates of survival than untreated controls when challenged with WSSV (Chang *et al.*, 2003). In a recent study, Chang *et al.* (2012) reported the immunostimulatory effect of zingerone, the active principle in ginger that has antioxidant and anti-inflammatory properties, and its effect on the growth, immunity and disease resistance of juvenile Pacific white shrimp (*L. vannamei*). They observed significant weight gain in shrimps fed with 1, 2.5 and 5 mg of zingerone (per kg diet) incorporated in the feed and given for 56 days in comparison with the control diet. They also observed increased levels of phenoloxidase, lysozyme and phagocytic activities in the animals fed on zingerone-incorporated diets, and higher survival rates when challenged with pathogenic *V. alginolyticus*. Methanolic extracts of herbal immunostimulants such as *Acalypha indica, Cynodon dactylon, Picrorrhiza kurrooa, Withania somnifera,* and *Zingiber officinalis*, incorporated in the diet of the tiger shrimp, *P. monodon* showed improvement of their immune system as seen in the hematological, biochemical and other immune response parameters, and also improved survival when challenged with WSSV in comparison with a control diet without herbal extracts (Yogeeswaran *et al.*, 2012). In conclusion, there is much scope and promise for novel immunostimulatory products that can result in overexpression of innate molecules involved in defense against pathogen invasion in crustaceans.

30.4 ACKNOWLEDGEMENTS

The authors are grateful to the Department of Biotechnology, Government of India, and the Indian Council of Agriculture Research for the funding support towards some of their published work on crustacean immunity cited in this article.

REFERENCES

Adams, A. 1991. Response of penaeid shrimp to exposure to *Vibrio* sp. *Fish Shellfish Immunol* **1**: 59–70.

Aguirre-Guzman, G., Sanchez-Martinez, J.G., Campa-Cordova, A., *et al.*, 2009. Penaeid shrimp immune system. *Thai J Vet Med* **39**: 205–15.

Albores, V.F., Hernández-Lopez, J., Gollas-Galván, T., *et al.*, 1998. Activation of shrimp cellular defense functions by microbial products, in *Advances in Shrimp Biotechnology* (ed. T.W. Flegal). Bangkok, National Center for Genetic Engineering and Biotechnology, 161–6.

Amparyup, P., Donpudsa, S. and Tassanakajon, A. 2008. Shrimp single WAP domain (SWD)-containing protein exhibits proteinase inhibitory and antimicrobial activities. *Dev Comp Immunol* **32**: 1497–1509.

Amparyup, P., Sutthangkul, J., Charoensapsri, W. and Tassanakajon, A. 2012. Pattern recognition protein binds to lipopolysaccharide and β-1,3-glucan and activates shrimp prophenoloxidase system. *J Biol Chem* **287**: 10060–69.

Amparyup, P., Charoensapsri, W. and Tassanakajon, A. 2013. Prophenoloxidase system and its role in shrimp immune responses against major pathogens. *Fish Shellfish Immunol* **34**: 990–1001.

Anas, A., Lowmann, D.W., Williams, D., *et al.*, 2009. Alkali insoluble glucan extracted from *Acremonium diospyri* is a more potent immunostimulants in the Indian White Shrimp, *Fenneropenaeus indicus* than soluble glucan. *Aquac Res* **40**: 1320–27.

Anderson, D.P. 1992. Immunostimulants, adjuvants, and vaccine carriers in fish: application to aquaculture. *Annu Rev Fish Dis* **2**: 281–307.

Antony, S.P., Singh, I.S.B., Sudheer, N.S., *et al.*, 2011. Molecular characterization of a crustin-like antimicrobial peptide in the giant tiger shrimp, *Penaeus monodon*, and its expression profile in response to various immunostimulants and challenge with WSSV. *Immunobiology* **216**: 184–94.

Aspan, A. and Söderhäll, K. 1991. Purification of phenol oxidase from crayfish blood cells and its activation by an endogenous serine proteinase. *Insect Biochem* **21**: 363–73.

Aspan, A., Huang, T.S., Cerenius, L. and Söderhäll, K. 1995. cDNA cloning of prophenoloxidase from the freshwater crayfish *Pacifastacus leniusculus* and its activation. *Proc Natl Acad Sci USA* **92**: 939–43.

Assavalapsakul, W. and Panyim, S. 2012. Molecular cloning and tissue distribution of the Toll receptor in the black tiger shrimp, *Penaeus monodon*. *Genet Mol Res* **11**: 484–93.

Babu, D.T., Antony, S.P., Joseph, S.P., *et al.*, 2013. Marine yeast *Candida aquaetextoris* S527 as a potential immunostimulant in black tiger shrimp *Penaeus monodon*. *J Invertebr Pathol* **112**: 243–52.

Bachere, E., Mialhe, E. and Rodriguez, J. 1995. Identification of defence effectors in the hemolymph of crustaceans with particular reference to the shrimp *Penaeus japonicus* (Bate): prospects and applications. *Fish Shellfish Immunol* **5**: 597–612.

Bai, N., Zhang, W., Mai, K., *et al.*, 2010. Effects of discontinuous administration of β-glucan and glycyrrhizin on the growth and immunity of white shrimp *Litopenaeus vannamei*. *Aquaculture* **306**: 218–24.

Boman, H. 1995. Peptide antibiotics and their role in innate immunity. *Annu Rev Immunol* **13**: 61–92.

Bowie, A. and O'Neill, L.A.J. 2000. The interleukin-1 receptor/Toll-like receptor superfamily: signal generators for pro-inflammatory interleukins and microbial products. *J Leukoc Biol* **67**: 508–14.

Bricknell, I. and Dalmo, R.A. 2005. The use of immunostimulants in fish larval aquaculture. *Fish Shellfish Immunol* **19**: 457–72.

Campa-Cordova, A.I., Hernandez-Saavedra, N.Y., de Philippis, R. and Ascencio, F. 2002. Generation of superoxide anion and SOD activity in haemocytes and muscle of American White shrimp (*Litopenaeus vannamei*) as a response to β-glucan and sulphated polysaccharide. *Fish Shellfish Immunol* **12**: 353–66.

Cerenius, L., Lee, B.L. and Söderhäll, K. 2008. The proPO-system: pros and cons for its role in invertebrate immunity. *Trends Immunol* **29**: 263–71.

Chang, C.F., Chen, H.Y., Su, M.S. and Liao, I.C. 2000. Immunomodulation of dietary β-1,3-glucan in the brooders of the black tiger shrimp *Penaeus monodon*. *Fish Shellfish Immunol* **10**: 505–14.

Chang, C.F., Su, M.S., Chen, H.Y. and Liao, I.C. 2003. Dietary beta-1,3-glucan effectively improves immunity and survival of *Penaeus monodon* challenged with white spot syndrome virus. *Fish Shellfish Immunol* **15**: 297–310.

Chang, Y.P., Liu, C.H., Wu, C.C., *et al.*, 2012. Dietary administration of zingerone to enhance growth, non-specific immune response, and resistance to *Vibrio alginolyticus* in Pacific white shrimp (*Litopenaeus vannamei*) juveniles. *Fish Shellfish Immunol* **32**: 284–90.

Cheng, W., Liu, C.H., Tsai, C.H. and Chen, J.C. 2005. Molecular cloning and characterisation of a pattern recognition molecule, lipopolysaccharide- and beta-1,3-glucan binding protein (LGBP) from the white shrimp *Litopenaeus vannamei*. *Fish Shellfish Immunol* **18**: 297–310.

Chotigeat, W., Deachamag, P. and Phongdara, A. 2007. Identification of a protein binding to the phagocytosis activating protein (PAP) in immunized black tiger shrimp. *Aquaculture* **271**: 112–20.

Chotikachinda, R., Lapjatupon, W., Chaisilapasung, S., *et al.*, 2008. Effect of inactive yeast cell wall on growth performance, survival rate and immune parameters in Pacific white shrimp, (*Litopenaeus vannamei*). *Songklanakarin J Sci Technol* **22**: 677–88.

Chou, P.H., Chang, H.S., Chen, I.T., *et al.*, 2009. The putative invertebrate adaptive immune protein *Litopenaeus vannamei* Dscam (LvDscam) is the first reported Dscam to lack a transmembrane domain and cytoplasmic tail. *Dev Comp Immunol* **33**: 1258–67.

Chou, P.H., Chang, H.S., Chen, I.T., *et al.*, 2011. *Penaeus monodon* Dscam (PmDscam) has a highly diverse cytoplasmic tail and is the first membrane-bound shrimp Dscam to be reported. *Fish Shellfish Immunol* **30**: 1109–23.

Chuang, K.H., Ho, S.H. and Song, Y.L. 2007. Cloning and expression analysis of heat shock cognate 70 gene promoter in tiger shrimp (*Penaeus monodon*). *Gene* **405**: 10–18.

Cuthbertson, B.J., Shepard, E.F., Chapman, R.W. and Gross, P.S. 2002. Diversity of the penaeidin antimicrobial peptides in two shrimp species. *Immunogenetics* **54**: 442–5.

Danielli, E., Ferro, E.A. and Marzoni, R. 1989. Antibacterial activity and induced immunological responses in *Squilla mantis* (Crustacea, stomatopoda) hemolymph. *Eur Aquac Soc Publ* **10**: 81–2.

Daquing, A.C., Sato, T., Koda, H., *et al.*, 1999. A novel endogenous inhibitor of phenoloxidase form *Musca domestica* has a cystine motif commonly found in snail and spider toxins. *Biochemistry* **38**: 2179–88.

Da Silva, C.C.A. 2002. Activation of prophenoloxidase and removal of *Bacillus subtilis* from the hemolymph of *Acheta domesticus* L. Orthoptera: Gryllidae. *Neotrop Entomol* **31**: 487–91.

Deachamag, P., Intaraphad, U., Phongdara, A. and Chotigeat, W. 2006. Expression of a phagocytosis activating protein (PAP) gene in immunized black tiger shrimp. *Aquaculture* **255**: 165–72.

Dechklar, M,, Udomkit, A. and Panyim, S. 2008. Characterization of Argonaute cDNA from *Penaeus monodon* and implication of its role in RNA interference. *Biochem Biophys Res Commun* **367**: 768–74.

Destoumieux, D., Bulet, P., Loew, D., *et al.*, 1997. Penaeidins, a new family of antimicrobial peptides isolated from the shrimp *Penaeus vannamei* (Decapoda). *J Biol Chem* **272**: 28398–406.

Devaraja, T.N., Otta, S.K., Shubha, G., *et al.*, 1998. Immunostimulation of shrimp through oral administration of *Vibrio* bacterin and yeast glucan, in *Advances in Shrimp Biotechnology* (ed. T.W. Flegal). Bangkok, National Center for Genetic Engineering and Biotechnology, 167–70.

Dong, Y., Taylor, H.E. and Dimopoulos, G. 2006. AgDscam, a hypervariable immunoglobulin domain containing receptor of the *Anopheles gambiae* innate immune system. *PLoS Biol* **4**: e229.

Epand, R. and Vogel, H. 1999. Diversity of antimicrobial peptides and their mechanisms of action. *Biochim Biophys Acta* **1462**: 11–28.

Evans, E.E., Weinheimer, P.F., Painty, B., *et al.*, 1969. Secondary and tertiary responses of induced bactericidin from West Indian spiny lobster *Panulirus argus*. *J Bacteriol* **98**: 943–6.

FAO. 2012. *FAO Yearbook 2010. Fishery and Aquaculture Statistics*. Rome, Food and Agriculture Organization of United Nations.

Flegel, T.W. 2012. Historic emergence, impact and current status of shrimp pathogens in Asia. *J Invertebr Pathol* **110**: 166–73

Hsieh, S.L., Chiu, Y.C. and Kuo, C.M. 2006. Molecular cloning and tissue distribution of ferritin in Pacific white shrimp (*Litopenaeus vannamei*). *Fish Shellfish Immunol* **21**: 279–83.

Itami, T., Takahashi, Y. and Nakamura, Y. 1989. Efficacy of vaccination against vibriosis in cultured Kuruma prawn *Penaeus japonicus*. *J Aquat Animal Health* **1**: 238–42.

Itami, T., Takahashi, Y., Tsuchihira, E., *et al.*, 1994. Enhancement of disease resistance of kuruma prawn *Penaeus japonicus* and increase in phagocytic activity of prawn hemocytes after oral administration of β-1,3–glucan (Schizophyllan), in *Proceedings of the 3rd Asian Fisheries Forum, Singapore 1992* (eds L.M. Chou, A.D. Munro, T.J. Lam *et al.*,). Manila, Asian Fisheries Society, 375–8.

Itami, T., Kubono, K., Asano, M., *et al.*, 1998a. Enhanced disease resistances of Kuruma shrimp *Penaeus japonicus* after oral administration of peptidoglycan derived from *Bifidobacterium thermophilum*. *Aquaculture* **164**: 277–88.

Itami, T., Maeda, M., Suzuki, N., *et al.*, 1998b. Possible prevention of white spot syndrome (WSS) in kuruma shrimp, *Penaeus japonicus* in Japan, in *Advances in Shrimp Biotechnology* (ed. T.W. Flegal). Bangkok, National Center for Genetic Engineering and Biotechnology, 291–5.

Janeway, C.A. and Medzhitov, R. 2002. Innate immune recognition. *Annu Rev Immunol* **20**: 197–216.

Jiravanichpaisal, P., Lee, S.Y., Kim, Y.A., *et al.*, 2007. Antibacterial peptides in hemocytes and hematopoietic tissue from freshwater crayfish *Pacifastacus leniusculus*: characterization and expression pattern. *Dev Comp Immunol* **31**: 441–55.

Johansson, M.W. 1999. Cell adhesion molecules in invertebrate immunity. *Dev Comp Immunol* **23**: 303–15.

Kanost, M.R. 1999. Serine proteinase inhibitors in arthropod immunity. *Dev Comp Immunol* **23**: 291–301.

Karunasagar, I. and Karunasagar, I. 1999. Diagnosis, treatment and prevention of microbial diseases of fish and shell fish. *Curr Sci* **76**: 387–99.

Karunasagar, I., Pai, R., Malathi, G.R. and Karunasagar, I. 1994. Mass mortality of *Penaeus monodon* due to antibiotic resistant *Vibrio harveyi* infection. *Aquaculture* **128**: 203–9.

Kurtz, J. and Franz, K. 2003. Evidence for memory in invertebrate immunity. *Nature* **425**: 37–8.

Lai, X., Kong, J., Wang, Q., *et al.*, 2011. Cloning and characterization of a β-1,3-glucan-binding protein from shrimp *Fenneropenaeus chinensis*. *Mol Biol Rep* **38**: 4527–35.

Lee, S.Y., Wang, R. and Söderhäll, K. 2000. A lipopolysaccharide- and beta-1,3-glucanbinding protein from hemocytes of the freshwater crayfish *Pacifastacus leniusculus*. Purification, characterization, and cDNA cloning. *J Biol Chem* **275**: 1337–43.

Lehnert, S.A. and Johnson, S.E. 2002. Expression of hemocyanin and digestive enzyme messenger RNAs in the hepatopancreas of the black tiger shrimp *Penaeus monodon*. *J Comp Biochem Physiol B Biochem Mol Biol* **133**: 163–71.

Liang, Z., Sottrup-Jensen, L., Aspan, A., *et al.*, 1997. Pacifastin, a novel 155-kDa heterodimeric proteinase inhibitor containing a unique transferrin chain. *Proc Natl Acad Sci USA* **94**: 6682–7.

Lightner, D.V. 2011. Virus diseases of farmed shrimp in the Western Hemisphere (the Americas): a review. *J Invertebr Pathol* **106**: 110–30.

Lin, C.Y., Hu, K.Y., Ho, S.H. and Song, Y.L. 2006. Cloning and characterization of a shrimp clip domain serine protease homolog (c-SPH) as a cell adhesion molecule. *Dev Comp Immunol* **30**: 1132–44.
Lin, Y.C., Vaseeharan, B., Ko, C.F., *et al.*, 2007. Molecular cloning and characterization of a proteinase inhibitor, alpha 2-macroglobulin (alpha2-M) from the haemocytes of tiger shrimp *Penaeus monodon*. *Mol Immunol* **44**: 1065–74.
Little, T.J., O'Connor, B., Colegrave, N., *et al.*, 2003. Maternal transfer of strain-specific immunity in an invertebrate. *Curr Opin Biol* **13**: 489–92.
Liu, C.H., Tseng, M.C. and Cheng, W. 2007. Identification and cloning of the antioxidant enzyme, glutathione peroxidase, of white shrimp, *Litopenaeus vannamei*, and its expression following *Vibrio alginolyticus* infection. *Fish Shellfish Immunol* **23**: 34–45.
Liu, H., Jiravanichpaisal, P., Söderhäll, I., *et al.*, 2006. Antilipopolysaccharide factor interferes with white spot syndrome virus replication *in vitro* and *in vivo* in the crayfish *Pacifastacus leniusculus*. *J Virol* **80**: 10365–71.
Luo, T., Yang, H., Li, F., *et al.*, 2006. Purification, characterization and cDNA cloning of a novel lipopolysaccharide-binding lectin from the shrimp *Penaeus monodon*. *Dev Comp Immunol* **30**: 607–17.
Luo, T., Li, F., Lei, K. and Xu, X. 2007. Genomic organization, promoter characterization and expression profiles of an antiviral gene *PmAV* from the shrimp *Penaeus monodon*. *Molecular Immunol* **44**: 1516–23.
Maheswari, R., Mullainadhan, P. and Arumugam, M. 2002. Isolation and characterization of an acetyl group-recognizing agglutinin from the serum of the Indian white shrimp *Fenneropenaeus indicus*. *Arch Biochem Biophys* **402**: 65–76.
Maiti, B., Khushiramani, R., Tyagi, A., *et al.*, 2010. Recombinant ferritin protein protects *Penaeus monodon* infected by pathogenic *Vibrio harveyi*. *Dis Aquat Org* **88**: 99–105.
Mustaq, S.S. and Kwang, J. 2011. Oral vaccination of baculovirus-expressed VP28 displays enhanced protection against white spot syndrome virus in *Penaeus monodon*. *PloS One* **6**: e26428.
Patat, S.A., Carnegie, R.B., Kingsbury, C., *et al.*, 2004. Antimicrobial activity of histones from hemocytes of the Pacific white shrimp. *Eur J Biochem* **271**: 4825–33.
Perazzolo, L.M. and Barracco, M.A. 1997. The prophenoloxidase activating system of the shrimp, *Penaeus paulensis* and associated factors. *Dev Comp Immunol* **21**: 385–95.
Phongdara, A., Laoong-u-thai, Y. and Wanna, W. 2007. Cloning of eIF5A from shrimp *Penaeus monodon*, a highly expressed protein involved in the survival of WSSV-infected shrimp. *Aquaculture* **265**: 16–26.
Ponprateep, S., Tassanakajon, A. and Rimphanitchayakit, V. 2011. A Kazal type serine proteinase SPIPm2 from the black tiger shrimp *Penaeus monodon* is capable of neutralization and protection of hemocytes from the white spot syndrome virus. *Fish Shellfish Immunol* **31**: 1179–85.
Ponprateep, S., Tharntada, S., Somboonwiwat, K. and Tassanakajon, A. 2012. Gene silencing reveals a crucial role for anti-lipopolysaccharide factors from *Penaeus monodon* in the protection against microbial infections. *Fish Shellfish Immunol* **32**: 26–34.
Qiu, L., Jiang, S., Huang, J., *et al.*, 2009. Molecular cloning and mRNA expression of cyclophilin A gene in black tiger shrimp (*Penaeus monodon*). *Fish Shellfish Immunol* **26**: 115–21.
Ren, Q., Xu, Z.L., Wang, X.W., *et al.*, 2009. Clip domain serine protease and its homolog respond to *Vibrio* challenge in Chinese white shrimp, *Fenneropenaeus chinensis*. *Fish Shellfish Immunol* **26**: 787–98.
Ren, Q., Du, Z.Q., Li, M., *et al.*, 2012. Cloning and expression analysis of an anti-lipopolysaccharide factor from giant freshwater prawn, *Macrobrachium rosenbergii*. *Mol Biol Rep* **39**: 7673–80.
Rimphanitchayakit, V. and Tassanakajon, A. 2010. Structure and function of invertebrate Kazal-type serine proteinase inhibitors. *Dev Comp Immunol* **34**: 377–86.
Rosa, R.D., Bandeira, P.T. and Barracco, M.A. 2007. Molecular cloning of crustins from the hemocytes of Brazilian penaeid shrimps. *FEMS Microbiol Lett* **274**: 287–90.
Rusaini and Owens, L. 2010. Insight into the lymphoid organ of penaeid prawns: a review. *Fish Shellfish Immunol* **29**: 367–77.
Sakai, M. 1999. Current research status of fish immunostimulants. *Aquaculture* **172**: 63–92.
Shanthi, S. and Vaseeharan, B. 2012. cDNA cloning, characterization and expression analysis of a novel antimicrobial peptide gene penaeidin-3 (Fi-Pen3) from the haemocytes of Indian white shrimp *Fenneropenaeus indicus*. *Microbiol Res* **167**: 127–34.
Smith, V.J. and Söderhäll, K. 1983. β-1,3-glucan activation of crustacean hemocytes *in vitro* and *in vivo*. *Biol Bull* **164**: 299–314.
Smith, V.J., Brown, J.H. and Hauton, C. 2003. Immunostimulation in crustaceans: does it really protect against infection? *Fish Shellfish Immunol* **15**: 71–90.

Snieszko, S.T. 1974. The effect of environmental stress on outbreak on infectious diseases of fishes. *J Fish Biol* **6**: 197–208.

Söderhäll, K. and Smith, V.J. 1986. Prophenoloxidase-activating cascade as a recognition and defense system in arthropods, in *Hemocytic and Humoral Immunity in Arthropods* (ed. A.P. Gupta). New York, John Wiley and Sons, Ltd., 251–86.

Söderhäll, K. and Cerenius, L. 1992. Crustacean immunity. *Annu Rev Fish Dis* **2**: 3–23.

Söderhäll, K. and Cerenius, L. 1998. Role of the prophenoloxidase activating system in invertebrate immunity. *Curr Opin Immunol* **10**: 23–8.

Söderhäll, I., Kim, Y.A., Jiravanichpaisal, P., *et al.*, 2005. An ancient role for a prokineticin domain in invertebrate hematopoiesis. *J Immunol* **174**: 6153–60.

Söderhäll, I., Wu, C., Novotny, M., *et al.*, 2009. A novel protein acts as a negative regulator of proPO activation and melanization in the freshwater crayfish *Pacifastacus leniusculus*. *J Biol Chem* **284**: 6301–10.

Somnuk, S., Tassanakajon, A. and Rimphanitchayakit, V. 2012. Gene expression and characterization of a serine proteinase inhibitor PmSERPIN8 from the black tiger shrimp *Penaeus monodon*. *Fish Shellfish Immunol* **33**: 332–41.

Song, Y. and Hsieh, Y. 1994. Immunostimulation of tiger shrimp (*Penaeus monodon*) hemocytes for generation of microbicidal substances: analysis of reactive oxygen species. *Dev Comp Immunol* **18**: 201–9.

Sricharoen, S., Kim, J.J., Tunkijjanukij, S. and Söderhäll, I. 2005. Exocytosis and proteomic analysis of the vesicle content of granular hemocytes from a crayfish. *Dev Comp Immunol* **29**: 1017–31.

Sritunyalucksana, K., Cerenius, L. and Söderhäll, K. 1999. Molecular cloning and characterization of prophenoloxidase in the black tiger shrimp, *Penaeus monodon*. *Dev Comp Immunol* **23**: 179–86.

Sritunyalucksana, K., Wongsuebsantati, K., Johansson, M.W. and Söderhäll, K. 2001. Peroxinectin, a cell adhesive protein associated with the proPO system from the black tiger shrimp, *Penaeus monodon*. *Dev Comp Immunol* **25**: 353–63.

Sritunyalucksana, K., Wannapapho, W., Lo, C.F. and Flegel, T.W. 2006. PmRab7 is a VP28-binding protein involved in white spot syndrome virus infection in shrimp. *J Virol* **80**: 10734–42.

Sugumaran, M. 1996. Roles of the insect cuticle in host defense reactions, in *New Directions in Invertebrate Immunology* (eds K. Söderhäll, S. Iwanaga and G.R. Vasta). Fair Haven, New Jersey, SOS Publications, 355–74.

Sugumaran, M. and Nellaiappan, K. 2000. Characterization of new phenoloxidase inhibitor from the cuticle of *Manduca sexta*. *Biochem Biophys Res Commun* **268**: 379–83.

Sun, C., Du, X.J., Xu, W.T., *et al.*, 2010. Molecular cloning and characterization of three crustins from the Chinese white shrimp, *Fenneropenaeus chinensis*. *Fish Shellfish Immunol* **28**: 517–24.

Sung, H.H., Kou, G.H. and Song, Y.L. 1994. Vibriosis resistance induced by glucan treatment in tiger shrimp (*Penaeus monodon*). *Fish Pathol* **29**: 11–17.

Sung, H.H., Yang, Y.L. and Song, Y.L. 1996. Enhancement of microbial activity in the tiger shrimp *Penaeus monodon* via immunostimulation. *J Crustacean Biol* **16**: 278–84.

Supungul, P., Klinbunga, S., Pichyangkura, R., *et al.*, 2004. Antimicrobial peptides discovered in the black tiger shrimp *Penaeus monodon* using the EST approach. *Dis Aquat Org* **61**: 123–35.

Takahashi Y, Uehara K, Watanabe R, *et al.*, 1998. Efficacy of oral administration of fucoidan, a sulphated polysaccharide in controlling white spot syndrome in kuruma shrimp in Japan, in *Advances in Shrimp Biotechnology* (ed. T.W. Flegal). Bangkok, National Center for Genetic Engineering and Biotechnology, 171–3.

Tam, J., Lu, Y. and Yang, J. 2000. Marked increase in membranolytic selectivity of novel cyclic tachyplesins constrained with an antiparallel two-B strand cysteine knot framework. *Biochem Biophys Res Commun* **267**: 783–90.

Tan, S.H., Degnan, B.M. and Lehnert, S.A. 2000. The *Penaeus monodon* chitinase 1 gene is differentially expressed in the hepatopancreas during the molt cycle. *Mar Biotechnol* **2**: 126–35.

Tassanakajon, A., Amparyup, P., Somboonwiwat, K. and Supungul, P. 2010. Cationic antimicrobial peptides in penaeid shrimp. *Mar Biotechnol* **12**: 487–505.

Thanardkit, P., Khunrae, P., Suphantharika, M. and Verduyn, C. 2002. Glucan from brewer's yeast: preparation, analysis and use as a potential immunostimulants in shrimp feed. *World J Microbiol Biotechnol* **18**: 527–39.

Tonganunt, M., Phongdara, A., Chotigeat, W. and Fujise, K. 2005. Identification and characterization of syntenin binding protein in the black tiger shrimp *Penaeus monodon*. *J Biotechnol* **120**: 135–45.

Tonganunt, M., Saelee, N., Chotigeat, W. and Phongdara, A. 2009. Identification of a receptor for activated protein kinase C1(Pm-RACK1), a cellular gene product from black tiger shrimp (*Penaeus monodon*) interacts with a protein, VP9 from the white spot syndrome virus. *Fish Shellfish Immunol* **26**: 509–14.

Tyagi, A., Khushiramani, R., Karunasagar, I. and Karunasagar, I. 2007. Antivibrio activity of recombinant lysozyme expressed from black tiger shrimp, *Penaeus monodon*. *Aquaculture* **272**: 246–53.

Venegas, C.A., Nonaka, L., Mushiake, K., *et al*., 2000. Quasi-immune response of *Penaeus japonicus* to penaeid rod-shaped DNA virus (PRDV). *Dis Aquat Org* **42**: 83–9.

Wang, R., Liang, Z., Hal, M. and Söderhäll, K. 2001a. A transglutaminase involved in the coagulation system of the freshwater crayfish, *Pacifastacus leniusculus*. Tissue localisation and cDNA cloning. *Fish Shellfish Immunol* **11**: 623–37.

Wang, R., Lee, S.Y., Cerenius, L. and Söderhäll, K. 2001b. Properties of the prophenoloxidase activating enzyme of the freshwater crayfish, *Pacifastacus leniusculus*. *Eur J Biochem* **268**: 895–902.

Wang, X. and Wang, J. 2013a. Pattern recognition receptors acting in innate immune system of shrimp against pathogen infections. *Fish Shellfish Immunol* **34**: 981–9.

Wang, X.W. and Wang, J.X. 2013b. Diversity and multiple functions of lectins in shrimp immunity. *Dev Comp Immunol* **39**: 27–38.

Wang, Y.C., Chang, P.S. and Chen, H.Y. 2008. Differential time-series expression of immune-related genes of Pacific white shrimp *Litopenaeus vannamei* in response to dietary inclusion of beta-1,3-glucan. *Fish Shellfish Immunol* **24**: 113–21.

Wedde, M., Weise, C., Kopacek, P., *et al*., 1998. Purification and characterization of an inducible metalloprotease inhibitor from the hemolymph of greater wax moth larvae, *Galleria mellonella*. *Eur J Biochem* **225**: 535–43.

Wongprasert, K., Sangsuriya, P., Phongdara, A. and Senapin, S. 2007. Cloning and characterization of a caspase gene from black tiger shrimp (*Penaeus monodon*) infected with white spot syndrome virus (WSSV). *J Biotechnol* **131**: 9–19.

Yeh, M.S., Kao, L.R., Huang, C.J. and Tsai, I.H. 2006. Biochemical characterization and cloning of transglutaminases responsible for hemolymph clotting in *Penaeus monodon* and *Marsupenaeus japonicus*. *Biochim Biophys Acta* **1764**: 1167–78.

Yogeeswaran, A., Velmurugan, S., Punitha, S.M., *et al*., 2012. Protection of *Penaeus monodon* against white spot syndrome virus by inactivated vaccine with herbal immunostimulants. *Fish Shellfish Immunol* **32**: 1058–67.

Zhang, J., Li, F., Wang, Z., *et al*., 2006. Cloning, expression and identification of ferritin from Chinese shrimp, *Fenneropenaeus chinensis*. *J Biotechnol* **125**: 173–84.

Zhao, D., Chen, L., Qin, C., *et al*., 2009. Molecular cloning and characterization of the lipopolysaccharide and β-1,3-glucan binding protein in Chinese mitten crab (*Eriocheir sinensis*). *Comp Biochem Physiol B Biochem Mol Biol* **154**: 17–24.

Index

Fish Vaccination, First Edition. Edited by Roar Gudding, Atle Lillehaug and Øystein Evensen.